Dietary Sugars and Health

edited by
Michael I. Goran
Professor of Preventive Medicine and Pediatrics
Keck School of Medicine
University of Southern California, Los Angeles

Luc Tappy
Professor of Physiology
Lausanne University School of Biology and Medicine, Switzerland

Kim-Anne Lê
Research Scientist,
Dept. of Nutrition and Health
Nestle Research Center, Nestec Ltd.

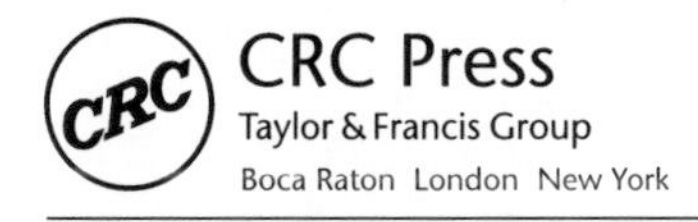
CRC Press
Taylor & Francis Group
Boca Raton London New York

CRC Press is an imprint of the
Taylor & Francis Group, an **informa** business

CRC Press
Taylor & Francis Group
6000 Broken Sound Parkway NW, Suite 300
Boca Raton, FL 33487-2742

Printed on acid-free paper
Version Date: 20141118

International Standard Book Number-13: 978-1-4665-9377-0 (Hardback)

Library of Congress Cataloging-in-Publication Data

Dietary sugars and health / editors, Michael I. Goran, Luc Tappy, Kim-Anne L?, Stanley Ulijaszek.
p. ; cm.
Includes bibliographical references and index.
ISBN 978-1-4665-9377-0 (hardcover : alk. paper)
I. Goran, Michael I., editor. II. Tappy, Luc, editor. III. L?, Kim-Anne, editor. IV. Ulijaszek, Stanley J., editor.
[DNLM: 1. Dietary Sucrose--adverse effects. 2. Dietary Sucrose--metabolism. 3. Metabolic Diseases--etiology. 4. Obesity--etiology. QU 83]

QP702.S8
612.3'96--dc23 2014043754

Visit the Taylor & Francis Web site at
http://www.taylorandfrancis.com

and the CRC Press Web site at
http://www.crcpress.com

Contents

Editors

Michael I. Goran, PhD, is a professor of preventive medicine and pediatrics at the Keck School of Medicine, University of Southern California in Los Angeles. He is the founding director of the USC Childhood Obesity Research Center and holds the Dr. Robert C. and Veronica Atkins Endowed Chair in Childhood Obesity and Diabetes. Dr. Goran also serves as co-director of the USC Diabetes and Obesity Research Institute. He is a native of Glasgow, Scotland, and earned his PhD from the University of Manchester, UK (1986). His research has focused on the causes and consequences of childhood obesity for over 25 years. His work is focused on understanding the metabolic and nutritional factors linking obesity to increased disease risk during growth and development and using this information as a basis for developing interventions for prevention and risk reduction. He has published over 300 professional peer-reviewed articles and reviews and is the co-editor of *Handbook of Pediatric Obesity*. He has been the recipient of a number of awards including, The Nutrition Society Medal for Research (1996), The Lilly Award for Scientific Achievement in Obesity (2006), and the Bar-Or Award for Excellence in Pediatric Obesity Research (2009).

Kim-Anne Lê, PhD, has been studying the effects of sugars and fructose on cardiometabolic risk markers over the past 10 years. She earned her PhD at the Department of Physiology of Lausanne University, Switzerland and completed a postdoctoral fellowship at the Childhood Obesity Research Center at University of Southern California in Los Angeles. She has received research support from the Swiss National Foundation for Science for these activities, and is presently a research scientist at Nestec Ltd, Nestlé Research Center, Lausanne, Switzerland.

Luc Tappy, MD, is a professor of physiology at the Lausanne University School of Biology and Medicine, and an associate physician in the service of endocrinology, diabetes and metabolism at the Lausanne University Hospital. He has extensively studied the metabolic fate of fructose in healthy humans and in patients with metabolic disorders with the use of tracer methods. As a physician, he has been mainly involved in the dietary management and surgical treatment of obese patients. His research has been supported by grants from the Swiss National Science Foundation and has included research projects funded by Nestlé SA, Vevey, Switzerland, and by the Ajinomoto Co., Inc., Japan.

Contributors

Eva Arrigoni
Agroscope Research Station
Wädenswil, Switzerland

France Bellisle
Unité de Recherche en Epidémiologie Nutritionnelle
Université Paris
Bobigny, France

Lim Wen Bin
Clinical Nutrition Research Centre
Singapore Institute for Clinical Sciences
Singapore

Claire D. Brindis
Philip R. Lee Institute for Health Policy Studies
and
Department of Pediatrics
University of California
San Francisco, California

Rebecca J. Brown
Section on Pediatric Diabetes and Metabolism
National Institute of Diabetes and Digestive and Kidney Diseases
National Institutes of Health
Bethesda, Maryland

Victoria J. Burley
Nutritional Epidemiology Group
School of Food Science and Nutrition
University of Leeds
Leeds, United Kingdom

Janet E. Cade
Nutritional Epidemiology Group
School of Food Science & Nutrition
University of Leeds
Leeds, United Kingdom

Vivian L. Choo
Toronto 3D Knowledge Synthesis and Clinical Trials Unit
St. Michael's Hospital
and
Department of Nutritional Sciences
University of Toronto
Toronto, Ontario, Canada

Kimberly Cox-York
Department of Food Science and Human Nutrition
Colorado State University
Fort Collins, Colorado

Adrian I. Cozma
Toronto 3D Knowledge Synthesis and Clinical Trials Unit
St. Michael's Hospital
and
Undergraduate Medical Education
Faculty of Medicine
University of Toronto
Toronto, Ontario, Canada

Jaimie N. Davis
Department of Nutritional Sciences
The University of Texas at Austin
Austin, Texas

Russell J. de Souza
Toronto 3D Knowledge Synthesis and Clinical Trials Unit
St. Michael's Hospital
Toronto, Ontario, Canada

and

Department of Clinical Epidemiology and Biostatistics
McMaster University
Hamilton, Ontario, Canada

Adam Drewnowski
Center for Public Health Nutrition
and
Department of Epidemiology
University of Washington
Seattle, Washington

Karin Eli
Unit for Biocultural Variation and Obesity
Institute of Social and Cultural Anthropology
University of Oxford
Oxford, United Kingdom

Mary Chong Foong Fong
Clinical Nutrition Research Centre
Singapore Institute for Clinical Sciences
and
Department of Paediatrics
Yong Loo Lin School of Medicine
National University of Singapore
Singapore

Michael I. Goran
Department of Preventive Medicine
and
Childhood Obesity Research Center
University of Southern California
Los Angeles, California

Vanessa Ha
Toronto 3D Knowledge Synthesis and Clinical Trials Unit
St. Michael's Hospital
Toronto, Ontario, Canada

and

Department of Clinical Epidemiology and Biostatistics
Faculty of Health Sciences
McMaster University
Hamilton, Ontario, Canada

Peter J. Havel
Department of Molecular Biosciences
School of Veterinary Medicine
and
Department of Nutrition
University of California
Davis, California

Frank B. Hu
Department of Nutrition
Harvard School of Public Health
and
Harvard Medical School
Boston, Massachusetts

Qiong Hu
Department of Nutrition and Exercise Physiology
University of Missouri
Columbia, Missouri

Yeo Shi Hui
Clinical Nutrition Research Centre
Singapore Institute for Clinical Sciences
Singapore

Viranda H. Jayalath
Toronto 3D Knowledge Synthesis and Clinical Trials Unit
St. Michael's Hospital
Toronto, Ontario, Canada

and

Department of Human Health and Nutrition
University of Guelph
Guelph, Ontario, Canada

Asker E. Jeukendrup
Gatorade Sports Science Institute
Barrington, Illinois

and

School of Sport and Exercise and Health Sciences
Loughborough University
Loughborough, United Kingdom

Richard J. Johnson
Division of Renal Diseases and Hypertension
University of Colorado
Denver, Colorado

Sára Karjalainen
Department of Pediatric Dentistry
University of Turku
Turku, Finland

Christina Kast
Agroscope Research Station
Bern, Switzerland

Kim-Anne Lê
Nestlé Research Center
Nestec Ltd.
Lausanne, Switzerland

Stacey Lee
Department of Nutritional Sciences
The University of Texas at Austin
Austin, Texas

Laura Gabriela Sánchez Lozada
Laboratory of Renal Physiopathology
and
Department of Nephrology
INC Ignacio Chávez
Mexico City, Mexico

Adrian Lussi
Department of Preventive, Restorative and Pediatric Dentistry
University of Bern
Bern, Switzerland

Robert H. Lustig
Philip R. Lee Institute for Health Policy Studies
and
Department of Pediatrics
University of California
San Francisco, California

Magdalena Madero
Department of Nephrology
INC Ignacio Chávez
Mexico City, Mexico

Vasanti S. Malik
Department of Nutrition
Harvard School of Public Health
and
Harvard Medical School
Boston, Massachusetts

Bernadette P. Marriott
Department of Medicine
Medical University of South Carolina
Charleston, South Carolina

Amy K. McLennan
Unit for Biocultural Variation and Obesity
Institute of Social and Cultural Anthropology
University of Oxford
Oxford, United Kingdom

Timothy H. Moran
Department of Psychiatry and Behavioral Sciences
Johns Hopkins University School of Medicine
Baltimore, Maryland

Michael Pagliassotti
Department of Food Science and Human Nutrition
Colorado State University
Fort Collins, Colorado

Elizabeth J. Parks
Department of Nutrition and Exercise Physiology
University of Missouri
Columbia, Missouri

Vishala Parmasad
Department of Anthropology
University of British Columbia
Vancouver, British Columbia, Canada

Anisha I. Patel
Philip R. Lee Institute for Health Policy Studies
and
Department of Pediatrics
Benioff Children's Hospital
University of California
San Francisco, California

Barry M. Popkin
Department of Nutrition
School of Public Health
University of North Carolina
Chapel Hill, North Carolina

Jonathan Q. Purnell
The Knight Cardiovascular Institute
Division of Endocrinology, Diabetes, and Clinical Nutrition
and
The Bob and Charlee Moore Institute for Nutrition and Wellness
Oregon Health and Science University
Portland, Oregon

Sirirat Reungjui
Division of Nephrology
Khon Kaen University
Thailand

Kristina I. Rother
Section on Pediatric Diabetes and Metabolism
National Institute of Diabetes and Digestive and Kidney Diseases
National Institutes of Health
Bethesda, Maryland

Laura A. Schmidt
Philip R. Lee Institute for Health Policy Studies
University of California
San Francisco, California

Laura Shumow
National Confectioners Association
Washington, DC

John L. Sievenpiper
Toronto 3D Knowledge Synthesis and Clinical Trials Unit
and
Li Ka Shing Knowledge Institute
St. Michael's Hospital
Toronto, Ontario, Canada

Eva Söderling
Institute of Dentistry
University of Turku
Turku, Finland

Kimber L. Stanhope
Department of Molecular Biosciences
University of California
Davis, California

Allison C. Sylvetsky
Section on Pediatric Diabetes and Metabolism
National Institute of Diabetes and Digestive and Kidney Diseases
National Institutes of Health
Bethesda, Maryland

Luc Tappy
Department of Physiology
University of Lausanne
Lausanne, Switzerland

Yada Treesukosol
Department of Psychiatry and Behavioral Sciences
Johns Hopkins University School of Medicine
Baltimore, Maryland

Stanley J. Ulijaszek
Unit for Biocultural Variation and Obesity
Institute of Social and Cultural Anthropology
University of Oxford
Oxford, United Kingdom

Effie Viguiliouk
Toronto 3D Knowledge Synthesis and Clinical Trials Unit
and
Department of Nutritional Sciences
University of Toronto
Toronto, Ontario, Canada

Barbara Walther
Agroscope Research Station
Bern, Switzerland

Tiffany Weir
Department of Food Science and Human Nutrition
Colorado State University
Fort Collins, Colorado

John S. White
White Technical Research
Argenta, Illinois

Marisa Wilson
Institute of Geography and the Lived Environment
University of Edinburgh
Edinburgh, United Kingdom

Introduction

The hypothesis that dietary sugars play a major contributing role in the links between diet, obesity, and metabolic disease outcomes has gained considerable attention over the past decades. This attention has generated interest across the globe from all walks of life including the public, academia, the food and beverage industry, the media, public health advocates, and policy-makers. Consumption of sugars is currently suspected to play an important role in the pathogenesis of not only obesity, but also of noncommunicable disorders at large, including diabetes, cardiovascular disorders, fatty liver disease, and some forms of cancers as well as oral health. There is indeed compelling evidence that consumption of sugars, either as sucrose or from added sugars and sweeteners such as high-fructose corn syrup, has increased continuously over the past 50 years, contributes in the region of 15–20% of total energy intake in several North American and European countries, and rises toward this level in many developing countries. Even though some data suggest a recent decline, there is no argument that current levels of consumption of dietary sugars at all stages of life far exceed those of previous generations and of numerous health recommendations. In addition, sugars and sweeteners have rapidly proliferated in our food supply. Over the same period, the prevalence of obesity and associated metabolic diseases has increased dramatically. Cause or correlation? The age-old question. Given that obesity results from an imbalance between energy intake and energy expenditure, and the large contribution of sugars to our daily energy intake, there is no doubt that sugar calories make a significant contribution to this pathogenesis. The overall purpose of this book is to review the wide variety of evidence and approaches that have been used to study these connections.

A wide range of research approaches are currently being used to examine the links between dietary sugars, obesity, and disease risk. These approaches include ecological studies across populations, epidemiological studies, human clinical investigations, and animal models using high-sucrose or high-fructose diets as a means of obtaining animal models of obesity and metabolic disorders. This broad variety of studies has led to the collection of a large amount of human data as well as experimental evidence showing that sugars can indeed induce hyperphagia, visceral obesity, insulin resistance, dyslipidemia, hepatic steatosis, and many other features relevant to human diseases. This body of work has also produced a vast amount of new information regarding possible molecular mechanisms underlying the metabolic effects of sugars that might explain its pathogenic role. In humans, many cohort studies provide compelling evidence for a relationship between dietary sugars, obesity, and chronic diseases. In contrast, human mechanistic studies providing mechanistic information are relatively scarce, and, for obvious ethical and practical reasons, mainly address the effects of short-term dietary intervention.

The actual scientific issue regarding the ultimate health effects of sugars is, however, more complex than recognizing sugar as one of several energy-dense nutrients responsible for body weight gain. First, there is an additional concern that dietary sugars, especially added sugars, and sugary beverages, in particular, may be important factors responsible for driving excessive food intake. In addition to the obvious caloric effects, new emerging data show that the consequences of the way sugars are metabolized can also contribute independently to metabolic disease risk—the noncaloric effects of sugars. This concern is based on the possibility that sugar calories may differ from calories from other nutrients by exerting specific deleterious effects based on the metabolic pathways involved. This suspected effect of sugar is not shared by all carbohydrates, since whole cereals, consisting mainly of starch associated with dietary fibers, are generally considered beneficial to health. Starch from whole cereal will be degraded in the gut by the joined actions of pancreatic and brush border intestinal enzymes and will eventually be absorbed as glucose. In contrast, table sugar, made up of one molecule of glucose linked with one molecule of fructose, will be split by intestinal disaccharidase and will result in the absorption of both glucose and fructose. The fructose component of sucrose makes up for the major difference between sugars in terms of actual substrates absorbed in the portal blood. This has logically led to new research that focuses on specific pathways used for fructose metabolism and how they may be involved in the pathogenesis of chronic diseases associated with obesity.

Fructose research in humans was very active in the 1980s, but was mainly focused on the hypothesis that fructose could be a first choice sweetener for diabetic patients. Such studies provided strong evidence that replacing sucrose or starch with fructose actually reduced postprandial glycemia and HbA1c in diabetic patients. However, these studies also documented that increasing fructose consumption may be associated with an increase in blood triglyceride concentration. This raised concern regarding the long-term effects of pure fructose for cardiovascular health, and the interest for fructose as a dietary product for diabetics rapidly decreased. These studies provide much useful information, but were not really designed to address our current concerns, which are mainly questions such as: Does consumption of high sugars increase overall energy intake through inadequate satiating effects? Does an excess of dietary sugars cause more adverse health effects than other calorie sources? Does a high intake of sugars represent a health hazard for normal-weight subjects in energy balance, or when present in a isocaloric, weight-maintenance diets? Are the potential negative effects of dietary sugars exacerbated in the obese individual? Are the effects of dietary sugars on obesity and health outcomes more pronounced at different stages of the life-cycle? Are all sugars equal in their obesogenic effects or are the differences in the way glucose and fructose are metabolized in the body significant in terms of chronic disease risk?

The answers to these questions are obviously of utmost importance for public health. Specific public health policies and even litigation regarding sugar consumption are strongly advocated by some as a means of tackling the epidemics of obesity and related metabolic diseases. Such actions have an ethical dimension that must be taken into consideration. For example, public health policies could constitute, to some extent, a means of forcefully limiting sugar consumption to obtain health benefits. Such action, however, transgresses the right of individuals to self-determination, which is one of the pillars of ethics, and can be justified only if one has strong evidence that sugar is indeed a special nutrient and constitutes a specific health hazard, and that the proposed policies and litigations will actually be effective in attaining a significant improvement of health-related outcomes in the population. This is hotly debated today and needs indeed to be settled urgently.

Given the large amount of emerging experimental, clinical, and population data relevant to the health effects of sugars, which encompass a wide array of approaches, ranging from molecular biology to clinical science and epidemiology, it is difficult, even for expert scientists in the field, to get a global, integrated, and balanced view of the "known knowns" as well as the "known unknowns" in this complex and rapidly evolving area of investigation. Our aim, when we decided to work on this book, was to gather together the most up-to-date and relevant information regarding all aspects of dietary sugars relating to health outcomes. Since we were committed to a balanced approach, we solicited contributions from all relevant sectors ranging from the food and beverage industry, food science, biology, pathophysiology, clinical medicine, and finally public health. For each topic, we actively recruited contributions from world-renowned experts and asked them to contribute concise, yet complete overviews of the state of the art in their specific fields of expertise. This effort led to the generation of an impressive amount of information on sugars and their relation to health, resulting in this comprehensive textbook. We were particularly interested in achieving a balance of contributions from a variety of perspectives including global (contributing authors represent a wide variety of countries), discipline (from experimental studies to public health policy), and sector (from academia to the food and beverage industry). We even solicited chapters from contributors with known opposing views because we wanted this book to be complete, unbiased, and all encompassing. However, we recognize that in no way does this body of work solve many of the ongoing debates, such as: Is sugar a toxic nutrient or merely part of our total energy overload? Are all sugars equal in their effects on the body? Do sugars cause obesity and/or associated metabolic conditions?

However, we believe the information presented is complete, up-to-date, balanced, and unbiased providing the information for you, the reader, to digest and develop your own opinion. When selecting topics and experts, we were careful to provide information as objective and balanced as possible. Personal conclusions of contributors show wide variations, and their statements reflect their own interpretation of the data, irrespective of our own interpretations and beliefs as editors. We feel that this approach was very successful, and we hope that you, the readers of this book, will find here enough information to come to your own conclusions on the many unanswered questions and critical needs for future investigation. One thing we do know and hope that we would all agree upon is that this is a critically important area of public health research and requires our utmost attention and careful, unbiased studies of the highest scientific standard and integrity. We hope you enjoy reading this work and that it benefits your world in some way whether a student, researcher, food scientist, public health advocate, politician, or food consumer.

1 Social Aspects of Dietary Sugars

Amy K. McLennan, Stanley J. Ulijaszek, and Karin Eli

CONTENTS

KEY POINTS

- Introduction
  - Begins with Mintz's [1] landmark work on sugar.
  - Three decades later, sugary products are now consumer items in the contemporary era of global food corporations, mass consumption, and food marketing.
  - This chapter considers the experiences that sugary products evoke via sensory and social meanings.
  - This is done by paying attention to advertising slogans and campaigns of well-known sugary consumer products.
- The experience of sugars: space, time, and reward
  - Meaning in sugary foods is often implicitly created and communicated through slogans, labels, and placement of foods.
  - These foods can either create time or save time, evoke the local or the exotic.
  - The feeling sugars inspire can be interpreted as refreshing, enjoyable, satiating or rewarding (sugar-free equivalents are less-commonly advertised in this way).
- Sugars and identity: clear brands, ambivalent consumption
  - Products can reinforce identity and status.
  - Sugars have ambiguous positions; use of sugars as a reward can be considered good or bad parenting; sugars may be framed as natural and synthetic/refined; shared and secretive.
- Conclusion
  - Our preference for sugars and sweetness is linked to biological and social factors.
  - When Mintz wrote in 1985, meanings were created at the intersections between consumers and larger political forces.
  - Today these meanings are more often created by corporations for the purposes of selling food products.

INTRODUCTION

Sugars may create feeling, but people create meaning. As Sidney Mintz [1] demonstrated in his landmark monograph, *Sweetness and Power*, the taste and desire for sugars and sweetness is not wholly biological or innate. Arguing that the rapid incorporation of sugar into the English diet in the nineteenth century reflected much more than the human preference for sweetness, he suggested that sugar consumption was mediated by, and in turn affected, the dynamics of its production. He argued, moreover, that consumption and production themselves were influenced by the changing social meanings and consumer uses of sugar and that the use and meanings attached to sugar likewise fed back into patterns of consumption and production. Sugar implicated slave labor and colonial domination, industrialization, and urbanization, and was, according to Mintz, not merely a bearer of sweetness but a profoundly social substance.

In the 29 years since Mintz's monograph was published, the "social" in food—and of sugar therein—has been subject to the accelerating forces of globalization, including the emergence and spread of new information and communication technologies. Like sweetened tea in the nineteenth century [1], readymade sugary products are centrally placed consumer items in the contemporary era of global food corporations, mass consumption, and the near-ubiquity of food-marketing messages. In this chapter, we examine several social aspects of sugar production and consumption linked to the marketing of corporate branded sugary and sweet products in the last three decades. We pay specific attention to the experiences and identities to which sugars are linked. The commercial world of food products on which we focus, and of which sugars are a key component, was only just emerging at the time Mintz produced *Sweetness and Power*.

Products which contain dietary sugars generally fall into the broad category of "fast moving consumer goods," along with other products such as toiletries, that are sold quickly, are relatively cheap, and are consumed frequently [2]. Such products are consumed both culturally and physiologically. Physiologically, sugars are a source of dietary energy, but one that, as reviewed in Chapter 15, may be addictive [3]; the release of opioids and dopamine upon the consumption of sugars supports this view [4]. Beverages sweetened by various added sugars are perhaps consumed more culturally than physiologically, but can be ingested in great quantity. Carbohydrates consumed in liquid form induce lower satiety than those consumed in solid form [5], making high intake of such beverages a determinant for obesity [6]. In fulfilling sweet cravings yet producing limited satiety, dietary sugars transform edible products into the commodities of modern mass consumption—quickly consumed objects for which there is a ready market demand.

As anthropological and sociological studies have shown, food holds meanings that surpass nutritional and economic factors. From taboos to cuisines, food is used to draw distinctions between social classes [7], national identities [8], and ethnic, religious, and gender groups [9,10]. The sensory qualities of food are central to its social meanings, in evoking memory and community, and in making experience. Food can invoke sensory experiences that transcend eating in the present tense, including collective, national memories [11,12], imagined connections to ancestral communities [13], and feelings of belonging or foreignness [14]. Sweet products implicate (and are designed and used to evoke) particular social meanings, experiences, and identities. Sweetness is closely associated with the experience of reward, both direct, through the taste of sweetness, and indirect, through making time and space for its consumption. It is also associated with the marking of group belonging, and with ambivalent consumer identity, both conformist and subversive, an issue that will be elaborated later in this chapter.

Such meanings are not uncomplicated reflections of sweetness as a taste, but are linked to the commodification of sweetness and to the corporate branding of specific products that carry added sugars or sweet tastes. Sugars can take many forms—being included in products as diverse as drinks, confectioneries, cookies, breads, and fast foods—and readily transform into a wide range of products, often changing inedible or unpalatable forms into edible ones. Sugars are also hidden in products where sweetness is seemingly absent; processed food products almost universally contain large amounts of sugars regardless of whether consumers might consider them "sweet" or "savory." Moreover, packaged food products often mask tactile and visual qualities that consumers might associate with sugars, especially stickiness and a glazed appearance. Thus, in the process of meaning-making, the products themselves are more important than the sugars that sweeten them. Yet dietary sugars, even when hidden, are implicated in the evocation and promulgation of these social meanings.

EXPERIENCE OF SUGARS: SPACE, TIME, AND REWARD

Consumers of sugary products—whether they are sweetened soft drinks, chocolates, fast foods, or snacks—take in not only sugar, but also an experience that the product provides. Part of this experience may be related to the physiological response to the products' ingestion. However, most of the neurotransmitters involved are not specific to particular emotions [15], and what the ingestion of a sugary product means to a consumer depends on prior individual experience and memory as well as broader social context. Mintz [1] suggests that this meaning-making in the case of sugar is derived from the intersection of "outside" and "inside" influences. Outside meanings reflect the place of this commodity in colonial history, commerce, politics, law, and policymaking. Thus, the outside meaning of sugar varies between countries: in the UK, sugar is deeply embedded in British colonial history and has been naturalized across more than 200 years of commercial activity involving the production of sugar as a commodity and its transformation into a wide range of products including confectionaries, pickles, and alcoholic spirits made from residues of sugar production. In the USA, a colonial junior partner to the UK in the sugar industry, sugar is less culturally embedded than the idea of sweetness, which is now produced in enormous quantity by transforming a commodity that is closer to the American heart, corn, into high-fructose corn syrup. Inside meanings are generated by imitation of elite practices by the general population. Historically, sugar was consumed by the wealthy and powerful; when industrial production made it generally affordable, the general population quickly took it on as something for general consumption. During the industrialization of Britain, even poor laborers sought and enjoyed sugar in their cups of tea [1]. Nowadays, people in power are, in part, responsible for both the presence of new products and for their meanings. Inside meanings are created by the consumers of sugar-based and sugar-containing products, but are also built into products by their producers: they are overtly stated on packaging and in advertisements.

Improvements to communication technologies, including televisions, telephones, computers, and the world wide web, have facilitated the spread of meanings and messages on a global scale in the past three decades. The meanings inherent in sugars and sugary products surround us every day: they are spelled out in advertising campaigns and slogans, or subtly hinted at through product placement or label design. These outside meanings are reinforced by inside meanings associated with the sensory pleasure elicited by sugars. The links between sensory experience, emotion, and memory are key to transforming the meanings embedded in sugary products into experience [16]. This is where the advertising of sugary products comes into play. Table 1.1 lists a number of advertising slogans used in the promotion of sugary products, and we discuss these further in the following paragraphs. Although we cite the year of release for each of the slogans, it is important to note that many of these slogans are long-running, have been recycled and redeployed by companies, or have re-emerged on video-sharing sites where they enjoy a virtual following. Some of these slogans have become iconic and form an inherent part of the products' identities.

Sugary products, like cigarettes before them, are marketed by some companies as creating time in the day—not unlike the tea break that Mintz documented—when a well-earned break can be enjoyed. A long-running Nestlé slogan suggests that consumers should "Have a Break ... Have a Kit Kat;" the company later attempted to patent the first part of the slogan in a 9-year court battle with Mars, which underlines the importance of this advertising idea to Nestlé. Coca-Cola has previously been sold as "The Pause That Refreshes," while a widespread McDonalds trademark and advertising campaign featured the slogan and song lyrics "You Deserve a Break Today." The images and

TABLE 1.1
Advertising Slogans Referred to in this Chapter (In Order of Appearance)

Product Name	Producer (Parent Company)	Slogan/Advertisement Name	Slogan/Advertisement Date(s) and Details	Link (Accessed 27 June 2013)
Kit Kat	Nestlé	Have a break … have a Kit Kat	1958: Launched in the UK 1970s: Expanded to Europe, Japan, and the USA 1990s: Expanded to Malaysia, India, and China 2000s: Expanded to Bulgaria, Russia, Turkey, and Venezuela	About Kit Kat! www.kitkat.com
Coca-Cola	Coca-Cola	The Pause That Refreshes Pause For Refreshment	1929: Created 1939: Altered and re-released	History of Coca-Cola slogans www.coca-cola.co.uk/about-us/heritage/history-of-coca-cola-slogans.html
McDonalds	McDonalds	You Deserve a Break Today	1971–1975, 1980–1984: Owned by the company for print and television in Australia, Canada, USA, the Netherlands, UK, Puerto Rico 1989–1990: Canada, US, UK, Puerto Rico	Trademark Information www.mcdonalds.com/us/en/terms_conditions.html
Oikos	Dannon	Possibly the best yoghurt in the world	2012: Featured at the US Superbowl	The Oikos Secret www.oikosyogurt.com/what-is-greek-yogurt/oikos-secret.aspx
Coca-Cola	Coca-Cola	Share a Coke with …	2011: Launched in Australia 2013: Launched in 20 further countries, including Brazil, China and across the UK, and Europe	Coca-Cola named creative marketer of the year www.coca-colacompany.com/stories/work-that-matters-coca-cola-named-creative-marketer-of-the-year-wins-20-additional-cannes-lions
Nutri-Grain	Kellogg's	Fuel On	Reference to food, fuel, and athletic performance has been a central part of this brand in Australia since 1984 [17]	Kellogg's Nutri-Grain Fuel On www.nutrigrain.com.au/
Nutri-Grain cereal bars	Kellogg's	Nutri-Grain helps take care of you so you can take care of everything	1990s: Rose to popularity in the UK, US, Canada, and Ireland	Kellogg's Nutri-Grain Cereal Bars www.nutrigrain.com/
Lucozade	GlaxoSmithKline	Replaces Lost Energy Aids Recovery	1927: Product launched as an aid to recovery from illness 1983: Rebranded as an energy drink	Lucozade www.gsk.com/products/our-consumer-healthcare-products/lucozade.html

Pepsi	Pepsico	The Choice of a New Generation	1984: Launched and trademarked; marketed heavily until 1991 through a range of well-known entertainment personalities 2012: Trademark lapsed and purchased by an oatmeal company	Business Insider: Pepsi let trademark lapse www.businessinsider.com/better-oats-uses-pepsis-tagline-in-new-campaign-2012-3?op=1
Red Bull	Red Bull GmbH	It Gives You Wings!	1987: Launched in Austria with reference to flying 1992: Cartoon advertisements that accompanied slogan launched 1994: Began to move into international markets, beginning with Hungary	Red Bull Milestones http://energydrink.redbull.com/red-bull-history
Mars	Mars	Work, Rest and Play	1959: Launched as the product was adapted from a war-time food for soldiers to a snack (confectionery rationing in the UK was lifted in 1953)	Our History www.marsbar.co.uk/default.aspx
Snack	Cadbury (Kraft)	Bridge That Gap	1960s: Launched 1973: Revived 1998: Revived	Campaign: Cadbury's revives "gap" line www.campaignlive.co.uk/news/22727/ UK television adverts 1955–1990 www.headington.org.uk/adverts/chocolate_sweets.htm
Bounty	Mars	The Taste of Paradise	Currently used; no information on slogan history available	Mars Chocolate www.mars.com/global/brands/chocolate.aspx
Mounds and Almond Joy	Hershey's	Unwrap Paradise	1988: Products moved under Hershey Foods and re-launched	Almond Joy and Mounds www.hersheys.com/almondjoy-mounds.aspx
Burger King	Burger King	We Do It Like You'd Do It	1988: Launched	Burger King "Our History" www.bk.com/en/us/company-info/about-bk.html
Sara Lee	Sara Lee	The Joy of Eating	2006: Launched following company restructuring	Welcome to Sara Lee www.thejoyofeating.com/
Sprite	Coca-Cola	Obey Your Thirst	1994: Launched 2003: Re-launched for the product Sprite	The Coca-Cola Company: Obey Your Thirst campaign [21]
7-Up	PepsiCo	Now that's refreshing	1990s: Launched 2010: Expanded into the Pepsi Refresh Project of small grant funding	Pepsico Media: The Pepsi Refresh Project Awards www.pepsico.com/PressRelease/The-Pepsi-Refresh-Project-Awards-13-Million-to-Support-the-Publics-Favorite-Idea03222010.html
Snickers	Mars	Hungry? Why wait? Grab a Snickers! Don't let hunger happen to you Snickers really satisfies	A long history of advertisements relating to satisfaction of hunger; no specific information on slogan history available	Snickers www.snickers.com/

continued

TABLE 1.1 (continued)
Advertising Slogans Referred to in this Chapter (In Order of Appearance)

Product Name	Producer (Parent Company)	Slogan/Advertisement Name	Slogan/Advertisement Date(s) and Details	Link (Accessed 27 June 2013)
Diet Coke	Coca-Cola	Just for the Taste of it Just for the Fun of it	1987–1989: Launched in the USA	The Diet Coke Story www.dietcoke.com/about-diet-coke/our-story.jsp
Diet Coke	Coca-Cola	♥ No sugar. No calories	2006: Appeared on Coca-Cola Light cans in continental Europe 2013: Linked with a video advertising campaign in the USA and UK	Link to 2013 video advertisement: http://www.youtube.com/watch?v=HuHV4gwSXn4
Diet Pepsi	Pepsico	Get the Skinny		Media Press Release www.pepsico.com/PressRelease/Diet-Pepsi-Debuts-its-Sleek-New-Look-at-Mercedes-Benz-Fashion-Week02082011.html
Milky Way	Mars	The sweet you can eat between meals without ruining your appetite	1970s: Slogan launched, used for several decades [38]	Mars wins over ITC in Milky Way ads battle www.accessmylibrary.com/article-1G1-11754235/mars-wins-over-itc.html
Belvita Breakfast Biscuits	Mondelez International (Kraft Foods)	Biscuits specially designed for breakfast	2011: First marketed in Europe 2012: Expanded to the USA, Brazil, and Canada	US: Kraft to launch Belvita biscuits in the USA www.just-food.com/news/kraft-to-launch-belvita-biscuits-in-the-us_id117760.aspx
Coca-Cola	Coca-Cola	Charity	1998: Global Muslim market	http://memory.loc.gov/cgi-bin/query/r?ammem/cola:@field%28DOCID+@lit%28kocx761n%29%29
Coca-Cola	Coca-Cola	First experience	1999: Morocco	http://memory.loc.gov/cgi-bin/query/r?ammem/cola:@field%28DOCID+@lit%28kocx93n7%29%29
Coca-Cola	Coca-Cola	Snowflakes	1999: Italy	http://memory.loc.gov/cgi-bin/query/r?ammem/cola:@field%28DOCID+@lit%28kocx9364%29%29
Breyers' Ice Cream	Unilever	All-natural ice cream	1997: United States (variations on this theme appeared as early as 1983)	http://www.youtube.com/watch?v=bWB2T_dDuUA
Reese's Peanut Butter Cups	Hershey's	Three-way	2007: United States	http://www.youtube.com/watch?v=RhfD4nwruRY
Milano Cookies	Pepperidge Farm (Campbell Soup Company subsidiary)	Chocolate: The highlight of my night	2013: United States	http://www.youtube.com/watch?v=OeFhyMeys0o

television commercials that accompanied the slogan over the years very rarely featured any food, instead depicting couples or families gathered together laughing or chatting. Such campaigns readily convince consumers that they need and deserve a break in their hurried lives and demonstrate how processed products are a work-free means of achieving it. Time out can be spent alone or with friends; an advertisement for sweetened Oikos yoghurt shown during the 2012 US Superbowl depicted a woman knocking her partner unconscious so she could enjoy eating the sweet, rich product by herself, while a multinational Coca-Cola campaign encouraged consumers to "Share a Coke with …" the person whose name was printed on the bottle. Through such meaning-filled slogans and images, the sensory reward from consuming foods/beverages high in sugars can be extended to the rewards of relaxation or social connection, inspiring memories of blissful moments of independent contemplation or conversation with friends, and respite from the stresses of the day.

Alternatively, sugary products have been marketed as helping consumers use their time more efficiently. Here, the meaning-making metaphors are those that evoke energy, fuel, and activity. In Australia, New Zealand, and South Africa, a Kellogg's Nutri-Grain commercial urges consumers to "Fuel On" with the breakfast cereal; the same brand in the UK produces cereal bars and asserts that "Nutri-Grain helps take care of you so you can take care of everything" [see also Reference 17]. Similarly, the sports drink Lucozade "Replaces Lost Energy." Calorie-dense foods are particularly targeted by marketers at people who consider themselves to have an active or busy lifestyle: a hallmark of the contemporary consumer-citizen. Such products can be consumed without the need for preparation, enabling consumers to live effortlessly effervescent lives without losing time in eating and drinking. This culture of fast food emerged in the USA in the 1930s [18] and developed iteratively with the snack foods that filled spaces between meals. Cool sugary drinks can be gulped, chocolate bars munched out of individual packages, and fast food obtained at a moment's notice. Such food products are cheap vehicles for sugar that are targeted by the producers to provide a low-cost energy boost to help consumers to focus and achieve a high level of daily activity; these products were initially developed in the USA, a nation that greatly values industriousness. With some products, companies have also created and filled the space between making time and saving time. The widespread Mars Bar slogan gives us the option to "Work, Rest and Play," while "Bridge That Gap" is a registered trademark for Cadbury's Snack in the UK.

Some sugary products have been developed that call on imagination and corporeal memory to transport consumers to another place. One can close one's eyes and find "The Taste of Paradise," the theme of a long-running television and cinema advertisement for the Bounty chocolate-covered coconut bar sold by Mars across the European Union. Mounds and Almond Joy, similar products marketed by Hershey's in the USA, are advertised sitting prominently on a pristine white beach with coconut palms overhead accompanied by the slogan "Unwrap Paradise." These products are not chosen by consumers for their sugar content. Rather they are chosen for the taste and experience they elicit, both of which are facilitated by sugar. Sugar hides in the background and serves to emphasize not only the flavor of coconut but also the imagined or remembered experience of a warm, sunny vacation. For those who prefer the comforts of the local, there are products that urge consumers to remember home-cooked cakes and cookies filled not only with sugar, but also with sweet love and affection. Appealing to this sense, Burger King launched the advertising campaign stating, "We Do It Like You'd Do It," likening its food to backyard barbeques and home-style devotion to cooking. The use of such imaginative geographies is also linked to cultural capital [19], to which we turn in the following section.

Fast foods, including sugary foods and drinks, are marketed as being associated with fun, happiness, satiation/satisfaction, and positive experiences [20]. For instance, the Sara Lee brand slogan, "The Joy of Eating," encourages consumers to remember, anticipate, and seek the pleasurable feeling that processed food consumption elicits. The lemon-lime drink Sprite emphasizes the importance of satiating the feeling of desire, urging consumers to "Obey Your Thirst" [21], while Seven-Up instead calls on the consumer to imagine what drinking it might feel like: "Now that's refreshing." Snickers' series of advertising campaigns calls attention to the experience of consumption, from hunger and anticipation to consumption and satiation: "Hungry? Why wait? Grab a Snickers!," "Don't let hunger happen to you," and "Snickers Really Satisfies." The psychological complexities of the use of sugary confectionery as a reward for behavior, a treat for special occasions or for celebrating key dates, and in memory and emotion, are reviewed by Albon [22]. The producers and marketers of these sugary products do not promote them on the basis of their sweetness; when sweetness abounds, how can any product gain distinction in the marketplace on the basis of sweetness alone? Rather, sweetness is a given, and marketing translates sweetness into bodily and social experience, to the extent that even if a product has never been tried before, it is easy to imagine what eating it might feel like.

The importance of the intersection of the physiological effects of sugar and meaning-making around sugar-containing products can be examined through a comparison of sugar with nonsugar consumer goods. The most obvious of these, insofar as they deliberately and explicitly avoid the inclusion of sugar, are foods sweetened with noncaloric sweeteners. Such products fill the only niche of people's lives that sugar cannot arguably fill: the health-related demand for sweetness-without-calories. Synthetic noncaloric sweeteners have been discovered or synthesized to fill this niche, although they do not adequately fill the place of experience and meaning. Sugar-free products such as Diet Coke use slogans such as "Just for the Taste of it" or "Just for the Fun of it." In 2011, Diet Pepsi released a smaller-diameter package paired with the highly controversial slogan "Get the Skinny," and the implied message that skinnier is better, at New York City's Fall Fashion Week. Products containing calorie-free sweeteners frequently attempt to appeal to the rationally thinking dieting consumer who seeks the taste of sugar and the body shape that dieting—abstaining from sugar—is purported to bring. Notably, the slogans promoting such products frequently reduce their experiential dimensions to focus on qualities of physical appearance (lightness, slenderness), mimicry of sugar (taste without the calories), or the lifestyle that a slender body type is purported to bring (such as fun). They rarely evoke the social, sensory, and emotional experiences invoked in the marketing of their sugary equivalents. Sweet products without sugar are, at the same time, much harder to sell [23,24], possibly in part because the feeling that sugar gives when consumed in a product is more effective in the generation of experience, emotion, and meaning-making, than are noncaloric sweeteners.

SUGARS AND IDENTITY: CLEAR BRANDS, AMBIVALENT CONSUMPTION

Sugars tend to be hidden in the products that are consumed, and identity interlocks not with sugar itself but with the foods in which it is embedded, and, by extension, the ways in which sugary foods are packaged and marketed. As a key ingredient of fast food products that offer a "break"—that suggest (or sell) a desired lifestyle—sugar is bound up with brands. Food brands, laden with taglines that offer readymade identities, encourage consumption practices that emphasize self-image, status, and peer group belonging. Food brand consciousness, which influences consumption of easily identifiable products, constitutes a barrier to healthy eating among teenagers insofar as those who do not participate in branded food consumption risk social ostracism [25]. The selective incorporation of these products into the body then becomes a statement of social self-awareness. But food brands also have a strong bearing on identity beyond the context of teenage sociality. The iconicity of Coca-Cola, with its free market connotations, has played out differently in diverging political–economic contexts, highlighting the conflict between the brand's self-promoted association with freedom, on the one hand, and its part in extending neoliberal ideology through globalization, on the other hand. Thus, while in the former East Germany Coca-Cola was associated with status consumption [26] as capitalism arrived at the end of the Cold War, in both Turkey [27,28] and Peru [29], local brands of cola were marketed as national alternatives to the US brand, as an aspect of resistance to globalization.

In advertising to international markets, the Coca-Cola Company has explicitly evoked the identity-making qualities associated with sensory remembrance. For example, in three very different Coca-Cola advertisements—directed at the Italian (Snowflakes (1999)), Moroccan (First Experience (1999)), and the global Muslim (Charity (1998)) markets—nostalgic images of children consuming the product were used to situate the brand as bringing together past and present, connecting adults with their childhood selves and linking generations and communities through a shared, timeless taste. All three advertisements are featured on a Library of Congress web page which delineates the history of Coca-Cola television advertisements through archival material. As portrayed on the web page, the shifting themes and styles of Coca-Cola advertisements reflect the cultural zeitgeist of their respective eras. Coca-Cola, then, becomes a stand-in for US cultural identity [30].

Yet, while sugary food brands may provide the clarity of copywritten messages, sugar-containing products remain ambivalent. Both desired and spurned, lavished and withheld, sugars occupy conflicted space in contemporary food terrains. Albon [22] suggests that sweets and confectionery are located at the intersection of food and "cultural artefact," positioned outside the realms of nourishment and meals but constituting an important category of consumption, especially for children to whom many products are advertised [22,31]. This is not an accident: in many industrialized countries, it was more advantageous for emerging food corporations to create a new market for processed foods rather than attempt to replace existing food practices and meals with new products [18]. Snack foods thus appropriated the spaces between meals, especially in countries such as the US [1], and could both "ruin" a person's appetite for a meal or sustain a person between meals. At once acknowledging the former and appealing to the latter, a long-running slogan of the Milky Way chocolate bar in Australia and the UK was "The sweet you can eat between meals without ruining your appetite." The use of the slogan on television was the subject of a complaint by the Health Education Authority and antisugar lobbyists, who contended that it was unhealthy to encourage such snacking between meals. However, the Independent Television Commission which reviewed the case agreed with the producer, Mars, that the advertisements actually encouraged restrained eating.

Sugar-containing products are ambivalent in other ways as well. Rewarding children with sweets and limiting children's sugar consumption are both considered acts of "good" parenting, depending on the context [22,32,33]. The provision and withholding of sugary foods are thus ambivalently linked with relational identities within families and peer groups. Psychological ambivalence may also facilitate the consumption of sugary and fatty foods [34] and contribute to obesity [35].

Sugar, a versatile, hidden substance, can be framed as "good" or "bad," "natural" or "refined," sought after or avoided: all in service of the sweet product being sold. According to Mintz [36], "'New' foods replace 'old, outdated' foods. 'Pure' foods replace what are called 'impure' foods. 'Science' triumphs. Soon enough, of course, the old foods will reappear, in attractive, modern, and expensive packages, whereupon they will be touted as 'natural.' Thus the market triumphs again" (p. 10). Two examples illustrate the extreme flexibility in the marketing of sugar-containing products. Breyers' (Unilever) iconic 1997 television commercial for the US market urges consumers to buy "taste, not technology," by portraying a preschool-age child reading the brand's vanilla ice cream ingredient list with ease: "milk, cream, sugar, and vanilla." The ingredients are recognizably sourced from the natural world, and it is easy to overlook the industrial processes that are realistically used in the production of each ingredient, especially in sugar refining. The advertisement appeals to consumers who are sceptical about comparatively unnatural industrially produced synthetic sweeteners, which once positively signaled advanced industrialization but are today also associated with corporate domination. Cane sugar, which is natural insofar as it is less associated with these scientific processes, appears relatively politically benign. By contrast, a 2013 UK fashion magazine (*InStyle*) full-page advertisement for Diet Coke, which features a can glistening with beads of moisture and hovering weightlessly over blades of grass, states: "♥ No sugar. No calories." According to the advertising, this product contains no naturally occurring impurities but rather is designed to give the consumer the body they desire. Both advertisements emphasize the simplicity of their products, while appealing to (albeit different) constructions of the "natural."

Divergent messages about sugar, however, often appear within the same advertisement; indeed, the ambivalent status of sugar constitutes the core of many marketing campaigns for sugar-containing products. Sugar might be dangerous to health, but it is also a reward: a happy, sometime secretive, indulgence. "Subversive" eating, as Albon [22] argues, is a central motivation for children's consumption of "bad for you" sugary foods. Sustained into adulthood, this sense of "subversiveness," or "naughtiness" [33,37], is then exploited, and even promoted, in the marketing of sugary products. Thus, in a 2007 US television advertisement, Hershey's informs viewers that a Reese's Peanut Butter Cup is "the perfect three-way: milk chocolate, Reese's peanut butter, and you," to the sounds of Chromeo's "Needy Girl," inviting the consumer to partake in a clandestine assignation with their proxy-lovers, milk chocolate and peanut butter. And a recent (2013) US television advertisement for Pepperidge Farm's Milano Cookies portrays a married upper-middle-class couple clandestinely binging on biscuits for emotional support, with the tagline "my yummy secret."

CONCLUSION

As Mintz [1] demonstrated, the preference for sugar and sweetness is linked both to biological and social factors. In the UK, across recent centuries, sugars have grown "more important in people's consciousness, in family budgets, and in the economic, social, and political life of the nation" (p. 167). The commercial world of food products on which we focus in this chapter, and to which sugar is a vital component, was only just emerging at the time Mintz produced *Sweetness and Power*. However, sweetness and power remain entangled, with sugary food products and corporate producers succeeding sugar and governments. When Mintz wrote about sugar in 1985, he described the way in which it was produced by colonial powers and slave labor, and sold back to people as a new commodity. The process of meaning-making was situated in the space between producers and consumers. The locus of meaning-making around sugar and sweet foods has shifted in recent decades, with producers—no longer the government, but instead processors, packagers, distributors, and marketers—filling a wide range of products with both sugar and meaning. There is much less space for consumers to create meaning, other than through the consumption of specific brands. Now, sugar is not only spooned into tea, but is hidden in food during production, and its meaning is much less negotiated between consumers and producers, but more created through branding and labeling.

REFERENCES

1. Mintz SW. Sweetness and Power: *The Place of Sugar in Modern History*. New York: Penguin Books; 1985.
2. Çelen A, Erdoğan T, Taymaz E. *Fast Moving Consumer Goods: Competitive Conditions and Policies*. Ankara: Economic Research Center, Middle East Technical University; 2005.
3. Drewnowski A, Bellisle F. Liquid calories, sugar, and body weight. *Am J Clin Nutr*. 2007;85(3):651–61. Available from: http://www.ncbi.nlm.nih.gov/pubmed/17344485
4. Avena NM, Rada P, Hoebel BG. Evidence for sugar addiction: Behavioral and neurochemical effects of intermittent, excessive sugar intake. *Neurosci Biobehav Rev*. 2008;32(1):20–39.
5. Pan A, Hu FB. Effects of carbohydrates on satiety: Differences between liquid and solid food. *Curr Opin Clin Nutr Metab Care*. 2011;14(4):385–90.
6. Olsen NJ, Heitmann BL. Intake of calorically sweetened beverages and obesity. *Obes Rev*. 2009;10(1):68–75. Available from: http://www.ncbi.nlm.nih.gov/pubmed/18764885 [accessed 24 May 2013].
7. Bourdieu P. *Distinction: A Social Critique of the Judgement of Taste*, 1984th ed. Cambridge: Harvard University Press; 1979.
8. Appadurai A. How to make a national cuisine: Cookbooks in contemporary India. *Comp Stud Soc Hist*. 1988;30(1):3–24.
9. Bahloul J. From a Muslim banquet to a Jewish seder: Foodways and ethnicity among North African Jews. In: Cohen MR, Udovitch AL, editors. *Jew Among Arabs: Contacts and Boundaries*. Princeton, NJ: Darwin; 1989. p. 85–96.
10. Counihan CM, Kaplan S. *Food and Gender: Identity and Power*. Reading, MA: Harwood Academic Publishers; 1998.
11. Seremetakis CN. *The Senses Still: Perception and Memory as Material Culture in Modernity*. Chicago, IL: University of Chicago Press; 1996.
12. Holtzman JD. Food and memory. *Annu Rev Anthropol*. 2006;35:361–78.

13. Sutton DE. *Remembrance of Repasts: An Anthropology of Food and Memory*. Oxford: Berg; 2001.
14. Law L. *Home Cooking: Filipino Women and Geographies of the Senses in Hong Kong. Empire of the Senses*. Oxford: Berg; 2005.
15. Netter P. Health and pleasure. In: Warburton DM, Sherwood N, editors. *Pleasure and Quality of Life*. Chichester, NY: Wiley; 1996. p. 81–9.
16. Ferzacca S. Lived food and judgments of taste at a time of disease. *Med Anthropol*. 2004;23(1):41–67. Available from: http://www.ncbi.nlm.nih.gov/pubmed/14754667 [accessed 21 July 2011].
17. Harrison P, Chalmers K, D'Souza S, Coveney J, Ward P, Mehta K et al. *Targeting Children with Integrated Marketing Communications: Children and Food Marketing Project Report*. Adelaide: SA Health; 2010.
18. Levenstein HA. *Paradox of Plenty: A Social History of Eating in Modern America*. Oxford: Oxford University Press; 1993.
19. May J. "A little taste of something more exotic": The imaginitive geographies of everyday life. *Geography*. 1996;81(1):57–64.
20. Harris JL, Pomeranz JL, Lobstein T, Brownell KD. A crisis in the marketplace: How food marketing contributes to childhood obesity and what can be done. *Annu Rev Public Health*. 2009;30:211–25. Available from: http://www.ncbi.nlm.nih.gov/pubmed/18976142 [accessed 25 May 2013].
21. Teague K. The Coca-Cola Company: Obey your thirst campaign (2004). In: Riggs T, editor. *Encyclopedia of Major Marketing Campaigns (Volume 2)*. Farmington Hills: Thomson Gale; 2006. p. 347–50.
22. Albon DJ. Approaches to the study of children, food and sweet eating: A review of the literature. *Early Child Dev Care*. 2005;175(5):407–17. Available from: http://www.tandfonline.com/doi/abs/10.1080/0300443042000244055[accessed 17 May 2013].
23. Duffey KJ, Popkin BM. Shifts in patterns and consumption of beverages between 1965 and 2002. *Obesity*. 2007;15(11):2739–47. Available from: http://www.ncbi.nlm.nih.gov/pubmed/18070765
24. Popkin BM, Nielsen SJ. The sweetening of the world's diet. *Obes Res*. 2003;11(11):1325–32.
25. Stead M, McDermott L, MacKintosh AM, Adamson A. Why healthy eating is bad for young people's health: Identity, belonging and food. *Soc Sci Med*. 2011;72:1131–1139.
26. Veenis M. Cola in the German Democratic Republic: East German fantasies on Western consumption. *Enterp Soc*. 2011;12(3):489–524.
27. Foster RJ, Özkan D. Consumer citizenship, nationalism, and neoliberal globalization in Turkey: The advertising launch of Cola Turka. *Advert Soc Rev*. 2005;6(3). Available from: http://muse.jhu.edu/journals/advertising_and_society_review/v006/6.3ozkan_foster.html [accessed 24 July 2014].
28. Ogan CL, Filiz C, Kaptan Y. Reverse glocalization? Marketing a Turkish cola in the shadow of a giant. *J Arab Muslim Media Res*. 2007;1(1):47–62.
29. Alcalde MC. Between Incas and Indians: Inca Kola and the construction of a Peruvian-global modernity. *J Consum Cult*. 2009;9(1):31–54.
30. Library of Congress. Highlights in the history of Coca-Cola television advertising. 2000. Available from: http://memory.loc.gov/ammem/ccmphtml/colahist.html [accessed 11 May 2013].
31. James A. The good, the bad and the delicious: The role of confectionery in British society. *Sociol Rev*. 1990;38(4):666–88.
32. Fischler C. Learned versus "spontaneous" dietetics: French mothers' views of what children should eat. *Soc Sci Inf*. 1986;25(4):945–65.
33. Lupton D. Food, memory and meaning: The symbolic and social nature of food events. *Sociol Rev*. 1994;42(4):664–85.
34. Maio GR, Haddock GG, Jarman HL. Social psychological factors in tackling obesity. *Obes Rev*. 2007;8(S1):123–5.
35. Butland B, Jebb S, Kopelman P, McPherson K, Thomas S, Mardell J et al. *FORESIGHT. Tackling Obesities: Future Choices—Project Report*, 2nd ed. Foresight. London: UK Government Office for Science; 2007.
36. Mintz SW. Sugar: Old champion, new contenders. *Food Ethics*. 2009;4(2):5–10.
37. Trostle J. Comments on defining the shape of biocultural studies. *Med Anthropol Q*. 1990;4(3):371–4.
38. Johnson M. Mars wins over ITC in Milky Way ads battle (December 19, 1991). Press release archived by AccessMyLibrary. Available from: http://archive.today/Y8ew [accessed 24 July 2014].

2 Political Economies of Sugar
Views from a Former Sugarcane Industry

Marisa Wilson and Vishala Parmasad

CONTENTS

KEY POINTS

- Part I: Questioning the neoliberal market in sugar
  - International political economies of sugar are shaped by long-term power relations between former colonies and former colonizers. In line with other food regimes, international political economies of sugar are increasingly influenced by neoliberal discourses of development.
  - British colonialism and industrialized food led to mass appropriations of land, labor, knowledge, and lives from the colonies by planter-colonists and later multinational corporations (MNCs).
  - The World Trade Organization's (WTO) model of trade liberalization is based on an ahistorical, apolitical discourse of a uniform global market in which all states (and firms) compete on an equal playing field.
- Part II: Material and discursive shifts in West Indian sugar
  - After colonialism, attempts to redress historical injustices in ex-sugar colonies resulted in preferential markets being established between Britain (and later the EU) and Commonwealth countries. Uneven trade liberalizations undermined these preferential markets but not others.
  - The neoliberal discourse of competitiveness obscures the persistence of protected markets for sugar produced by sugarcane and beet farmers in wealthier countries. The power of sugar MNCs derived from the very protections the ex-colonies are now being denied.
  - Farmers from former colonies must compete on the global market and the resulting price squeeze has led to the closure of sugar industries in some countries. The closure

of the Trinidadian sugar industry transformed local foodways as co-existing subsistence agriculture was hindered.
- Part III: Case study of the sugar industry in Trinidad
  - Trinidad was a British sugar colony to which African slaves (until 1838) and Indian indentured servants (1845–1917) were imported as labor. During the later years of colonialism, the sugar industry was consolidated under the MNC Tate & Lyle, which received preferential protection from Britain. After independence in 1962, the sugar industry was nationalized as the state-owned enterprise Caroni (1975) Ltd. Oil and gas laborers (predominantly Afro-Trinidadian) and sugarcane workers/farmers (predominantly Indo-Trinidadians) had been pitted against each other since the colonial period.
  - International Monetary Fund-led restructuring of the "uncompetitive" Trinidadian sugar industry began in the 1980s, and minimal efforts were made to diversify away from sugarcane. In 2003, Caroni (1975) Ltd was closed down and its 9000 former employees were required to accept "Voluntary Separation [severance] Packages".
  - As the majority of Caroni (1975) Ltd's lands were cultivated by independent small farmers, many lost their agricultural livelihoods. The restructuring of Caroni (1975) Ltd and closure of its last subsidiary in 2007 signaled the demise of agriculture in Trinidad since the company constituted the backbone of all its agricultural production. The voices of interviewed Indo-Trinidadian farmers confirm that the closure of the sugar industry in Trinidad was devastating for agricultural livelihoods.

INTRODUCTION

> One important phenomenon is that the sugar workers has [*sic.*] almost a second economy. He earns his living out of the industry, but because he finishes work at nine o'clock in the day he goes home and almost starts a second industry, a kitchen garden or an animal farm or something like that .... There is a sugar culture and change—change must be made in the context of this culture. ([44]: p. 17–18).

After years of escalating debt and losses, in 2003 the Trinidadian sugarcane industry was deemed uncompetitive by neoliberal-leaning analysts and closed down. From as early as the 1980s, the International Monetary Fund (IMF) had made recommendations in its Country Reports for restructuring Caroni (1975) Limited Company (Ltd), a state-owned sugar corporation and mill located on the island of Trinidad, the larger island of the two-island state, Trinidad and Tobago. The IMF's recommendations were consistent with its Structural Adjustment Programs elsewhere* and closely adhered to by Trinidadian policymakers. By contrast, ex-workers and sharecrop sugarcane farmers argued that the so-called "restructuring" of Caroni was actually a euphemism for its closure, a politically motivated attack on the lives of thousands of Trinidadians of Indian descent: "For a government to pursue a national policy in one area [oil and gas] … and to abandon it in others is to compromise the neutrality of the state" ([30]: p. 37). Underlying the issue of Caroni (1975) Ltd is a fundamental tension in Trinidadian society between industrial and agricultural models for development, and between competing political interests of Trinidadians of African origin and those of Indian origin. The class and racially charged politics and economics of sugarcane in Trinidad and Tobago affected people and environments in very place-based ways, but the fate of the Trinidadian sugar industry is also tied to long-term "pathways of power" [56] that reach beyond the borders of the nation state.

This chapter seeks to reveal how international political economies of sugar in the past established pathways of power traceable to the present, if increasingly under the material and discursive influence

* Such policies include privatization and deregulation, export-promotion to obtain foreign exchange, currency devaluation, cutting spending on social services such as healthcare and education, eliminating barriers to foreign multinationals and trade, decreasing wages and restricting credit, and raising interest rates.

of neoliberal models for development. These "power geometries" [33,34] are present both within and between countries, though global institutions such as the IMF and the World Trade Organization (WTO) set the rules for global market entry which are often more amenable to countries of a more "developed" status [12]. The chapter illustrates continuities and changes in political economies and cultures of sugar, with a brief review of current research on international political economies of sugar (Part I), which we then relate to regional (Part II) and national/localized (Part III) political economies and cultures of sugar in the West Indies and Trinidad, respectively. By comparing interconnected scales of sugar production and consumption, we offer a more empirical view of the history, economics, and politics of sugar than more market-based accounts of sugar's political economy.

QUESTIONING THE NEOLIBERAL MARKET IN SUGAR

Richardson* has conducted what is perhaps the most comprehensive research on the international political economy of sugar [46–49]. He explains uneven pathways of power that underpin the sugar industry by drawing from an older Marxist literature on food regimes developed by sociologists Friedmann and McMichael.† Like geographers Drummond and Marston [14], Richardson uses the theory of food regimes to argue that the international political economy of sugar has shifted from a *colonial regime*, characterized by mercantilist protections, to a postwar *national regime*, which prioritized national food security in the USA and Europe (and India, Japan, and China), to the present *corporate regime*, which favors transnational firms like Tate & Lyle‡ (see Box 2.1). In line with geographers of "neoliberalization,"§ Richardson ([45]: p. 4) argues against an inevitable or uniform neoliberal globalization of sugar, claiming that elements of all three regimes (and their social and environmental counterparts) continue to shape present political economies of sugar:

> While the objective of liberalization was entrenched [in recent international negotiations on sugar, see below] various provisions were made for specific types of protectionism, meaning vestiges of the national regime, and within this legacies of the colonial regime, could still be seen. ([45]: p. 91)

BOX 2.1 THE THREE FOOD REGIMES AND EXAMPLES ([45]: P. 64; OUR TABLE)

Colonial regime	The Commonwealth Sugar Agreement (1951) established preferential trade relations between Britain and its sugar colonies and ex-colonies
	The US Sugar Act (1764) was originally established between Britain and her US colonies for trade in molasses and raw sugar. The act later established colonial-like trade relations between the USA and Cuba, the Philippines, Mexico, and other countries
National regimes	Britain: 1925 subsidies for beet growers, 1936 subsidies for processors of sugar beet through the British Growers Association
	United States: 1934 Jones-Costigan Act controlled imports of sugarcane and regulated prices and supports for US farmers
	India: 1932 Sugar Industry Protection Act established national protections (through guaranteed prices and quotas) for sugar processors
Corporate regime	See Box 2.2

---

* Ben Richardson is an assistant professor in International Political Economy at the University of Warwick.

† See References 17–21, 36, and 53. For an alternative perspective on sugar and food regimes, particularly in relation to affluent cultures of consumption, see [15].

‡ Formed in 1921, Tate & Lyle is a British-based multinational corporation that specialized in sugar refining until 2010, when it diversified to sweeteners and other markets. Tate & Lyle owned the sugar industry in Trinidad and Tobago until 1975, when it was nationalized.

§ See References 5, 9–11, 26, 31, 32, and 42.

The present international political economy of sugar has various precedents, and there is a broad literature that addresses its uneven and brutal history (i.e., [1–3,22,38]; for a full review, see [45]: p. 6–10). Our present concern is to trace long-term pathways of power that perpetuate certain kinds of political economic formations over others, affecting places like the West Indies and, more specifically, Trinidad and Tobago, in particular. As Mintz [38,39] has shown (and as further elaborated by Ulijaszek, this volume), the successful path towards British industrialization was partly sustained through the production of working-class foods with high sugar content such as marmalade. Industrial food production in Britain led to the mass appropriation of land, labor, knowledge, and often lives from the colonies, first by planter-colonists and later by multinational corporations (MNCs) such as Tate & Lyle. A counterpart to export crops produced as monocultures was the transformation of local foodways, as the "merchant-planter elite" ([14]: p. 133) and, later, MNCs "suppress[ed] particularities of time and place in both agriculture and diets" ([19]: p. 379).

These long-term pathways of power partially explain why islands like Trinidad, which had long produced sugarcane for export (along with some subsistence farming carried out by what Mintz calls "reconstituted peasants"; [37]), had trouble diversifying their agricultural economies after the restructuring/closure of Caroni.* As we shall see later in this chapter, the sugar industry in Trinidad was embedded in complex and powerful national and international networks which, after the demise of the industry, continued the trend towards land appropriation and industrialization, hindering alternative forms of agriculture that had emerged alongside large-scale sugarcane production.

Coexistence of Neoliberalism and Protectionism in the International Political Economy of Sugar

In the twentieth century, the international landscape of sugar (including both sugarcane and sugar beet) was characterized by not one but *three* interconnected markets, which roughly correspond to the three regimes outlined in Box 2.1. The first two were established on a preferential basis, whereas the third was the so-called "world" market. The latter was (and is) what Drummond and Marston ([14]: p. 88) call a "thin" market, largely comprised of cheap leftover sugar that escaped the other two protected markets. At present, one of these two protected markets (corresponding to the US/EU national regime) continues to boost the incomes of farmers and sugar processors in the USA and the European Union. The other protected market, which was geared toward the former colonies in African, Caribbean, and Pacific countries (ACP), was recently eliminated in the name of global liberalization (see Box 2.3). While wealthier countries and regions continue to benefit from protectionism, newly liberalized ACP countries face an ongoing price squeeze driven by powerful MNCs such as those listed in Box 2.2, who often buy sugar at low prices in the global market to produce mass amounts of cheap industrial foodstuffs for that same market, boosting their countries' gross domestic product in the process.

Thus, the protectionism that remains in the international political economy of sugar favors public–private alliances that formed in the very countries that instituted the national regime in agriculture: the USA and the UK (and the other wealthy countries in the European Union such as France and Germany).† For instance, the 1992 Agreement on Agriculture‡ and subsequent international

* Compare their plight to former sugar-beet farmers in the European Union (EU), many of whom were able to switch to other crops after recent reforms to the EU's Common Agriculture Policy ([16]: p. 1).

† Industrial-state alliances are also forming for the production, refining, and manufacturing of sugar and their byproducts in non-Western countries such as Brazil, India, and Thailand, though often with supply chains linked to MNCs based in Europe or the USA. Other countries with significant sugar industries are China, Mexico, Pakistan, Colombia, Australia, and Indonesia.

‡ The Agreement on Agriculture was a treaty signed as part of the WTO Uruguay Round (1986–1994) of the General Agreement on Tariffs and Trade (GATT).

BOX 2.2 EUROPEAN MNCs INVOLVED IN THE PRODUCTION AND/OR PROCESSING OF SUGAR [23]

Company	Countries
Associated British Foods (UK)	China, Malawi, Mali, Mozambique, Swaziland, South Africa, Tanzania, Zambia
Tereos (France)	Mozambique, Brazil
Sudzucker (Germany)	Mauritius
JL Vilgrain (France)	Cameroon, Chad, Republic of the Congo
Tate & Lyle (UK)	Egypt, Laos, Zimbabwe
AlcoGroup (Belgium)	Brazil, Mauritius

agricultural trade policies include various loopholes that allow for continued tariffs on nonquota* imports of sugar into the USA, while permitting US food industries to import nonquota sugar duty-free as long as they re-export their final products onto the world market ([45]: p. 87–91). A similar provision exists for sugar refiners in the European Union, who may import raw sugarcane duty-free as long as they re-export the refined sugar to non-EU markets (though this is not always profitable; see http://saveoursugar.eu/wp-content/uploads/2012/09/Myths-and-Misconceptions-26-July.pdf). During the WTO Doha Round negotiations of 2004–2005, such protections were further institutionalized as sugar became listed as a "sensitive product," exempt from tariff reductions ([45]: p. 170–200). Moreover, through government procurement schemes [55], public bodies in places like the USA and UK determine a quota of sugar to be purchased at inflated prices from domestic sugarcane and/or beet producers (or ethanol producers)† to the detriment of most nondomestic producers who must compete with "unnaturally" low prices on the global market.

Such policies not only lead to gluts in "the" global market for sugar and sugar-laden food products, depressing prices and providing cheap, obesogenic food for the world's hungry, but also perpetuate inequalities between sugarcane farmers in poorer countries and beet and cane farmers in wealthier countries. National (or, in the case of the European Union, regional) protections such as government procurement, tariffs, and subsidized quotas persist because of powerful ties between private cane and beet farmers and corporations and their public representatives, public–private alliances that formed in some places and not others. The US sugar industry, for example, donates more money to US presidential campaigns than the entire US agricultural sector ([45]: p. 132–3). Such "state-market condominiums" [51,52] did not emerge in the former colonial world, where sugarcane "farmers" were actually laborers working for capitalist interests generated from without (assisted by elites from within), and where the clientelistic politics of postcolonial nation-building was "disarticulated" from the interests of those working in the land [13]. In the rest of this chapter, we will argue with a regional and national case study that the present neoliberal agenda for sugar conceals enduring protections in wealthy countries but also eclipses fundamental relations between land, labor, and capital (and, in the case of Trinidad, race), which were established during the time of colonialism. An ironic counterpart to the brutal history of Caribbean sugar, also concealed in neoliberal accounts, is sugar's connection to rural lifeways and livelihoods.

* To meet the WTO obligations, the USA (and EU) must allow for the duty-free import of a minimum quantity (presently 1.3 million tons) of raw sugar cane from about 40 countries who share this small quota. Under US law, the amount imported under this scheme (called tariff rate quotas) cannot exceed 15% of US demand in sugar; the rest (85%) is guaranteed at higher prices to US sugar producers. The scheme does not include sugar imported duty-free by US companies under the re-export policies referred to in this paragraph.

† Provisions for the production of ethanol from sugar beet or cane produced in the USA were made in an amendment to the 2008 Farm Bill and renewed in the 2013 Farm Bill. Called the Feedstock Flexibility Program, the policy covers the extra costs of producing ethanol from sugar (rather than from corn, which is cheaper) and provides tax credits for ethanol production ([45]: p.130).

MATERIAL AND DISCURSIVE SHIFTS IN WEST INDIAN SUGAR: SITUATING TRINIDADIAN "DEVELOPMENT"

Neoliberal ideas of development underpinned by words like "competition" imply a kind of *El Dorado*, an "ideal and impossible vantage point of totally liberalized world economy" ([45]: p. 178). By contrast, and as indicated in the previous section, the current corporate sugar regime prioritizes MNCs and large industrial farmers from wealthy countries like the USA, the UK, Germany, and France (and MNCs from New Agricultural Countries like Brazil* and Thailand), at the expense of peoples and environments in many former sugarcane colonies. Recent transformations of sugar landscapes in the West Indies have accompanied ideological shifts in discussions of development and trade, as trade blocs like the Forum of the Caribbean Group of African, Caribbean and Pacific (ACP) States (CARIFORUM),† and countries like Trinidad and Tobago are drawn into the global race for the so-called sustainable economic development [6].

In this section, we explain how discourses of neoliberalization have altered the agenda for sugar in the West Indies, leading to the restructuring (Barbados, Jamaica, Guyana, Belize) and closure (Trinidad and Tobago, St. Kitts, and Nevis) of the sugar industry on individual islands. While the focus will ultimately center on recent debates about sugar in Trinidad leading up to and following the closure of the industry, we will begin with a brief overview of changes to the colonial regime between the European Union and the CARIFORUM. As we argue, official justifications for the gradual liberalization of trade eclipse historical and present-day inequalities that stem from the persistence of preferential markets in the EU and the USA *and* from the lasting political economic power of elites *within* former colonies such as Trinidad. New advocates of neoliberal "development" in the Caribbean also undermine alternative views of agri*culture* and socioeconomic well-being, which are given voice through ethnographic data presented in the final part of the chapter.

The modern counterpart of the colonial sugar regime emerged in 1951, when Britain and its major sugar colonies [i.e., Australia, British Guiana (now Guyana), Fiji, Mauritius, and South Africa] signed the Commonwealth Sugar Agreement (CSA). In 1958, a special provision called the Sugar Protocol was made for colonies and ex-colonies of what became known as the ACP, a grouping of the so-called underdeveloped Commonwealth countries that excluded Australia ([14]: p. 90). Like preferential markets between the USA and Cuba (that arguably had a similar colonial-type relationship until 1959), the Sugar Protocol guaranteed a market for sugar produced in the West Indies and other regions in the ACP. Through tariffs on refined sugar (which continue to the present), it also boosted the refining capacity and capital accumulation of British corporations such as Tate & Lyle.

When Britain joined the European Community in 1973, the latter agreed to continue preferences instituted by the Sugar Protocol through the Lomé Convention of 1975, which included a special annex for the Protocol. The Lomé provided each country in the ACP quotas for duty-free access to the EU market along with development aid (through the Georgetown Agreement; see Box 2.3) until the late 1990s, when New Agricultural Countries such as Brazil began to complain to the WTO of "unfair competition" under the WTO's "nondiscrimination" principle. Preferential trade in sugar continued through the Cotonou Agreement, which replaced the Lomé Convention and continued until December 2007, when the WTO waiver on preferences ended.

The colonial regime in sugar was replaced by a policy for the gradual liberalization of trade between the West Indies and the European Union. On 15 October 2008, the newly established CARIFORUM signed an Economic Partnership Agreement (EPA) with the EU, which not only eliminated preferential access to EU markets, but also mandated the gradual elimination of tariffs and other protections on sugar produced and refined in the Caribbean over a period of 25

* For a case study of sugar and uneven development in Brazil, see Reference 47.

† CARIFORUM is a group of 16 Caribbean states established in 1992 as a political forum for consultation on regional integration, cooperation, and trade (see http://www.caricom.org/jsp/community_organs/cariforum/cariforum_main_page.jsp?menu = cob, accessed 15 August 2013).

BOX 2.3 TIMELINE OF SUGAR TRADE AGREEMENTS BETWEEN EUROPEAN AND ACP/CARIBBEAN COUNTRIES

Year	Action	Parties	Description/Implications
1951	CSA	UK and British West Indies, Australia, Fiji, East Africa, South Africa, Mauritius	Purchasing commitments established between the UK and ex-colonies
1975	Georgetown Agreement	Formation of the ACP	Aid provided for development and poverty reduction in member states and greater integration into world economy
1975	Lomé Convention & Sugar Protocol	European Economic Community (EEC) and the ACP	Aid and trade enabled new forms of cooperation, especially with former British, Dutch, Belgian, and French colonies. Duty-free access for most ACP agricultural and mineral exports to enter the EEC. Preferential access based on quotas for products such as sugar and beef, in competition with EC agriculture. Committed the EEC to 3 billion in aid and investment in ACP countries. Sugar Protocol established as a separate annex for an "indefinite period"
1994	WTO	128 country signatories by end of 1994	Agriculture entered multilateral trading system with nondiscrimination principle between countries. Weakening of pre-existing Lomé Convention
2000	Cotonou Agreement	EU and the ACP	ACP fragmented into regional blocks with move towards free trade. ACP pushed for a longer implementation period for Cotonou before reciprocal trade liberalization
2001	Everything But Arms Agreement	EU and Least Developed Countries (LDCs)	Duties abolished for quotas on all products for LDCs. Decreased ACP's ability to construct unified negotiating position. Decreased EU's ability to manage imports
2007	Unilateral Denunciation of Sugar Protocol	WTO's Dispute Settlement Mechanism	Phrase "indefinite period" understood as a means of ending the protocol at a specified date. Sugar Protocol deemed incompatible with WTO commitments
2008	EPA	EU and CARIFORUM (including the Dominican Republic, Haiti, Surinam)	Ended the Commonwealth/colonial dimension of the EU-Caribbean sugar trade. Replicated the terms of the Everything But Arms Agreement (duty-free, quota-free access to EU markets), but with no guarantees on prices or market share. Gradual liberalization of trade between CARIFORUM and the EU

Source: Richardson B, Richardson-Ngwenya P. *Bulletin of Latin American Research*. 2013; 32(3): 1–16.

years. Though this gradual time frame for liberalization is "unprecedented in any trade agreement" ([6]: p. 11), the idea that trade between the West Indies and the EU *will* eventually be liberalized hinges on a particular spatial imaginary—a uniform, global market economy—which conceals the persistence of protected markets in the USA and the European Union.

In line with neoliberally minded analysts from the EU and elsewhere [40], Jamaican Richard Bernal (the Caribbean's Executive Director of the Inter-American Development Bank) has argued that the West Indies needs to adopt a policy of "global repositioning" and that the EPA between CARIFORUM and the EU will enable a kind of "sustainable economic development" in line with this outward focus. According to Bernal ([6]: p. 20, 7), the major obstacle to making the region globally competitive in sugar is psychological: "Why does the region take for granted that it can and will produce world class performers and indeed world champions in every field of sport and the creative arts but doubt that our entrepreneurs and workers cannot be internationally competitive?" His discourse of the Caribbean's faulty collective psychology is consistent with the ahistorical and apolitical neoliberal model, which emphasizes current and future "competitiveness" rather than past injustices, starting from the assumption that all economies compete on an equal playing field. Such discourses reflect what Richardson and Ngwenya ([49]: p. 7) call an "inversion of meaning" from the previous sugar regime, which had emphasized the need to redress historical injustices by providing a guaranteed market for West Indian sugar. In the post-Cold War age, when rich countries no longer need to "buy allegiance" or quell "colonial guilt" with trade preferences ([24]: p. 59), the colonial regime is being replaced by a corporate neoliberal regime, which is, like any other economic model, full of inconsistencies and gaps, exemplified by the kinds of protections described earlier. Historically a dumping ground for excess sugar that escaped preferential markets, the present "global" market is still isolated from controlled sugar markets that persist in places like the US and the EU. Yet, it is in this market that the remaining West Indian sugar producers must (eventually) compete, along with MNCs like Tate & Lyle, whose present "competitiveness" was engendered by the very kinds of protections described above:* "Instead of firms responding to competition through adjustment, or paying the ultimate price in a Darwinian economic universe, they responded by shaping the terms of competition in their own favour" ([52]: p. 769).

While the IMF-led policy for restructuring the state-owned sugar company in Trinidad and Tobago was hailed by the World Bank as a neoliberal victory ([49]: p. 10), it led to drastic shifts (but also continuities) in long-established relations between land, labor, and capital in Trinidad. The biggest losers were sugarcane workers and sharecrop farmers, who lost their incomes and, at least in some cases, the land on which subsistence agriculture was once practiced. The biggest winners were political and economic elites in Trinidad, who capitalized on former Caroni lands: "There has been a marked tendency for workers and small farmers [in Trinidad] to experience difficulty in accessing stable jobs and land, whilst wealthy investors seem to effortlessly consume vast swaths of former sugar lands for golf courses and large hotel complexes" ([49]: p. 13).

Trinidadians who benefitted from the closure of the sugarcane industry were largely in favor of the EPA between the European Union and the West Indies, for many had established their wealth by importing cheap food manufactures from Britain and, later, the USA: "many state ministers and technocrats had more interest in gaining easy access for the region's professional class to the EU and cheaper imports for its tourist businesses" ([49]: p. 8). Public–private alliances in Trinidad differ markedly from the "state-market condominiums" in the USA and the EU, however. For instead of political and financial ties between politicians and farmers/corporations (exemplified by the US sugar lobby), elites in Trinidad are empowered through *externally* oriented relations with MNCs like Nestlé and Czarnikow. Rather than relying on the "uncompetitive" (and now defunct) Trinidadian sugar industry, Czarnikow now imports cheap raw and refined sugar so that the food manufacturing industry in Trinidad may produce inexpensive soft drinks and other sugary products, contributing to unprecedented levels of obesity in the country.

SUGAR IN TRINIDAD

This final section seeks to provide a more nuanced and empirical understanding of the sugar industry in Trinidad than dominant neoliberal discourses of global competitiveness, which ignore the social, ecological, and bodily effects of cheap sugar. Alternative economies of subsistence-level

* Along with such protections are complex policy instruments like the WTO's Agreement on Trade-Related Investment Measures (TRIMs) and its Agreement on Subsidies and Countervailing Measures (SCMs), which generally favor countries of a more "developed" status [54].

agriculture, routes to political empowerment, and notions of autonomy are all drawn out from interviews with those most affected by the closure of Caroni (1975) Ltd: its previous sharecrop farmers. But before we introduce their perspective, it is important to provide a brief historical overview of the sugar industry in Trinidad.

Historical Background

Unlike most other Caribbean sugar colonies, large-scale sugar production in Trinidad began only in the second half of the eighteenth century. Though a Spanish colony at that time, it was largely through the efforts of the French planters who settled there from the mid-1800s that sugarcane became Trinidad's most important crop and, except for a few brief periods of rivalry with cocoa, its major export [8]. Sugar production increased after Spain ceded the colony to the British in 1797. Over the course of the nineteenth century, the number of sugarcane estates, companies, and factories consolidated from more than 200 estates and companies in 1807 to 50 by 1900, 8 by 1950, and only 4 in 1975 [43]. In 1937, Tate & Lyle purchased and incorporated two medium-sized sugar companies under a company named Caroni Limited. By 1962, Caroni Ltd had acquired most of the land under cane cultivation in Trinidad. Its landholdings extended to over 73,000 acres of land, and its milling operations processed nearly 90% of Trinidadian sugar.* In 1970, the Trinidad and Tobago government purchased 51% of the ordinary stock of Caroni Ltd (increasing to 100% by 1976) and began to consolidate smaller sugar production companies into what was to become the state-owned Caroni (1975) Ltd. From 1978 to 2003, Caroni (1975) Ltd was the major agricultural employer in Trinidad, controlling the largest area of agricultural lands.

Labor in the Trinidadian sugarcane industry had first been provided by slaves, whose emancipation in 1838 resulted in an acute labor shortage. To fill the gap, the British brought over 143,000 Indians as indentured laborers to Trinidad in the period 1845–1917 [8]. Many ex-indentured Indians and their descendants settled in Trinidad on the margins of estates, though only a minority received lands promised in lieu of a return passage to India. Indian farmers and laborers were separated from the political mainstream by their rural location, differences in religion (being Hindus and Muslims), and language (most immigrants spoke Bhojpuri or another Indian language and only learned the local English dialect after years of residence). They continued to be marginalized in the postindenture period [8].

The rise of the trade union movement from the 1920s provided an alternative route to representation for all workers in Trinidad, including sugar workers and cane farmers. Efforts to unify labor interests were undermined by the colonial authorities and local elites, whose economic interests and peaceful rule were threatened by the empowerment and political leverage of a united working class [35]. As opposed to the politics of Afro-Trinidadians, who were identified with the oil and gas industry, Indo-Trinidadian political interests were shaped around sugar and agriculture. Because the two unions were separated by occupation as well as race,† it was easy to pit one against the other. Social divisions became solidified as political divisions in the postindependence (1962) period, after the People's National Movement came to the fore as the face of Afro-Trinidadian political representation.

Caroni (1975) Ltd and Livelihood Practices

Caroni (1975) Ltd was a major focal point around which the agricultural livelihoods of "reconstituted" Indo-Trinidadian peasants centered. Deep affective linkages to the company and to the land

* Caroni Ltd (1972) *Spotlight on Caroni Limited.* Voice & Vision (Caribbean) Ltd.

† In the 1930s, two unions were established: the Oil Field Workers' Trade Union, comprising the mainly African-Trinidadian petroleum workers, and the All Trinidad Sugar Estates and Factories Workers' Trade Union, comprising the mainly Indian-Trinidadian sugar workers and cane farmers.

were consistently referenced in interviews conducted by Parmasad in 2013 and for the Caroni Sugar Museum and Heritage Site Project in 2010 and 2011. While these interviews described farming life as "hard," many also illustrated attachments to the notion of self-sufficiency and autonomy:

> Long-time [long ago], life was hard, and we didn't have money …. I used to have to make clothes for the children out of flour-sack, but we had a garden out in the back and we could always pick something to eat even if we didn't have any money … once you have garden to grow ting, you could survive.
>
> **Former sugarcane farmer (male), 80 years old**

> We start[ed] planting cane after we married … we start up with one acre we rent from his uncle who was renting from Caroni … we eh [didn't] have no money, and as we plant and we get pay we used to save up five dollars, ten dollars … we work hard, we never had to take money from nobody, I learn sewing and used to sew in the evening by flambeaux [temporary kerosene torches in glass bottles] and then wake up in the morning to go in the caneland to plant or to weed and then in the evening is time for we own garden … we had baigan [aubergine], ochro [okra], pumpkin, aloo [potato], dasheen, eddoes [both tubers, the former with edible leaves used to make callaloo, a thick vegetable soup] … whatever in season we used to have … and on a weekend I selling in the market whatever we eh eat out … and we had the rice box in the corner too … we was poor too bad, but we children never starve.
>
> **Former sugarcane farmer (male), 88 years old**

As opposed to a view of the Trinidadian sugar industry as a purely export-driven enterprise, large-scale sugarcane cultivation under Caroni (1975) Ltd had long facilitated subsistence farming for households and produce for local markets. Moreover, from the 1980s, Caroni (1975) Ltd diversified into the cultivation of citrus, rice, beef, and dairy farming, largely for domestic consumption. The company's research station developed variations of anti-insecticides based on locally available raw materials and performed scientific research into potential varieties of crops that could be grown locally. Caroni (1975) Ltd also sold weedicides, fertilizers, and other agricultural necessities at subsidized prices, which farmers used for both sugarcane and subsistence production. Many sugarcane farmers had household gardens, where root and vegetable crops were grown for subsistence and additional income. Extensive rice cultivation also took place across the marshy lands of the agricultural belt.

> Every house in the village used to grow rice and have a rice box to have the rice secure for the year … when you cut and beat the rice and bring it home, you used to have to dry it and keep it somewhere, and that was the rice box. And that used to stay for two years and three years and ting, when it well properly dry. And when you want to eat, or you want to sell a little bit, you had to dry it back, and mill it. They used to have a mill by the neighbour up the road … and then you sell it. … But then when Caroni closed down, the price of rice was too low, and the cost of labour too high, so people stop planting rice when they stopped planting cane.
>
> **Former sugarcane farmer (male), 58 years old**

While Caroni (1975) Ltd did manage to diversify to a limited degree, large-scale plans for diversification never materialized. Rather than emphasizing the multifunctional nature of the sugar industry in Trinidad, local discourses in the media and Parliament centered on the company's overall unprofitability, in line with IMF reports that recommended privatization. A 1999 IMF Country Report noted that Caroni (1975) Ltd had "intractable problems" such as the "need to retrain or reduce a largely unmechanized workforce" that was paid more than cane farmers in other countries, such as Brazil.*

* IMF Staff Country Report No. 99/48, Trinidad and Tobago: Staff Report for the Article IV Consultation, IMF, Washington, DC; IMF Country Report No. 03/232, July 2003, Trinidad and Tobago: 2003; Article IV Consultation-Staff Report; Public Information Notice on the Executive Board Discussion; Statement by the Executive Director for Trinidad and Tobago.

Rather than simply a restructuring exercise, however, the company's closure was seen as a direct attack on the Indo-Trinidadian population and on the agricultural sector, in general. The closure of Caroni (1975) Ltd led to a deep sense of hurt and disenfranchisement on the part of Indo-Trinidadians.

> There is more to it than the closure of Caroni. ... This is a country where if you stick your finger in the ground, it will grow. We have been farmers for centuries .... Before the great oil came in 1907, what did this country rely on for its exports? It was all agriculture. All agriculture. We ate locally. Now ... US $600 million worth of food is imported! ([4]: p. 1)

This sense of betrayal and victimization underlies specific grievances of the ex-Caroni employees, which continue to the present. Along with a number of disputes over the so-called Voluntary Separation [severance] Packages (VSEP; see Box 2.4), former sharecrop farmers and employees of Caroni (1975) Ltd complained that they received no share in the multi-million dollar financial aid package provided by the European Union for agricultural development. Controversy continues over whether the funds were allocated to be paid to cane farmers seeking to continue in agriculture following the closure of Caroni (1975) Ltd or for the government to disburse as it chooses. As of

BOX 2.4 GRIEVANCES OF EX-CARONI EMPLOYEES

Lack of dialogue	Government did not consult concerned parties or enter into any negotiations with union representatives before presenting Caroni (1975) Ltd employees with nonnegotiable conditions for their effective retrenchment
Lack of transparency to the proposed restructuring	Little or no information was made available to ex-employees or the public about potential future employment under the restructured Caroni companies
Reneging on financial promises by government-backed bodies	In 2003, the Agricultural Development Bank of Trinidad (ADB) and the Unit Trust Corporation (UTC, a mutual fund company affiliated with the Central Bank of Trinidad and Tobago) offered a "cane sweetener loan" to all former Caroni employees. Ex-employees were advised to invest their VSEP in a 6-year investment scheme from the UTC's Individual Retirement Unit Account (IRUA) and were guaranteed at least a doubling of their investments in 6 years if the fund continued earning at half the rate it was then earning (26.12%). The principal of the investment was immediately available to investors as a loan at 8% per annum, minus a 2% management fee, and no loan instalments were to be paid until the investment doubled. Six years later, the investment had earned only 48%, of which the ADB took all, including dividend payout, blaming the global financial crisis. The ADB offered 0% for the entire 6 years. Ex-employees initially received a letter informing them they were in arrears for the principal and 8% interest on the "loans" they had received. After threatened legal action against the UTC and ADB, in October 2009 the workers' debts to the ADB were cancelled as a result of an agreement between the UTC and the ADB [25,28]. No dividends were received by the workers
Lack of transparency in offers of agricultural lands	Obscurity in the number of land leases (through the VSEP) disbursed and made available, and reasons for this delay
Uncertainty and delay in receipt of pensions	The legal documents to ensure payment of pension benefits were only signed in 2009, 6 years after the VSEP packages were received [50]
Unfair treatment in land distribution	Ex-employees who had received assurances of preferential treatment in receipt of lands continued to await leases for years, while residential and agricultural squatters on Caroni lands have been regularized
Unfair disbursement of EU funds	Farmers received no share in the multimillion dollar financial aid package made available by the EU to Trinidad and Tobago for agricultural development [29]

the time of writing, the government has used a majority of the EU funds to set up massive farms of monocultures largely geared towards exports (e.g., hot peppers) [29].

The case study of sugar in Trinidad reveals a power-laden history with implications that are both country-specific and tied to past and present international political economies of sugar. The multiple functions of the sugar industry in Trinidad are eclipsed by neoliberal discourses that demand quantification of global competitiveness. Trinidad is but one example of the place-based, historical nature of sugar production, which must be considered for all countries that have produced and continue to produce sugar.

CONCLUSION

The closure Caroni (1975) Ltd exemplifies the ways in which dominant discourses of global competitiveness undermine more localized human and nonhuman relations, political economies, and ecologies that remain influential in the very places where the international political economy of sugar first took root. Accounts of sugar as either internationally "competitive" or "uncompetitive" simplify complex political economic and historical relations, "establish[ing] some kinds of connection while denying others" ([30]: p. 237). As Jackson and Ward [27] argue, global frameworks for the sugar industry eclipse socionatural formations that work at other scales, such as the national or the local. Present emphases on "getting the [WTO] rules right" ([45]: p. 119–22) conceal long-term state-market relations that have made some "globals" and "locals" more formidable than others [34]. The now-prevalent discourse of a single, uniform "world" market, perpetuated by institutions such as the WTO, not only disregards persistent inequalities within and between countries, but overrides development alternatives that frame sugar as both multifunctional and *agricultural* [42].

In this chapter, we have argued that neoliberal depictions of the Trinidadian sugar industry discount alternative polities and economies of food production that formed over time in Indo-Trinidadian agricultural communities, ways of life that would change dramatically after the Trinidadian government decided to adopt an industrial development strategy based on oil and gas. Similar to the global textile industry [52], the main players in the international political economy of sugar continue to benefit from national protections, whilst taking advantage of transnational capitalist networks, some of which stem from the time of colonialism. In no other region in the world is this more true than the Caribbean, where the capitalist production of sugarcane established associations between land, labor, capital, and race that continue to orient the region away from domestic agriculture despite ongoing efforts to diversify agricultural production, now in the name of food and nutrition security.

REFERENCES

1. Abbott GC. *Sugar*. London: Routledge; 1990.
2. Albert B, Graves A (eds.). *Crisis and Change in the International Sugar Economy, 1860–1914*. Norwich and Edinburgh: ISC Press; 1984.
3. Albert B, Graves A (eds.). *The World Sugar Economy in War and Depression, 1914–40*. London: Routledge; 1988.
4. Bagoo A. The closure of Caroni (1975) Limited. *Trinidad and Tobago News*, 18 May 2013. http://www.trinidadandtobagonews.com/blog/?p=7553#more-7553 (accessed 19 July 2013).
5. Barnett C. The consolation of 'neoliberalism'. *Geoforum*. 2005; 36(1): 7–12.
6. Bernal R. *Globalization: Everything but Alms. The EPA and Economic Development*. Grace Kennedy Foundation Lecture. Kingston: Grace Kennedy Foundation; 2008.
7. Bernal R. Cariforum–EU Economic Partnership Agreement negotiations: Why and how. *Journal of Eastern Caribbean Studies*. 2008; 33(2): 1–21.
8. Brereton B. *A History of Modern Trinidad, 1783–1962*. Portsmouth: Heinemann; 1981.
9. Castree N. From neoliberalism to neoliberalisation: Consolations, confusions and necessary illusions. *Environment and Planning A*. 2006; 38(1): 1–6.

10. Castree N. Neoliberalising nature: Processes, effects, and evaluations. *Environment and Planning A*. 2008; 40(1): 153–73.
11. Castree N. Crisis, continuity and change: Neoliberalism, the left and the future of capitalism. *Antipode*. 2010; 41(s1): 185–213.
12. Chang H. *Kicking Away the Ladder: Development Strategy in Historical Perspective*. London: Anthem Press; 2002.
13. De Janvry A. *The Agrarian Question and Reformism in Latin America*. Baltimore, MD: Johns Hopkins University Press; 1981.
14. Drummond I, Marston T. *The Condition of Sustainability*. Routledge: London; 1999.
15. Fine B, Heasman M, Wright J. *Consumption in the Age of Affluence: The World of Food*. London: Routledge/Chapman & Hall; 1996.
16. Fischer Boel M. Sugar reform: The view from Europe. In: Food Ethics Council (ed.). *Sugar. A Bitter Pill?* London: Food Ethics Council, p. 1–3; 2009.
17. Friedmann H. The political economy of food: The rise and fall of the postwar international food order. *American Journal of Sociology*. 1982; 88(supplement): S248–86.
18. Friedmann H. International regimes of food and agriculture since 1870. In: Shanin T (ed.). *Peasants and Peasant Societies*. Oxford: Basil Blackwell. 1987; p. 258–76.
19. Friedmann H. Distance and durability: Shaky foundations of the world food economy. *Third World Quarterly*. 1992; 13(2): 371–83.
20. Friedmann H. Premature rigour: Or can Ben Fine have his contingency and eat it too? *Review of International Political Economy*. 1994; 1(3): 553–61.
21. Friedmann H, McMichael P. Agriculture and the state system: The rise and fall of national agricultures, 1870 to the present. *Sociologia Ruralis*. 1987; 29 (2): 93–117.
22. Galloway J. *The Sugar Cane Industry: An Historical Geography from its Origins to 1914*. Cambridge: Cambridge University Press; 1989.
23. GRAIN. Corporate candyland: The looming GM sugar cane invasion. 2009; http://www.grain.org/system/old/seedling_files/seed-09-04-1.pdf (accessed 26 August 2013).
24. Harrison M. *King Sugar: Jamaica, the Caribbean, and the World Sugar Industry*. New York: New York University Press; 2001.
25. Hassanali S. VSEP sweetener turns sour for former Caroni workers. *Trinidad Guardian*; 14 October 2012.
26. Heynen N, McCarthy J, Prudham S, Robbins P. *Neoliberal Environments: False Promises and Unnatural Consequences*. London: Routledge; 2007.
27. Jackson P, Ward N. Connections and responsibilities: The moral geographies of sugar. In: Nutzenadel A, Trentmann N (eds.). *Food and Globalization*. Oxford: Berg; 2008. p. 235–52.
28. Jankie A. Where's the money? Investors to take ADB, UTC to court. *Trinidad Express*; 5 February 2011.
29. Julien J. Cane farmers still hoping to collect $414 m from EU. *Trinidad Express*; 6 February 2011.
30. LaGuerre J. Sociological impact of changes at Caroni (1975) Ltd. In: Sanatan Dharma Maha Sabha (ed.). *Future of the Caroni (1975) Ltd: A Position Document*. Caroni, Trinidad and Tobago: Sanatan Dharma Maha Sabha; 1989. p. 35–40.
31. Larner W. Neoliberalism? *Environment and Planning D*. 2003; 21(4): 509–12.
32. Leitner H, Jamie P, Sheppard ES (eds.). *Contesting Neoliberalism: Urban Frontiers*. New York: Guilford; 2007.
33. Massey D. A global sense of place. *Marxism Today*. 1991; 38: 24–9.
34. Massey D. *For Space*. London: Sage; 2005.
35. Meighoo K. *Politics in a Half Made Society: Trinidad and Tobago, 1925–2002*. Princeton, NJ: Markus Wiener Publishers; 2003.
36. McMichael P. A food regime genealogy. *Journal of Peasant Studies*. 2009; 36(1): 139–69.
37. Mintz S. A note on the definition of peasantries. *Journal of Peasant Studies*. 1973; 1(1): 96–106.
38. Mintz S. *Sweetness and Power: The Place of Sugar in Modern History*. New York: Viking Penguin; 1985.
39. Mintz S. Sugar. Old champion, new contenders. In: Food Ethics Council (ed.). *Sugar. A Bitter Pill?* London: Food Ethics Council, p. 1–3; 2009.
40. Payne A, Sutton, P. Repositioning the Caribbean within globalisation. *The Caribbean Papers, a Project on Caribbean Economic Governance*. Waterloo, Canada: The Centre for International Governance Innovation; 2007.
41. Peck J. *Constructions of Neoliberal Reason*. Oxford: Oxford University Press; 2010.
42. Pretty J. *Agri-Culture: Reconnecting People, Land and Nature*. London: Earthscan; 2002.
43. Public Relations Department, Caroni (1975) Limited. Caroni, Trinidad and Tobago: Public Relations Department of Caroni Limited; 1988. p. 1–50.

44. Ramlogan V. The future of Caroni (1975) Ltd. In: Sanatan Dharma Maha Sabha (ed.). *Future of the Caroni (1975) Ltd: A Position Document*. Caroni, Trinidad and Tobago: Sanatan Dharma Maha Sabha; 1989. p. 11–22.
45. Richardson B. *Sugar: Refined Power in a Global Regime*. New York: Palgrave Macmillan; 2009.
46. Richardson B. Restructuring the EU-ACP sugar regime: Out of the strong there came forth sweetness. *Review of International Political Economy*. 2009; 16(4): 673–97.
47. Richardson B (with Lehtonen M, McGrath S). *An exclusive engine of growth: The development model of Brazilian sugar cane*. Ethical Sugar Discussion Paper. London: Ethical Sugar; 2009. p. 1–36.
48. Richardson B. Refined power: The political economy of sugar in the 21st century. In: Food Ethics Council (ed.). *Sugar. A Bitter Pill?* London: Food Ethics Council; 2009. p. 1–3.
49. Richardson B, Richardson-Ngwenya P. Cut loose in the Caribbean: Neoliberalism and the demise of the Commonwealth sugar trade. *Bulletin of Latin American Research*. 2013; 32(3): 1–16.
50. Sorias L. Caroni ex-workers to get pension. *Trinidad Guardian*; 16 May 2009.
51. Underhill GRD. State, market and global political economy: Geneology of an (inter-?) discipline. *International Affairs (Royal Institute of International Affairs 1944-)*. 2000; 76(4): 805–24.
52. Underhill GRD. States, markets and governance for emerging market economies: Private interests, the public good and the legitimacy of the development process. *International Affairs (Royal Institute of International Affairs 1944-)*. 2003; 79(4): 755–81.
53. Weis T. *The Global Food Economy: The Battle for the Future of Farming*. London: Zed Books; 2007.
54. Weiss L. Global governance, national strategies: How industrialized states make room to move under the WTO. *Review of International Political Economy*. 2005; 12(5): 723–49.
55. Weiss L, Thurbon E. The business of buying American: Public procurement as trade strategy in the USA. *Review of International Political Economy*. 2006; 13(5): 701–24.
56. Wolf E (with Silverman S). *Pathways of Power: Building an Anthropology of the Modern World*. Berkeley, CA: The University of California Press; 2001.

3 Sugars in Beverages and Body Weight

France Bellisle

CONTENTS

KEY POINTS

- There is considerable variability not only in conclusions about sugar-containing beverages and body weight, but also in study designs, definitions of outcome measures, and even definitions of sugar-containing beverages themselves. Establishing standards in this field of study might reduce the high level of discordance.
- Imposed, mandatory intake of extra calories in the form of sugar-sweetened beverages is likely to induce weight gain. This nonsurprising observation confirms that the capacity for compensation or adjustment for repeated administration of energy loads is limited, particularly for beverage energy. Overconsumption of energy, particularly, but not only in beverage form, should be prevented or discouraged.
- The significant adverse effects reported in susceptible individuals or persons with high intakes deserve further attention. While numerous healthy, normal weight individuals seem capable of integrating energy-containing beverages of various kinds into their daily diet, other persons are at risk. The recently reported interaction between genetic predisposition and level of intake is a promising area for further investigation.

- Consumption of sugar-sweetened beverages does not happen in isolation. A high intake of sugar-sweetened beverages might be a marker of a generally unhealthy lifestyle characterized by a high-total-energy intake, a nutritionally poor diet, little exercise, smoking, among other risk factors. The importance of context should not be overlooked.
- If the energy intake from beverages is high, it could interfere with the body energy balance, facilitating chronic overconsumption and weight gain.
- Energy intake from beverages seems to induce little satiation: the intake of solid foods does not decrease when accompanied by the intake of energy-containing beverages. Energy from beverages induces less satiety than energy from solids, as assessed by postingestive hunger and satiety feelings, or by energy intake recorded at later eating occasions.
- Various hypotheses have been proposed to explain the satiety deficit of beverage energy: cognitive, sensory, metabolic, etc.

INTRODUCTION

In addition to the sugars ingested in solid foods, sugars are also present in many popular drinks. As with solids, sugars in beverages contribute to palatability, texture, mouth feel, and to energy content. Ingesting energy from beverages constitutes a relatively recent shift of dietary practice for mankind [1]. During the evolution of the human species, water remained the sole source of fluid for millennia (from 200,000 BC), in addition to maternal milk for infants [1]. Juice, wine, beer, and animals' milk were introduced in the human diet from about 9000 to 4000 years BC. Herbal infusions, tea, coffee, to which the consumer can add varying amounts of sweetener, are more recent options. From the beginning of the twentieth century, sweet drinks were developed intensively by the food industry. Drinks that contribute energy to the diet (from sugars and/or other nutrients) have gained much popularity in recent years, in all parts of the world, where fruit, dairy, and other types of drinks have been consumed in increasing amounts by both children and adults [2].

Drinking is essential for survival. Fluid has to be ingested in order to compensate for the obligatory fluid losses in urine, perspiration, and breathing. The daily losses in sedentary adults range from 1300 to 3450 mL [2,3]. If fluid intake does not match losses, then dehydration occurs. Acute dehydration, even modest (corresponding to 1–2% body weight loss), results in impaired cognition, moodiness, headaches, poor thermoregulation, reduced cardiovascular function, and impaired physical capacity [4]. Higher levels of dehydration can rapidly induce major physical and mental symptoms, potentially lethal [5].

A large proportion of daily fluid needs should be covered by drinking, and the rest by the water contained in solid foods [2]. While plain water could fulfil all fluid needs of healthy individuals, contributing no energy, most people select a variety of energy-containing beverages on a daily basis. Thus, beverage intake contributes not only to the body fluid homeostasis, but also to the energy balance, with potential consequences on body weight control. According to the US "Beverage Guidance Panel" [3], all beverages combined should contribute at most 14% of the total caloric intake.

National surveys reveal that drinks supply around 10% of the total daily energy in the diet of adults in France [6] and 18% in Great Britain [7]. In Americans, this proportion is about 21% [3]. Such figures suggest that energy intake from beverages might be problematic in some populations or individuals.

In recent decades, epidemiological evidence has raised the question of a potential role for energy-containing beverages in the global increase in obesity frequency. The major emphasis is on sugar-sweetened beverages and, particularly in the American context, on high-fructose corn syrup (HFCS)-sweetened beverages. Overweight and obesity in America have reached unprecedented peaks in recent years (66 and 33%, respectively, in 2005–2006) [8]. The steep rise in overweight and obesity in America paralleled the increase in consumption of sugar and particularly the rise in consumption of sweetened beverages from the late 1970s to the end of the century [9]. In 2009–2010, American children and adults consumed over 151 kcal a day from sugar-containing beverages

[10]. These figures show a decrease from data reported in 1999–2000 (68 kcal in children and 45 kcal in adults) and reflect a reduced soda and fruit drink consumption, marginally compensated by increases in sports and energy drinks and sweetened tea and coffee [10]. Similarly, increases in sugar-sweetened beverage consumption have paralleled increase in overweight and obesity rates in other countries, for example, Great Britain [7] and Mexico [11].

In addition to obesity, intake of sweetened beverages has been associated with increased risk of type 2 diabetes [8,12], metabolic syndrome [8], hypertriglyceridemia [13,14], coronary heart disease [15,16], high blood pressure [17], ovarian dysfunction [18], and dental erosion [19] as reviewed in more detail in later chapters. A recent editorial of the scientific journal *Public Health Nutrition* presented soft drinks as the dietary version of the cigarette [20]. This view, however, is not universally accepted and many experts question the role of sugar-sweetened beverages in weight and health issues [21]. This chapter will briefly review the vast literature published in this area and focus mainly on the energy regulation/body weight control literature.

SUGAR-CONTAINING BEVERAGES

Sugar-containing beverages are a subset of the many energy-containing drinks available to consumers. Some bring only energy from sugars (sweetened tea and coffee, fruit juices, soft drinks) and their energy content is determined by the amount of natural or added sugar. Other beverages contain protein, fat, or a combination of nutrients whose concentration determines the final composition and energy content. Other energy-providing beverages are alcoholic drinks (beer, wine, cider, liquor) that also can contribute a substantial amount to the daily energy load. The present chapter will concentrate on nonalcoholic beverages that are marketed with sugar.

Juice is the liquid part that can be extracted from plants, often from fruits. Presently, juices are available in various forms. In certain parts of the world, for example, in Europe, regulatory texts define pure juices, juices made from concentrates, and nectars, all of which contain only fruit and water without added sugar [22]. Some juices are at times fortified with health additives such as calcium and vitamin. Fruit juices bring between 20 (tomato) and 70 kcal (grapes) per 100 mL. Beverages made of water, sugar, and fruit aromas are not legally referred to as "juices," but simply as "fruit drinks." Their energy load mainly depends on their sugar content.

Fizzy soft drink production started with the intention of making water safer, as the use of naturally carbonated waters was intended to eliminate water-borne pathogens at the origin of diseases. Carbonation techniques developed and soda water was sold from the end of the eighteenth century [23]. Flavors were then added to carbonated water and effervescent drinks gained worldwide popularity in the last century. In the early days, many carbonated beverages were marketed as "tonic" [24], particularly the "cola" products that contained coca, a stimulant plant from South America. One important ingredient in such products is the sweetening agent, generally sucrose, glucose or, in America, HFCS. These sugars bring 4 kcal/g and their concentration in soft drinks is about 10–15%.

ENERGY FROM BEVERAGES AND ENERGY BALANCE

During a meal, the intake of beverages, whether or not they contain energy, does not affect the intake of solid foods either under laboratory settings [25,26] or in free-living persons [27]. Actually, in free-living conditions, beverages are rarely ingested without any food [6,27–30]. The intake of solid foods does not decrease when the meal is accompanied by an energy-yielding beverage (sugar-sweetened, milk, alcohol, or else) so that energy-containing beverages simply add their calories to those of the solid foods ingested in meals and snacks [27,31]. In addition, consumption of energy-yielding beverages leads to similar reductions of experienced thirst as drinking water but does not reduce hunger [29]. These observations suggest that the intake of energy from beverages is poorly recognized by the body appetite/satiety systems (compared to energy ingested in solid form) and might therefore induce "passive overconsumption" of energy, facilitating weight gain on the long term.

This clearly important dietary issue has stimulated a host of scientific investigations. The potentially causal association between consumption of sugar-containing beverages and body adiposity has been extensively researched in subjects of all ages. The sugar-containing beverages considered in these studies include several types: fruit drinks, sodas, tea, coffee, plus local varieties. Methodologies, including definitions of factors and outcome measures, are extremely diverse and the results reported are largely discordant.

Cross-Sectional Studies

Cross-sectional studies look at associations between aspects of diet or lifestyle and outcomes such as health and weight parameters at one point of time. They can, in no way, identify causal relationships and their usefulness in the present controversy has been questioned [32]. In children and adults, some cross-sectional studies have reported positive associations between body adiposity measures and intake of sugar-containing beverages (e.g., [13,33–37]). In contrast, some did not find any significant relationship between these variables (e.g., [38–42]). Among others, the national CSFII and NHANES studies, that collected data in 38,409 American adults from 1989 to 2002, observed that the risk of obesity increased with many factors (age, sex, television watching time, fat intake) but not with the intake of sugar-containing beverages [43]. Finally, other studies reported ambiguous findings, with significant associations found only in age, sex, or socioeconomic subgroups [44,45].

Prospective Cohort Studies

In prospective cohort studies, participants are followed over a number of years and associations are examined between certain aspects of diet or lifestyle and changes in outcomes of interest, for example, body weight or risk of becoming obese. Numerous prospective cohort studies of the association between consumption of sugar-containing beverages and body adiposity have been carried out. They vary broadly in their methods and yield inconsistent results.

Studies ranging from a few weeks to a few years reported that the intake of sugar-added beverages was associated with total energy intake and/or weight gain in children [46–50]. Large cohort studies in American adults have established that a high intake of sugar-sweetened beverages is associated with an increased risk of weight gain [51], coronary heart disease [52], and type 2 diabetes [8]. Among others, the American Nurses' Study (91,249 women) reported a positive association between intake of sugar-sweetened drinks and both an increase in body weight and incidence of type 2 diabetes [53]. At the outset of this study, body mass index (BMI) was not different according to the level of daily intake of sodas. A larger increase in BMI over the years was reported in women whose consumption changed from below one soda per month to more than one a day but not in women with high but stable intake. Similarly, in a follow-up of Spanish adults, a positive association between intake of sugar drinks and body weight appeared only in subjects who had gained more than 3 kg in the previous 5 years, suggesting vulnerability in this group [54].

By contrast, no association was found between consumption of sugar-sweetened beverages and longitudinal changes in BMI in cohorts of children [55–57] and adults [58,59]. Ambiguous results were reported in cohorts of German [60] and Australian children and adolescents [15,61], with associations appearing only in subgroups of the population.

The relationship between consumption of sugar-containing beverages and body weight might be modulated by genetic factors. A "genetic-predisposition score" was computed on the basis of 32 BMI-associated genetic variants in participants of large-scale prospective cohort studies [62]. Both the increases in BMI over time and the risk of incident obesity associated with various levels of genetic predisposition (per increment of 10 risk alleles) were higher in participants with higher intake of sugar-sweetened beverages.

Interventions and Randomized Control Trials

Interventions and randomized controlled trials (RCTs) have been conducted to investigate the impact of ingesting sugar-containing drinks on weight outcomes. Generally such studies aim at reducing consumption of sugary drinks in children and adults, but a few studies have also looked at the effects of experimentally induced increases in intake. In a school-based intervention conducted among British children aiming at reducing the intake of sodas [63,64], a decrease in the risk of overweight was observed after 1 year but was not confirmed at the 3-year follow-up. In American teenagers with a daily intake of sugar-containing beverages reaching at least 360 mL, energy-free beverages were supplied for 25 weeks. In the total group of participants, this strategy did not induce any change in body weight; however, a significant decrease in BMI was reported in obese subjects (BMI >30 kg/m²) [65]. In American overweight or obese adolescents with a regular consumption of sugar-sweetened beverages, an intervention decreased reported consumption down to nearly 0 after 1 year and induced a reduced intake in the next year of follow-up, compared to intake in the control group [66]. In spite of these changes in intake, BMI did not differ between the intervention and control groups at the end of follow-up. Once again, a significant between-group difference in the change in BMI at 1 year was reported only in a subgroup of subjects (participants of Hispanic origin).

Some experimental studies examined the effects of imposed ingestion of sugar-containing foods or beverages. When participants were required to drink 1150 g of sugar-containing soda (530 kcal) per day for 3 weeks, a weight gain of almost 1 kg was observed in women, but not in men [67]. By contrast, no significant weight changes were observed in normal weight or obese women following 4 weeks of imposed daily intake of sugar beverages (430 kcal/day) [68,69] or in postmenopausal women following 1 year of imposed daily intake of 150–250 kcal/day in the form of calcium-fortified energy-containing drinks [70]. In overweight adults, the free delivery of sugar-containing foods and drinks for 10 weeks led to an increase in body weight and body fat mass [71]. Much of the increase in energy intake in this study was due to the sugar-containing beverages. During an 18-month trial, normal weight children (4–12 years of age) were randomly assigned to receive and consume 250 mL/day of either a sugar-containing beverage or a similar artificially sweetened beverage [72]. Attrition was high (26%). Weight, body fat mass, and waist-to-hip ratio increased significantly less in the sugar-free group than in the sugar-beverage group, suggesting that the extra calories brought by the sugar beverage (104 kcal) were not compensated for by adjusting intake of other energy sources.

Systematic Reviews and Meta-Analyses

The results of cross-sectional and longitudinal observations, as well as those of interventions and RCTs are clearly inconsistent, in children and adults. Systematic reviews and meta-analyses have been published in order to make sense of this inconclusive literature [32,73–82]. Each of these review papers selected a subset of the literature in order to answer specific questions of interest. Their selection criteria could specify a minimal duration of follow-up, the type of experimental design, the variables reported, or the type of control for confounders. As could be expected, systematic reviews and meta-analyses also reached discordant conclusions depending on the subset of studies included. For Forshee et al. [74], the association is close to zero, while Olsen and Heitmann [78] view the association as "possible."

A recent systematic review and meta-analysis including only RCTs and prospective cohort studies examined the body weight effects associated with sugar consumption in children and adults [80]. Among the 30 RCT (minimum of 2-week duration) and 38 cohort studies (minimum of 1-year duration) considered in this work, a majority focused mainly or exclusively on sugar consumed through beverages. RCTs in adults showed that experimentally decreasing or increasing sugar intake led to changes in body weight consistent with the induced changes in energy intake. A quantitative meta-analysis based on five cohort studies showed a significantly increased risk of being overweight in children with at least one serving a day versus children with no or very little intake of sugar-sweetened beverages (odds ratio 1.55; 95% CI 1.32–1.82). This particular article sheds light on some potential reasons for the cacophony observed in the relevant literature. The large differences in methodologies clearly make convergent results difficult to obtain. It is noteworthy, however, that many of the studies reported only partly positive results, applying to subsets of the populations or particular conditions but not others: discordant results do not only appear between different studies using different methods, but also within studies applying a consistent protocol. When measurable changes (increases or decreases) in sugar intake were obtained via experimental interventions, the changes in body weight that resulted were entirely consistent with an energy balance hypothesis: sugar in beverages affected weight in direct relation to its energy content. Nonetheless, decreases in sugar intake were difficult to obtain especially in children in whom compliance was poor. In spite of a generally positive association between intake of sugar and weight, the meta-regression of RCTs conducted in adults showed no evidence of a dose–response association between sugar intake and body weight. A consistent effect in cohorts appeared mainly when comparing groups with the highest intakes of sugars versus those with the lowest intakes.

ENERGY FROM DRINKS AND BODY WEIGHT: THE "SATIETY DEFICIT HYPOTHESIS"

Why should energy ingested in beverages raise a specific threat for body weight control? One hypothesis posits that the energy load of beverages (from sugar or other nutrients) might exert less satiating power than the energy obtained from solid foods, thereby facilitating overconsumption [83]. Two aspects of the satiating power are classically discriminated in experimental designs: satiation (inhibition of eating that occurs during one ingestive event) and satiety (inhibition of further eating following the end of one ingestive event).

Satiation Studies

Experimental protocols carried out under laboratory conditions have addressed the satiating potency of beverages versus solid sources of energy within one eating event. Table 3.1 lists a number of experimental studies directly comparing solid foods and beverages, with brief descriptions of their design and results. Overall, this literature suggests that energy ingested at meal time from beverages contributes less to satiation than comparable energy loads from solids [84–87].

Satiety Studies

Satiety studies using the preload and supplementation paradigms were conducted to examine various aspects of postmeal satiety. One important aspect of preload studies is the demonstration of compensation or adjustment in the subsequent ingestive episodes for the energy consumed in the preload: do beverage preloads induce equal compensation for their energy value as do solid foods? In this field, a rare occurrence in nutrition research, the experimental results are largely consistent in spite of differences in protocols. Table 3.2 presents a number of influential reports directly comparing beverages and solid foods. The overwhelming conclusion is: solid foods have higher satiety potency than beverages, whether the difference is expressed in terms of experienced satiety, compensatory reductions of intake at later eating occasions, or total daily intake [88–97].

A few discordant reports exist. Soda and cookies suppressed hunger equally during the interval between a 300 kcal load and lunch [98]. Drinking yoghurts (regular or fiber-enriched) induced higher satiety sensations and more adequate compensation at the next meal than solid foods such as bananas or crackers, suggesting moderating effect of nutrient content [99]. Numerous reports

TABLE 3.1
Beverages versus Solids: Comparisons of Immediate Satiation Effects Measured under Laboratory Conditions

Reference	Design	Observations
Lavin et al. [86]	Three 60 kcal sugar-containing stimuli: a pastille (chewed for 10 min), a gel (eaten in 5 min), a beverage (drunk in 2 min), consumed 5 min before lunch	No difference in hunger and satiation ratings Lower energy intake at meal following pastille than beverage
De Wijk et al. [84]	Chocolate-flavored dairy drink versus semisolid food, sipped through a straw Crossover	47% more liquid needed to reach satiation. After standardization of sipping effort and oral processing, same amount of both products produce same satiation
Zijlstra et al. [87]	Chocolate-flavored milk-based liquid, semiliquid, or semisolid	Higher intake of liquid needed to reach satiation than semiliquid (14%) and semisolid (30%). Standardizing eating rate decreased differences. Viscosity crucial factor
Flood-Obaggy and Rolls [85]	Apple juice, versus apple sauce versus apple; 125 kcal preloads consumed 15 min before lunch	Apple decreased meal intake more than juice and sauce Fullness ratings: apple larger than sauce larger than juice Adequate energy compensation after all preloads

exist in the literature about successful weight loss associated with the intake of liquid meal replacers [100]. These products are sugar solutions supplemented with protein, fiber, and micronutrients. No major problem with satiety or hunger has been reported with such diets. It might be that liquid sources of energy can exert a satisfactory satiety effect when used as a major source of energy in replacement of solid meals, particularly in motivated dieters. This hypothesis remains to be confirmed by further investigation. Whatever the outcome of this research, however, direct comparison studies have established that the satiating potency of liquid meal replacers is lower than that of equivalent solid meal replacement products, which induce lower ratings of hunger and desire to eat and lower insulin and ghrelin levels in the postingestive hours [101,102].

Comparison of Nutrients Ingested in Beverage Form

It has been proposed that the macronutrients, such as protein, CHO, and fat, might exert different satiety effects when they are ingested in beverages, as they do when ingested in solid foods [103]. More precisely, it has been hypothesized that humans may lack a physiological mechanism for adequately processing CHO or alcoholic calories in beverages because only breast milk and water were available while Homo Sapiens evolved between 100,000 and 200,000 years ago [1].

The role of nutrient composition on the satiety effects of beverages has been examined. Greater satiety was experienced following breakfast served with a glass of milk than after the same breakfast served with an isocaloric fruit drink [104]. Increasing the protein content of beverages enhanced experienced satiety and/or decreased intake at a meal presented 30–120 min later [105–107]. Once again, contradictory observations exist: a glass of milk, a fruit juice, and a soda, either presented as a preload before a meal [108] or as a beverage ingested with a meal [25], produced identical effects on later hunger and intake. In a cross-over study, 300 kcal dietary challenges were administered in the form of solid and liquefied versions of identical foods high in protein, fat, or CHO [95]: for all macronutrients, beverages had lower satiety effects than solid foods but the results showed no evidence of macronutrient-related differences. While these data do not support the hypothesis of a specific deficit in satiety for CHO in beverage form, they do suggest that increasing the protein content might improve the generally low satiating value of beverages.

TABLE 3.2
Satiety Effects after Solid versus Beverage Preloads

Reference	Design	Observations
Bolton et al. [89]	Grape and orange juices versus grapes and oranges	Satiety ratings higher after solid foods Intake not measured
Tournier and Louis-Sylvestre [97]	Tomato juice or soup versus tomato juice or soup plus gelatin at lunch Test meal after 4 h delay	Higher daily intake after beverage preload on the same day
Hulshof et al. [93]	Liquid formula versus formula plus gum Test meal after 3.5 h delay Three energy levels: 100, 400, and 800 kcal	Satiety ratings higher for solid No difference in energy intake on same day No difference in energy intake on the next day
Haber et al. [91]	Apple juice versus apple puree No test meal	Satiety ratings higher after solid preload Intake not measured
DiMeglio and Mattes [90]	Forced intake of soda or jelly beans through the day; 450 kcal/day; 4 weeks Crossover design	No change in motivational ratings Energy intake lower in solid than liquid weeks. Energy compensation 118% for solids versus −17% for beverage Spontaneous time of intake was different for liquids and solids
Almiron-Roig et al. [98]	Soda versus cookies, 300 kcal Delay: 20 or 120 min	No difference in satiety between solid and liquid preload. Soda but not cookies decreased thirst sensations. Lower energy intake at lunch when preload was ingested 20 min before meal versus 120 min
Mourao et al. [122]	Liquid versus solid sources of CHO, protein, and fat eaten with lunch. Crossover	Daily intake higher on days beverages were ingested No effect on appetite ratings Duration of postlunch satiety not different Little difference between lean and obese subjects
Mattes [95]	Crossover dietary challenge at lunch: 300 kcal solid, liquid (soup), or beverage form High CHO, protein, or fat	Soups and solid foods affected appetite ratings equally Beverage (apple juice) had lowest effects on ratings Daily energy intake lowest after soup, highest after beverage
Almiron-Roig et al. [99]	Four 111 kcal preloads: drinking yoghurt, fiber-enriched drinking yoghurt, crackers, banana, versus isometric volume of water Delay: 60 min	Yoghurts and banana produced higher satiety scores than crackers. Adequate compensation at meal for yoghurts, lower compensation for banana and crackers
Mattes and Campbell [96]	Crossover, 300 kcal loads of solid (apple), semisolid (apple sauce), and beverage (apple juice) either with a meal or as a snack	Beverage elicited weakest effect on appetite ratings Interval to next meal was shortest after beverage No difference on daily energy intake
Apolzan et al. [88]	Nutritional supplement in liquid or solid form 4 h follow-up	Fullness ratings higher with solid No difference in food intake Postingestive glucose, insulin, and CCK higher with solid
Houchins et al. [92]	Forced intake of energy matched beverages versus solid form fruit and vegetables 400–550 kcal/day Crossover, 8 weeks	Beverage elicited 53% energy compensation Solid elicited 78% energy compensation Lower compensation in obese than normal weight subjects Body weight increased in obese during beverage and solid phases Body weight increased in normal weight subjects during beverage phase only

TABLE 3.2
Satiety Effects after Solid versus Beverage Preloads

Reference	Design	Observations
Leidy et al. [94]	Liquid versus solid meal Elderly subjects (over 72 years) 4 h follow-up	Hunger and desire to eat were higher after beverage than solid Fullness was higher after solid than beverage
Martens et al. [123]	Chicken breast plus water (15% daily energy) Solid or liquefied 3 h follow-up	Solid protein suppressed hunger and desire to eat more than liquid protein
Martens et al. [112]	Peaches and water Solid or liquefied	No difference in postingestive sensations after liquid or solid CHO
Cassady et al. [111]	Liquid and solid preloads expected to turn either liquid or solid in the stomach Test meal after 4 h delay	Liquid preloads (oral and/or gastric) induced higher hunger, lower fullness, more rapid gastric emptying and oro-cecal transit, lower insulin and GLP-1, lower ghrelin suppression, and higher intake
Akhavan et al. [124]	Liquid versus solid preloads of gelatin, sucrose and whey protein 1 h follow-up Cross-over	No difference in hunger or food intake following liquid versus solid sugar preloads. Solid whey protein and gelatin induced greater experienced satiety than liquid forms. Solid and liquid whey protein equally suppressed intake at test meal

Physical Phase as a Critical Factor of Satiety and Compensation

A recently published systematic review of the very heterogeneous literature on energy compensation [109] examined the impact of factors that can affect the ultimate level of compensation for ingested energy. Forty-eight controlled laboratory studies were included, from which data were extracted for 253 interventions. This review confirmed the significant influence of two key variables: time delay between preload and test meal and physical form of the preload. Completeness of compensation decreases with increasing intermeal interval time (very poor compensation beyond 120 min), and liquid state of the preload induces significantly less compensation than preloads in solid form. The median energy compensation for liquids is 43%, while it reaches 83% for solids. Overall, this review confirms the reported weak satiating effects of beverages and the inadequate compensation for their energy content.

THE SATIETY DEFICIT: SOME EXPLANATORY MECHANISMS

A variety of mechanisms have been suggested to explain the satiety deficit observed following the intake of energy in beverage form.

Cognitive Influences (Attention, Memory, Perception, and Learned Attitudes)

In everyday life, consumers have expectations about the satiation/satiety that is likely to develop after consuming particular foods. The notion of "expected satiety" has been proposed in recent reports [110] and evidence suggests that expected satiety might be lower for liquids. Adult subjects participated in a cross-over study in which liquid and solid preloads were ingested 4 h before a test meal [111]. Through cognitive manipulation, the participants were led to believe that the preloads would be either liquid or solid not only in the mouth, but also in the stomach after being ingested. Oral liquid preloads and preloads expected to be liquid in the stomach elicited greater hunger and lower fullness, more rapid gastric-emptying and oro-cecal transit times, lower insulin and GLP-1 release, and lower ghrelin suppression than did oral solid preloads and preloads expected to be solid in the stomach. Subsequent energy intake at the test meal was higher following preloads expected to be liquid in the stomach. Over the remainder of the test days, the preloads expected to turn liquid in the stomach were associated with 21.8% higher intake than were the preloads expected to be solid in the stomach.

The attention paid to foods during eating is higher than that paid to beverages for many reasons. Visual cues are minimized with beverages, whereas they are important guides of behavior when ingesting solid foods from a plate. The act of chewing and the various oro-sensory cues it produces are thought to be crucially involved in satiation and satiety [86]. A laboratory study confirmed this notion: a variety of liquid foods were either drunk (from glass) or eaten (served in bowl, eaten with spoon) and compared to equivalent solid foods, controlled for energy and nutrient content [112]. After "drinking" a food, most subjects (80%) wished to consume more of the same food in order to alleviate hunger and thirst. After "eating" an identical amount of the same liquid food, the proportion was only 5%. This observation suggests that the act of drinking might generate insufficient cues (visual, olfactory, gustatory, or somesthetic) to support efficient satiety. In agreement with these notions, one liquid (or semisolid) food, soup, which is usually eaten from a bowl using a spoon, has been consistently shown to exert very strong satiating effects, at times stronger than solid foods, in sharp contrast with liquids ingested as beverages [95].

Oral Processing Time

The apparent satiety deficit of beverages versus solids might result from the difference in oral processing time between liquids and solids. The rate of ingestion is indeed a powerful determinant of satiation affecting solid foods as well as liquid ones: eating quickly could facilitate overconsumption [113,114]. One factor that can affect ingestion rate and satiation/satiety is beverage viscosity [84,87,115]. The viscosity of otherwise identical milkshakes was found inversely related to postprandial hunger ratings; however, it did not affect the subject-determined time interval until the next eating event, nor the total energy intake over 24 h [116].

Post-Oral Factors

It has been suggested that differences in digestive responses for solids and liquids might affect satiating power. In particular, responses of the "cephalic phase of digestion" might be critically different [111,113]. While solid foods trigger anticipatory secretion of pancreatic polypeptide (PP) and insulin, liquids are inadequate stimuli to evoke such cephalic-phase responses [117]. However, since drinking rarely occurs in the absence of eating [6,28], the contemporary intake of fluids and solids at meal times should trigger a complete cephalic-phase response and associated satiation/satiety effects. This could not explain the often reported "satiety deficit" of beverages consumed in the context of mixed meals although it might contribute to the deficit observed following liquid preloads.

Gastric cues have long been hypothesized to contribute significantly to hunger, satiation, and satiety [118]. Tests of gastric emptying times showed that liquids empty from the stomach more rapidly than do solids [119]. Viscosity not only affects oral processing time, but also gastric dilution and gastric emptying, as shown in a study using magnetic resonance imaging techniques [120]. In this study, the fullness ratings followed for 80 min after the ingestion of liquid mixed-nutrient formulas were correlated to total gastric volumes and, for a given gastric volume, were higher for high viscosity than low viscosity meals.

The glycemic index (GI) of many CHO-bearing beverages (particularly sodas) has been hypothesized to contribute to their low satiety effect. This hypothesis, however, is not consistent with GI data: soft drinks and other CHO-bearing liquids such as fruit juices, for example, have moderate rather than high GI values [121]; in addition, since beverages are consumed mainly during meals, the total GI value of the meal has to be considered, rather than the specific GI values of individual meal components.

CONCLUSIONS

Fluid homeostasis is essential to life: adequate amounts of fluid have to be ingested daily in order to match the obligatory losses. "Adequate" amounts can vary between 2 and 6 l a day, or even more, in adults, depending on numerous factors including body size, physical activity level, and temperature, among others [2]. Drinking should supply a large proportion (as much as 80%) of the daily needs in fluid, and the rest should be obtained from the water contained in solid foods. Although pure water could fulfil all physiological needs, most people choose to consume a variety of beverages each day, many of which bringing energy as well as fluid. While drinking decreases thirst, it does not decrease hunger and it has often been reported that the energy ingested in beverage form does not induce adequate satiety: the energy ingested in drinks simply adds to energy consumed in solid form. Many reports suggest that energy-containing beverages, particularly sugar-containing beverages, could be one important factor inducing excessive energy intake and, on the long-term, facilitating the acquisition of excessive body adiposity levels.

This issue has generated a vast and discordant literature giving rise to a long-standing controversy. While numerous epidemiological or interventions studies have shown no association between intake of sugar-sweetened beverages and body adiposity in subjects of all ages, a number of other studies have indeed established cross-sectional or longitudinal links between them. Systematic reviews reflect the same inconsistencies. While large differences in methods could account for discordant results between studies, it is often seen that within studies, the same protocol yields significant effects in subgroups of participants and not in others. The consumption of sugar-sweetened beverages does not appear to be associated with adverse effects in large segments of the population, perhaps due to a moderate level of consumption, adequate levels of physical activity, and/or favorable genetic makeup. Deleterious effects, however, have been demonstrated in other consumers. Subjects with weight control difficulties, as evidenced by changing BMI before or during the studies, or subjects with very high (highest tertiles or quintiles) or increasing consumption levels, seem more likely to exhibit vulnerability to the effects of high intake of sugar-containing beverages than more stable groups. Genetic predisposition is a key factor in determining individual vulnerability, but socioeconomic influences could also play a major role.

The low satiety efficiency of beverages, as compared to solid foods, is now well documented. The exact mechanism of the satiety deficit associated with consumption of energy from beverages remains to be elucidated. Many aspects of the act of ingestion likely contribute to it as well as postingestive factors. Recent mechanistic studies suggest that the satiety deficit of beverages might be a drinking/eating issue as much as, or perhaps rather than, a liquid/solid issue. The relative contributions of cognitive factors at the time of intake, as well as expectations formed by previous experience, appear as novel areas for investigation. It remains to be established if and under what conditions postingestive influences, such as the reflexes of the cephalic-phase of digestion, do in fact contribute to the low satiety power of beverages.

For all people with health and weight control concerns, it is highly important to realize that a substantial proportion of the present-day energy intake comes from beverages that are likely to have poor satiating efficiency in the circumstances of daily life. Energy-containing drinks of all nutrient compositions can easily facilitate a form of "passive overconsumption" in "unknowing" consumers although, clearly, not all consumption is overconsumption. It might be possible to prevent or limit beverage-induced overconsumption by facilitating consumer awareness, even if the physiological responses to energy in beverage form cannot be changed.

Obviously "knowing" is not sufficient to modify behaviors. Intervention studies aiming at reducing the consumption of sugar-energy beverages have revealed poor compliance, particularly in children, and yielded modest results in terms of body weight change. Research has shown that consumption of sugar-sweetened beverages does not happen in isolation. A high intake of sugar-sweetened beverages might be a marker of a generally unhealthy lifestyle characterized by a high-total-energy intake, a nutritionally poor diet, little exercise, smoking, among other risk factors.

In the strategy to prevent or limit the overconsumption induced by energy-containing beverages, the importance of context should not be overlooked.

CONFLICTS OF INTEREST

The author is a member of a number of scientific advisory committees for the food and beverage industry, including General Mills, Coca Cola, and the EUFIC. The author has also received honoraria for conferences and articles, in particular, from the International Sweetener Association and Mondelez International.

REFERENCES

1. Wolf A, Bray GA, Popkin BM. A short history of beverages and how our body treats them. *Obes Rev* 2007; 9: 151–64.
2. Benelam B, Wyness L. Hydration and health: A review. *Br Nutr Found Nutr Bull* 2010; 35: 3–25.
3. Popkin BMP, Armstrong LE, Bray GM, Caballero B, Frei B, Willett WC. A new proposed guidance system for beverage consumption in the United States. *Am J Clin Nutr* 2006; 83: 529–42.
4. Ritz P, Berrut G. The importance of good hydration for day-to-day health. *Nutr Rev* 2005; 63 (Part II): S6–13.
5. Lieberman HR. Hydration and cognition: A critical review and recommendations for future research. *J Am Coll Nutr* 2007; 26: 555S–61S.
6. Bellisle F, Thornton SN, Hébel P, Denizeau M, Tahiri M. A study of fluid intake from beverages in a sample of healthy French children, adolescents and adults. *Am J Clin Nutr* 2010; 64: 350–5.
7. Ng SW, Mhurchu CN, Jebb SA, Popkin BM. Patterns and trends of beverage consumption among children and adults in Great Britain. *Br J Nutr* 2012; 108: 536–51.
8. Hu FB, Malik VS. Sugar-sweetened beverages and risk of obesity and type 2 diabetes: Epidemiologic evidence. *Physiol Behav* 2010; 100: 47–54.
9. Drewnowski A. The real contribution of added sugars and fats to obesity. *Epidemiol Rev* 2007; 29: 160–71.
10. Kit BK, Fakhouri TH, Park S, Nielsen SJ, Ogden CL. Trends in sugar-sweetened beverage consumption among youth and adults in the United States: 1999–2010. *Am J Clin Nutr* 2013; 98: 180–8.
11. Barquera S, Campirano F, Bonvecchio A. Caloric beverage consumption patterns in Mexican children. *Nutr J* 2010; 9: 47.
12. Fagherazzi G, Vilier A, Saez Sartorelli D, Lajous M, Balkau B, Clavel-Chapelon F. Consumption of artificially and sugar-sweetened beverages and incident type 2 diabetes in the Etude Epidémiologique auprès des femmes de la Mutuelle Générale de l'Education Nationale—European Prospective Investigation into Cancer and Nutrition cohort. *Am J Clin Nutr* 2013. doi:10.3945/ajcn.112.050997.
13. Dhingra R, Sullivan L, Jacques PF et al. Soft drink consumption and risk of developing cardiometabolic risk factors and the metabolic syndrome in middle-aged adults in the community. *Circulation* 2007; 116: 480–8.
14. Nettleton JA, Lutsey PI, Wang Y, Lima JA, Michos ED, Jacobs Jr JR. Diet soda intake and risk of incident metabolic syndrome and type 2 diabetes in the Multi-Ethnic Study of Atherosclerosis (MESA). *Diab Care* 2009; 32: 688–94.
15. Ambrosini GL, Oddy WH, Huang RC, Mori TA, Beilin LJ. Prospective associations between sugar-sweetened beverage intakes and cardiometabolic risk factors in adolescents. *Am J Clin Nutr* 2013; 98: 327–34.
16. Fung TT, Malik V, Rexrode KM, Manson JE, Willett WC, Hu FB. Sweetened beverage consumption and risk of coronary heart disease in women. *Am J Clin Nutr* 2009; 89: 1037–42.
17. Chen L, Caballero B, Mitchell DC et al. Reducing consumption of sugar-sweetened beverages is associated with reduced blood pressure: A prospective study among United States adults. *Circulation* 2010; 121: 2398–406.
18. Schliep KC, Schisterman EF, Mumford SL et al. Energy-containing beverages: Reproductive hormones and ovarian function in the BioCycle study. *Am J Clin Nutr* 2013; 97: 621–30.
19. Kaplowitz GJ. An update on the dangers of soda pop. *Dent Assist* 2011; 80: 18–20.
20. Yngve A, Haapala I, Hodge A, McNeill G, Tseng M. Making soft drinks the dietary version of the cigarette. *Public Heath Nutr* 2012; 15: 1329–30.
21. Sievenpiper JL, de Souza RJ. Are sugar-sweetened beverages the whole story? *Am J Clin Nutr* 2013; 98: 261–3.

22. Braesco V, Gauthier T, Bellisle F. Jus de fruits et nectars. *Cah Nutr Diet* 2013; 48: 248–56.
23. Riley JJ. *A History of the American Soft Drink Industry: Bottled Carbonated Beverages, 1807–1957.* Washington: American Bottlers of Carbonated Beverages, 1958.
24. Emmins C. Soft drinks. In *The Cambridge World History of Food* (Cambridge: Cambridge University Press, 2000), 702–12.
25. DellaValle DM, Roe LS, Rolls BJ. Does the consumption of caloric and non-caloric beverages with a meal affect energy intake? *Appetite* 2005; 44: 187–93.
26. Rolls BJ, Bell EA, Thorwart ML. Water incorporated into a food but not served with a food decreased energy intake in lean women. *Am J Clin Nutr* 1999; 85: 351–61.
27. De Castro JM. The effects of spontaneous ingestion of particular foods or beverages on the mal patterns and overall nutrient intake of humans. *Physiol Behav* 1993; 53: 1133–44.
28. De Castro JM. A microregulatory analysis of spontaneous fluid intake by humans: Evidence that the amount of liquid ingested and its timing is mainly governed by feeding. *Physiol Behav* 1988; 43: 705–14.
29. McKiernan F, Houchins JA, Mattes RD. Relationships between human thirst, hunger, drinking, and feeding. *Physiol Behav* 2008; 94: 700–8.
30. McKiernan F, Hollis JH, McCabe G, Mattes RD. Thirst-drinking, hunger-eating: Tight coupling? *J Am Diet Assoc* 2009; 109: 486–90.
31. De Castro JM, Orozco S. Moderate alcohol intake and spontaneous eating patterns of humans: Evidence of unregulated supplementation. *Am J Clin Nutr* 1990; 52: 246–53.
32. Allison DB, Mattes RD. Nutritively sweetened beverage consumption and obesity: The need for solid evidence on a fluid issue. *JAMA* 2009; 301: 318–20.
33. Ariza AJ, Chen EH, Binns HJ, Christoffel KK. Risk factors for overweight in five- to six-year-old Hispanic-American children: A pilot study. *J Urban Health* 2004; 81: 150–61.
34. Giammattei J, Blix G, Marshak HH, Wollitzer AO, Pettitt DJ. Television watching and soft drink consumption: Association with obesity in 11- to 13-year-old schoolchildren. *Arch Pediatr Adoles Med* 2003; 157: 882–6.
35. Gillis LJ, Bar-Or O. Food away from home, sugar-sweetened drink consumption and juvenile obesity. *J Am Coll Nutr* 2003; 22: 539–45.
36. Liebman M, Pelican S, Moore SA et al. Dietary intake, eating behavior, and physical activity-related determinants of high body mass index in rural communities in Wyoming, Montana, and Idaho. *Int J Obes Relat Metab Disord* 2003; 27: 684–92.
37. Nicklas TA, Yang SJ, Baranowski T, Zakeri I, Berenson G. Eating patterns and obesity in children. The Bogalusa Heart Study. *Am J Prev Med* 2003; 25: 9–16.
38. Andersen LF, Lillegaard IT, Overby N, Lytle L, Klepp KI, Johansson L. Overweight and obesity among Norwegian schoolchildren: Changes from 1993 to 2000. *Scand J Public Health* 2005; 33: 99–106.
39. Bandini LG, Vu D, Must A, Cyr H, Goldberg A, Dietz WH. 1999.Comparison of high-calorie, low-nutrient-dense food consumption among obese and non-obese adolescents. *Obes Res* 1999; 7: 438–43.
40. Forshee RA, Storey ML. Total beverage consumption and beverage choices among children and adolescents. *Int J Food Sci Nutr* 2003; 54: 297–307.
41. Gibson S, Neate D. Sugar intake, soft drink consumption and body weight among British children: Further analysis of National Diet and Nutrition Survey data with adjustment for under-reporting and physical activity. *Int J Food Sci Nutr* 2007; 58: 445–60.
42. O'Connor TM, Yang SJ, Niclas TA. Beverage intake among preschool children and its effect on weight status. *Pediatrics* 2006; 118: e1010–8.
43. Sun SZ, Empie MW. Lack of findings for the association between obesity risk and usual sugar-sweetened beverage consumption in adults—A primary analysis of databases of CSFII-1989–1991, CSFII-1994–1998, NHANES III, and combined NHANES 1999–2002. *Food Chem Toxicol* 2007; 45: 1523–36.
44. Overby NC, Lillegaard IT, Johansson L, Andersen LF. High intake of added sugar among Norwegian children and adolescents. *Public Health Nutr* 2004; 7: 285–93.
45. Rodriguez-Artalejo F, Garcia EL, Gorgojo L et al. Consumption of bakery products, sweetened soft drinks and yogurt among children aged 6–7 years: Association with nutrient intake and overall diet quality. *Br J Nutr* 2003; 89: 419–49.
46. Berkey CS, Rockett HR, Field AE, Gillman MW, Colditz GA. Sugar-added beverages and adolescent weight change. *Obes Res* 2004; 12: 778–88.
47. Dubois L, Farmer A, Girard M, Peterson K. Regular sugar-sweetened beverage consumption between meals increases risk of overweight among preschool-aged children. *J Am Diet Assoc* 2007; 107: 924–34.
48. Ludwig DS, Peterson KE, Gortmaker SL. Relation between consumption of sugar-sweetened drinks and childhood obesity: A prospective, observational analysis. *Lancet* 2001; 357: 505–8.

49. Mrdjenovic G, Levitsky DA. Nutritional and energetic consequences of sweetened drink consumption in 6- to 13-year-old children. *J Pediatr* 2003; 142: 606–10.
50. Welsh JA, Cogswell ME, Rogers S, Rockett H, Mei Z, Grummer-Strawn LM. Overweight among low-income preschool children associated with the consumption of sweet drinks: Missouri, 1999–2002. *Pediatrics* 2005; 15: e223–9.
51. Mozaffarian D, Tao T, Rimm EB, Willett WC, Hu FB. Changes in diet and lifestyle and long-term weight gain in women and men. *N Engl J Med* 2011: 364: 2392–404.
52. De Koning L, Malik VS, Kellogg MD, Rimm EB, Willett WC, Hu FB. Sweetened beverages consumption, incident coronary heart disease, and biomarkers of risk in men. *Circulation* 2012; 125: 1735–41.
53. Schulze MB, Manson JE, Ludwig DS, Colditz GA, Stampfer MJ, Willett WC. Sugar-sweetened beverages, weight gain, and incidence of type 2 diabetes in young and middle-aged women. *JAMA* 2004; 292: 927–34.
54. Bes-Rastrollo M, Sanchez-Villegas A, Gomez-Gracia E, Martines JA, Pajares RM, Martinez-Gonzales MA. Predictors of weight gain in a Mediterranean cohort: The Seguimiento Universidad de Navarra Study. *Am J Clin Nutr* 2006; 83: 362–70.
55. Blum JW, Jacobsen DJ, Donnelly JE. Beverage consumption patterns in elementary school aged children across a two year period. *J Am Coll Nutr* 2005; 24: 93–8.
56. Johnson L, Mander AP, Jones LR, Emmett PM, Jebb SA. Is sugar-sweetened beverage consumption associated with increased fatness in children? *Nutrition* 2007; 23: 557–63.
57. Newby PK, Peterson KE, Berkey CS, Leppert J, Willett WC, Colditz GA. Beverage consumption is not associated with changes in weight and body weight and body mass index among low-income preschool children in North Dakota. *J Am Diet Assoc* 2004; 104: 1086–94.
58. French SA, Jeffery RW, Forster JL, McGovern PG, Kelder SH, Baxter JE. Predictors of weight change over two years among a population of working adults: The Healthy Worker Project. *Int J Obes Relat Metab Disord* 1994; 18: 145–54.
59. Kvaavik E, Andersen LF, Klepp KL. The stability of soft drinks intake from adolescence to adult age and the association between long-term consumption of soft drinks and lifestyle factors and body weight. *Public Health Res* 2005; 8: 149–57.
60. Libuda L, Alexy U, Sichert-Hellert W et al. Pattern of beverage consumption and long-term association with body-weight status in German adolescents—Results from the DONALD study. *Br J Nutr* 2008; 99: 1370–9.
61. Jensen BW, Nichols M, Allender S et al. Inconsistent associations between sweet drink intake and a 2-year change in BMI among Victorian children and adolescents. *Pediatric Obesity* 2013. doi:10.1111/j.2047-6310.2013.00174.x
62. Qi Q, Chu AY, Kang JH et al. Sugar-sweetened beverages and generic risk of obesity. *N Engl J Med* 2012; 367: 1387–96.
63. James J, Thomas P, Cavan D, Kerr D. Preventing childhood obesity by reducing consumption of carbonated drinks: Cluster randomised controlled trial. *BMJ* 2004; 328: 1237.
64. James J, Thomas P, Kerr D. Preventing childhood obesity: Two year follow-up results from the Christchurch obesity prevention programme in schools (CHOPPS). *BMJ* 2007; 335: 732.
65. Ebbeling CB, Fledman HA, Osganian SK, Chomitz VR, Ellenbogen SJ, Ludwig DS. Effects of decreasing sugar-sweetened beverage consumption on body weight in adolescents: A randomized, controlled pilot study. *Pediatrics* 2006; 117: 673–80.
66. Ebbeling CB, Feldman HA, Chomitz VR et al. A randomized trial of sugar-sweetened beverages and adolescent body weight. *N Engl J Med* 2012; 367: 1407–16.
67. Tordoff MG, Alleva AM. Effect of drinking soda sweetened with aspartame or high-fructose corn syrup on food intake and body weight. *Am J Clin Nutr* 1990; 51: 963–9.
68. Reid M, Hammersley R, Hill AJ, Skidmore P. Long-term dietary compensation for added sugar: Effects of supplementary sucrose drinks over a 4-week period. *Br J Nutr* 2007; 97: 193–203.
69. Reid M, Hammersley R, Duffy M. Effects of sucrose drinks on macronutrient intake, body weight, and mood state in overweight women over 4 weeks. *Appetite* 2010; 55: 130–6.
70. Haub MD, Simons TR, Cook CM, Remig VM, Al-Tamimi EK, Holcomb CA. Calcium-fortified beverage supplementation on body composition in postmenopausal women. *Nutr J* 2005; 4: 21.
71. Raben A, Vasilaras TH, Moller AC, Astrup A. Sucrose compared with artificial sweeteners: Different effects on ad libitum food intake and body weight after 10 wk of supplementation in overweight subjects. *Am J Clin Nutr* 2002; 76: 721–9.
72. de Ruyter JC, Olthof MR, Seidell JC, Katan MB. A trial of sugar-free or sugar-sweetened beverages and body weight in children. *N Engl J Med* 2012; 367: 1397–406.

73. Drewnowski A, Bellisle F. Liquid calories, sugar, and body weight. *Am J Clin Nutr* 2007; 85: 651–61.
74. Forshee RA, Anderson PA, Storey ML. Sugar-sweetened beverages and body mass index in children and adolescents: A meta-analysis. *Am J Clin Nutr* 2008; 87: 1662–71.
75. Malik VS, Schulze MB, Hu FB. Intake of sugar-sweetened beverage and weight gain: A systematic review. *Am J Clin Nutr* 2006; 84: 274–88.
76. Malik VS, Willett WC, Hu FB. Sugar-sweetened beverages and BMI in children and adolescents: Reanalysis of a meta-analysis. *Am J Clin Nutr* 2009; 89: 438–9.
77. Mattes RD, Shikany JM, Kaiser KA, Allison DB. Nutritively sweetened beverage consumption and body weight: A systematic review and meta-analysis of randomized experiments. *Obes Rev* 2011; 12: 346–65.
78. Olsen NJ, Heitmann BL. Intake of calorically sweetened beverages and obesity. *Obes Rev* 2009; 10: 68–75.
79. Pereira MA. The possible role of sugar-sweetened beverages in obesity etiology: A review of the evidence. *Int J Obes* 2006; 30: S28–36.
80. Te Morenga L, Mallard S, Mann J. Dietary sugars and body weight: Systematic review and meta-analyses of randomised controlled trials and cohort studies. *BMJ* 2012; 345: e7492. doi:0.11/bmj.e7492.
81. Van Baak MA, Astrup A. Consumption of sugars and body weight. *Obes Rev* 2009; 10 (Suppl. 1): 9–23.
82. Vartanian LR, Schwartz MB, Brownell KD. Effects of soft drink consumption on nutrition and health: A systematic review and meta-analysis. *Am J Public Health* 2007; 97: 667–75.
83. Mattes RD. Beverages and positive energy balance: The menace is the medium. *Int J Obes* 2006; 30: S60–5.
84. De Wijk RA, Zijlstra N, Mars M, de Graaf C, Prinz JF. The effects of food viscosity on bite size, bite effort and food intake. *Physiol Behav* 2008; 95: 527–32.
85. Flood-Obaggy JE, Rolls BJ. The effect of fruit in different forms on energy intake and satiety at a meal. *Appetite* 2009; 52: 416–22.
86. Lavin JH, French SJ, Ruxton CHS, Read NW. An investigation of the role of oro-sensory stimulation in sugar satiety. *Int J Obes* 2002; 26: 384–8.
87. Zijlstra N, Mars M, de Wijk RA, Westerterp-Plantenga MS, de Graaf C. The effect of viscosity on ad libitum intake. *Int J Obes* 2008; 32: 676–83.
88. Apolzan JW, Leidy HJ, Mattes RD, Campbell WW. Effects of food form on food intake and postprandial appetite sensations, glucose and endocrine responses, and energy expenditure in resistance trained v. sedentary older adults. *Br J Nutr* 2011; 106: 1107–16.
89. Bolton RP, Heaton KW, Burroughs LF. The role of dietary fiber in satiety, glucose, and insulin: Studies with fruit and fruit juice. *Am J Clin Nutr* 1981; 34: 211–7.
90. DiMeglio DP, Mattes RD. Liquid versus solid carbohydrate: Effects on food intake and body weight. *Int J Obes Relat Metab* 2000; 24: 794–800.
91. Haber GB, Heaton KW, Murphy D, Burroughs LF. Depletion and disruption of dietary fibre: Effects on satiety, plasma-glucose, and serum-insulin. *Lancet* 1997; 8040: 679–62.
92. Houchins JA, Burgess JR, Campbell WW et al. Beverage vs. solid fruits and vegetables: Effects on energy intake and body weight. *Obesity* 2011. doi:10.1038/oby.2011.192
93. Hulshof T, de Graaf C, Weststrate JA. The effects of preloads varying in physical state and fat content on satiety and energy intake. *Appetite* 1993; 21: 273–86.
94. Leidy HJ, Apolzan JW, Mattes RD, Campbell WW. Food form and portion size affect postprandial appetite sensations and hormonal responses in healthy, nonobese, older adults. *Obesity* 2010; 18: 293–9.
95. Mattes RD. Soup and satiety. *Physiol Behav* 2005; 83: 739–47.
96. Mattes RD, Campbell WW. Effects of food form and timing of ingestion on appetite and energy intake in lean young adults and in young adults with obesity. *J Am Diet Assoc* 2009; 109: 430–7.
97. Tournier A, Louis-Sylvestre J. Effect of the physical state of a food on subsequent intake in human subjects. *Appetite* 1991; 16: 17–24.
98. Almiron-Roig E, Flores SY, Drewnowski A. No difference in satiety or in subsequent energy intakes between a beverage and a solid food. *Physiol Behav* 2004; 82: 671–7.
99. Almiron-Roig E, Grathwohl D, Green H, Erkner A. Impact of some isoenergetic snacks on satiety and next meal intake in healthy adults. *J Hum Nutr Diet* 2009; 22: 469–74.
100. Heymsfield SB, van Mierlo CAJ, van der Knaap HCM, Heo M, Frier HI. Weight management using a meal replacement strategy: Meta and pooling analysis from six studies. *Int J Obes Relat Disord* 2003; 27: 537–49.
101. Rothacker DQ, Watemberg S. Short-term hunger intensity changes following ingestion of a meal replacement bar for weight control. *Int J Food Sci Nutr* 2004; 55: 223–6.

102. Tieken SM, Leidy HJ, Stull AJ, Mattes RD, Schuster RA, Campbell WW. Effects of solid versus liquid meal-replacement products of similar energy content on hunger, satiety, and appetite-regulating hormones in older adults. *Horm Metab Res* 2007; 39: 389–94.
103. Blundell JE, Rogers PJ. Satiating power of food. In *Encyclopedia of Human Biology*, Vol. 6, 723–33. London: Academic Press, 1991.
104. Dove ER, Hodgson JM, Puddey IB, Bellin LJ, Lee YP, Mori TA. 2009. Skim milk compared with a fruit drink acutely reduces appetite and energy intake in overweight men and women. *Am J Clin Nutr* 2009; 90: 70–5.
105. Bertenshaw EJ, Lluch A, Yeomans MR. Satiating effects of protein but not carbohydrate consumed in a between-meal beverage context. *Physiol Behav* 2008; 93: 427–36.
106. Bertenshaw EJ, Lluch A, Yeomans MR. Dose-dependent effects of beverage protein content upon short-term intake. *Appetite* 2009; 52: 580–7.
107. Tsuchiya A, Almiron-Roig A, Lluch A, Guyonnet D, Drewnowski A. Higher satiety ratings following yogurt consumption relative to fruit drink or dairy fruit drink. *J Am Diet Assoc* 2006; 106: 550–7.
108. Almiron-Roig E, Drewnowski A. Hunger, thirst, and energy intakes following the consumption of caloric beverages. *Physiol Behav* 2003; 79: 767–73.
109. Almiron-Roig E, Palla L, Guest K et al. Factors that determine energy compensation: A systematic review of preload studies. *Nutrition Rev* 2013. doi:10.1111/nure.12048.
110. Brunstrom JM. The control of meal size in human subjects: A role for expected satiety, expected satiation and premeal planning. *Proc Nutr Soc* 2011; 70: 155–61.
111. Cassady BA, Considine RV, Mattes RD. Beverage consumption, appetite, and energy intake: What did you expect? *Am J Clin Nutr* 2012. doi:10.3945/ajcn.111.025437.
112. Martens MJI, Westerterp-Plantenga MS. Mode of consumption plays a role in alleviating hunger and thirst. *Obesity* 2012; 20: 517–24.
113. De Graaf C. Texture and satiation: The role of oro-sensory exposure time. *Physiol Behav* 2012; 107: 496–501.
114. De Graaf C, Kok FJ. Slow food, fast food and the control of food intake. *Nat Rev Endocrinol* 2010; 6: 290–3.
115. Zijlstra N, Mars M, de Wijk RA, Westerterp-Plantenga MS, Holst JJ, de Graaf C. Effect of viscosity on appetite and gastro-intestinal hormones. *Physiol Behav* 2009; 97: 68–75.
116. Mattes RD, Rothacker D. Beverage viscosity is inversely related to postprandial hunger in humans. *Physiol Behav* 2001; 74: 551–7.
117. Teff KL. Cephalic phase pancreatic polypeptide responses to liquid and solid stimuli in humans. *Physiol Behav* 2010; 99: 317–23.
118. Cannon WB, Washburn AL. An explanation of hunger. *Am J Physiol* 1912; 29: 441–54.
119. Fisher RS, Malmud LS, Bandini P, Rock E. Gastric emptying of a physiologic mixed solid–liquid meal. *Clin Nucl Med* 1982; 7: 215–21.
120. Marciani L, Gowland PA, Spiller RC et al. Effect of meal viscosity and nutrients on satiety, intragastric dilution, and emptying assessed by MRI. *Am J Physiol Gastrointest Liver Physiol* 2001; 2082: G1227–33.
121. Atkinson FS, Foster-Powell K, Brand-Miller JC. International tables of glycemic index and glycemic load values. *Diab Care* 2008; 31: 2281–3.
122. Mourao DM, Bressan J, Campbell WW, Mattes RD. Effects of food form on appetite and energy intake in lean and obese young adults. *Int J Obes* 2007; 31: 1688–95.
123. Martens MJI, Lemmens SGT, Born JM, Westerterp-Plantenga MS. A solid high-protein meal evokes stronger hunger suppression than a liquefied high-protein meal. *Obesity* 2011; 19: 522–7.
124. Akhavan T, Luhovyy BL, Anderson GH. Effect of drinking compared with eating sugars or whey protein on short-term appetite and food intake. *Int J Obes* 2011; 35: 562–9.

4 Sugars in Confectionery Products

Technical Functions and Links to Health Outcomes

Laura Shumow

CONTENTS

KEY POINTS

- A number of different types of sugars are used in confectionery products, but sucrose and glucose syrup are currently the two most common sweeteners.
- The ability of sugars to crystallize, form a glass, and undergo the chemical reactions Maillard browning and caramelization is key to the texture and flavor of common candy products.
- While limited research exists on the impact of candy on health, evidence to date suggests that candy consumption is not linked to obesity and chronic disease.
- Candy-eating behavior is a promising research opportunity area and the public would benefit from understanding how to promote balanced moderate enjoyment of treats.
- There is an interesting emerging body of evidence on cocoa flavanols and chocolate demonstrating a positive impact on cardiovascular health with promising research questions for the future.

INTRODUCTION

Confections, also known as candy, are a broad category of sweet foods with a long and rich history. The earliest records of candy and candy-making techniques date back to 2000 BC where they were inscribed in hieroglyphics on walls of Egyptian tombs and ancient rolls of papyrus [1]. In fact, the word "candy" is derived from the ancient Arabian word, "qandi," which means something made with sugar. Sugar has always and continues to be essential to the composition of candy products. The unique properties of sugars are what make the production of candy possible. The sweetness of sugar and the ability of sugars to crystalize, become a glass, and undergo chemical reactions are critical to the essence of candy. Additionally sugars are important for the microbiological safety and quality of candy products.

Before the widespread availability of sugar from cane, honey was typically used to make sweet confectionery products. Fruits, nuts, grains, and seeds were coated with honey, not only for sweetness and flavor, but also as a preservative. These ancient candies included pastes of nuts and honey resembling marzipan and an early type of hard candy made from boiled barley and water which was then typically rolled in sesame seeds.

Candies were also historically used for medicinal purposes. For example, licorice, which is derived from a root, dates back to the early times of humans and was believed to promote health [1]. Physicians often added honey to their medicinal herbs to mask the unpleasant flavor. Limited research exists on candy and health today, however recent data suggest that candy consumption is not associated with risk of obesity or chronic disease. It is unclear why this is, but is perhaps due to the small contribution of candy to the overall diet. There is a greater body of evidence on chocolate and health, which suggests that intrinsic components of cocoa, the main ingredient in chocolate, may promote cardiovascular health.

The story of chocolate is its own fascinating and enchanting tale. The cocoa tree, which can only be grown in a narrow band 20° north and south of the equator, originated in equatorial Central America and produces a fruit called the cocoa pod. Cocoa beans are the seeds of the cocoa fruit. The indigenous Mayans are thought to have celebrated cocoa at least 2000 years ago, demonstrated by carved images of cocoa pods on the walls of their elaborate stone temples. The subsequently dominant Aztec culture left evidence of cocoa reverence in writings referring to cocoa as a gift from the gods. In the 1600s, European explorers brought cocoa back to Europe and added sugar to create a sweet drink. Later, solid chocolate was developed by the Dutchman Coenraad Van Houten through the addition of fat and sugar [2].

Today, candy is popular across the globe, although different regions have their own unique preferences. The confectionery industry is more diverse than most food sectors in that it encompasses both small retail manufacturers as well as large global manufacturers. Unlike much of the food produced for larger regional distribution, a great deal of candy is still made to satisfy local traditions and flavors. Due to its popularity and reflection of unique cultural differences, candy is often given as a gift. Most people consider candy to be a treat that is consumed for its pleasurable qualities. Candy has been considered a special treat and played an important role in cultural traditions and celebrations for thousands of years and continues to be associated with holidays and traditions.

TYPES OF SUGARS USED IN CONFECTIONERY PRODUCTS

A variety of different types of monosaccharides and disaccharides, or sugars, are commonly used, often in combination, in confectionery products. The physicochemical properties of each type of sugar contribute to the unique properties of the confectionery products from which they are made. The main sugars used in candy are sucrose, glucose syrups, and invert sugar, and the distinct properties of these sugars in confectionery are summarized in Table 4.1. However, a multitude of other sugars may also be used in various applications including glucose (dextrose), fructose, maltose, and lactose. Less refined forms of sugars including honey, maple syrup, and molasses are used in a small number of products; however these ingredients are challenging due to higher cost and natural impurities. Alternative sweeteners are used to varying degrees to create sugar-free options of most types of confections.

Reducing Sugars

An important classification of sugars used in confectionery products is whether or not they are characterized as "reducing sugars." Reducing sugars have a free aldehyde group that is available to become oxidized to a carboxylic acid. A free aldehyde group is necessary for a sugar to react in the Maillard browning reaction, which is one of the most important chemical reactions that occurs during cooking of candy and any food. The disaccharide sucrose is not a reducing sugar; however, the monosaccharides glucose and fructose, as well as disaccharides maltose and lactose are reducing sugars.

Sucrose

Sucrose (table sugar) is the leading sweetener used in the candy industry. In the USA alone, the confectionery industry uses approximately 10 million tons of sucrose annually [3]. Sucrose is naturally present in a wide range of plants, but is sourced commercially from both sugar beets and sugarcane.

TABLE 4.1
Distinct Properties of Common Sweeteners Used in Confectionery Products

Sugar Type	Key Properties in Confectionery
Sucrose	Promotes crystallization
	Not a reducing sugar, therefore more resistant to browning
	Contributes sweetness
	Enhances flavor release
Glucose syrup	Prevents crystallization
	Contains reducing sugars that can undergo browning
	Controls viscosity
	Controls uptake of moisture from the air
	Modifies high sweetness from sucrose
Invert sugar	Prevents crystallization
	Contains reducing sugars

Use of sucrose sourced from beets versus sugarcane results virtually in no difference in the end confectionery products as long as the sugar is well refined. Confectioners use sucrose in multiple forms, but most commonly in a granulated form. Granulated sugar is available in different sizes of particles ranging from large crystals of over 2000 μm, which are used as a surface decoration to fine powder with particles of less than 20 μm, which are used as seed crystals [4]. Additionally, liquid sucrose, a saturated solution of sucrose and water, is used by some candy manufactures for convenience.

Sucrose is a disaccharide consisting of one glucose unit and one fructose unit with a molecular weight of 341. While sucrose is not a reducing sugar, the subcomponent parts, fructose and glucose, are classified as reducing sugars. Sucrose does not have reducing capacity because the glucose–fructose bond ties up the otherwise free aldehyde group. Sucrose has a solubility limit of 67% in water at room temperature [5]. This solubility is the driving force behind crystallization and also impacts the ability of a candy to release flavors in the mouth. The unique solubility and crystallization chemistry of sucrose, which is discussed in greater detail in "Basic Functionality of Sugars in Confectionery Products and Desserts", is what makes it possible to create many kinds of candy.

Glucose Syrup

Glucose syrups of starches are another essential sweetener used in candy products. In the USA, glucose syrups are almost exclusively made from corn, whereas in Europe most glucose syrups are typically derived from wheat. The US confectionery industry uses approximately 400,000 tons of glucose syrups from corn annually [4].

Glucose syrups play a number of roles in confectionery products, but one of the most important roles is the prevention of unwanted sucrose crystallization or "graining." Partial crystallization (graining) results in a change in the appearance of a candy product as well as a rough texture. Confectioners use the term "doctoring" to refer to the addition of a solution of saccharides other than sucrose, such as glucose syrup or invert sugar to prevent this undesirable physical change in confections during storage. The term dextrose equivalents (DEs) refers to the amount of the reducing sugar capacity present in a given glucose syrup. This factor is key to selecting a glucose syrup that will function appropriately in a given formulation. The DE is linked to molecular weight, which influences the solubility, crystallization inhibition, viscosity, and hygroscopicity of the glucose syrup. The most common glucose syrup used in confectionery is 42 DE, which consists mostly of maltose and also contains larger chain polymers and is less sweet than sucrose. Higher DE glucose syrups are also used in some formulations of confectionery products, such as some caramels and fillings.

Invert Sugar

Invert sugar is a syrup of sucrose that has been broken down from a disaccharide of glucose (dextrose) and fructose (levulose) to the free subcomponent parts. The result is a product of reducing sugars that is 50% glucose and 50% fructose. Inversion of sucrose occurs naturally by heating and is accelerated by the addition of acids or can be manufactured with the use of enzymes. While inversion of sugar occurs naturally under the conditions of candy making, invert sugar can also be bought and used as an ingredient. Invert sugar has similar functions to glucose syrup in confectionery products in controlling the "grain" or crystallization of sucrose. Prior to widespread availability of glucose syrup, inversion of sugar was the primary method that candy makers used to control sucrose crystallization, but use has now significantly declined due to the low cost of glucose syrup.

Alternative Sweeteners

Reduced sugar or sugar-free options are available on the market for most types of confections. For example, the majority of the gum market is now sugar-free. However, for most traditional confections, consumers typically prefer the taste of sugars and while sugar-free alternatives for many candies are available, they have not been embraced by the broader candy-consuming public.

A range of alternative sweeteners are used in the category of sugar-free confectionery products. The most common bulk sugar substitutes are the sugar alcohols or polyols, including sorbitol, maltitol, erythritol, isomalt, and lactitol, which are only partially absorbed in the human gastrointestinal tract and thus contribute fewer calories than sugar. One significant drawback of polyols is that they typically have a laxative effect. This category of sweeteners helps mimic the textural properties of sugar, but is generally not very sweet and must also be combined with a high-intensity sweetener.

High-intensity sweeteners present notable challenges for confectioners including flavor, consumer acceptability, regulatory, and safety considerations. Several high-intensity sweeteners are used in sugar-free confectionery products including aspartame, acesulfame potassium, saccharin, and sucralose. In recent years, there has been development in natural high-intensity sweeteners such as stevial glycosides, which has attracted significant consumer interest. High-intensity sweeteners are further discussed in Chapter 7.

BASIC FUNCTIONALITY OF SUGARS IN CONFECTIONERY PRODUCTS AND DESSERTS

Sugars are an essential ingredient in candy, and the specific chemical properties of individual sugars are exploited to create many of the important technical characteristics of confections. In addition to providing sweetness, sugars act as flavor and color precursors, determine crystallization and texture, and act as a bulking agent. Through influencing water activity, sugars help control microbiological growth and quality attributes over the course of a candy product's shelf life. Furthermore, each sugar has its own unique chemical properties, and much of the equipment to manufacture confectionery products has been designed to optimize these characteristics. Regulatory considerations also influence the use of sugars in confectionery products. Not all sugar substitutes are approved for use in confectionery, and different countries and regulatory bodies have different rules regarding the use of these ingredients. The main functions of sugars in confectionery are summarized in Table 4.2.

Sweetness, Flavor, and Color

Unsurprisingly, providing sweetness is the most basic function of sugars in candy products. Sweetness is one of the five tastes and is detected by receptors on human taste cells that bind to various sugars and sugar substitutes. Analytical methods are not usually used to measure sweetness; rather, sweetness is measured through human sensory panels. Different sugars contribute varying degrees of sweetness and are all compared relative to sucrose as a reference point. For example, most glucose syrups used in confectionery products are about half the sweetness of sucrose, while high-intensity sweeteners such as aspartame are up to 200 times sweeter than sucrose [2].

Beyond simple sweetness, flavor is an extremely important attribute in confectionery products. Flavor often comes from added natural or artificial flavorings; however, flavor compounds may also

TABLE 4.2
Key Functions of Sugars in Confectionery Products

Key Functions of Sugars in Confectionery Products
Sweetness and precursors for flavor and color compounds
Bulk and determines the texture and structure
Controls crystallization
Impacts processing and regulatory requirements
Increases microbiological safety and shelf life through control of water

be formed naturally by the breakdown of sugars in the candy-making process. There are two main chemical reactions involving sugars that give rise to flavor development of candy. These reactions occur naturally, as a result of typical traditional preparation methods, and are essential to the desirable characteristics of many confectionery products including the flavor and color of chocolate and cocoa products, caramels, toffees, brittles, and nougats.

Maillard Browning

Maillard browning is one of the most common chemical reactions that occur in confectionery and other heat-treated foods. Along with caramelization, Maillard browning is essential to the flavor of caramels, toffees, and butterscotch. Also, the flavor development in roasted nuts and roasted cocoa beans (ultimately processed into chocolate) are largely due to these reactions. While this color and flavor development is desirable in these cases, it is unfavorable in other applications where different colors and flavors are desired such as hard candy, gummies, and aerated candies.

Maillard browning occurs at a wide range of temperatures; however the familiar caramel flavor development occurs between 100 and 180°C when a reducing sugar reacts with any protein or free amino acids [4]. This reaction leads to the transformation of the sugar and amino acid reactants into a wide range of products including a host of color and flavor compounds. This process is limited by the amount of "free amines" which are supplied by the protein. The reducing potential of different proteins varies depending on their amino acid composition. The amount and nature of the specific end products depends on the concentration and reactivity of sugars, the amount of free amines, the processing time, the temperature of the process, the pH of the product, and the water content of the product.

Caramelization

Another example of a flavor development process that occurs naturally from candy processing is caramelization, which happens when sugars are heated to temperatures around 160°C. Caramelization is a set of multifaceted chemical reactions that lead to the degradation of sugars. Unlike Maillard browning which is the reaction between an amino acid and a reducing sugar, caramelization is the pyrolytic decomposition of sugars and is aided by salts and acids. So, while sucrose cannot participate in Maillard browning, it will undergo caramelization. The reaction results in the breakdown of sucrose and other sugars into many different chemical products including complex nutty and bitter flavors and dark brown color compounds. Caramelization reactions are time- and temperature-dependent and are also influenced by pH and salinity.

Water Content and Activity

Candy tends to be very stable and microbiologically safe with a typical shelf life of 6 months to 2 years. Sensory and quality factors, rather than safety, determine the end of most candy products' shelf life. The water content of different confectionery products varies from a low 1–2% in a very hard candy to upwards of 30% moisture in a syrup filling. Water content is important to a confection's texture; however, in terms of determining shelf life and microbiological safety, a more relevant measure than water content is water activity [6]:

$$a_w = p/p_0,$$

where a_w is water activity, p the vapor pressure of water in the product, and p_0 the vapor pressure of water at the same temperature.

Water activity refers to the amount of water that is free to react and is measured by the ratio of the relative vapor pressures of the food to the vapor pressure of water. Water activity is the ratio of

TABLE 4.3
Water Activity of Common Candies

Confectionery	Water Activity
Jam	0.8–0.85
Fondants and creams	0.65–0.8
Marshmallow	0.6–0.75
Gummy and jelly candies	0.5–0.75
Nougat	0.4–0.65
Chewy candies, caramel, and fudge	0.45–0.6
Hard candy, brittles	0.25–0.4

the vapor pressure of the material to the vapor pressure of pure water. It is expressed as a number between 0 and 1, with 0 referring to a theoretical solution that contains no free water and 1 referring to the water activity of 100% pure water. Water activity is reduced by solutes, such as salts, sugars, and proteins and is also impacted by a number of factors, including concentration and type of solute as well as the temperature.

Water activity is a key determinant of food safety. Sugars in confectionery products bind water and make it unavailable to participate in reactions or support microbiological growth. Bacteria cannot thrive at water activity level below 0.85 and molds and yeasts cannot grow at a range of lower water activities, but absolutely not below 0.60. Water activity is also relevant to measures of quality. For example, water activity determines the likelihood of moisture migration between a candy product and the environment where a product is held or different components of a candy product. The relative humidity of the environment and the water activity will determine the direction of the moisture migration. A product with a relatively low water activity is more likely to take up humidity from the air and become sticky or soft and a product with high water activity is more likely to lose water to the air, becoming hard and dry. Water activities of common confectionery products are shown in Table 4.3 [6].

Texture and Structure

Sugars contribute a great deal of the body and bulk of confectionery products, although vary in the percent contribution by specific type of candy. For example, white and milk chocolate typically contain about 50–75% sugar, while dark chocolates typically have less sugar. Dark chocolate can contain as much as 65% sugar or as little as less than 10% sugar. Lower-percent sugar chocolate products are becoming more popular as consumers become interested in very-high-percent cocoa dark chocolates. Nonchocolate candy is comprised mostly of sugar, with hard candies consisting of up to 95% sugars.

Beyond simply making up the bulk of a candy product, the state of the sugar contributes to the textural qualities in candy. Sugars may take several physical forms that impact the texture and the appearance of the finished product. Sugars may be dissolved in solution, present in a crystalline form or as an amorphous or glassy state. Candy may also contain sugars in more than one state within a given product. Examples of candies in these various physical forms are discussed in "Sugars in Crystalline Candy."

One of the factors that dictates the physical state is solubility of a sugar. Solubility is the maximum concentration of particles that are able to dissolve in a given amount of water. The solubility is limited by molecular interactions of the particles with water molecules. Solubility is one of the parameters that influences the type and quality of candy products that can be made from certain ingredients. Based on their size, configuration, and chemical potential for hydrogen bonding, different sugars have different inherent solubility limits, which all increase in a temperature-dependent manner. When the solubility limit is reached, the solution is said to be saturated. It is possible to drive solubility beyond the saturation point to a "supersaturated" solution through heating the solution to increase the solubility point and cooling without agitation. This principle is used to produce certain crystalline candies such as "rock candy."

A crystalline structure is comprised of a highly organized chemical matrix of sugar molecules lined up in the form of a lattice. Due to the thermodynamically stable nature of the crystalline form, there is a latent heat of fusion or a release of energy in the form of heat when the crystals form. Noncrystalline structures, such as glasses, are characterized by more random orientations of sugar molecules. A glass is not technically a solid in thermodynamic terms, but a liquid that is so heavily saturated and thick that it does not flow at room temperature. A glass transition temperature is used to measure the temperature at which the solution transitions from being fluid-like to so viscous that the molecules are immobilized. For example, a candy product with a glass transition temperature of 30°C would be a solid-like product at temperatures of 30° and below, but would melt above this temperature.

Controlling crystallization is an important element in confectionery manufacturing. Some candies are exclusively crystalline (e.g., rock candy, tableted candies); other candies are exclusively noncrystalline (e.g., hard candy, cotton candy), while many candies are partially crystalline, or "grained" (fondants, nougats, marshmallows, fudge/caramels). Crystallization causes a rough grainy texture and an opaque color, while glasses are hard, smooth, and translucent. The likelihood of a solution undergoing crystallization and the nature of crystallization that occurs is influenced by a number of factors including formulation and processing conditions.

Nucleation refers to the formation of new crystals in a solution. Nucleation occurs only in a supersaturated solution. The addition of a "seed crystal" as well as agitation will promote nucleation. Growth of crystals occurs at lower degrees of sugar saturation. The presence of other molecules will prevent sugar molecules from coming together to form crystals. For example, long-chain polysaccharides such as those in low-DE glucose syrup and starch and large protein and fat molecules found in dairy ingredients result in a higher viscosity as well as lower amount of free water, which reduces the mobility of sucrose molecules and inhibits crystallization. Additionally, monosaccharides bond free water, preventing crystallization.

Functions of Sugars in Specific Confectionery Products

The confectionery category includes a wide range of sweet products including hard and soft candies, chocolate, and gum. All of these products contain sweeteners, such as sugars, syrups, or honey, in addition to other ingredients including spices, flavorings, gelling agents, colorings, and acids. Some candy also contains dairy products, milk fat, cocoa butter, other fats, dried fruits, nuts, and seeds.

The general process of making candy is quite simple. Sugars are mixed with water and heated. Heating causes water to evaporate from the mixture. As water evaporates, the percent solids in the mixture increases, which causes an elevation of the boiling point of the solution. The phenomenon of boiling point elevation allows the confectioner to control the moisture content and thus textural qualities of the product. Boiling point elevation is determined by the number of particles present in the solution. Once the appropriate boiling point is reached, the sugar mixture is then cooled and processed to promote the desired physical state by using various processing techniques specific to each product. For example, whipping and gelling agents are used to promote aeration in a marshmallow and addition of gelling agents and depositing into molds is necessary for gummies. For many candies, flavors, colors, acids, and other inclusions may be added at this point in the process. Finally, the product is cut and packaged.

Prior to the availability of thermometers, which allow control of the final product by the measure of boiling point elevation, confectioners used the "cold water test" and developed terms such as "soft ball" and "hard crack" to describe the consistency of the sugar solutions cooked to certain moisture contents. These terms are still used today and are shown in Table 4.4 with the

TABLE 4.4
Boiling Point and Moisture Content of Common Confectionery Products

Boiling Temperature (°C)	Moisture Content (%)	Description	Confectionery Products
110–116	15–20	Soft ball	Gummies, fondant, creams
117–120	10–15	Firm ball	Caramel, marshmallow
121–130	5–10	Hard ball	Nougat
130–145	3–5	Soft crack	Butterscotch, taffy
145–155	1–3	Hard crack	Hard candy, brittles

corresponding approximate boiling points and moisture contents [6]. Also, while candy was traditionally prepared under atmospheric pressure, newer models of equipment cook sugar solutions under vacuum. The effect of this reduction of pressure is more efficient evaporation of moisture and reduced reactivity of sugars in chemical reactions such as Maillard browning, caramelization, and inversion. The vacuum also allows confectioners to better control foaming that occurs during heating of sugars.

Functions of Sugars in Noncrystalline Confectionaries

Hard Candies/Boiled Sweets

Hard candy or "boiled sweets" are characterized as an amorphous solid or "glass." They are smooth, hard, translucent, and available in a range of shapes and types, including lollipops, candy canes, filled, and solid pieces. Hard candy is made by cooking a sugar solution to a high temperature, resulting in a very low-moisture content (typically less than 4%). Hard candies are made from a combination of sucrose and glucose syrup (or invert sugar) ranging from 70% sucrose and 30% glucose syrup to 45% sucrose and 65% glucose syrup [7]. The exact ratio is optimized for the equipment and type of cooking process used by the confectioner. Flavors, colors, and acids are also added to most hard candies. Brittles and butterscotch are hard candies that contain dairy fat and nuts.

The glucose syrup (or alternatively invert sugar) in the hard candy formulation is used to prevent crystallization of sucrose, which is considered a defect in hard candy. However, the glucose syrup also presents problems throughout the shelf life of the product. The low molecular weights of the monosaccharides in the glucose syrup or invert sugar are hygroscopic and therefore attract water. When humidity is absorbed from the air, the product becomes sticky. Furthermore, the absorbed water acts as a plasticizer and drives down the glass transition temperature of the hard candy which ultimately promotes crystallization.

Gummies and Aerated Candies

Gummies, jellies, and aerated candies are uniquely textured products that come in a range of shapes and sizes. They include marshmallows, Turkish delight, fruit leathers, taffy, the centers of jelly beans, gummy bears, etc. These products are noncrystalline sugar syrups that are stabilized by a hydrocolloid agent. Hydrocolloid agents are gelling and thickening agents including starch, gelatin, carrageenan, and pectin. The specific formulation of hydrocolloids is the critical factor in manipulating the texture of the end product. For example, while gummies made with gelatin result in a long flexible elastic texture, starch gelled gummies have a short chewy texture. Pectin results in a short brittle clean bite. By binding water and increasing the viscosity, gelling agents also have an important function of inhibiting sucrose crystallization.

Gummies were traditionally made by heating the sugar hydrocolloid solutions in copper kettles over an open flame, but are now made under vacuum in pressure cookers with steam injection. The cooked solution is deposited into starch molds, which was traditionally done by hand but is now automated by a machine called a mogul. Following depositing, the gummies take hours to days to reach moisture equilibration. Some gummies are finished by "sanding" or coating in sugar, while others are covered in oil or wax for a smooth texture. Aerated candies, such as marshmallow and nougat, are soft fluffy candies made from a stabilized foamed sugar solution. The foam is created by mechanically whipping air into the simple sugar solution. The suspended air bubbles are stabilized with a hydrocolloid such as egg albumin or gelatin. Nougat requires the addition of fat for its chewy texture.

Sugars in Crystalline Candy

Most crystalline candies are made through careful control of crystallization to promote the formation of very small consistent crystals. A notable exception to processing that promotes small crystals is the manufacture of rock candy, which intentionally yields the formation of large sugar crystals. The large sugar crystals in rock candy are formed by use of a rough surface that provides a site for crystal formation. Slow evaporation of a cooled supersaturated sucrose solution results in growth of the sugar crystals.

Several types of candy may either be noncrystalline or partially crystalline ("grained") and the degree of graining is inherent to the product's quality. For example, one type of caramel may be smooth and runny, while another caramel product may be firm and chewy. This is due to multiple formulation and processing factors, including fat and protein content, cooking temperature, and degree of sugar crystallization. There are varying degrees of graining in marshmallows, caramels, cream centers, and nougats. This is often accomplished through use of fondants as an ingredient in many partially crystalline confections.

Fondants consist of tiny recrystallized sugar crystals that are ideally so small they cannot be detected by the tongue and are suspended in a dense liquid sugar syrup. The crystals are approximately 5–15 μm in size. Fondants are made by first heating a 60–80% sucrose and 7–30% glucose syrup water along with water to 115–120°C. The sugar solution is then allowed to cool to 40–50°C. Vigorous stirring initiates crystallization of sucrose. Cream centers are made by mixing fondant with a "frappe," which is an aerated sugar solution, and a sugar solution usually containing more water than the fondant called "bob syrup." The frappe adds levity to the cream center, and the bob syrup is used to control the viscosity.

Another type of crystalline confection is tableted candies, such as pressed mints. These candies are made by compressing a free-flowing solution of a suitable sugar (or sugar alcohol) and binders under high pressure in a mould. Sucrose, fructose, glucose, maltitol, sorbitol, and xylitol are commonly used in tableted confections. Under pressure, the sugar or sugar alcohol molecules fracture, stretch, and re-bond strongly to one another.

Panned confectionaries are a type of candy with a hard or soft candy coating made by building up layers of coating in a rotating pan. Hard panning refers to a process whereby a hard crystalline shell is formed around a center. Examples of hard panned candies include candy-coated chocolate pieces, Jordan almonds, and jaw breakers. Soft panned products, such as jelly beans, have a softer crystalline shell. This process takes a long time as many layers are needed to form a sugar shell that is a desirable thickness. Chocolate panned products are candies coated in chocolate using similar equipment. These include chocolate-covered nuts, for example.

Function of Sugars in Chocolates

The primary ingredients in chocolate are derived from cocoa beans, which are the seeds of the fruit produced by the cacao tree. Cocoa beans are fermented and then dried. Beans are then moved to a processing facility where they are roasted and shelled. The removal of the shell results in "nibs," which are ground into a smooth paste, referred to as "chocolate liquor," which is the essential ingredient of chocolate. Chocolate liquor can either be pressed to release cocoa butter and cocoa powder or used directly in finished chocolate. To produce finished chocolate, chocolate liquor is mixed with varying amounts of cocoa butter and sugar.

Chocolate liquor is very bitter and the addition of sugar makes it palatable. When first added to the chocolate mixture, the sucrose particles are large. The smooth creamy texture of chocolate is produced by breaking up the sugar particles through a process called conching. Conching is a mechanical kneading of the chocolate liquor–sugar mixture resulting in the fracture of sugar particles into smaller components and can take hours to days. The length of conching determines the ultimate particle size of the sucrose molecules in the chocolate and the smoothness of the chocolate. Emulsifiers, such as lecithin, are added to prolong the shelf life and prevent fat crystallization, known as "bloom." Flavors such as vanilla are added to compliment the inherent cocoa flavor. Not surprisingly, the addition of milk solids creates milk chocolate.

Chocolate is the only confectionery product subject to national and international standards of identity. Many countries, as well as the international regulatory body Codex Alimentarius, have standards of identity for chocolate. Chocolate standards of identity are mostly intended to ensure that the fat content and quality of chocolate products meet a threshold level, specifically ensuring a certain level of cocoa butter. US standards of identity also require that sweet and semisweet chocolate (also known as dark chocolate) and milk chocolate contain a nutritive sweetener.

TYPICAL CANDY CONSUMPTION

Candy is considered a sweet treat in most cultures. The majority of people report eating candy; however the quantity of candy most people consume may actually be lower than expected. In fact, in a recent government survey of Americans, 97% of adults reported consuming candy at least once over the course of the year [8]. Inconsistent definitions of candy present a challenge to understanding exactly how much candy people typically eat; however, candy intake generally accounts for only a small percentage of total caloric intake and added sugars in the US diet. In the US population, per capita candy consumption accounts for approximately 2.2% of total energy intake [8]. Average candy intake in the USA has been reported to be less than 50 kcal per person per day [8]. This amount is equivalent to a small piece of chocolate, several hard candies, a string of licorice, or a small handful of jellybeans.

While most people eat candy throughout the year, usually people do not eat candy every day. US Department of Agriculture data have shown that the average American, ages 2 years and older, consumes candy on 138.7 eating occasions per year, or about 2–3 times per week [9]. Data collected from market data sources indicate Americans consume candy slightly more frequently, 153.3 eating occasions per year or closer to three times per week [9].

The contribution of candy to added sugar intake of Americans older than 2 years in the USA is moderate at only approximately 5 g/day or about 6% of total added sugar [10]. Typical sugar contribution of common confectionery products is shown in Table 4.5 [11]. Given its relatively modest contribution of added sugars, candy ranks fifth as a source of added sugars in the US diet, after sugary drinks (soda/energy/sports/sweetened bottled water drinks; 35.7%), grain-based desserts (12.9%),

TABLE 4.5
Calories and Sugars in Popular Candies

Product	Calories (kcal)	Sugars* (g)	Calories from Sugars (kcal)
Milk chocolate bar, 43 g	235	23	91
Dark chocolate bar, 41 g	230	19	78
Snack size bar, chocolate covered caramel w/nuts, 14 g	70	7	30
Candies, milk chocolate coated peanuts, 46 g	240	22	87
Hard candies, four pieces, 14 g	60	9	36
Jelly beans, 10 large, 28 g	105	20	80
Chewing gum, sugarless, 2 g	5	0	0

sugar-sweetened fruit drinks (10.5%), and dairy-based desserts (6.6%) [10]. Likewise, candy is not a leading contributor of solid fats in the diet of Americans (2 years and older) contributing 3.1% to total saturated fat intake [10].

CANDY AND HEALTH

Safety of Candy

Generally, candy products are quite safe. Due to the low water activity of confectionery products, the presence of pathogenic bacteria is not a widespread problem, especially for nonchocolate sugar candy. Recent outbreaks associated with *Salmonella* in nuts have raised concerns about the safety of high-fat, low-moisture products. As a result, manufacturers that use these products have strengthened their safety standards and several governments including the USA and China have updated their food safety regulations. Confectioners use validated roasting methods to control this risk in chocolate liquor and nuts. Since many confectioners use allergens such as nuts, milk, and wheat, and process on shared equipment, allergen management is the number one food safety and regulatory concern for confectioners. Confectionery manufactures manage allergens through good manufacturing practices and accurate labeling of allergens. Furthermore, confectioners carefully monitor their supply chain to prevent using ingredients that may contain contaminants.

Oral Health

Today, dental hygiene practices have a more significant impact on improving dental health than changes in diet. Nonetheless, dietary habits remain an area of interest by dental health authorities, and typical recommendations include reducing the frequency of eating and drinking between meals as well as reducing the duration that fermentable carbohydrates are in the mouth. While frequency of eating is the main dietary factor for dental health, candies are one of several foods and drinks associated with increased risk for dental caries, along with sugar-sweetened beverages, sticky foods, sugary-starchy snacks, and simple sugars such as sucrose, honey, and molasses [12].

Cariogenicity, or the likelihood of a substance to induce dental caries, is associated with the total amount of fermentable carbohydrates in a food, but cannot be determined by the sugar or carbohydrate content alone. Noncarbohydrate characteristics of a food, such as the texture and other nutrients (fat, minerals, etc.) modify cariogenicity, as can the circumstances of food consumption such as drinking water while eating or the combination of foods consumed together [13]. Related to texture, the retention time of food on the teeth is also a very important factor. Perhaps surprisingly, chocolate has been shown to clear from the mouth rapidly, which is likely due to the high fat content.

Interestingly, despite the sugar content, a couple of classic studies suggest that chocolate consumption may not lead to the formation of dental caries. In his study of 436 individuals over 5 years in the 1950s, Gustofason et al. showed that people who ate chocolate were not more likely to develop dental caries than those who consumed no snacks [13]. Similarly in 1988, Yankell et al. [14] found that exposure to mixtures of chocolate ingredients did not increase risk factors for the development of dental caries. Furthermore, more recent evidence suggests that certain naturally occurring cocoa components may inhibit dental plaque formation in rodents.

There is a well-developed body of research demonstrating the impact of sugar-free chewing gum on oral health. Sugar-free chewing gum typically contains sugar alcohols such as xylitol and sorbitol, which are noncariogenic because plaque-forming bacteria cannot metabolize them. The chewing process stimulates saliva, which increases oral clearance of sugars, acids, and food debris from the mouth. The increased salivary flow also leads to neutralization and buffering of plaque acids and remineralization of tooth enamel [15]. Several clinical trials have shown that chewing sugar-free gum reduces the incidence of cavities. For example, Szöke et al. [16] showed that chewing sugar-free gum three times a day for 2 years resulted in a 38.7% reduction in dental caries.

Candy and Obesity, Chronic Health

There is limited research on the specific impact of candy consumption on chronic health. Generally, health professionals and authorities recognize that while it is most important to manage calories and the balance of nutrients, consumers can enjoy small amounts of their favorite treats as part of a healthy and balanced diet and lifestyle. Additionally, several recently published cross-sectional studies have shown that candy and chocolate consumption in children and adults is not associated with increased weight, BMI, or waist circumference. These cross-sectional data have also shown that candy consumption is not associated with risk of metabolic syndrome in adults.

Specifically, O'Neil et al.'s 2011 study [17] examining the association of candy consumption with total energy intake, weight status, and cardiovascular disease (CVD) risk factors in more than 15,000 US adults showed that, while candy contributed modestly to caloric intake, there was no association of candy intake with increased weight/body mass index. Another O'Neil et al. [18] study in 2012 of 11,182 US children and adolescents showed that while children and adolescent candy consumers had slightly higher intakes of total energy and added sugars, they were less likely to be overweight or obese than noncandy consumers. There were no associations between candy consumption and cardiovascular risk factors, including no difference in blood pressure or blood lipid levels [17,18]. Likewise and also in 2012, Golomb et al. [19] published a study of approximately 1000 adults that showed those who ate chocolate more frequently had a lower body mass index than those who ate chocolate less often. This occurred despite the fact that those who ate chocolate more often did not eat fewer calories, nor exercise more frequently than those who ate chocolate less frequently. Similarly, Murphy et al. [20] found in 2013 that frequency of candy intake was not associated with increased weight status or CVD risk factors in adults. A longitudinal study, which measured candy consumption and health characteristics at baseline in 10-year olds and at follow up 10–20 years later, found no relationship between baseline candy consumption and body mass index or CVD risk factors in young adults [21].

This evidence is interesting but of limited use to our understanding of the impact of candy consumption on public health due to its cross-sectional design. However, the studies seem to suggest that many people are able to include candy as part of an overall balanced lifestyle. The consumption data show that candy is a relatively minor contributor to overall calories, which may explain the lack of association between consumption and weight despite the high energy density of the products. Additionally, behavioral research suggests that learning how to include favorite foods, such as chocolate, may play an important role in achieving and sustaining healthy eating behaviors. This is supported by a small pilot study by Piehowski et al. [22] in 2012 on the effects of consuming either a chocolate treat or other sweet snack daily on measures of weight loss in women following a reduced-calorie diet. Researchers found that incorporating a sweet snack daily as part of an overall reduced calorie diet does not inhibit positive changes in body weight and body fat percentage and helped reduce cravings for additional sweets. Furthermore, several recent studies have shown that candy consumption may lead to improved mood and greater likelihood to help others. For example, Meier et al. [23] found that consuming sweet foods increased agreeableness and pro-social behavior.

More research is needed in this area to understand the impact of consuming confections on overall health, wellness, and dietary patterns. Behavioral research investigating how to promote moderate consumption of treats would be especially useful for health professionals to help their clients develop strategies to manage treat intake.

Chocolate and Health

Over the past decade, evidence from numerous population-based studies supports an association between the consumption of modest amounts of cocoa and chocolate and a range of positive effects on cardiovascular health. One of the first studies that investigated the impact of cocoa on cardiovascular health was Hollenberg et al.'s [24] study of the Kuna Indians, an indigenous people that live on a group of islands off the coast of Panama. The Kuna were observed to have very low blood pressure, which was particularly surprising due to the relatively high salt content of their diets. Furthermore, the Kuna did not develop the typical age-related rise in blood pressure that is observed in Western countries and more importantly, the Kuna were observed to have a very low incidence of CVD mortality. Yet, when the Kuna moved from their island home to Western countries, they experienced a rise in blood pressure and risk of CVD, thus ruling out a genetic predisposition to lower blood pressure. An investigation of the differences between the traditional Kuna lifestyle versus Western lifestyle uncovered that the Kuna drink on average five cups of cocoa per day or more. Beyond the Kuna, studies of numerous populations including large samples of Americans and Europeans, men and women, diseased and healthy individuals, have shown an association between cocoa and chocolate consumption with markers of cardiovascular health.

Following the interesting epidemiological findings, clinical trials were conducted to investigate the impact of chocolate on CVD risk factors. These intervention studies indicate that consumption of flavanol-containing dark chocolate and cocoa products may improve the function of the cardiovascular system and reduce blood pressure and cardiovascular risk factors, reduce the reactivity of platelets making them less prone to form clots, and improve markers of inflammation. Clinical research also links the regular consumption of products rich in cocoa flavanols to lowered blood pressure. Recent meta-analyses of 66 randomized clinical trials found consistent short- and long-term improvements in blood pressure, insulin resistance, lipid profiles, and vascular dilation associated with chocolate and cocoa consumption [25,26].

These health effects have largely been attributed to cocoa flavanols. Flavanols are part of a broader class of phytochemical compounds called flavonoids. Flavonoids are potent, naturally occurring compounds found in a wide range of plant-based foods and in recent years, these natural compounds have widely been studied for their ability to confer important health benefits. Flavanols are prevalent in commonly consumed foods including cocoa, chocolate, tea, apples, grapes, and red wine. The probable mechanism by which flavanols improve vascular function has been described by Schroeter et al. [27]. Schroeter's study showed that flavanol-rich cocoa induced the nitric oxide pathway, which is known to mediate blood flow. Administration of the specific flavanol (–)-epicatechin resulted in a comparable rise in nitric oxide and is therefore thought to be the chemical responsible for the vascular benefits of cocoa [27].

More recently, preliminary evidence is pointing to an association of cocoa flavanols with brain function and cognition. Desideri et al. [28] reported that regular consumption of dietary cocoa flavanols improved cognitive function in elderly subjects with early memory decline. Other recent studies indicate potential effects on anxiety and mood [29]. Strandberg et al. [30] found that elderly men who reported a preference for chocolate exercised more, had lower BMIs, and also reported greater feelings of wellbeing.

The science surrounding the potential health benefits of cocoa and chocolate is growing steadily. While more research is needed to confirm and extend these findings, the clinical investigations on cocoa-based flavanols support the inclusion of cocoa and chocolate, balanced with calorie intake, as part of a dietary approach to help maintain, and support cardiovascular health.

SUMMARY

Since the advent of the first primitive candies, sugars have been essential to the definition and formation of candy products. A number of different types of sugars are used in confectionery products, but sucrose and glucose syrup are currently the two most common sweeteners. The ability of sugars to crystallize, form a glass, and undergo the chemical reactions Maillard browning and caramelization is key to the texture and flavor of common candy products. There is interest by the confectionery industry in expanded use of alternative sweeteners to create new products, and great advancements have already been made in this area in recent years; however, there are significant hurdles to further development including regulatory considerations, safety concerns, and consumer acceptance.

Candy is typically very safe and tends to be consumed in moderate amounts. While limited research exists on the impact of candy on health, evidence to date suggests that candy consumption is not linked to obesity and chronic disease. Health authorities recognize that there is a role for all foods including candy in a healthy happy life. In fact, restrictive practices may be detrimental to eating habits and wellbeing. Candy-eating behavior is a promising research opportunity area and the public would benefit from understanding how to promote balanced moderate enjoyment of treats. There is an interesting emerging body of evidence on cocoa flavanols and chocolate, demonstrating a positive impact on cardiovascular health with promising research questions for the future.

CONFLICTS OF INTEREST

Laura Shumow is Director of Scientific and Regulatory Affairs at the National Confectioners Association. NCA is the not-for-profit trade association representing the interests of the US confectionery industry. Outside of her employment with the association, Ms. Shumow has not received payment from any organization to work on this article.

REFERENCES

1. Gott P, Van Houton LF. *All About Candy and Chocolate*. Chicago: National Confectioners Association of the United States, Inc.; 1958.
2. Beckett ST. *Industrial Chocolate Manufacture and Use*, 3rd Edition. Osney Mead, Oxford: Blackwell Science; 1999.
3. USDA. *Historical Sweetener Market Data*. United States Departments of Agriculture Farm Service Agency; 2013.
4. Edwards WP. *The Science of Sugar Confectionery*. Cambridge: The Royal Society of Chemistry; 2000.
5. Jackson EB. *Sugar Confectionery Manufacture*. New York: Blackie; 1990.
6. Barnett C. *The Science & Art of Candy Manufacturing*. Duluth: Magazines for Industry; 1978.
7. Ergun R, Lietha R, Hartel RW. Moisture and shelf life in sugar confections. *Crit Rev Food Sci Nutr*. 2010;50(2):162–9.
8. Hornick B, Duyff R, Murphy M, Shumow L. Proposing a definition of candy in moderation. *Nutrition Today*. 2014;49(2):87–94.
9. Shumow L, Barraj L, Murphy M, Bi X, Bodor A. Candy consumption in the United States. *FASEB J* 2012;26:1005.3.
10. USDA. *Report of the Dietary Guidelines Advisory Committee on the Dietary Guidelines for Americans*. United States Department of Agriculture, Center for Nutrition Policy and Promotion; 2010.
11. USDA. *USDA National Nutrient Database for Standard Reference*, Release 22. United States Department of Agriculture, Agricultural Research Service. 2009.
12. Morrissey RB, Burkholder BD, Tarka Jr SM. The cariogenic potential of several snack foods. *J Am Dent Assoc*. 1984;109:589–91.
13. Gustofason B, Quensel CE, Lanke L et al. The Vipeholm dental caries study: The effect of different levels of carbohydrate intake on dental caries activity in 436 individuals observed for five years. *Acta Ondontol Scand*. 1954;11:232.
14. Yankell SL, Emling RC, Shi X, Greco MR. Low cariogenic potential of mixtures of sucrose and chocolate, cocoa or confectionery coatings. *J Clin Dent*. 1988;1:28–30.
15. Machiulskiene V, Nyvad B, Baelum V. Caries preventive effect of sugar-substituted chewing gum. *Community Dent Oral Epidemiol*. 2001;29:278–88.
16. Szöke J, Banoczy J, Proskin HM. Effect of after-meal sucrose-free gum-chewing on clinical caries. *J Dent Res*. 2001;80:1725–9.
17. O'Neil CE, Fulgoni VL, Nicklas TA. Candy consumption was not associated with body weight measures, risk factors for cardiovascular disease, or metabolic syndrome in US adults: NHANES 1999–2004. *Nutr Res*. 2011;31(2):122–30.
18. O'Neil CE, Fulgoni VL, Nicklas TA. Association of candy consumption with body weight measures, other health risk factors for cardiovascular disease, and diet quality in US children and adolescents: NHANES 1999–2004. *Food Nutr Res*. 2011;55. Epub ahead of print: doi: 10.3902/fnr.v5Sio.5794.

19. Golomb BA, Koperski S, White HL. Association between more frequent chocolate consumption and lower body mass index. *Arch Intern Med.* 2012;172(6):519–21.
20. Murphy M, Barraj LB, Bi X, Stettler N. Body weight status and cardiovascular risk factors in adults by frequency of candy consumption. *Nutrition J.* 2013;12:53.
21. O'Neil CE, Nicklas TA, Liu Y, Berenson GS. Candy consumption in childhood is not predictive of weight, adiposity measures or cardiovascular risk factors in young adults: The Bogalusa Heart Study. *J Hum Nutr Diet.* 2013. doi:10.1111/jhn.12200.
22. Piehowski KE, Preston AG, Miller DL, Nickols-Richardson SM. A reduced-calorie dietary pattern including a daily sweet snack promotes body weight reduction and body composition improvements in premenopausal women who are overweight and obese: A pilot study. *J Am Diet Assoc.* 2011;111:1198–203.
23. Meier B, Moller SK, Riemer-Peltz M, Robinson MD. Sweet taste preferences and experiences predict prosocial inferences, personalities, and behaviors. *J Pers Soc Psychol.* 2012;102(1):163–74.
24. Hollenberg NK, Fisher ND, McCullough ML. Flavanols, the Kuna, cocoa consumption, and nitric oxide. *J Am Soc Hypertens.* 2009;3(2):105–12.
25. Shrime MG, Bauer SR, McDonald AC, Chowdhury NH, Coltart CE, Ding EL. Flavonoid-rich cocoa consumption affects multiple cardiovascular risk factors in a meta-analysis of short-term studies. *J Nutr.* 2011;141:1982–8.
26. Hooper L, Kay C, Abdelhamid A et al. Effects of chocolate, cocoa, and flavan-3-ols on cardiovascular health: A systematic review and meta-analysis of randomized trials. *Am J Clin Nutr.* 2012;95(3):740–51.
27. Schroeter H, Heiss C, Balzer et al. (−)-Epicatechin mediates beneficial effects of flavanol-rich cocoa on vascular function. *Proc Natl Acad Sci.* 2006;103(4):1024–9.
28. Desideri G, Kwik-Uribe C, Grassi D et al. Benefits in cognitive function, blood pressure, and insulin resistance through cocoa flavanol consumption in elderly subjects with mild cognitive impairment: The Cocoa, Cognition, and Aging (CoCoA) study. *Hypertension.* 2012;60(3):794–801.
29. Pase MP, Scholey AB, Pipingas A et al. Cocoa polyphenols enhance positive mood states but not cognitive performance: A randomized, placebo-controlled trial. *J Psychopharmacol.* 2013;27(5):451–8.
30. Strandberg TE, Strandberg AY, Pitkälä K, Salomaa VV, Tilvis RS, Miettinen TA. Chocolate, well-being and health among elderly men. *Eur J Clin Nutr.* 2008;62(2):247–53.

5 Effects of Dietary Sugars from Natural Sources on Health Outcomes

Eva Arrigoni, Christina Kast, and Barbara Walther

CONTENTS

KEY POINTS

- Dietary sugars derived from fruits do not play an important role in health promotion per se, whereas the synergy of secondary plant metabolites, dietary fiber, and vitamin C are responsible for the potential beneficial effects of fruits.
- Energy in fruit is mainly derived from the sugars glucose, fructose, and sucrose, but the glucose-to-fructose ratio varies between fruit types.
- The preventive effects of fruits can be optimized when their consumption is part of an overall healthy lifestyle.
- The beneficial effect of honey on many health outcomes has not exclusively been related to its sugar composition, but to its numerous additional compounds, such as enzymes, flavonoids, and polyphenols.
- Honey is a complex food and its composition varies greatly depending on its geographical and botanical origin. This could be one of the major reasons for the often controversial results of numerous investigations using honey to treat various medical conditions.
- In both diabetic patients and healthy people, honey has been found to positively impact blood glucose levels and insulin production due to its lower GI compared to sucrose.

- The main components of honey are fructose, glucose, and water. Minor components are, for example, oligosaccharides, flavonoids, polyphenols, organic acids, and antimicrobials.
- Honey due to its antimicrobial properties promotes wound healing, which is especially well documented for burns.

INTRODUCTION

Naturally occurring sugars in food are comprised of the monosaccharides glucose and fructose as well as the disaccharides sucrose and lactose. Other constituents such as galactose and maltose are mainly liberated during the hydrolysis of lactose and starch, respectively. Although glucose and fructose are present in most plants, only fruits and honey contain them in nutritionally relevant quantities. Sucrose can be found in high amounts in sugarcane and sugar beets, both of which serve as sources for sugar extraction. Moreover, some fruits contain appreciable amounts of sucrose as well. Lactose, on the other hand, is exclusively present in milk and represents the sole carbohydrate source for human nutrition during the first phase of life.

FRUITS

Together with vegetables, fruits are an essential part of the human diet. Botanically, a fruit is defined as the reproductive morphological part of a flowering plant in which seeds are formed and developed [1]. In culinary practice and food processing, however, fruits generally refer to any edible part of a plant with a sweet taste and pleasant flavor. This corresponds to most edible fleshy fruits in the botanical sense that can generally be eaten raw, but does not include nuts, legumes, or wild fruits. From a nutritional point of view, fruits are commonly classified as pomaceous fruits (the most often consumed being apples and pears), stone fruits (peaches followed by apricots and cherries), berries (grapes, strawberries, and currants), citrus fruits (such as oranges), and other tropical/subtropical fruits, with bananas being the most consumed fruit worldwide followed by melons which botanically are vegetables [2].

Table 5.1 represents a selection of the most often consumed fruits worldwide and some fruit products. In general, fruits are characterized by a water content of 80–90% and thus are low in energy, except for bananas. Energy is mainly derived from available carbohydrates which vary from 3 to 15% in fruit. The higher carbohydrate level in bananas is partly due to starch which is present at levels of 3% or more even in ripe bananas [3], whereas the starch content decreases to negligible levels during ripening in all other types of fruits [2]. Both proteins and fats are present in very low concentrations in fruits, but they are good sources of dietary fiber (especially when they are consumed unpeeled), particularly soluble fiber due to their high pectin content. The fact that berries contain an elevated amount of dietary fiber can be explained by the higher proportion of fiber-rich morphological compartments such as skin and seeds. Organic acids as well as the sugar-to-acid ratio are key determinants of taste. Major acids are malic, citric, and tartaric acids [1]. Although malic acid is predominant in pomaceous fruits and bananas, the main organic acid in citrus and tropical/subtropical fruits, as well as in most berries, is citric acid. Grapes, on the other hand, are characterized by high amounts of tartaric acid. In general, the acid level decreases during ripening, but it also differs considerably depending on the type of fruit (Table 5.1).

In addition, fruits are important sources of micronutrients. Their mineral content generally varies between 0.3 and 1.0% [4]. In particular, they have high levels of potassium and magnesium [5]. Moreover, many fruits are important sources of vitamin C. Similar amounts as in citrus fruits (approximately 40–50 mg/100 g edible portion) can be found in strawberries and red currants as well as in kiwi fruits and mangoes, whereas black currants contain up to 200 mg/100 g edible portion [2,3]. Pomaceous and stone fruits, on the other hand, contain roughly 5–15 mg vitamin C. Apricots, peaches, and cantaloupe melons additionally contain β-carotene (pro-vitamin A) in substantial amounts.

Secondary plant metabolites have been recognized rather recently as dietary compounds that may have a considerable impact on human health. They are ubiquitous in plants to protect them

TABLE 5.1
Average Energy Content/100 g Edible Portion and Composition (g/100 g Edible Portion) of Fruits and Fruit Products

	Kcal	kJ	Water	CHO	Pro	Fat	Fiber	Organic Acids
Fruits								
Apples	54	228	84.9	11.4	0.3	0.6	2.0	0.5
Apricots	43	183	85.3	8.5	0.9	0.1	1.5	1.4
Bananas	88	374	73.9	20.0	1.2	0.2	1.8	0.6
Blueberries	36	153	84.6	6.1	0.6	0.6	4.9	1.4
Cherries, sweet	62	265	82.8	13.3	0.9	0.3	1.3	1.0
Cherries, tart	53	225	84.8	9.9	0.9	0.5	1.0	1.8
Cranberries	35	148	87.4	6.2	0.3	0.5	2.9	1.4
Currants, black	39	168	81.2	6.1	1.3	0.2	6.8	2.6
Currants, red	33	139	84.7	4.8	1.1	0.2	3.5	2.3
Grapefruit	38	161	88.4	7.4	0.6	0.2	1.6	1.5
Grapes	67	286	81.1	15.2	0.7	0.3	1.5	0.9
Kiwi fruit	51	215	83.0	9.1	1.0	0.6	2.1	1.5
Lemons	35	151	90.2	3.2	0.7	0.6	N/A	4.9
Mandarins	46	195	86.5	10.1	0.7	0.3	1.7	N/A
Mangoes	57	243	82.0	12.4	0.6	0.5	1.7	0.3
Melons, cantaloupe	54	231	85.4	12.4	0.9	0.1	0.7	0.1
Melons, water	37	159	90.3	8.3	0.6	0.2	0.2	N/A
Oranges	42	179	85.7	8.3	1.0	0.2	1.6	1.1
Papayas	32	134	87.9	7.1	0.5	0.1	1.9	0.1
Peaches	41	176	87.3	8.9	0.8	0.1	1.9	0.6
Pears	55	233	82.9	12.4	0.5	0.3	3.3	0.3
Pineapples	55	234	84.9	12.4	0.5	0.2	1.0	0.7
Plums	48	205	83.7	10.2	0.6	0.2	1.6	1.3
Raspberries	34	143	81.4	4.8	1.3	0.3	4.7	2.1
Strawberries	32	136	89.5	5.5	0.8	0.4	1.6	1.0
Fruit products								
Apple juice, commercial	48	203	88.1	11.1	0.1	N/A	N/A	0.7
Orange juice, commercial	42	178	89.5	8.7	0.7	0.1	0.4	1.0
Orange marmalade	258	1098	35.0	63.6	0.4	N/A	N/A	0.9
Strawberry jam	256	1088	35.0	62.5	0.3	0.2	N/A	0.9
Apples, dried	248	1054	26.7	55.4	1.4	1.6	11.2	2.2
Apricots, dried	240	1019	17.6	47.9	5.0	0.5	17.6	7.9
Dates, dried	276	1174	20.2	65.1	1.9	0.5	8.7	1.3
Raisins	291	1238	15.7	68.0	2.5	0.6	5.2	1.6

Source: Souci SW, Fachmann W, Kraut H. *Die Zusammensetzung der Lebensmittel, Nährwert-Tabellen,* 7th ed. Stuttgart: medpharm GmbH Scientific Publishers; 2013.
Note: N/A, data not available.

against herbivores and microbial infections as well as from ultraviolet light and to attract pollinators and seed-dispersing animals [6]. They can be divided into three main groups: flavonoids including phenolic and polyphenolic compounds; terpenoids with carotenoids being the best-known members of this family; and alkaloids plus sulfur-containing compounds [6]. Although some groups such as flavonoids, phenolic acids, and carotenoids are abundant in almost all plant groups, others are present in specific botanical families (e.g. glucosinolates in cabbage vegetables, phytoestrogens in soy and cereals, or monoterpenes in citrus fruits and herbs) [7].

Fruits are largely eaten fresh, but they can also be transformed into various products. This may lead to shifts in composition as shown in Table 5.1 for some representative examples. Apples and oranges are primarily processed into juice, whereby mainly bioactive substances such as dietary fiber and secondary plant metabolites remain largely in the pomace, and vitamin C is mostly destroyed. However, the latter is often re-added afterwards. Drying which is very popular for apricots, dates, or raisins has a high impact on composition. Water removal leads to a significant increase in energy, macronutrient, mineral, and dietary fiber content, but vitamin C is lost to a great extent [2]. A clear shift in composition is also seen in jams or jellies due to the addition of high amounts of sugar. This results in a distinct reduction of water, macro-, and micronutrients as well as bioactive substances.

Available carbohydrates are mainly the two monosaccharides glucose and fructose as well as the disaccharide sucrose. Other mono- to oligosaccharides are only present in trace amounts [2]. Table 5.2 shows the sugar composition as it varies between fruits and selected fruit products. It should be noted, however, that the sugar content can vary depending on the cultivar. Moreover, it might also be influenced to some extent by other preharvest factors such as exposure to sunlight or temperature as well as by the stage of ripeness when picked and storage conditions [8].

The glucose-to-fructose ratio can be used as a characteristic for distinguishing fruit types. Pomaceous fruits, for example, are characterized by much higher fructose levels than glucose, whereas stone fruits generally contain somewhat higher glucose levels than fructose. For berries and citrus fruits, the ratio is approximately equal with a tendency toward slightly higher fructose concentrations. Sucrose is very dominant in many tropical/subtropical fruits and some stone fruits (except cherries), but it is found in very low levels in various berries including grapes [9].

In addition to sugars, the potential laxative sorbitol is abundant in pomaceous and stone fruits. Berries may also contain trace amounts [9], whereas this sugar alcohol is not present in citrus fruits and tropical/subtropical fruits. As can be seen in Table 5.2, pears contain even more sorbitol than glucose and fructose.

NUTRITIONAL ASPECTS OF FRUIT

Fruits are generally low in energy density [5]. Moreover, the World Health Organization has described all fruits as being nutrient-dense, whereas according to the United States Department of Agriculture's MyPyramid processed fruits and fruit juices are also included in this category [10]. This difference demonstrates the various perspectives used to calculate nutrient density. Shrapnel and Noakes [11] reported recently that nutrient density scores for fruits vary widely and that dried fruits and fruit juices are characterized by lower scores. According to their model, fresh fruits should therefore be preferred to dried fruits and whole fruits to fruit juices.

In addition, the physical form of fruits is of importance. Whole fruits have a higher satiety effect than fruit purées, and purées have higher satiety ratings than fruit juices [12]. This is mainly due to the consecutive removal of dietary fiber and associated substances during processing. Since price is an important determinant from a consumer's point of view, it is important to note that fruits (and vegetables) provide vitamins, minerals, and other key nutrients at reasonable costs despite being relatively costly as an energy source [13].

Based on their high nutrient density, fruits are often good sources of dietary fiber and some micronutrients. In the USA, they provide 11% of the total dietary fiber supply, but provide only 3% of food energy and 6% of carbohydrates [14]. Moreover, fruits are the major contributors of vitamin C (41%) and an important source of potassium (11%), vitamin B6 (9%), carotenoids (8%), folate (6%), and magnesium (6%) [14].

The contribution to macro- and micronutrient intake from fruits differs somewhat between countries, as recently published values for Switzerland show. Compared to the USA, Schmid et al. [15]

TABLE 5.2
Sugar Composition and Sorbitol Content (g/100 g Edible Portion) of Fruits and Fruit Products

	Glucose	Fructose	Sucrose	Sorbitol
Fruits				
Apples	2.0	5.7	2.5	0.51
Apricots	1.7	0.9	5.1	0.82
Bananas	3.5	3.4	10.3	N/A
Blueberries	2.5	3.3	0.2	0.00
Cherries, sweet	7.1	6.3	0.2	0.76[a]
Cherries, tart	5.2	4.3	0.4	1.17[a]
Cranberries	3.0	2.9	0.1	N/A
Currants, black	2.4	3.2	0.7	N/A
Currants, red	2.0	2.5	0.3	N/A
Grapefruit	2.4	2.1	2.9	N/A
Grapes	7.1	7.1	0.4	0.20
Kiwi fruit	4.3	4.6	0.2	N/A
Lemons	1.4	1.4	0.4	N/A
Mandarins	1.7	1.3	7.1	N/A
Mangoes	0.9	2.6	9.0	N/A
Melons, cantaloupe	1.6	1.3	9.5	N/A
Melons, water	2.0	3.9	2.4	N/A
Oranges	2.3	2.6	3.4	N/A
Papayas	3.6	3.5	N/A	N/A
Peaches	1.0	1.2	5.7	0.89
Pears	1.7	6.7	1.8	2.17
Pineapples	2.1	2.4	7.8	N/A
Plums	3.4	2.0	3.4	1.41
Raspberries	1.8	2.1	1.0	0.00
Strawberries	2.2	2.2	1.0	0.03
Fruits products				
Apple juice, commercial	2.4	6.4	1.7	0.56
Orange juice, commercial	2.6	2.5	3.4	N/A
Orange marmalade	17.4	15.4	27.1	N/A
Strawberry jam	21.9	18.7	13.5	N/A
Apples, dried	9.8	27.8	12.3	2.49
Apricots, dried	9.7	4.9	28.7	4.60
Dates, dried	25.0	24.9	13.8	1.35
Raisins	32.0	33.2	1.9	0.89

Source: Souci SW, Fachmann W, Kraut H. *Die Zusammensetzung der Lebensmittel, Nährwert-Tabellen,* 7th ed. Stuttgart: medpharm GmbH Scientific Publishers; 2013.

Note: N/A, data not available.

[a] Most values refer to Souci et al. [3] except Reference [93].

reported a higher contribution to the dietary fiber intake (approximately 16%) and a slightly higher contribution to carbohydrates (approximately 8%) at a comparable energy intake (approximately 4%). Vitamin C contribution seems to be somewhat lower with approximately 35%, whereas values for folate and carotenoids were reported to be higher in Switzerland (both approximately 15%). Vitamin B6 (approximately 11%), potassium (approximately 13%), and magnesium (approximately 8%) were stated to be in a similar range as in the USA [15].

According to the German Consumption Study II [16], there are gender-specific differences. Since women were reported to consume more fruit than men, the contribution of fruits to the intake of the above-mentioned nutrients is approximately 20–30% higher for women. Overall, the data reported for Germany were slightly higher than those reported for the USA and Switzerland, since German values refer to the intake of fruits plus fruit products, the latter adding approximately 10% to the overall fruit consumption. The only exception was vitamin C. It was found that 26 and 31% of its total intake for men and women, respectively, came from fruit [16].

Data based on the European Prospective Investigation into Cancer and Nutrition (EPIC) cohorts have also revealed some gender-specific differences, but even more distinct variations among countries. Dietary fiber intake from fruits ranged from 12 to 34% in men and 16 to 38% in women, respectively, with highest percentages found in Spain, France, and Italy and the lowest found in the UK [17]. Similar observations were made for vitamin C. Fruits contributed 23–55% and 30–59% of vitamin C intake in men and women, respectively, with the highest amounts in Italy and Spain and the lowest in Sweden and the UK [18]. In the UK, however, fruit juices additionally contributed 14–24% and 13–23% to the daily intake of vitamin C of men and women, respectively. This is in agreement with Caswell [19], who reported that up to 25% of the daily vitamin C comes from fruit juices in the UK, particularly for teenagers and young adults, who are known to consume less fruits [16]. Moreover, fruit juices contribute 3–9% to the daily sugar intake, but nothing to the fiber intake [19]. Vitamin B6 intakes from fruits varied from 7 to 19% in men and 11 to 23% in women in the EPIC countries; these percentages were by far the highest in Italy and the lowest again in Sweden and the UK, particularly in men [18]. As for β-carotene, variations among intake levels in the EPIC countries were found to be even higher, ranging between 2 and 30% in men and 2 and 35% in women [20], again by far the highest in Italy and the lowest in the Northern countries as well as in the UK and Greece, where vegetables are responsible for at least 80% of the β-carotene intake. The contribution of fruits to potassium intake varied from 6% in Denmark to 19% in Italy for men and from 10% in Norway to 21% in Italy for women [21]. Similarly, regarding the magnesium intake, fruits contributed from 4% in Denmark to 11% in Italy for men and from 7% in Denmark to 14% in Spain for women [21]. In Europe, overall, a north-to-south gradient for the contribution of fruits to the above-mentioned nutrients was observed. This is consistent with a higher energy intake from fruits [22] and a lower energy contribution from highly processed foods in Southern countries [23].

LINKS BETWEEN FRUIT INTAKE AND HEALTH OUTCOMES

The consumption of fruits and vegetables as low glycemic index (GI) foods has been recommended for weight loss and diabetic management [24]. Indeed, it has been recognized for a long time that foods rich in dietary sugars usually have lower GI values than common starchy foods [25]. Table 5.3 gives an overview of the GI and glycemic load (GL) values of fruits and selected fruit products. Among them, the majority are considered to be low GI foods [11,26]. Glucose, fructose, and sucrose do not only determine the sweetness of fruits, but also affect plasma glucose levels in different ways [25].

According to the International Tables of Glycaemic Index and Glycaemic Load Values, the mean GI values of glucose, fructose, and sucrose are reported to be 92 ± 2 ($n = 4$ studies), 15 ($n = 3$ studies), and 65 ± 4 ($n = 6$ studies), respectively [26]. Correspondingly, GL values of 9, 2, and 7 are stated. These differences between the three main sugars as well as the high variability in their content (see Table 5.2) clearly affect the GI and, accordingly, the GL of fruits. However, other constituents may also have an impact on GI values of fruits.

Trout and Behall [27] observed that the so-called acidic fruits, such as apples, apricots, or oranges, with pH values of 3.2–4.2 had lower GI values than what were expected based on their sugar composition, whereas the so-called near-neutral fruits, such as various melons and papaya, with pH 5.3–6.5 were characterized by GI values similar or even higher to what was calculated based on the sugar composition of these fruits. These researchers proposed a model that organic acids and their acidic anions slow down gastric emptying, thereby lowering the GI. They found a significant correlation between measured GI values and fruit pH, but a less strong association with acids [27]. This latter finding can be explained by the fact that other fruit components, such as potassium or proteins, affect the pH value. In addition, dietary fiber and cell wall structures are known to influence GI and GL. This is also seen by the higher GI values for juices and jams compared to the corresponding whole fruits (Table 5.3). For dried fruits, however, no such effect is seen, since they still contain dietary fiber. As mentioned above, however, they are considered to be low in nutrient density. Therefore, Shrapnel and Noakes [11] have suggested to rank the nutritional quality of carbohydrate-rich foods, including fruits, by incorporating both GI and nutrient density. Similarly, Atkinson et al. [26] recommended not using the GI in isolation, but rather taking the energy density and the macronutrient profile of foods into consideration as well.

TABLE 5.3
GI (Mean Values ± SEM; Glucose = 100%) and GL Values of Fruits and Fruit Products Determined in Subjects with Normal Glucose Tolerance

	GI	GL
Fruits		
Apples	36 ± 2[a]	6
Apricots	34 ± 3	3
Bananas	51 ± 3[a]	11
Blueberries, wild	53 ± 7	5
Cherries, dark, pitted[b]	63 ± 6	9
Grapes, black	59	11
Kiwi fruit[c]	58 ± 7	7
Mangoes[c]	51 ± 5[a]	8
Melons, cantaloupe	65 ± 9	4
Melons, water	76 ± 4[a]	N/A
Oranges	43 ± 3[a]	3
Papayas[c]	66 ± 7	6
Pineapples[c]	59 ± 8[a]	6
Strawberries	40 ± 7	1
Fruit products		
Apple juice	41 ± 2[a]	N/A
Orange juice[d]	50 ± 2	12
Orange marmalade	48 ± 9	9
Strawberry jam	49 ± 3[a]	10
Apples, dried	29 ± 5	11
Apricots, dried[e]	31	7
Dates[f]	42 ± 4	18
Raisins	64 ± 11	28

Source: Atkinson FS, Foster-Powell K, Brand-Miller JC. *Diabetes Care* 2008;31:2281–3.
Note: Unless otherwise stated, portions contained 50 g of carbohydrates. GL values are estimated by multiplying GI by listed g carbohydrates/serving and dividing by 100. N/A, data not available.
[a] Average of all available data.
[b] Portion of fruit and reference contained 20 g carbohydrates.
[c] Portion of fruit and reference contained 25 g carbohydrates.
[d] $n = 4$.
[e] $n = 3$.
[f] $n = 5$.

As for GL, it becomes obvious that values are mostly higher for fruit products than for whole fruits. This is mainly due to the fact that their total sugar content in one serving is higher. A serving of fruit juice (250 mL) or a serving of dried fruits (60 g) contains roughly twice as much sugar as a serving of fruit (120 g), whereas a 30 g serving of jam or marmalade may even contain three to four times as much sugar as the corresponding fruit.

The amount of fruits consumed influences their contribution to the daily GL. As outlined above, fruit consumption across Europe varies considerably. Correspondingly, the relative contribution of fruits to the overall GL has found to vary from approximately 5% in Sweden to approximately 15% in Spain for men and from approximately 9% in Sweden and Denmark to approximately 17% in Spain for women [28].

It is widely accepted that fruit and vegetable intake is related to good health. Moreover, they have shown a disease-preventive potential. Beneficial effects are mainly due to the low energy density, the high nutrient density, and the presence of bioactive substances. Reviews reporting associations between fruit and vegetable consumption altogether and various diseases or their biomarkers are relatively abundant [12,29–33], whereas studies differentiating between fruit and vegetable intake as well as investigations on individual fruits are scarce.

However, some of the above-mentioned reviews report several effects as a result of fruit intake only. In general, total fruit consumption was not shown to significantly affect diabetes incidence [29,30]. As for cardiovascular diseases, subanalyses of vegetable and fruit studies have revealed significant inverse relations of fruit consumption and both coronary heart disease and stroke, whereas the protective effect of fruit on cancer was less convincing [29].

The relation of low GI fruit consumption to glycemic control and risk factors for coronary heart disease in type 2 diabetes has recently been investigated. For this purpose, data of a previously published study assessing the role of a low GI diet [34] were re-examined for the effect of low GI fruit consumption [35]. Pomaceous, citrus, and stone fruits as well as classic berries were classified as low GI fruits, whereas tropical fruits such as bananas and mangoes, different melons as well as grapes were considered to be high GI fruits. At the baseline, the low GI fruits accounted for 0.7 servings/day in both the low GI fruit and the high cereal fiber intervention group. After 6 months, the consumption in the low GI fruit group increased to 1.3 servings/day, whereas it decreased in the high cereal fiber group to 0.3 servings/day. Total fruit intake, however, remained constant at 2 servings/day in both groups. Overall, the highest quartile of low GI fruits intake showed a significant benefit on glycemic control, blood lipids, and blood pressure compared to the lowest quartile. Regarding individual fruits, citrus fruit and berry consumption was found to be related to an HbA_{1c} (a long-term indicator of average plasma glucose concentration) reduction as the primary outcome; apple consumption was correlated negatively with triglycerides and coronary heart disease risk and positively with high-density lipoprotein (HDL) cholesterol; and berry intake was negatively correlated with glucose and blood pressure, but positively correlated with triglycerides. No significant relations were observed with pears and stone fruits [35]. It was concluded that further studies are needed to determine the optimal levels of fruit consumption in order to maximize glycemic control.

While several studies have focused on individual secondary plant metabolites such as resveratrol [36], anthocyanins [37], and ellagitannins [38], studies on the beneficial effects of corresponding fruits (grapes, cherries, strawberries, and raspberries, respectively) are scarce [39–41] or even missing [42]. In the following section, health-related effects of specific fruits or fruit juices consumed in physiologically reasonable amounts are summarized.

EFFECTS OF SPECIFIC FRUITS ON HEALTH OUTCOMES

Apples: Studies on relationships between apples and human health have been reviewed by Hyson [43]. It has been found that consuming one or more medium-sized apple/day was associated with a reduction in cancer risk at several sites compared to consuming less than one apple/day. Moreover, apple and pear intake at the highest two quintiles (averages of 93.5 and 164.9 g/day, respectively) showed a significant inverse relation to lung cancer compared to the lowest quintile (43 g/day). An inverse association between apple intake and coronary mortality was observed in Finnish women (more than 71 g of apple/day) and elderly Dutch men (an average of 69 g/day) compared to persons consuming no apples. In addition, apple consumption has been found to increase antioxidative enzymes that serve as biomarkers related to cardiovascular risk. Recent investigations have also suggested a beneficial effect of apple consumption on asthma and pulmonary function, type 2 diabetes, weight management, and bone health despite some inconsistencies and the need for further studies [43].

Grapes: Grapes and wine, in particular, have been studied in relation to the French paradox: the consumption of red wine has been proposed to be responsible for the low incidence of cardiovascular diseases despite the high amount of fat in the French diet. Studies on grapes and grape juices have suggested cardiovascular benefits as well via decreased platelet aggregation, improved endothelial function, and reduced blood pressure [41], whereby these positive effects were mainly attributed to the grape seeds and skin [44]. However, there is little epidemiologic evidence that grapes play a unique role in disease prevention [5].

Berries: Studies on the effect of berries on cardiovascular diseases have been summarized by Basu et al. [45], who reported that epidemiological data showing an inverse association between berry consumption and cardiovascular risk factors are limited, although some interventions in healthy and at risk humans showed a significant decrease of these risk factors. These effects need to be further investigated. Moreover, these researchers have recommended consuming berries fresh or frozen rather than processed due to the changes in their nutritional profile as discussed above. In terms of specific berries, cranberries have been studied more extensively with a focus on using cranberry juice to prevent and treat urinary tract infections [46].

Citrus fruits: Inconsistent results have been reported in an Australian review of more than 100 studies that investigated the association of citrus fruit intake and cancer risk. Only 48% showed an inverse association, whereas in 52% of these studies, no association was found [47]. Similarly, a review evaluating the impact of food groups on stroke risk revealed that citrus fruits led to a significant reduction in stroke risk in three out of six prospective cohort studies [48]. In addition, a similar effect was observed for total fruit intake in five of these studies.

Fruit juices: Due to their lower nutrient density and larger serving size, the health effects of fruit juices are presumed to be somewhat weaker than those of whole fruits. Moreover, the fact that fruit juices contain similar amounts of sugar as soda beverages might affect metabolic health negatively. Nevertheless, when reviewing the health effects of consuming fruit juices, in general, Caswell [19] found no association between fruit juice consumption and weight status or body mass index, but evidence from epidemiological and clinical studies that fruit juice consumption reduces the coronary heart disease risk. This is in agreement with the fact that orange juice has been found to increase HDL cholesterol and reduce blood pressure [49]. Evidence of a protective effect of fruit juice on cancer was not strong [19]. Moreover, studies looking at different types of fruit juices and their health effects are largely lacking. It has only been reported that cranberry juice may decrease the number of urinary tract infections (see above) and that purple grape juice may improve endothelial function and platelet aggregation [19].

HONEY

Honey produced by honeybees has served as a natural sweetener since ancient times and was the major sweetener for food until sugar began to be produced in large amounts from other sources. Nowadays, honey is still highly valued for food flavoring and sweetening and is also often used for medical purposes, as will be detailed below. Worldwide, about 1.2 million tons of honey are produced annually [50]. The major honey-producing countries are China, Turkey, the USA, Ukraine, Mexico, and Argentina [51,52]. Although China and Argentina produce a large amount of honey, the annual consumption in these countries is low (0.1–0.2 kg per capita per year) compared to other countries, such as the USA, Canada, and Australia (0.6–0.8 kg per capita per year). In European countries, such as Italy, France, Great Britain, and Denmark, 0.3–0.4 kg of honey are annually consumed per person, while the consumption of honey is highest in Germany, Austria, Switzerland, Hungary, and Greece (1.0–1.8 kg per capita per year) [50,51].

The Codex Alimentarius [53] sets global quality standards for food products that are traded internationally. Within these standards, honey is defined as "the natural sweet substance produced by honeybees from the nectar of plants or from the secretions of living parts of plants or excretions of plant sucking insects on the living parts of plants, which the bees collect, transform by combining with specific substances of their own, deposit, dehydrate, store and leave in the honey comb to ripen and mature." Blossom honey comes from nectars of plants, while honeydew honey comes mainly from the excretions of insects that suck on the living parts of plants (*Hemiptera*) or the secretions of the living parts of plants [53].

The composition of honey is listed in Table 5.4. Honey consists primarily of sugars (60.5–82.5%) and water (usually between 15% and 20%). The predominant sugars are the monosaccharides fructose and glucose. Furthermore, di-, tri-, or higher oligosaccharides may be found in honey. Blossom honey from the nectar of plants contains only low amounts of trisaccharides, while honeydew honey that comes from the excretion of plant-sucking insects may contain higher amounts of melezitose. About 25 minor oligosaccharides have been characterized in honey, such as panose, 1-kestose, 6-kestose, and palatinose, which presumably have prebiotic effects [54].

Small amounts of minerals are found in honey. The mineral content of honey (which is measured as electrical conductivity) is an important characteristic for the determination of its botanical origin.

TABLE 5.4
Composition of Blossom and Honeydew Honey

	Blossom Honey		Honeydew Honey	
	Average (g/100 g)	Range (g/100 g)	Average (g/100 g)	Range (g/100 g)
Water		15–20[a]		15–20[a]
Monosaccharides				
Fructose	39.6[a]	32.5–45.2	33.8[b]	28.3–39.8
Glucose	30.9[a]	24.3–39.9	23.9[a]	19.0–31.5
Disaccharides				
Sucrose	0.7[a]	0.05–6.2	0.5[a]	0.05–1.0
Maltose	0.6[a]	0.1–2.3	1.4[a]	0.5–2.5
Turanose	1.4[a]	0.8–2.9	1.8[a]	0.5–2.5
Trehalose	0.3[a]	0.05–1.5	1.1[a]	0.1–2.4
Isomaltose	0.3[a]	0.2–2.2	0.3[a]	0.1–10.8
Other disaccharides	2.3[a]	1.1–5.5	1.8[a]	0.5–5.0
Trisaccharides				
Melezitose	0.2[a]	0.1–1.0	5.3[a]	0.3–22.0
Erlose	0.7[a]	0.1–6.0	1.4[a]	0.1–5.3
Other trisaccharides	0.5[c]	0.5–1.0	3.0[c]	0.1–6.0
Unknown, higher oligosaccharides		1.0–3.0[a]		1.0–3.0[a]
Total sugars	77.0[a]	61.5–82.5	70.4[a]	60.5–81.0
Minerals	0.2[c]	0.1–0.5	0.9[c]	0.6–2.0
Amino acids, proteins	0.3[c]	0.2–0.4	0.6[c]	0.4–0.7
Organic acids	0.5[c]	0.2–0.8	1.1[c]	0.8–1.5

[a] Reference [94].
[b] Reference [95].
[c] Reference [50].

The nutritional value of these minerals is low, however, considering the small amount of honey that is usually consumed per day.

The main enzymes that can be found in honey are diastase (amylase), which reduces glycogen into smaller sugar units, and invertase (alpha-1,4-glucosidase), which metabolizes sucrose into the two monosaccharides fructose and glucose, as well as the enzyme glucose oxidase, which produces the disinfectant hydrogen peroxide. The bees add these enzymes from their pharyngeal glands during the process of honey production. These enzymes are heat- and light-sensitive, and therefore honey preferentially should not be heated and should be stored in the dark at low temperatures. Measuring the activity of these enzymes is often used for testing honey quality with respect to heat and/or storage damage.

Additional compounds can be found in honey in low amounts, including numerous aroma components that define the characteristic taste of a particular honey. These components are characteristic for the botanical origin of the honey and often are the main criterion for customers when choosing a particular type. To preserve these mostly volatile aroma components as much as possible, it is best to store honey at low temperatures. Honey can also contain up to 500 mg/kg total polyphenols, such as flavonoids (quercetin, luteolin, kaempferol, apigenin, chrysin, and galangin) or phenolic acids and their derivatives [50]. These components are known for their antioxidant activities.

CHARACTERISTICS OF VARIOUS TYPES OF HONEY

Worldwide, a vast variety of unifloral honeys are produced with very characteristic flavors and aromas. Due to a unique botanical environment, some unifloral honeys may only be produced in certain regions of the world, such as the manuka honey that is produced in New Zealand and in some regions of Australia. Unifloral honeys vary to a great extent in color, aroma, sugar composition, and mineral- and organic acid content. Bee keepers can often market unifloral honey at a higher price compared to polyfloral honey, and consumers expect a defined, typical taste when they buy honey from a specific botanical origin. Honey can be labeled as unifloral honey if it primarily originates from a single botanical source and shows the typical sensory and physicochemical characteristics of the corresponding type of honey. For example, robinia honey (often wrongly labeled as acacia honey) has a very low mineral content, a high fructose, and a low glucose content. The sweetness of fructose is higher than glucose, and therefore robinia honey is perceived as sweeter than other types of honey with a higher glucose content (e.g. rape honey). Due to the high fructose-to-glucose ratio, robinia honey has a relatively low GI and may be suitable as a sweetener for people with an impaired glucose tolerance. In general, honeydew honeys contain a higher amount of minerals compared to blossom honeys (with some exceptions, e.g., chestnut honey). An electrical conductivity of more than 0.8 mS/cm is characteristic for honeydew honeys, while floral honeys typically have an electrical conductivity of less than 0.5 mS/cm. In between these values are floral honeys mixed with honeydew. The requirements for various unifloral honeys have been summarized by the International Honey Commission [55], by Beckh and Camps [56], and in the German Honey Directive [57]. Examples of unifloral honeys are listed in Tables 5.5 and 5.6 and Figure 5.1.

Unifloral honeys are well-defined and more uniform than polyfloral honeys, since they need to comply with strict criteria for sensory, physicochemical, and pollen analysis, while polyfloral honeys vary depending on the ratio of the floral or honeydew sources. Therefore, well-defined honeys with respect to their geographical origin, as well as their sensorial and physicochemical characteristics, such as unifloral honeys, should preferably be used for studying the medical effects related to honey.

TABLE 5.5
Physicochemical Characteristics of Selected Unifloral Honeys

Honey Type	Electrical Conductivity (mS/cm)	Fructose (g/100 g)	Glucose (g/100 g)
Chestnut (*Castanea sativa*)	1.38 ± 0.27[a]	40.8 ± 2.6[a]	27.9 ± 2.5[a]
Citrus (*Citrus* spp.)	0.19 ± 0.06[a]	38.7 ± 2.6[a]	31.4 ± 2.1[a]
Clover (*Trifolium*, *Melilotus*, or *Lotus* spp.)	Max. 0.2[b,c,d]	Fructose/glucose max. 1.3[c]	
Dandelion (*Taraxacum officinale*)	0.51 ± 0.07[a]	37.4 ± 1.8[a]	38.0 ± 2.8[a]
Eucalyptus (*Eucalyptus* spp.)	0.48 ± 0.06[a]	39.1 ± 2.2[a]	33.0 ± 1.9[a]
Leatherwood/Ulmo (*Eucryphia* spp.)	>0.5[d]	Fructose/glucose >1.15[d]	
Manuka (*Leptospermum scoparium*)	>0.5[d]	Fructose/glucose 1.12–1.47[d]	
Rape (*Brassica* spp.)	0.19 ± 0.05[a]	38.3 ± 1.7[a]	40.5 ± 2.6[a]
Robinia (*Robinia pseudoacacia* L.)	0.16 ± 0.04[a]	42.7 ± 2.3[a]	26.5 ± 1.7[a]
Sunflower (*Helianthus annuus* L.)	0.34 ± 0.08[a]	39.2 ± 1.6[a]	37.4 ± 1.5[a]
Tilia (*Tilia* spp.)	0.62 ± 0.12[a]	37.5 ± 2.9[a]	31.9 ± 2.5[a]
Honeydew	1.2 ± 0.22[a]	32.5 ± 1.9[a]	26.2 ± 2.5[a]

[a] Ref. [55].
[b] For honey from New Zealand, max. 0.3.
[c] Ref. [57].
[d] Ref. [56].

TABLE 5.6
Aroma Description of Selected Unifloral Honeys

Honey Type	Aroma	Further Features
Chestnut	Woody, chemical, warm, spoiled[a]	Strong, bitter taste
Citrus	Fresh (anise), floral-fresh fruit[a]	Methylanthranilate, min. 2 mg/kg[b]
Clover	Floral, weak aromatic[b]	
Dandelion	Woody, spoiled[a]	Odor strong and spoiled (cat urine)
Eucalyptus	Woody, warm, spoiled[a]	
Leatherwood	Perfumed, harsh[c]	
Ulmo	Weak floral[c]	
Manuka	Harsh[c], chemical	Thixotropy
Rape	Floral-fresh fruit, warm, spoiled, vegetal[a]	Odor of cabbage, fast crystallization
Robinia	Floral-fresh fruit, warm[a]	Strong sweetness, stays liquid for more than a year
Sunflower	Floral-fresh fruit, warm, vegetal[a]	
Tilia	Woody, chemical, fresh[a]	Odor strong and chemical (menthol)
Honeydew	Woody, warm[a]	Stays liquid for a long time

[a] Reference [55].
[b] Reference [57].
[c] Reference [56].

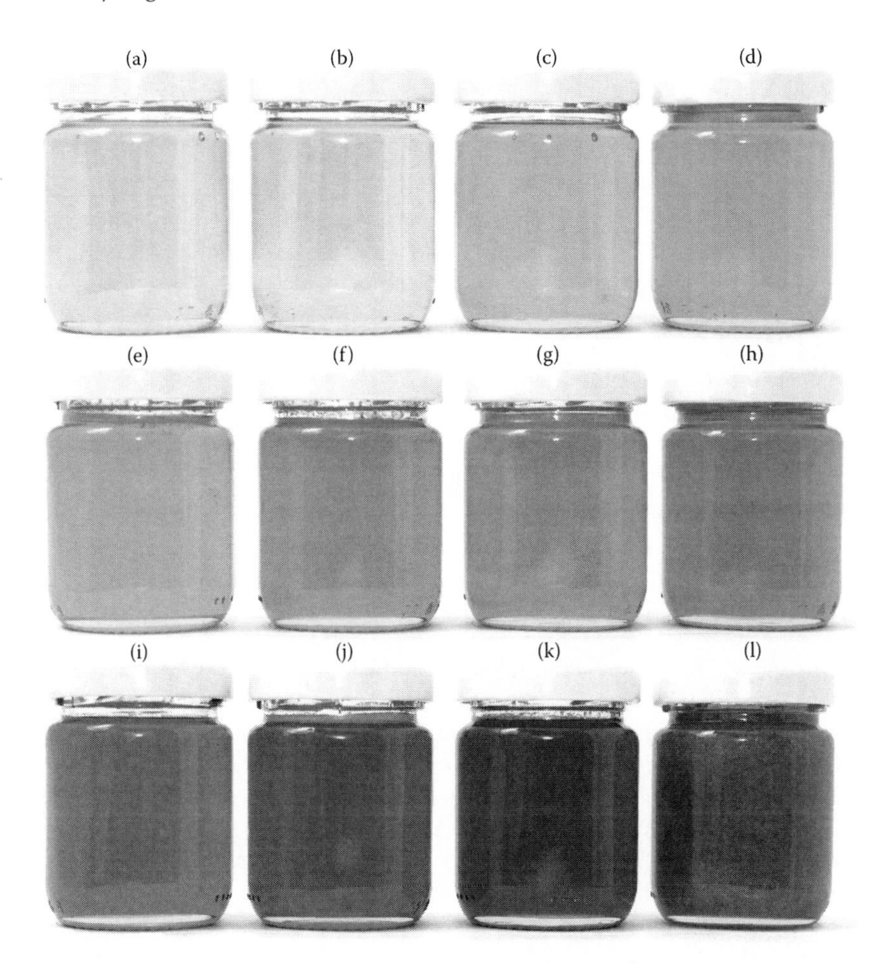

FIGURE 5.1 **(See color insert.)** Colors of unifloral honeys. Examples of unifloral honeys: (a) robinia, (b) citrus, (c) clover, (d) rape, (e) tilia, (f) leatherwood, (g) dandelion, (h) sunflower, (i) chestnut, (j) eucalyptus, (k) honeydew, (l) manuka. The honeys were liquefied (except manuka honey). The color of any type of unifloral honey may vary to a certain extent, especially when a honey crystallizes, for example, a crystallized rape honey is whitish-yellow.

QUALITY STANDARDS FOR HONEY

According to the Codex Alimentarius [53], no food ingredient or additive is allowed to be added to honey nor is any constituent particular to honey removed from the honey, such as pollen. Analysis of the different pollen types, which are generally found in a low amount in honey, is important for the identification of the botanical and geographical origin of the honey and also for testing for adulteration.

The Codex Alimentarius limits the moisture content to a maximum of 20% except for heather honey, which can contain up to 23% water. An elevated water content can speed up the fermentation process under unfavorable storage conditions. If yeasts multiply in honey, they metabolize sugars to alcohol and acetic acid, and these metabolic products change the honey taste in an unfavorable manner. Apart from the moisture content of honey, the risk for fermentation depends on the temperature at which the honey is stored and on its botanical origin, for example, honey derived from rape nectar often has a higher risk for fermentation than honey derived from other sources. For these types of honey, the moisture content of a honey should preferably be below 17% so that the risk for fermentation is also low.

Honey should not be heated or processed to such an extent that its quality is impaired. The determination of the hydroxymethylfurfural (HMF) content and/or enzyme activities (diastase or invertase) serve as analytical tests for freshness and for possible heat damage. Freshly harvested honey contains a very low amount of HMF and shows high enzyme activity (e.g. diastase activity, which is measured in Schade Units). If honey is heated, especially at temperatures higher than 55°C, the HMF concentration increases rapidly. During storage, the HMF concentration increases in relation to the surrounding temperature, the duration of storage, and the pH value. According to the Codex Alimentarius, HMF content of honey should not be more than 40 mg/kg, or 80 mg/kg in the case of honey of declared origin from tropical countries. A minimal amount of 8 Schade Units is required by the Codex Alimentarius for the diastase activity, except for honeys that have a naturally low enzyme content such as citrus or robinia honey.

Honey has also to comply with the maximum residue limits (MRLs) established by the Codex Alimentarius Commission. Bee keepers use veterinary drugs to control bee diseases and many chemicals, such as organic acids or coumaphos, flumethrin, and thymol, are approved for treatment of the mite *Varroa destructor.* If correctly applied, the risk is low that the MRLs in honey are exceeded.

LINKS BETWEEN HONEY AND HEALTH OUTCOMES

A high GI is expected for honey, since it consists primarily of sugars (60.5–82.5%). Some studies, however, showed a low GI, below 55, for some unifloral honeys, such as the Australian yellow box honey, stringybark honey, or German robinia honey [58,59]. Furthermore, several clinical studies have shown that the plasma glucose response to honey in comparison to glucose was significantly reduced depending on the honey type [58–64]. These researchers suggest that the reason for the attenuated rise of blood glucose after honey consumption could be due to the high proportion of fructose, which has a lower GI than glucose [59,64]. Comparisons of honeys with equal mixtures of fructose and glucose support this hypothesis to some extent.

Several factors could potentially explain the reduced hyperglycemia or glucose levels after consumption of honey. Fructose and palatinose may delay gastric emptying and digestion and slow down the rate of the intestinal absorption of glucose, whereas fructose absorption is enhanced in the presence of glucose. The mechanism remains unclear, but absorption of fructose is the greatest when equal amounts of glucose and fructose are ingested simultaneously [65]. It is hypothesized that fructose and oligosaccharides in honey might contribute to decreased food intake by enhancement of satiety and therefore play a role in weight management [66]. But the results of the studies investigating the influence of honey on weight management are not conclusive [67]. Due to its different sugar constituents, honey has a prebiotic effect on nonpathogenic or beneficial bacteria that is comparable to that of fructo- or galactooligosaccharides or inulin [54,68]. The latest findings on the systemic effect of intestinal microbiota suggest a possible link to diabetes mellitus and therefore a possible indirect influence of honey on glucose management through its restoring effect on imbalanced or altered gut microbiome and other not-yet-identified mechanisms [69,70].

Diabetes mellitus is commonly associated with an impaired lipid metabolism and hepatic dysfunctions or abnormalities. Honey supplementation enhances hepatic glucose uptake and glycogen synthesis and storage, which could improve glycemic control in diabetic patients. Furthermore, the antioxidant effects of honey might protect the liver and improve glucose homeostasis. Despite the evidence that fructose may have a detrimental effect on lipid metabolism when consumed in high doses, honey consumption has not been found to have a negative influence on the liver. On the one hand, fructose consumption from honey is relatively low compared to many sugar- or fructose-sweetened beverages, and, on the other hand, its numerous bioactive constituents may counteract the potential deleterious effect of fructose [67].

In an early study by Samanta et al. [71] with patients with type 1 diabetes mellitus, honey consistently produced a lower glycemic effect compared to glucose and sucrose when equivalent amounts of carbohydrates were consumed. Due to these findings, the metabolic effect of honey compared to pure glucose, fructose, and sugar in healthy people as well as diabetic patients was investigated in several studies, which were reviewed by Erejuwa et al. [67]. GI and the peak incremental index were found to be significantly lower in healthy people as well as in patients with diabetes type 1 after honey consumption compared to sucrose. In healthy people, insulin and C-peptide (a marker for insulin production) levels were lower after honey consumption compared to glucose consumption [67]. However, in another study, the level of C-peptide was found to be increased in both patients and controls after honey consumption. The researchers, therefore, suggested an improved endogenous insulin secretion [60].

In patients with diabetes mellitus type 2, the findings have been more controversial. The comparison of white bread, honey, and sucrose in a mixed breakfast showed no beneficial effects of honey in a group of type 2 diabetic patients [72]. These results were confirmed in an investigation of the metabolic effect of honey and white bread alone or in combination with other food, showing a similar degree of hyperglycemia in type 2 diabetics [73]. In addition, an increasing supplementation of the diet of diabetic patients with honey resulted in significantly increased HbA_{1c} after 8 weeks [74] compared to baseline hemoglobin and to the control group. However, the glucose content of the administered honey was unusually high with a fructose-to-glucose ratio of 0.46, which could explain the detrimental effect of the honey in this study combined with the high dose of honey at the end of the study. And in various experiments with type 2 diabetic patients performed by AL-Waili [75], the inhalation of honey significantly reduced elevated glucose levels and significantly improved glucose tolerance. The researchers therefore hypothesized that honey might affect glucose levels through its effect on prostaglandin and nitric oxide production. The fact that the effect was caused through intranasal inhalation supports the idea that specific ingredients in honey could penetrate the nose-to-brain barrier and directly stimulate glucose receptors, thereby provoking signals to increase insulin production [75]. When honey was compared to glucose, it was found to attenuate the postprandial glycemic response in all degrees of glucose intolerance, but it was most prominent in patients with a high degree of glucose intolerance or mild diabetes [76]. Most of the studies did not measure fructosamine or HbA_{1c} in diabetic patients. Thus, it is difficult to assess the long-term glycemic effect of honey in diabetic patients. Further clinical studies to ascertain these factors are needed [67].

Diabetic patients frequently suffer from impaired lipid metabolism such as elevated cholesterol and triglycerides, which are known factors for elevated risk of cardiovascular disease [77]. The results of both animal and human studies have suggested that honey supplementation could ameliorate impaired lipid metabolism by reducing triglycerides and low-density lipoprotein (LDL)- cholesterol as well as very-low-density lipoprotein (VLDL)-cholesterol and by increasing HDL-cholesterol [70,73,78–80].

Other Medical Uses/Applications of Honey

The medical use of honey has already been mentioned in the Bible, Koran, Torah, and Talmud, and since the ancient civilizations, a rich line-up of therapeutic effects of honey has been described. However, most evidence points to clinical use of honey for burns, wound care, and ulcers. Different properties of honey could explain the wound-healing effect. First of all, high sugar content reduces water availability and therefore inhibits the growth of microbes in the wound. Its acidity, with a pH value of below 5, is not favorable for microbial growth. The enzyme glucose-oxidase contained in honey produces hydrogen peroxide, which sanitizes the skin. Honey supports the healing process by facilitating an increase in lymphocytes and phagocytes and the release of cytokines and interleukins. Finally, the secondary plant metabolites with bactericidal properties contained in honey may play a beneficial role in wound healing [81].

Two recent reviews of the literature found over 50 studies related to the use of honey to treat burns, ulcers, and wounds with various etiologies. They investigated honey's antibacterial effect, wound-healing stimulating capacity, and anti-inflammatory, deodorizing and debridement properties [81,82].

However, several of the studies on wound healing were of poor quality, for example, the sample size was too small or the studies were not randomized or blinded. Two randomized controlled trials, however, were double- or single-blinded. Both of them investigated the effect of honey on wounds caused by partial or complete toenail removal and compared its effect to paraffin gauze and iodine dressing, respectively. The researchers concluded that there was no significant difference between honey and the paraffin dressing, while after total toenail removal, the iodine treatment was more effective in wound healing than honey [83,84].

Three studies examining the effect of honey on various skin conditions reported honey to be useful in managing seborrheic dermatitis, dandruff psoriasis, and various fungal conditions. However, these trials were not or only partially controlled [81].

The antibacterial effect of honey is best documented for burns. Thirteen clinical trials have investigated the efficacy of honey for healing burns in comparison to the therapy standard silver sulfadiazine (SSD), to polyurethane, to boiled potato peel, or to early tangential excision (TE) and skin grafting. Eight studies were performed by the same researchers using unprocessed undiluted honey. These studies reported better results for honey when compared to the other topical treatments, except for early TE and skin grafting. Five further studies compared honey to SSD or paraffin. Four were in favor of the honey, while one study found no difference between the honey and SSD. Therefore, honey may be a suitable alternative for treating burns. Compared to the studies on wound healing, the quality of these studies was better as they were randomized and the sample sizes were larger. Unfortunately, they were not blinded, and it was mostly unclear how the sample sizes were decided [81].

Wound healing is a known problem in cancer patients [85]. Although the quality of studies investigating the efficacy of honey in wound healing and infection inhibition in cancer patients is generally poor, a well-designed trial confirmed the positive results of these studies. According to that trial, honey reduced the severity and duration of radiation-induced oral mucositis, promoted wound healing, cleared infections, and reduced xerostomia (oral dryness symptom)-induced tooth decay [81].

For wound healing, honey may be a good alternative to other topical dressings, especially when all conventional therapies have failed, in cases of antibiotic resistance or in circumstances where the availability and cost of dressings are a problem. One main problem of even well-designed clinical trials is the fact that there is no consistency in the type, quality, and amount of the applied honey. Manuka honey from New Zealand or Australia is one of the best characterized and often used honeys [82] because of its high antibacterial capacity due to a high content of methylglyoxal. But other types of honey may also have an inhibitory effect on different bacterial strains responsible for infections and impaired healing of different wounds [86]. As mentioned before, the composition of the different types of honey varies greatly; therefore, their therapeutic effects depend on the concentration of special components. In general, it seems that darker colored honey has a higher antimicrobial activity than lighter colored honey [87]. Therefore, in future studies, a clear characterization of the honey used is essential for the interpretation of the results. Studying the antibacterial properties of honeys from various botanical origins may also lead to the discovery of further types of honeys that are well suited for wound healing.

Apart from the external application of honey on wounds, its antimicrobial activity has also been documented for treating bacterial gastroenteritis. Honey administered on the oral route was effective to treat infantile diarrhea and in vitro studies proved its bactericidal activity against several organisms causing gastrointestinal infections, including *Salmonella* and *Shigella* species, enteropathogenic *Escherischia coli* as well as *Helicobacter pylori* isolates which cause gastritis [88].

Additionally, gastric ulcers have been successfully treated using honey as a dietary supplement probably due to its gastroprotective anti-inflammatory properties [88].

Anticancer Effects of Honey

The in vitro and in vivo (in animal studies) treatment of cancer cells has indicated moderate antitumor and significant antimetastatic effects of honey as well as facilitation of the antitumor activity of certain chemotherapeutic drugs. The authors of these studies believe that the antitumor properties of honey could be attributed to the various polyphenols found in honey, such as caffeic acid, caffeic acid phenyl ester, chrysin, galangin, quercetin, acacetin, kaempferol, pinocembrin, pinobanksin, and apigenin. Single extracts of these polyphenols have shown promising pharmacological effects in different cancer cell lines tested in in vitro set-ups or in rat experiments [89]. However, their anticancer potential has not been tested in humans as either extracts or as natural constituent of honey. Therefore, further investigation is needed to clarify whether honey itself or the above-mentioned polyphenols in the concentrations measured in honey could be a successful anticancer treatment.

Antioxidant Effects of Honey

A short-term diet high in sucrose negatively affects the balance between free radical production and antioxidant defence, resulting in an increased lipid susceptibility to peroxidation. It has been suggested that the fructose moiety in the sucrose molecule is responsible for the pro-oxidant effect [90]. Fruits and vegetables are known to be rich sources of antioxidants, so it is not astonishing that honey originating from plant nectar has been reported to be rich in polyphenolic compounds [91]. Numerous investigations have found an antioxidant effect of honey on ameliorating oxidative stress in the gastrointestinal tract, pancreas, liver, kidney, reproductive organs, and plasma/serum. The fact that most of these results emanate from in vitro or animal studies indicates a need to investigate its antioxidant effect in humans suffering from chronic or degenerative diseases [91]. The few existing studies conducted on humans have indicated a beneficial effect on factors strongly related to coronary heart disease like hypertension or serum cholesterol levels [92], but better designed studies are needed to verify the potential and mechanism of honey to counteract oxidative stress and related chronic diseases.

CONCLUSION

In conclusion, it can be stated that sugars in fruits do not play an important role in health promotion per se. As a matter of fact, it is generally recognized that the synergy of secondary plant metabolites, dietary fiber, and vitamin C are responsible for the potential beneficial effects of fruits. However, there is a general consensus that further prospective studies and interventions are needed to strengthen these observations. Moreover, it should be noted that the preventive effects of fruits can be optimized when their consumption is part of an overall healthy lifestyle.

Likewise, the beneficial effect of honey on many health aspects has not exclusively been related to its sugar composition, but also to its numerous additional compounds, such as enzymes, flavonoids, and polyphenols. Honey is a complex food, and its composition varies greatly depending on its geographical and botanical origin. This could be one of the major reasons for the often controversial results of numerous investigations using honey to treat various medical conditions. The most benefit was found in its application to burns due to its antimicrobial effect. In both, diabetic patients and healthy people, honey has been found to positively impact blood glucose levels and insulin production due to its lower GI compared to sucrose.

REFERENCES

1. Li KT. Physiology and classification of fruits. In: Sinha NK, Sidhu JS, Barta J, Wu JSB, Pilar Cano M, editors. *Handbook of Fruits and Fruit Processing*, 2nd ed. Chichester, NY: Wiley-Blackwell; 2012. p. 3–12.
2. Belitz HD, Grosch W, Schieberle P. Fruits and fruit products. In: Belitz HD, Grosch W, Schieberle P, editors. *Food Chemistry*. Berlin: Springer; 2009. p. 807–61.
3. Souci SW, Fachmann W, Kraut H. *Die Zusammensetzung der Lebensmittel, Nährwert-Tabellen*, 7th ed. Stuttgart: medpharm GmbH Scientific Publishers; 2013.
4. Ebermann R, Elmadfa I, editors. Pflanzliche lebensmittel. *Lehrbuch Lebensmittelchemie und Ernährung*, 2nd corrected and extended ed. Wien: Springer; 2011. p. 337–550.
5. Slavin JL, Lloyd B. Health benefits of fruits and vegetables. *Advances in Nutrition* 2012;3:506–16.
6. Crozier A. Classification and biosynthesis of secondary plant products: An overview. In: Goldberg G, editor. *Plants: Diet and Health*. Oxford: Blackwell Publishing; 2003. p. 27–48.
7. Crozier A, Clifford MN, Ashihara H. *Plant Secondary Metabolites: Occurence, Structure and Role in Human Diet*. Oxford: Blackwell Publishing Ltd; 2006.
8. Moretti CL, Mattos LM, Calbo AG, Sargent SA. Climate changes and potential impacts on postharvest quality of fruit and vegetable crops: A review. *Food Research International* 2010;43:1824–32.
9. Herrmann K. *Inhaltsstoffe von Obst und Gemüse*. Stuttgart: Ulmer; 2001.
10. Drewnowski A, Fulgoni V. Nutrient profiling of foods: Creating a nutrient-rich food index. *Nutriton Review* 2008;66:23–39.
11. Shrapnel B, Noakes M. Discriminating between carbohydrate-rich foods: A model based on nutrient density and glycaemic index. *Nutrition & Dietetics* 2012;69:152–8.
12. Tohill BC, Seymour J, Serdula M, Kettel-Khan L, Rolls BJ. What epidemiologic studies tell us about the relationship between fruit and vegetable consumption and body weight. *Nutriton Review* 2004;62(10):365–74.
13. Darmon N, Darmon M, Maillot M, Drewnowski A. A nutrient density standard for vegetables and fruits: Nutrients per calorie and nutrients per unit cost. *Journal of the American Dietetic Association* 2005;105:1881–7.
14. Hiza HAB, Bente L, Fungwe T. Nutrient content of the U.S. food supply, 2005. *Home Economics Research Report* 2008;58:1–76.
15. Schmid A, Brombach C, Jacob S, Sieber R, Siegrist M. Ernährungssituation in der Schweiz. In: Keller U, Battaglia Richi E, Beer M, Darioli R, Meyer K, Renggli A et al., editors. *Sechster Schweizerischer Ernährungsbericht*. Bern: Bundesamt für Gesundheit; 2012. p. 49–126.
16. NVS II. Nationale Verzehrsstudie II—Ergebnisbericht Teil 2. Karlsruhe: Max-Rubner Institut; 2008.
17. Cust AE, Skilton MR, van Bakel MME, Halkjar J, Olsen A, Agnoli C et al. Total dietary carbohydrate, sugar, starch and fibre intakes in the European Prospective Investigation into Cancer and Nutrition. *European Journal of Clinical Nutrition* 2009;63:S37–60.
18. Olsen A, Halkjaer J, van Gils CH, Buijsse B, Verhagen H, Jenab M et al. Dietary intake of the water-soluble vitamins B1, B2, B6, B12 and C in 10 countries in the European Prospective Investigation into Cancer and Nutrition. *European Journal of Clinical Nutrition* 2009;63:S122–49.
19. Caswell H. The role of fruit juice in the diet: An overview. *Nutrition Bulletin* 2009;34:273–88.
20. Jenab M, Salvini S, van Gils CH, Brustad M, Shakya-Shrestha S, Buijsse B et al. Dietary intakes of retinol, [beta]-carotene, vitamin D and vitamin E in the European Prospective Investigation into Cancer and Nutrition cohort. *European Journal of Clinical Nutrition* 2009;63:S150–78.
21. Welch AA, Fransen H, Jenab M, Boutron-Ruault MC, Tumino R, Agnoli C et al. Variation in intakes of calcium, phosphorus, magnesium, iron and potassium in 10 countries in the European Prospective Investigation into Cancer and Nutrition study. *European Journal of Clinical Nutrition* 2009;63:S101–21.
22. Ocke MC, Larranaga N, Grioni S, van den Berg SW, Ferrari P, Salvini S et al. Energy intake and sources of energy intake in the European Prospective Investigation into Cancer and Nutrition. *European Journal of Clinical Nutrition* 2009;63:S3–15.
23. Margetts BM. Nutrient intake and patterns in the European Prospective Investigation into Cancer and Nutrition cohorts from 10 European countries. *European Journal of Clinical Nutrition* 2009;63:S1–2.
24. Afaghi A, Ziaee A, Kiaee SM, Hosseini N. Glycemic index and glycemic loads of variety of fruits: Clinical implementation of fruits' serving size in low glycemic load diet. *Current Topics in Nutraceutical Research* 2009;7:157–60.
25. Miller JB, Pang E, Broomhead L. The glycaemic index of foods containing sugars: Comparison of foods with naturally-occurring v. added sugars. *British Journal of Nutrition* 1995;73:613–23.

26. Atkinson FS, Foster-Powell K, Brand-Miller JC. International tables of glycemic index and glycemic load values: 2008. *Diabetes Care* 2008;31:2281–3.
27. Trout D, Behall KM. Prediction of glycemic index among high-sugar, low-starch foods. *International Journal of Food Sciences and Nutrition* 1999;50:135–44.
28. van Bakel MME, Kaaks R, Feskens EJM, Rohrmann S, Welch AA, Pala V et al. Dietary glycaemic index and glycaemic load in the European Prospective Investigation into Cancer and Nutrition. *European Journal of Clinical Nutrition* 2009;63:S188–205.
29. Boeing H, Bechthold A, Bub A, Ellinger S, Haller D, Kroke A et al. Critical review: Vegetables and fruit in the prevention of chronic diseases. *European Journal of Nutrition* 2012;51:637–63.
30. Carter P, Gray L, Troughton J, Khunti K, Davies MJ. Fruit and vegetable intake and incidence of type 2 diabetes mellitus: Systematic review and meta-analysis. *British Medical Journal* 2010;341:c4229.
31. Dauchet L, Amouyel P, Dallongeville J. Fruits, vegetables and coronary heart disease. *Nature Reviews Cardiology* 2009;6:599–608.
32. Key TJ. Fruit and vegetables and cancer risk. *British Journal of Cancer* 2011;104:6–11.
33. Ledoux TA, Hingle MD, Baranowski T. Relationship of fruit and vegetable intake with adiposity: A systematic review. *Obesity Reviews* 2011;12:e143–e150.
34. Jenkins DA, Kendall CC, McKeown-Eyssen G. Effect of a low-glycemic index or a high-cereal fiber diet on type 2 diabetes: A randomized trial. *Journal of the American Medical Association* 2008;300:2742–53.
35. Jenkins DJA, Srichaikul K, Kendall CWC, Sievenpiper JL, Abdulnour S, Mirrahimi A et al. The relation of low glycaemic index fruit consumption to glycaemic control and risk factors for coronary heart disease in type 2 diabetes. *Diabetologia* 2011;54:271–9.
36. Xu Q, Si LY. Resveratrol role in cardiovascular and metabolic health and potential mechanisms of action. *Nutrition Research* 2012;32(9):648–58.
37. Cassidy A, Mukamal KJ, Liu L, Franz M, Eliassen AH, Rimm EB. High anthocyanin intake is associated with a reduced risk of myocardial infarction in young and middle-aged women. *Circulation* 2013;127:188–96.
38. Landete JM. Ellagitannins, ellagic acid and their derived metabolites: A review about source, metabolism, functions and health. *Food Research International* 2011;44:1150–60.
39. Giampieri F, Tulipani S, Alvarez-Suarez JM, Quiles JL, Mezzetti B, Battino M. The strawberry: Composition, nutritional quality, and impact on human health. *Nutrition* 2012;28:9–19.
40. McCune LM, Kubota C, Stendell-Hollis NR, Thomson CA. Cherries and health: A review. *Critical Reviews in Food Science and Nutrition* 2011;51:1–12.
41. Pezzuto JM. Grapes and human health: A perspective. *Journal of Agricultural and Food Chemistry* 2008;56:6777–84.
42. Rao AV, Snyder DM. Raspberries and human health: A review. *Journal of Agricultural and Food Chemistry* 2010;58:3871–83.
43. Hyson DA. A comprehensive review of apples and apple components and their relationship to human health. *Advances in Nutrition* 2011;2:408–20.
44. Bertelli AAA, Das DK. Grapes, wines, resveratrol, and heart health. *Journal of Cardiovascular Pharmacology* 2009;54:468–76.
45. Basu A, Rhone M, Lyons TJ. Berries: Emerging impact on cardiovascular health. *Nutrition Review* 2010;68:168–77.
46. Côté J, Caillet S, Doyon G, Sylvain JF, Lacroix M. Bioactive compounds in cranberries and their biological properties. *Critical Reviews in Food Science and Nutrition* 2010;50:666–79.
47. Cuthrell K, Le Marchand L. Grapefruit and Cancer: A Review. *Potential Health Benefits of Citrus*, 936rd ed. Washington DC: American Chemical Society; 2006. p. 235–52.
48. Sherzai A, Heim LT, Boothby C, Sherzai AD. Stroke, food groups, and dietary patterns: A systematic review. *Nutrition Review* 2012;70:423–35.
49. Fujioka K, Lee MW. Obesity, metabolic syndrome, and the benefits of citrus. *Potential Health Benefits of Citrus*, 936th ed. Washington DC: American Chemical Society; 2006. p. 211–8.
50. Bogdanov S, Jurendic T, Sieber R, Gallmann P. Honey for nutrition and health: A review. *The Journal of the American College of Nutrition* 2008;27(6):677–89.
51. FAO Food and Agricultural Organization of the United Nations. Honey marketing and international trade. FAO Food and Agricultural Organization of the United Nations. Available from: ftp://ftp.fao.org/docrep/fao/012/i0842e/i0842e16.pdf (accessed on 31 March 2014).
52. World Trade Daily. Honey: World production, top exporters, top importers, and United States imports by country. World Trade Daily. Available from: http://worldtradedaily.com/2012/07/28/honey-world-production-top-exporters-top-importers-and-untied-states-imports-by-country/(accessed on 31 March 2014).

53. Codex Alimentarius. Codex Standard for Honey. Codex Alimentarius 2001; p. 1–8.
54. Sanz ML, Polemis N, Morales V, Corzo N, Drakoularakou A, Gibson GR et al. In vitro investigation into the potential prebiotic activity of honey oligosaccharides. *Journal of Agricultural and Food Chemistry* 2005;53(8):2914–21.
55. Persano Oddo L, Piro R. Main European unifloral honeys: Descriptive sheets. *Apidologie* 2004;35:S38–81.
56. Beckh G, Camps G. Neue Spezifikationen für Trachthonige. *Deutsche Lebensmittel-Rundschau* 2009;105(2):105–10.
57. Bundesministerium der Justiz. Deutsche Honigverordnung, Neufassung der Leitsätze. Bundesanzeiger 2011;111a:1–24. Available from: http://www.apis-ev.de/fileadmin/downloads/Leitsaetze_Honig_2011.pdf
58. Arcot J, Brand-Miller J. A preliminary assessment of the glycemic index of honey. A report for the Rural Industries Research and Development Corporation 2005; p. 1–24.
59. Deibert P, Konig D, Kloock B, Groenefeld M, Berg A. Glycaemic and insulinaemic properties of some German honey varieties. *European Journal of Clinical Nutrition* 2010;64(7):762–4.
60. Abdulrhman M, El HM, Ali R, Abdel HI, Abou El-Goud A, Refai D. Effects of honey, sucrose and glucose on blood glucose and C-peptide in patients with type 1 diabetes mellitus. *Complementary Therapies in Clinical Practice* 2013;19(1):15–9.
61. Ischayek JI, Kern M. US honeys varying in glucose and fructose content elicit similar glycemic indexes. *Journal of the American Dietetic Association* 2006;106(8):1260–2.
62. Münstedt K, Sheybani B, Hauenschild A, Brüggmann D, Bretzel RG, Winter D. Effects of basswood honey, honey-comparable glucose–fructose solution, and oral glucose tolerance test solution on serum insulin, glucose, and C-peptide concentrations in healthy subjects. *Journal of Medicinal Food* 2008;11(3):424–8.
63. Robert SD, Ismail AA. Two varieties of honey that are available in Malaysia gave intermediate glycemic index values when tested among healthy individuals. *Biomedical Papers of the Medical Faculty of the University Palacky, Olomouc, Czechoslovakia* 2009;153(2):145–7.
64. Shambaugh P, Worthington V, Herbert JH. Differential effects of honey, sucrose, and fructose on blood sugar levels. *Journal of Manipulative and Physiological Therapeutics* 1990;13(6):322–5.
65. Fujisawa T, Riby J, Kretchmer N. Intestinal absorption of fructose in the rat. *Gastroenterology* 1991;101(2):360–7.
66. Erejuwa OO, Sulaiman SA, Wahab MS. Fructose might contribute to the hypoglycemic effect of honey. *Molecules* 2012;17(2):1900–15.
67. Erejuwa OO, Sulaiman SA, Wahab MS. Honey—A novel antidiabetic agent. *International Journal of Biological Sciences* 2012;8(6):913–34.
68. Erejuwa OO, Sulaiman SA, Wahab MS. Oligosaccharides might contribute to the antidiabetic effect of honey: A review of the literature. *Molecules* 2012;17(1):248–66.
69. Cani PD, Neyrinck AM, Fava F, Knauf C, Burcelin RG, Tuohy KM et al. Selective increases of bifidobacteria in gut microflora improve high-fat-diet-induced diabetes in mice through a mechanism associated with endotoxaemia. *Diabetologia* 2007;50(11):2374–83.
70. Erejuwa OO, Sulaiman SA, Ab Wahab MS, Sirajudeen KNS, Salleh MSM, Gurtu S. Glibenclamide or metformin combined with honey improves glycemic control in streptozotocin-induced diabetic rats. *Journal of Clinical Pharmacology* 2011;50(9):1062.
71. Samanta A, Burden AC, Jones GR. Plasma glucose responses to glucose, sucrose, and honey in patients with diabetes mellitus: An analysis of glycaemic and peak incremental indices. *Diabetic Medicine* 1985;2(5):371–3.
72. Bornet F, Haardt MJ, Costagliola D, Blayo A, Slama G. Sucrose or honey at breakfast have no additional acute hyperglycaemic effect over an isoglucidic amount of bread in type 2 diabetic patients. *Diabetologia* 1985;28(4):213–7.
73. Katsilambros NL, Philippides P, Touliatou A, Georgakopoulos K, Kofotzouli L, Frangaki D et al. Metabolic effects of honey (alone or combined with other foods) in type II diabetics. *Acta Diabetologica Latina* 1988;25(3):197–203.
74. Bahrami M, Ataie-Jafari A, Hosseini S, Forouzanfar MH, Rahmani M, Pajouhi M. Effects of natural honey consumption in diabetic patients: An 8-week randomized clinical trial. *International Journal of Food Sciences and Nutrition* 2009;60(7):618–26.
75. AL-Waili NS. Intrapulmonary administration of natural honey solution, hyperosmolar dextrose or hypoosmolar distill water to normal individuals and to patients with type-2 diabetes mellitus or hypertension: Their effects on blood glucose level, plasma insulin and C-peptide, blood pressure and peaked expiratory flow rate. *European Journal of Medical Research* 2003;8(7):295–303.

76. Agrawal OP, Pachauri A, Yadav H, Urmila J, Goswamy HM, Chapperwal A et al. Subjects with impaired glucose tolerance exhibit a high degree of tolerance to honey. *Journal of Medicinal Food* 2007;10(3):473–8.
77. Kokil GR, Rewatkar PV, Verma A, Thareja S, Naik SR. Pharmacology and chemistry of diabetes mellitus and antidiabetic drugs: A critical review. *Current Medicinal Chemistry* 2010;17(35):4405–23.
78. AL-Waili NS. Natural honey lowers plasma glucose, C-reactive protein, homocysteine, and blood lipids in healthy, diabetic, and hyperlipidemic subjects: Comparison with dextrose and sucrose. *Journal of Medicinal Food* 2004;7(1):100–7.
79. Busserolles J, Gueux E, Rock E, Mazur A, Rayssiguier Y. Substituting honey for refined carbohydrates protects rats from hypertriglyceridemic and prooxidative effects of fructose. *Journal of Nutrition* 2002;132(11):3379–82.
80. Chepulis L, Starkey N. The long-term effects of feeding honey compared with sucrose and a sugar-free diet on weight gain, lipid profiles, and DEXA measurements in rats. *Journal of Food Science* 2008;73(1):1–7.
81. Bardy J, Slevin NJ, Mais KL, Molassiotis A. A systematic review of honey uses and its potential value within oncology care. *Journal of Clinical Nursing* 2008;17(19):2604–23.
82. Vandamme L, Heyneman A, Hoeksema H, Verbelen J, Monstrey S. Honey in modern wound care: A systematic review. *Burns* 2013;39(8):1514–25.
83. Mashall C, Queen J, Manjooran J. Honey vs povidone iodine following toenail surgery. *Wounds UK* 2005;1(1):10–8.
84. McIntosh CD, Thomson CE. Honey dressing versus paraffin tulle gras following toenail surgery. *Journal of Wound Care* 2006;15(3):133–6.
85. McNees P, Meneses KD. Pressure ulcers and other chronic wounds in patients with and patients without cancer: A retrospective, comparative analysis of healing patterns. *Ostomy Wound Manage* 2007;53(2):70–8.
86. Majtan J, Majtan V. Is manuka honey the best type of honey for wound care? *The Journal of Hospital Infection* 2010;74(3):305–6.
87. Taormina PJ, Niemira BA, Beuchat LR. Inhibitory activity of honey against foodborne pathogens as influenced by the presence of hydrogen peroxide and level of antioxidant power. *International Journal of Food Microbiology* 2001;69(3):217–25.
88. Jeffrey AE, Echazarreta CM. Medical use of honey. *Revista Biomédica* 1996;7:43–9.
89. Jaganathan SK, Mandal M. Antiproliferative effects of honey and of its polyphenols: A review. *Journal of Biomedicine and Biotechnology* 2009;2009:1–13.
90. Busserolles J, Rock E, Gueux E, Mazur A, Grolier P, Rayssiguier Y. Short-term consumption of a high-sucrose diet has a pro-oxidant effect in rats. *British Journal of Nutrition* 2002;87(4):337–42.
91. Erejuwa OO, Sulaiman SA, Ab Wahab MS. Honey: A novel antioxidant. *Molecules* 2012;17(4):4400–23.
92. Münstedt K, Hoffmann S, Hauenschild A, Bulte M, von Georgi R, Hackethal A. Effect of honey on serum cholesterol and lipid values. *Journal of Medicinal Food* 2009;12(3):624–8.
93. Stéger-Máté M. Physiology and classification of fruits. In: Sinha NK, Sidhu JS, Barta J, Wu JSB, Pilar Cano M, editors. *Handbook of Fruits and Fruit Processing*, 2nd ed. Chichester NY: Wiley-Blackwell; 2012. p. 433–66.
94. Bogdanov S, Bieri K, Gremaud G, Iff D, Känzig A, Seiler K, Stöckli H, Zürcher K. Bienenprodukte: 23 A Honig. *Swiss Food Manual* 2003;1–35.
95. Bogdanov S, Gfeller M. Classification of honeydew and blossom honeys by discriminant analysis. *ALP Science* 2006;500:1–9.

6 High-Fructose Syrup—So, What Is It Exactly?

John S. White

CONTENTS

KEY POINTS

- High-fructose syrup (HFS) comes from a botanical source, as do sucrose, fruit juice concentrates, and honey (indirectly).
- HFS and sucrose are highly refined, highly purified sweeteners that share common production processes.
- Composed of glucose and fructose, its composition is similar to sucrose and nearly identical to invert sugar.
- Sweetener individuality is lost after digestion—sucrose and HFS deliver the same sugars in nearly the same concentration to the bloodstream.

- HFS-55 was designed to be equally sweet with sucrose.
- HFS has functionality beyond sweetness, much of which is in common with sucrose.
- The rapid increase in HFS consumption occurred at the expense of sucrose, so fructose from added sugar was largely unchanged over the past 100 years.
- HFS consumption peaked in 1999 and has since been in decline.
- US consumption of sucrose is currently 50% more than HFS; global sucrose consumption is 10× HFS.
- There is no correlation between HFS or fructose with obesity in the USA; global correlation is unlikely due to scant use of sucrose.
- The significant increase in per capita daily energy intake in the USA over the past 40 years is more due to increased fat and cereal grains (glucose from starch) than added sugars, HFS, or fructose; dietary glucose exceeds fructose by more than 3:1 margin.
- Reactive dicarbonyl compounds (RDCs) and advanced glycosylation endproducts (AGEs) are ubiquitous in the environment and processed foods; sugars in HFS are not a unique or important source of dietary RDCs and AGEs; dietary sources are small compared to endogenous production.
- Reformulating foods and beverages from HFS to sucrose is a metabolic wash; the nutritional value does not change and is potentially misleading to consumers.

INTRODUCTION

Everyone on the planet, it seems, has heard of high-fructose syrup (HFS)—aka high-fructose corn syrup (HFCS), isoglucose, glucose–fructose syrup and fructose–glucose syrup. HFS enjoyed 35 successful and relatively quiet years as a liquid sweetener alternative to sucrose, widely understood to have the same sweetness, caloric value, composition, and functionality. HFS was abruptly thrust into the spotlight by a 2004 Commentary in the *American Journal of Clinical Nutrition* [1] showing an association between increased use of HFS between 1970 and 2000, and rising rates of obesity. Although the authors' hypothesis did not imply direct causation—"the overconsumption of HFCS in calorically sweetened beverages may play a role in the epidemic of obesity"—it had several significant consequences:

1. Attention was laser focused on HFS as a unique cause of obesity, while sucrose—with similar composition—became the preferred sweetener choice;
2. Fructose research was jump-started after a decade of inactivity; and
3. Many accepted the hypothesis without further proof and HFS became the poster child for poor nutrition and obesity.

Stories about it appear weekly in the media. It is a frequent topic of casual conversation; strangers and friends speak knowingly about it. We were told it is in every food, that it is *The One*, the dietary silver bullet that is single-handedly responsible for epidemics of obesity and related diseases in the USA. School districts and state legislatures call for its removal from school lunch programs, insisting manufacturers pull it out of food and beverage formulations and replace it with sugar (sugar!), ostensibly to improve nutritional quality. We were warned that developing countries and sugar-based economies should avoid its use. And if that were not enough, we were told it is toxic. *Toxic? Really?* A sweetener that has been used in foods and beverages for 45 years is toxic? The body count must be extraordinary. *How could that be?*

How could it not? We live in an era of instant transmission of unfiltered information, where opinion becomes fact, Blogger Kings and Queens dispense nutrition advice, and anyone caught introducing fact is exiled forthwith; where researchers side-step scientific debate for media limelight; where abstracts and press releases are used verbatim in news stories; where adequate fact-checking and peer review by journals and granting agencies seem to be relics of the past; and where common sense and perspective have been thrown out of the window.

HFS had the misfortune to catch the attention of the world at a time in history when half-truths, speculation, and half-baked science race so far ahead that fact and sound science have little hope of catching up.

A different view on HFS will be presented in this chapter [2–4]. You will find information that is missing from conversations, stories, papers, chapters, books, and other accounts you have encountered about HFS. This information is available to all, but overlooked, avoided, or discounted by most. For a balanced picture of HFS, compare what you read in other chapters of this textbook and elsewhere with information presented in this chapter.

A note of clarification: the term "high-fructose *corn* syrup" (HFCS) is commonly used in the USA, where cornstarch is the only raw material used in its production. By convention, the word "corn" is dropped when referring to the sweetener in a global context, acknowledging that additional agricultural crops ably supply the starch used for HFS production in other parts of the world. HFS will be used exclusively in this chapter except where specifically noted.

HFS ORIGINS

HFS was conceived as a liquid sweetener alternative to sucrose (table sugar) and was originally developed to satisfy two pressing needs in the USA. The first came from food manufacturers of sugar-based products. Sugarcane was traditionally grown in equatorial regions, many susceptible to both political and climatic upheaval. The availability and price of sugar fluctuated wildly in response to upsets in either one, disrupting food manufacturing until stability was restored. It was also recognized that sucrose hydrolyzes (inverts) in acidic systems [5], changing the sweetness and flavor characteristics of the product. And as a granular ingredient, sucrose must be dissolved in water before use in many applications, a labor- and energy-intensive process.

The second need came from the corn wet milling industry—millers of corn who use water to flow corn components through separation and refining processes—who had been successful sellers of cornstarch and corn syrup since the last half of the nineteenth century. Facing mature markets, the industry was looking for other uses of the starch raw material so abundant in Midwest corn. In particular, they sought a sweeter ingredient capable of competing head-on with sucrose in the vast number of applications for which existing corn-based products lacked sufficient sweetness.

Although regular corn syrup—containing glucose and glucose oligomers, but no fructose—is prized for its viscosity, sheen, humectancy, and solubility, it possesses less than half the sweetness of sucrose. This is a significant limitation in sweet applications, requiring twice the amount, cost and calories to deliver the same sweetness, and effectively excluded corn syrups from high-volume sucrose applications. It was well known that sucrose is a disaccharide of glucose and fructose. Invert sugar is a syrup sweetener in which the disaccharide bond in sucrose is hydrolyzed (inverted), releasing equal amounts of glucose and fructose. The corn wet milling industry believed a sweetener with the glucose/fructose composition, sweetness, and functional properties of invert sugar could be made by isomerizing plentiful glucose from their starch process to fructose. A confluence of technological developments made this belief a reality.

HFS became the sweetener that satisfied requirements of both food and corn wet milling industries: it was a stable, domestic sweetener comparable to sucrose in sweetness and it allowed the corn wet milling industry entrée to elusive sugar-sweetened products. HFS immediately proved itself an attractive alternative to sucrose, particularly in liquid applications, because it is stable in acidic foods and beverages. In its syrup form, HFS can be conveniently and economically pumped from truck or railcar delivery vehicles to customer storage and mixing tanks, where it requires only simple dilution before use. Because of favorable corn-growing conditions and plentiful farmland in the US Midwest, HFS has largely avoided the price and availability volatility of sucrose.* It was principally for these reasons that HFS was so readily accepted by the food industry and became one of the most successful food ingredients in modern history.

HFS PRODUCTION

Technology Development

Early development work on HFS was carried out in the 1950s and 1960s, with shipments of the first commercial product to the food industry occurring in the late 1960s. Two key developments made this possible: a clean and efficient means to convert low-sweetness glucose to higher-sweetness fructose (isomerization), and technology capable of separating the two.

By the 1950s, there were only three ways known to produce fructose: acid hydrolysis (inversion) of sucrose, a disaccharide of equal parts glucose and fructose; acid hydrolysis of the (natural) fructose polymer inulin, found in Jerusalem artichoke, chicory, and dahlia tubers; and alkaline isomerization of glucose, characterized by low yield and generation of unacceptable byproduct colors and flavors [6].

Akabori et al. [7] introduced a potentially cleaner and more efficient biochemical means of converting glucose to fructose in 1952, using an enzyme that catalyzed aldose–ketose isomerization without the need for regeneration of expensive cofactors. Marshall and Kooi of the Corn Products Company discovered a more cost-effective microbial xylose isomerase with affinity for glucose in 1957 [8]. Takasaki of the Japanese Agency of Industrial Science & Technology (AIST) later isolated a heat-stable version of the enzyme and then combined fermentation with enzyme immobilization to make a commercially viable isomerase [9]. Clinton Corn Processing Company and AIST teamed up to make the first commercial HFS (15% fructose) in 1966–1967.

Glucose isomerization is under thermodynamic control. With an equilibrium constant of ~1 at 60°C, a practical industrial processing temperature, roughly equimolar amounts of glucose and fructose can ultimately be produced. Thus, a 94% glucose syrup can produce about 47% fructose at equilibrium [10]. Lower yields are achieved in practice, however, necessitated by time and enzyme limitations. Clinton produced the first 42% fructose syrup ("first-generation" HFCS-42) in 1968. HFCS-42 was suitable for use in many food applications, but was less sweet than sucrose and unsuitable for use in products like carbonated beverages.

This product was called "high-fructose" corn syrup for two reasons: to distinguish it from regular corn syrup, which contained no fructose; and to ally it with fruit sugars, popular at the time and known to be rich sources of fructose. It turns out to have been an unwise choice of name, since HFCS is not high in fructose compared to other fructose sweeteners (sucrose, honey, fruit juice concentrates), some people find the chemical name "fructose" disconcerting in and of itself, and the name has contributed to the general misunderstanding about the sweetener.

A.E. Staley Manufacturing Company began manufacturing HFS-42 in 1968 under license from Clinton. Four years later, Clinton made HFS-42 using immobilized isomerase in the first continuous process. Around 1976, Staley's European partners, Amylum in Belgium and Tunnel Refineries in the UK, began producing HFS-42.

Efficient separation of glucose and fructose was the next hurdle to clear. Existing moving-bed, countercurrent chromatography was adapted to carbohydrate separation by Mitsubishi Chemical Industries in the mid-1970s. Japanese and US HFS producers licensed the technology and used it in 1978 to produce the first 55% fructose syrup, "second-generation" HFS-55.

After Staley researchers identified trace differences between HFS and sucrose in the early 1980s, industry-wide refining improvements eliminated the final barrier to full replacement of sucrose with HFS in carbonated beverages. Coca-Cola and Pepsi approved 100% use of HFS in 1984.

* It is a misconception that much of the US corn crop is used for HFS and that removing corn price supports will reduce HFS use. In reality, less than 4% of the crop was converted to HFS in 2011/2012 (USDA-ERS Feed Outlook: September 2013).

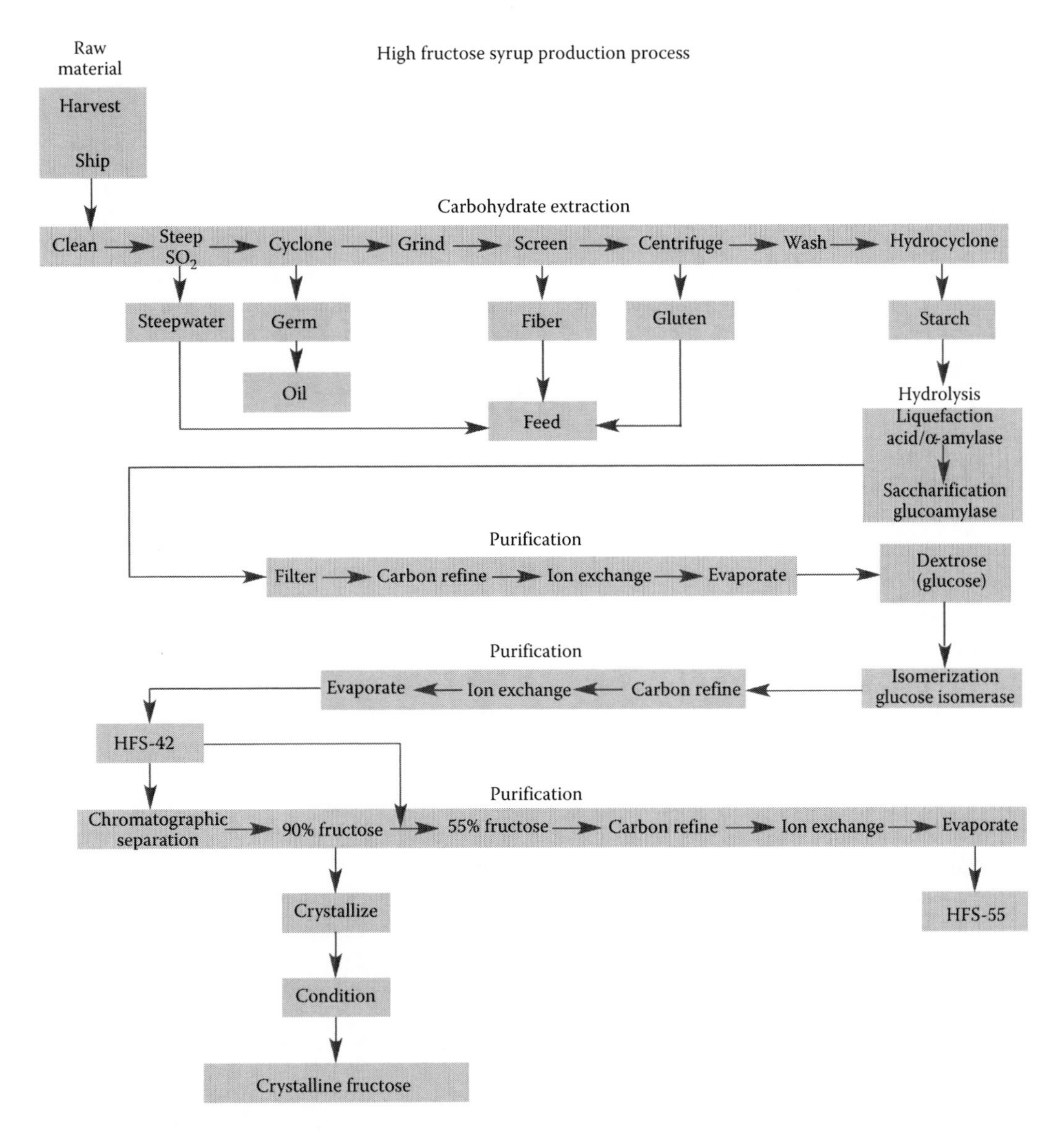

FIGURE 6.1 Typical HFS manufacturing process.

Additional information on the development of HFS is available in the more detailed discussions by White [11] and Hull [6].

Manufacturing Process

The basic sequence of steps required to produce HFS is depicted in Figure 6.1 and will be reviewed in several sections.

Raw Material

HFS manufacturing has two fundamental raw material requirements: a plentiful and consistent source of starch and abundant water. For this reason, many wet milling plants are sited in agricultural regions adjacent to rivers or lakes.

Corn is by and large the most commonly used starch in HFS production, not only in North America, but also in South America, Europe, and Asia. Potato starch is also used in Europe, but that starch composition is more difficult to work with. Asian processors also use some tapioca and rice starch. Wheat starch is commonly used in Europe, the Middle East, and Australia.

Carbohydrate Extraction

Once the raw agricultural feedstock material is cleaned, it must be treated to release the carbohydrate-containing starch from other material. For corn, this is achieved by steeping in a dilute solution of sulfur dioxide (SO_2) to soften the hull, control pH, and limit microbial growth and color formation during subsequent processing. SO_2 diffuses into the kernel and denatures the protein (corn gluten) matrix that fixes starch granules in place. Germ, fiber, and gluten fractions are sequentially removed through grinding, milling, screening, washing, filtration, and centrifugation until only starch remains. These fractions and steep water have nutritional value and are sold individually or incorporated into animal feed. Cornstarch can be physically or chemically treated to exhibit a host of functional characteristics, or used as the raw material for downstream maltodextrin, corn syrup, and dextrose (glucose) production.

Starch Hydrolysis

Starch is made up of densely packed crystals of high-molecular-weight glucose polymers. For downstream processing, these crystals must be hydrated to allow access by acid or hydrolytic enzymes to the polymer backbone. This is accomplished by "jetting" a slurry of starch and live steam through a high-pressure nozzle. Liquefaction (using acid or α-amylase enzyme) and saccharification (using glucoamylase enzyme) sequentially reduce the polymer length of starch molecules through hydrolysis of covalent bonds linking adjacent glucose molecules to produce first maltodextrins, then corn syrups, and finally monomeric dextrose (glucose). Each of these is an individual product class, and together they encompass scores of industrial and food ingredients. Impurities are removed through filtration, carbon and ion exchange treatments. Dextrose is valued not only as a food ingredient, but is further used within the corn wet milling industry as a fermentable sugar for production of ethanol, vitamins, amino acids, food acids, colorants, and organic intermediates for bioplastics and other synthetics. Outside corn wet milling, dextrose is a key ingredient in innumerable fermentation products, including foods and pharmaceuticals. But central to our focus in this chapter, dextrose (glucose) is also the feedstock for HFS production.

Isomerization, Fractionation, and Blending

Glucose-to-fructose isomerization takes place in large packed-bed reactors filled with immobilized glucose isomerase enzyme. High-concentration glucose syrup passes through the reactors in continuous flow. The product is collected as a mixture of glucose and fructose, which is further purified using carbon and ion exchange refining to produce HFS-42, "first-generation" HFS.

Enrichment of fructose is required for HFS-55, which is accomplished using moving-bed chromatography through a number of vessels linked in series. Fructose progress through the vessels is retarded by its high affinity for the calcium salt form of the strong-acid cation-exchange resin through which it passes. Recovery of a 90% fructose fraction is possible because of the relatively lower affinity and consequent faster progress of glucose through the resin. The 90% fructose fraction is blended with HFS-42 and then undergoes final purification treatment to produce HFS-55, "second-generation" HFS.

HFS-90 is found in some supplier catalogs, but in practice is used in minor amounts compared with HFS-42 and -55. HFS-90 also serves as the feedstock for crystalline fructose, a specialty sweetener introduced to the food and beverage industry in the late 1980s. Together, HFS-90 and crystalline fructose make up no more than a percent or two of aggregate fructose-containing corn sweeteners and mere fractions of a percent of total dietary sugars.

TABLE 6.1
Comparison of HFS and Sucrose Production Processes

Process	HFS	Sucrose
Botanical source	Corn	Cane or beet
Extraction	Steeping	Pulping
Purification—protein/fat removal	Wet milling—SO_2, mud filtration	Clarification—sulfitation, carbonatation, phosphatation
Enzymes	Depolymerization, isomerization	Filtration aid, inversion
Purification—trace contaminants	Carbon, ion exchange, centrifugation	Carbon, crystallization, centrifugation
Concentration	Evaporation	Evaporation, crystallization

HFS and Sucrose Use Common Manufacturing Processes

One of the myths surrounding HFS is that its manufacturing process is somehow more "industrial" and more complex than the "natural" and simpler processes for sucrose or other sweeteners and HFS is more "highly processed" than other sugars. Not really. Whether the botanical source is sugarcane and beets, cereal grain, or fruit, the goal of all sweetener manufacturing is the extraction and purification of desirable sugars away from the complex cellular and biochemical milieu—rich in undesirable colors, flavors, and aromas. Honey is given a free pass, since its unique characteristics are valued; however, this severely limits its use to products where consumers appreciate these attributes. And it is a closely held reality that fruit juice concentrates are first "stripped" of their color, flavor, and aroma by processing before they can be used in mainstream sweetener applications [12].

Table 6.1 presents a comparison of processes used in HFS and sucrose production. Note the parallels in processing from extraction to concentration. It is fair to conclude that both sweeteners employ sophisticated processing methods using good manufacturing practices to extract and purify sugars. There is no need to exalt or vilify either one.

One sticking point with some critics is the use of enzymes. While this is a well-publicized step in HFS production, it must be recognized that enzyme use is quite common throughout the food industry, including in sucrose and invert sugar manufacture. Enzymes are also accepted adjuncts in production of beer, wine and juices, dairy products, baked goods, and fermented foods and condiments; why not sweeteners as well?

COMPOSITION

The common nutritive sweeteners—sucrose, HFS, honey, and grape juice concentrate—contain fructose and glucose in near equal amounts. The composition of HFS is frequently confused with that of regular corn syrup and crystalline fructose, but as shown in Table 6.2 [13,14], there are stark

TABLE 6.2
Comparison of Sugars Composition of Common Nutritive Sweeteners

Component (% Total Sugars)	Corn Syrup	HFS-42	Sucrose	Total Invert	HFS-55	Crystalline Fructose
Sucrose			99.3	6		
Fructose	0	≥42	<0.01	47	≥55	≥99.9
Glucose	100	52	<0.01	47	41	0.1
Oligosaccharides		6			4	
Form	Syrup	Syrup	Dry	Syrup	Syrup	Dry

differences. As a hydrolysis product of starch, corn syrup is entirely composed of glucose and glucose oligomers of varying chain lengths, and contains no fructose. Entirely different in composition, crystalline fructose is highly purified fructose, containing no glucose. HFS-42 and -55 are mixtures of fructose (42 or 55%) and glucose, with a few percent of residual glucose oligosaccharides. Since salivary and intestinal amylases readily hydrolyze the oligosaccharides to their constituent glucose monomers during digestion, HFS is either 42% fructose and 58% glucose (HFS-42) or 55% fructose and 45% glucose (HFS-55). Thus, HFS-42 contains a bit less and HFS-55 a bit more fructose than sucrose.

Sucrose is a disaccharide comprising equal parts of glucose and fructose covalently linked together through a glycosidic bond (Figure 6.2, left-hand panel). Invert sugar is made by purposely hydrolyzing half (medium invert) or >90% (total invert) of the sucrose to glucose and fructose using acid or enzyme. But sucrose will also hydrolyze in low pH foods and beverages. For example, considerable inversion can occur in the low pH of carbonated beverages between bottling and consumption. It is somewhat ironic that soft drink purists who insist on sucrose-sweetened sodas are most likely drinking a sweetener composition more resembling invert sugar and HFS.

Though not included in Table 6.2, the sugar composition of honey and grape juice concentrate most closely resemble that of HFS, being largely monosaccharide glucose and fructose in roughly the same ratio. It is instructive to compare the fructose composition of nutritive sweeteners with that found in natural sources. More than 50 fruits, vegetables, and nuts fall within the 42–55% fructose composition range of HFS, sucrose, invert sugar, honey and grape juice concentrate. Apples and pears have the highest fructose percentage of any fruit (65 and 75%, respectively), a key reason apple and pear juice concentrates are so widely used to sweeten juice beverages.

Concern was recently raised by a 2011 paper purporting to show that HFS manufacturers and soft drink bottlers may be misleading the public by exceeding commonly assumed fructose percentages in HFS-55 [15]. The excess fructose vis-à-vis sucrose was promoted as a primary driver of unfavorable effects on metabolic health [16–19]. However, this paper may have been limited by use of inappropriate methodology since the authors employed an analytical method for honey, rather than one specifically optimized for HFCS [20].

HFS and Sucrose Individuality Is Lost Upon Digestion

A popular misconception about HFS is that its sugar constituents are somewhat different from those in sucrose and are therefore handled (metabolized) differently by the body. Not really. As depicted in the right-hand panel of Figure 6.2, HFS and sucrose are nearly equivalent in composition after digestion. The enzyme sucrase in the lumen of the small intestine hydrolyzes the glycosidic bond joining the α-D-glucopyranosyl form of glucose to the β-D-fructofuranoside form of fructose, releasing free monosaccharides that are transported into the portal blood. The residual oligosaccharides in HFS are hydrolyzed to monosaccharide glucose during digestion.

The free glucose and fructose appearing in the bloodstream from sucrose are chemically identical to those transported into the blood from monosaccharide food sources like HFS, honey, fruit juice concentrates, and scores of fruits, vegetables, and nuts. Thus, the sugars in HFS and sucrose lose their individuality once they are digested and are not differentiated by the body.

FUNCTIONALITY

HFS-55 and Sucrose Are Equally Sweet

A persistent myth about HFS is that it is sweeter than sucrose, thereby supposedly promoting overeating and concomitant obesity [1]. This myth is based on confusion of HFS—fructose *and* glucose—with pure crystalline fructose.

Table 6.3 compares the sweetness of fructose and glucose alone, and in combination as HFS and sucrose. Shallenberger and Acree [21] measured sweetness intensities of crystalline compounds and

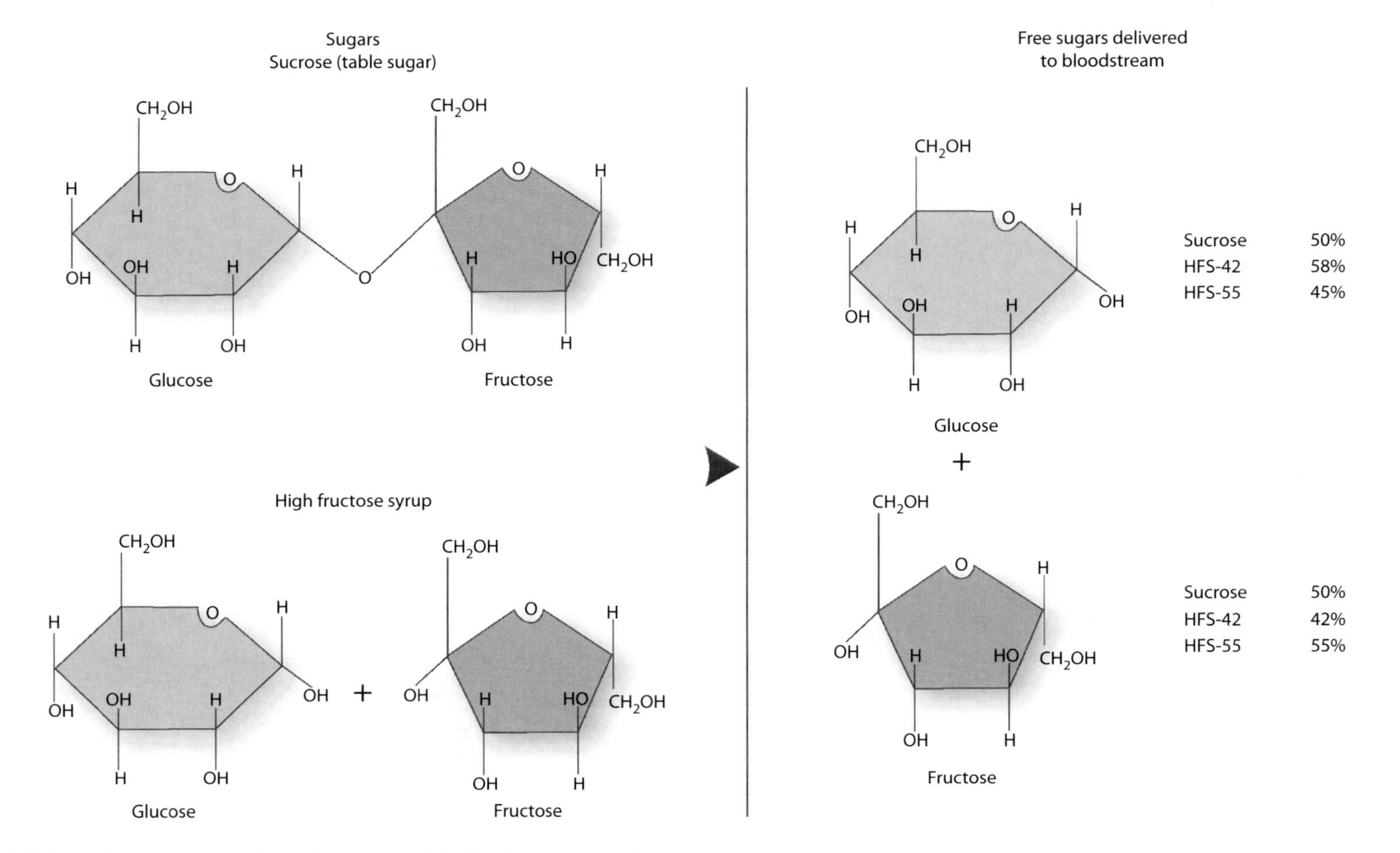

FIGURE 6.2 Structural comparison of sucrose and HFS before and after digestion.

TABLE 6.3
Sweetness Comparisons for Selected Nutritive Sweeteners

Sugars	Sweetness Intensity (Crystalline)	Relative Sweetness (10% Solution)
Fructose	180	117
Sucrose	100	100
HFS-55	—	99
HFS-42	—	90
Glucose	74–82	65

reported that fructose is 1.8 and 2.3 times sweeter than sucrose and glucose, respectively. Because HFS does not crystallize and is most often used in beverages at about 10% dry solids, White and Parke [22] compared the sweetness of sugars relative to sucrose at this concentration. They reported that pure fructose in solution is reduced to 1.2 times as sweet as sucrose, that HFS-55 and sucrose have equivalent sweetness, and that HFS-42 is 10% less sweet than sucrose.

HFS can be viewed as having the combined sweetness of fructose and glucose. Its sweeter fructose component is balanced by its much less sweet glucose component, resulting in HFS-55 having equivalent sweetness to sucrose. Thus, replacement of sucrose with HFS-55 did not lead to sweeter foods and beverages, and its sweetness should not be blamed for the epidemic of obesity.

HFS Adds Functionality Beyond Sweetness

An oft-heard misconception about HFS is that it is in *everything*. Not really, since 50% more sucrose is used in the USA than HFS. But the perception merits discussion since HFS sometimes appears unexpectedly in certain foods—often at low levels—because it adds functionality beyond sweetness.

Most of its functional attributes are due either to the unique chemical properties of free fructose or to the "reducing" nature of unbound fructose and glucose; these attributes are less pronounced or absent in sucrose. Beyond sweetness, the functional attributes of HFS include viscosity, fermentability, hygroscopicity (moisture attraction), and humectancy (moisture retention), resistance to crystallization (solubility), browning/flavor/aroma development, flavor enhancement, and colligative properties (osmotic pressure and freezing point depression).

This functionality translates to the following benefits in foods and beverages [23]:

- Sweetness—HFS provides sweetness intensity equivalent to sugar. HFS can replace sugar one-for-one on a dry solids basis.
- Flavor enhancement—the sweetness profile of HFS enhances many fruit, citrus, and spice flavors in beverages, bakery fillings, and dairy products.
- Freshness—HFS promotes freshness in several ways. It inhibits microbial spoilage by reducing water activity and extends shelf life through superior moisture control. Foods also taste fresh because HFS protects the firm texture of canned fruits and reduces freezer burn in frozen fruits.
- Soft texture—Chewy cookies, snack bars, and other baked goods derive their soft and moist texture from HFS, which retains moisture and resists crystallization after baking.
- Browning—HFS is a "reducing" sugar that gives superior browning, flavor, and aroma to baked goods and cooked meats.
- Stability—over time, HFS-sweetened products maintain sweetness and flavor with no quality loss due to storage temperature fluctuations or low product acidity. With HFS, product stability maintains the quality of carbonated and still beverages, as well as condiments like ketchup and fruit preserves.

- Pourability—HFS has a reduced freezing point, so "frozen" beverage concentrates have the added convenience of being pourable straight from the freezer and are easier for consumers to thaw and mix with water.
- Fermentability—about 96% of the sugars in HFS are fermentable. This is important in bread baking because HFS is more economical to use than sucrose.

Though there are functional differences both subtle and profound between HFS and sucrose, they perform similarly enough that they can be used interchangeably in a host of food and beverage applications where their functionalities overlap.

CONSUMPTION

As reviewed in more detail in Chapters 9 and 10, consumption of dietary sugars and HFS in the USA is estimated using two primary databases: USDA-ERS and NHANES. The US Department of Agriculture Economic Research Service (USDA-ERS) has collected considerable commodity production data, some for over a century. USDA reports consumption both as availability (gross production available for consumption) and loss-adjusted availability (a closer approximation of actual consumption, after correcting for losses between manufacturing/harvest and eating). The National Health and Nutrition Examination Survey (NHANES), conducted by the National Center for Health Statistics, has tracked changes in nutrient intake and public health through dietary surveys and physical examinations since 1971.

HFS and Fructose Are Not Predictive of US Obesity

USDA-ERS loss-adjusted commodity availability data [24] as proxy for sucrose, HFCS (note: US HFS) and fructose consumption are plotted in Figure 6.3 against recent US obesity statistics from the WHO Global InfoBase [25]. The following conclusions are supported by these data:

- Sucrose and HFS consumption curves are mirror images over the 1970–1985 period of rapid growth for HFS, suggesting a one-for-one replacement of sucrose with HFS and confirming functional similarities between the two sweeteners.
- HFS is not "in everything," another common misconception. Nearly 50% more sucrose than HFS is used in the USA today and the disparity appears to be growing.
- HFS consumption peaked in 1999 and has since been in steep decline. Consumption now is equivalent to 1984, the year US carbonated beverage manufacturers switched from sucrose to HFS.
- US obesity rates continued to climb beyond 1999. Although the Bray et al. HFS–obesity association appeared valid from 1970 to 1999, that association was lost before their commentary was published (2004) and certainly does not exist today.
- Fructose from added sugars changed very little over the past century, averaging 39 ± 4 g/day/capita since 1920. Fructose intake has also been decreasing since 1999 and is now equal to 1991 and 1927 levels. There is no association between fructose intake and obesity.
- Though not pictured here, White used USDA-ERS loss-adjusted availability data to demonstrate that total caloric sugars have also been in decline since 1999 [4].

Analysis of the NHANES database by Welsh et al. [26] confirmed downward trends in added sugars and, additionally, sugar-sweetened beverages after 1999–2000.

Sweeteners and Fructose Have Not Driven 40-Year US Energy Increase

Per capita daily energy intake has risen substantially since 1970, when HFS was first being used in US food products. If HFS and fructose truly are unique drivers of obesity and related diseases,

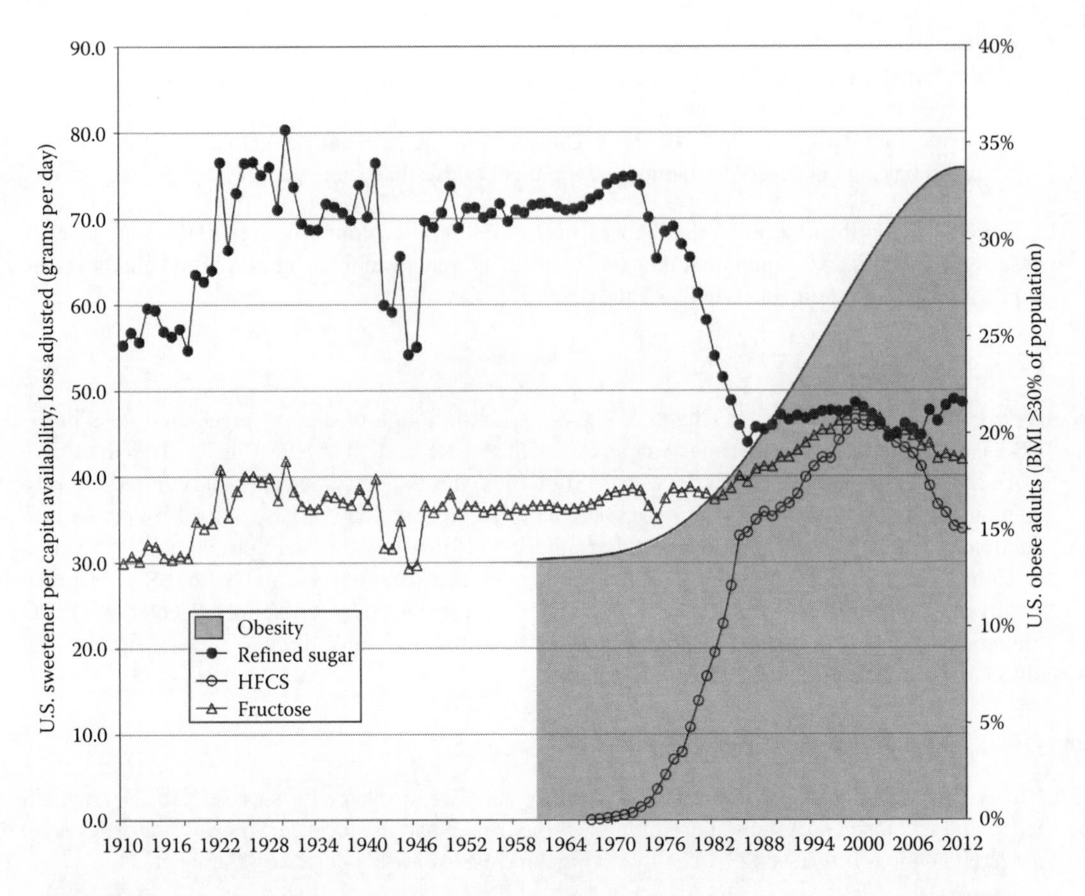

FIGURE 6.3 Historical comparison of US trends in consumption (availability) of sucrose, HFCS (note: US HFS) and fructose with rates of obesity in adults: 1910–2012.

their caloric contribution versus other dietary components over the intervening 40 years should have increased disproportionately. To test that proposition, White [2–4] and Carden et al. [27] independently analyzed USDA-ERS food and nutrient energy availability data and reported similar results.

The data of Carden et al. were adapted and summarized in Table 6.4. They drew several important conclusions that reinforce a null effect on obesity for fructose, in particular, and sweeteners, in general:

- Increased total energy intake was judged to be a significant contributor to increased obesity in the USA between 1970 and 2009.
- Increased consumption of foods providing glucose (primarily grain starches) and fat were significant drivers of increased total energy.
- Total fructose availability did not increase during this period and sweetener availability increased only slightly.
- Fructose was unlikely to have been a unique causal factor in the increased prevalence of obesity.

Thus, added sugars, HFS, fructose, and sugar-sweetened beverage intakes appear not to have increased meaningfully since HFS use began in the USA. This refutes the HFS and fructose hypotheses [2,3], which rely on disproportionate use of these sugars for validity. To blame contemporary health problems on HFS specifically, or caloric sweeteners generally, is not only unsupported by the data, it diverts attention from the most likely contributor to overweight and obesity: the imbalance between energy intake and expenditure.

TABLE 6.4
Cumulative Change in Food and Nutrient Energy Availability: 1970–2009

Dietary Component	Energy Available in 1970 (kcal/day)[a]	40-Year Net Energy Accumulation (kcal)[b]	% Change[c]
Food			
Sweeteners	410	212	1.3
Grains	404	3807	24.2
Fats and oils	368	3641	25.3
Nutrient			
Protein	276	486	4.7
Fat	751	4268	14.6
Carbohydrate (total)	1050	3915	9.8
Glucose	773	3915	13.0
Fructose	253	−0.7	0.0

[a] Values for 1970 were used to establish a constant baseline AUC for 1970–2009.
[b] Values represent actual AUC trends derived from annual data.
[c] Values were calculated from actual AUC compared to baseline AUC.

Dietary Glucose Dominates Fructose

Although the ratio of glucose-to-fructose is approximately 1:1 for most nutritive sweeteners, the ratio changes appreciably when the sugar composition of the whole diet is considered. Carden et al. used USDA loss-adjusted food availability data to calculate the amount of glucose and fructose available for absorption from all carbohydrate food sources [27]. They reported that glucose exceeded fructose by a ratio of 3:1, a value not dissimilar to the whole diet value of 5:1 estimated by White using similar methodology [4]. Sun et al. [28] used the 1999–2006 NHANES databases to compare fructose versus nonfructose intake patterns and concluded that the fructose energy contribution was lower than that of nonfructose sugars in more than 97% of the 25,000+ subjects studied.

These studies argue convincingly against the suitability of prevalent fructose-only study protocols for predicting metabolic outcomes in real-world diets.

HFS Is Not Predictive of Global Obesity

The International Sugar Organization (ISO) lists five prerequisites needed for successful development of an HFS industry [29]:

1. A domestic deficit of sugar and a high international sugar price
2. Sufficient supplies of low-cost starch
3. A well-developed food production and consumption infrastructure
4. Availability of capital for investment in research and development and plant and equipment
5. Favorable government policy.

It is because all five prerequisites coalesced in the USA in the 1960s and 1970s that HFS developed and flourished. One or more prerequisites are missing in most regions of the world.

Consequently, HFS is primarily a US sweetener, accounting for more than 60% of world production. On a global scale, however, HFS is dwarfed by sucrose, which accounts for 92% of combined sweetener consumption.

TABLE 6.5
Comparison of Global Sucrose and HFS Consumption: 2006–2012

	Consumption[a] (HFS % Share of [Sucrose + HFS])		
	Americas	**Asia and Oceania**	**Europe and Africa**
2006			
HFS	9.7 (21.8%)	1.9 (3%)	0.8 (2%)
Sucrose + HFS	44.5	63.2	43.3
2012			
HFS	9.4 (19.8%)	3.3 (4%)	1.0 (2%)
Sucrose + HFS	47.6	74.2	46.4
HFS % change, 2006–2012	–2%	+1%	+0%

[a] Million tonnes, white value and dry basis.

Accurate figures for global HFS consumption are difficult to come by; it is not clear in many cases whether they are based on actual intake or production. One such global comparison of sucrose and HFS consumption is presented in Table 6.5 [30]. It is not surprising that the HFS% share of total consumption (sucrose + HFS) is high in the Americas (~20%) and low in Asia/Oceania and Europe/Africa (2–3%), where sugar has been well entrenched for centuries and the ISO prerequisites are not easily met. From a global perspective, HFS is not gaining much traction against sucrose. Certainly HFS consumption is increasing in countries like Mexico, Argentina, and China; but this is more than offset by steep declines in the USA. And it should be noted that while HFS consumption surged in Mexico under the North American Free Trade Agreement (NAFTA), it appears to be leveling off after 3 years of gains.

LMC International tracks global production of HFS and other commodities [30]. The top HFS-producing countries/regions for 2012 were, in descending order: the USA, China, Japan, the European Union (EU), Argentina, Canada, South Korea, and Mexico. As a further test of whether HFS is a unique causal factor in global obesity, production numbers for the above countries were compared with their corresponding adult obesity prevalence rates reported in *The World Factbook* [31]. The resulting low coefficient of determination ($R^2 = 0.048$) indicates that HFS production (as proxy for consumption) is a poor predictor of global obesity.

Production can be a poor proxy for consumption in regions where manufacturing is centralized in a few countries, but exported for consumption to trade partners. Such is the case in the EU for HFS, where nine countries led by Hungary hold the quotas for all HFS production. It would be incorrect, for example, to assume that Hungarians consume the entire country's quota, since it is shared with other EU member countries through trade. This error was made in a recent paper seeking to correlate HFS consumption in the EU (and globally) with diabetes incidence [15]. It will be recognized that false-positive correlations would be calculated for HFS quota holders/exporters like Hungary, and false-negatives for HFS importers like the UK. The authors also argued that the +5% fructose differential in HFS versus sucrose was responsible for increased diabetes rates reported in HFS-producing countries. Their initial error was compounded when they failed to take into account the type of HFS made by each country: because of production and technological limitations, EU countries—and many others around the world—produce only HFS-42 [32], with an –8% fructose differential from sucrose. Had they been aware of this, one wonders if the authors would have encouraged production of *more* HFS in EU countries to stem the rise in diabetes.

HFS AND SUCROSE EQUIVALENCE

HFS and sucrose are similar in many ways: manufacturing, composition, caloric value, sweetness, functionality, and metabolism [33–37]. These similarities are compelling enough that five expert panels on HFS or fructose convened in the past two decades [38–42] and two prominent health professional organizations [43,44] concluded that HFS and sucrose are metabolically equivalent.

REACTIVE DICARBONYL COMPOUNDS AND ADVANCED GLYCATION ENDPRODUCTS

Concern was raised in 2008 that HFS in sugar-sweetened beverages was a unique contributor to the formation of RDCs and AGEs [45]. Though the concern was addressed [3], the issue occasionally resurfaces.

RDCs are intermediates in the Maillard reaction, a cascade of chemical reactions that takes place when sugars—especially monosaccharides—react with amines. Some compounds formed in the Maillard reaction are responsible for the pleasing colors, flavors, and aromas of baked and cooked foods, as discussed in more detail in Chapter 4. Others have been variously described as cytotoxic, mutagenic, carcinogenic, and pro-oxidant, but also demonstrated to have bactericidal, antiviral, antiparasitic, and antitumorigenic activities.

AGEs are formed when RDCs react with protein. These also have been characterized with contradictory properties: pro- and antioxidant, pro- and antimutagenic, toxic, and protective. As a matter of course, AGEs modify and crosslink most proteins in the body and affect their structure and function. This process is routinely controlled through continuous turnover of body proteins.

When considering whether or not HFS plays a unique role in RDCs and AGEs, the following points are useful to keep in mind [3]:

- RDCs are ubiquitous in the environment, appearing in the atmosphere, rivers, groundwater, drinking water, and household cleaners.
- RDCs and AGEs are produced from many simple sugars, including glucose and fructose.
- RDCs and AGEs are formed in common foods and beverages in the normal course of heating, cooking, baking, fermenting, and aging. HFS is not a unique and important contributor.
- RDCs and AGEs are continually produced in human metabolism. Although fructose is several times more reactive than glucose in these processes, it is rapidly taken up by the liver, so does not remain long in circulation; and once in the liver, it is quickly metabolized. The blood concentration of glucose is several times higher; it remains longer in circulation and has access to all body tissue.
- HFS is not a unique and important contributor of RDCs and AGEs to foods and beverages.
- Carbonated soft drinks do not contribute appreciably to endogenous RDC and AGE production. Eleven hundred twenty-nine (1129) servings of carbonated soft drink would need to be consumed to equal amounts produced by natural physiological processes in a single day.

OPEN QUESTIONS

HFS is frequently compared unfavorably to sucrose, but in truth, few researchers have evaluated HFS under real-world experimental conditions. The essential test is whether HFS poses a *unique* threat to public health *as commonly consumed.* It is imperative to evaluate its *uniqueness* against comparable sweeteners (i.e., sucrose or honey or grape juice concentrate). Glucose and starch *are not* comparable since they contain no fructose, are metabolized so differently, and are not functionally interchangeable with HFCS in foods and beverages. Likewise, fructose is a poor comparator since the isolated sugar is metabolized so differently from the glucose–fructose combination in HFS. And to be clinically important, effects unique to HFS must be proved within the range of normal human exposure and within the context of the whole diet, not at exaggerated levels or in isolation.

CONCLUSIONS

Despite the notoriety HFS has received in the past decade, it still remains a valued liquid sweetener to the food and beverage industry. It is hoped the information presented in this chapter will restore balance and perspective to the HFS/fructose debate and to other chapters in this textbook.

High fructose syrup—so, what is it exactly? It's a liquid sweetener alternative to sugar. No more and no less.

CONFLICTS OF INTEREST

As a consultant and advisor to the food and beverage industry in the area of nutritive sweeteners, the author receives compensation from scientific societies, research institutes, food industry councils, trade organizations, and individual companies. Past and present associations include the Calorie Control Council, the Corn Refiners Association, and the International Life Sciences Institute. Clients have an ongoing interest in nutritive sweetener research, development, production, applications, safety, nutrition, and education.

REFERENCES

1. Bray GA, Nielsen SJ, Popkin BM. Consumption of high-fructose corn syrup in beverages may play a role in the epidemic of obesity. *Am J Clin Nutr* 2004;79(4):537–43.
2. White JS. Straight talk about high-fructose corn syrup: What it is and what it ain't. *Am J Clin Nutr* 2008;88(6):1716S–21S.
3. White JS. Misconceptions about high-fructose corn syrup: Is it uniquely responsible for obesity, reactive dicarbonyl compounds, and advanced glycation endproducts? *J Nutr* 2009;139(6):1219S–27S.
4. White JS. Challenging the fructose hypothesis: New perspectives on fructose consumption and metabolism. *Adv Nutr* 2013;4(2):246–56.
5. Salomonsson I. http://www.danisco.com/cms/resources/file/eb241b041a6ed65/Shelf%20life.pdf (accessed 15 March 2007).
6. Hull P. Glucose syrups: Technology and applications. Chichester, UK/Ames, IA: Wiley-Blackwell, 2010.
7. Akabori S, Uehara K, Muramatsu I. On the biochemical formation of monosaccharides. *Proc Jpn Acad* 1952;28(1):39–43.
8. Marshall RO, Kooi ER, Moffett GM. Enzymatic conversion of D-glucose to D-fructose. *Science* 1957;125(3249):648–9.
9. Takasaki Y, Tanabe O. Enzyme method for converting glucose in glucose syrups to fructose. In: Office USP, ed. Agency of Industrial Science and Technology, Tokyo, Japan, 1971.
10. Lloyd N, Khaleeluddin K. A kinetic comparison of *Streptomyces* glucose isomerase in free solution and adsorbed on DEAE [diethylaminoethyl]-cellulose [Maize processing]. *Cereal Chem* 1976;53.
11. White JS. Fructose syrup: Production, properties, and applications. In: Schenck FW, Hebeda RE, eds. Starch Hydrolysis Products: Worldwide Technology, Production, and Application. New York: VCH, 1992: p. 177–99.
12. Thorn E. Internet: http://www.isnare.com/?aid=123197&ca=Wellness%2C+Fitness+and+Diet (accessed 28 February 2008).
13. Clarke MA. Cane sugar. In: Kroschwitz JI, ed. Kirk-Othmer Concise Encyclopedia of Chemical Technology, 4th Edition. New York: Wiley, 1999: p. 1915–7.
14. Buck AW. High fructose corn syrup. In: Nabors LO, ed. Alternative Sweeteners. Boca Raton, FL: CRC Press, 2012.
15. Ventura EE, Davis JN, Goran MI. Sugar content of popular sweetened beverages based on objective laboratory analysis: Focus on fructose content. *Obesity (Silver Spring)* 2011;19(4):868–74.
16. Goran MI, Ventura EE. Genetic predisposition and increasing dietary fructose exposure: The perfect storm for fatty liver disease in Hispanics in the U.S. *Dig Liver Dis* 2012;44(9):711–3.

17. Goran MI, Ulijaszek SJ, Ventura EE. High fructose corn syrup and diabetes prevalence: A global perspective. *Glob Public Health* 2013;8(1):55–64.
18. Goran MI, Dumke K, Bouret SG, Kayser B, Walker RW, Blumberg B. The obesogenic effect of high fructose exposure during early development. *Nature Rev Endocrinol* 2013;9(8):494–500.
19. Bray GA, Popkin BM. Calorie-sweetened beverages and fructose: What have we learned 10 years later. *Pediatric Obesity* 2013;8(4):242–8.
20. Hobbs LJ, Krueger D. Response to "Sugar content of popular sweetened beverages based on objective laboratory analysis: Focus on fructose content". *Obesity (Silver Spring)* 2011;19(4):687; author Goran reply-8; Hobbs & Krueger reply to Goran 8.
21. Shallenberger RS, Acree TE. Sugar Chemistry. Westport, CT: AVI Publishing Company, 1971.
22. White JS, Parke DW. Fructose adds variety to breakfast. *Cereal Foods World* 1989;34(5):392–8.
23. Corn Refiners Association. Questions & answers about high fructose corn syrup. Washington, DC, 2005.
24. USDA/Economic Research Service. USDA-ERS. Food Availability (Per capita) Data System: Food availability. Sugar and sweeteners (added), updated 20 August 2012.
25. World Health Organization (WHO). World Health Organization (WHO), Global database on body mass index. Global InfoBase. 21 August 2013 ed. apps.who.int/bmi/index.jsp (accessed 21 August 2013).
26. Welsh JA, Sharma AJ, Grellinger L, Vos MB. Consumption of added sugars is decreasing in the United States. *Am J Clin Nutr* 2011;94(3):726–34.
27. Carden TJ, Carr TP. Food availability of glucose and fat, but not fructose, increased in the US between 1970 and 2009: Analysis of the USDA food availability data system. *Nutr J* 2013;12(1):130.
28. Sun SZ, Anderson GH, Flickinger BD, Williamson-Hughes PS, Empie MW. Fructose and non-fructose sugar intakes in the US population and their associations with indicators of metabolic syndrome. *Food Chem Toxicol* 2011;49(11):2875–82.
29. ISO Market Evaluation Consumption and Statistics Committee. Alternative Sweeteners in a High Sugar Price Environment. London: International Sugar Organization, 2012.
30. LMC Sweetener Analysis. HFCS Annual Review. New York: LMC International, 2013.
31. CIA. The World Factbook: Obesity—Adult Prevalence Rate. U.S. Central Intelligence Agency, 2013.
32. Agrosynergie Groupement Europeen d'Interet Economique. Evaluation of CAP measures applied to the sugar sector. European Commission DG Agriculture and Rural Development, 2011.
33. Melanson KJ, Zukley L, Lowndes J, Nguyen V, Angelopoulos TJ, Rippe JM. Effects of high-fructose corn syrup and sucrose consumption on circulating glucose, insulin, leptin, and ghrelin and on appetite in normal-weight women. *Nutrition* 2007;23(2):103–12.
34. Soenen S, Westerterp-Plantenga MS. No differences in satiety or energy intake after high-fructose corn syrup, sucrose, or milk preloads. *Am J Clin Nutr* 2007;86(6):1586–94.
35. Stanhope KL, Griffen SC, Bair BR, Swarbrick MM, Keim NL, Havel PJ. Twenty-four-hour endocrine and metabolic profiles following consumption of high-fructose corn syrup-, sucrose-, fructose-, and glucose-sweetened beverages with meals. *Am J Clin Nutr* 2008;87(5):1194–203.
36. Angelopoulos TJ, Lowndes J, Zukley L et al. The effect of high-fructose corn syrup consumption on triglycerides and uric acid. *J Nutr* 2009;139(6):1242S–5S.
37. Rippe JM, Angelopoulos TJ. Sucrose, high-fructose corn syrup, and fructose, their metabolism and potential health effects: What do we really know? *Adv Nutr* 2013;4(2):236–45.
38. Glinsmann WH, Bowman BA. The public health significance of dietary fructose. *Am J Clin Nutr* 1993;58(5 Suppl):820S–3S.
39. Forshee RA, Storey ML, Allison DB et al. A critical examination of the evidence relating high fructose corn syrup and weight gain. *Crit Rev Food Sci Nutr* 2007;47(6):561–82.
40. Fulgoni III V. High-fructose corn syrup: Everything you wanted to know, but were afraid to ask. *Am J Clin Nutr* 2008;88(6):1715S.
41. Murphy SP. The state of the science on dietary sweeteners containing fructose: Summary and issues to be resolved. *J Nutr* 2009;139(6):1269S–70S.
42. Rippe JM, Kris Etherton PM. Fructose, sucrose, and high fructose corn syrup: Modern scientific findings and health implications. *Adv Nutr* 2012;3(5):739–40.
43. American Medical Association. Report 3 of the Council on Science and Public Health (A-08): The Health Effects of High Fructose Syrup. Chicago: American Medical Association, 2008.
44. Fitch C, Keim KS, Academy of Nutrition and Dietetics. Position of the Academy of Nutrition and Dietetics: Use of nutritive and nonnutritive sweeteners. *J Acad Nutr Diet* 2012;112(5):739–58.
45. Lo C-Y, Li S, Wang Y et al. Reactive dicarbonyl compounds and 5-(hydroxymethyl)-2-furfural in carbonated beverages containing high-fructose corn syrup. *Food Chem* 2008;107:1099–105.

7 Biological and Health Effects of Nonnutritive Sweeteners

Allison C. Sylvetsky, Rebecca J. Brown, and Kristina I. Rother

CONTENTS

KEY POINTS

- Nonnutritive sweeteners are sweet-tasting compounds that are hundreds or thousands of times sweeter than sucrose by weight and provide no or few calories when ingested.
- The approval and regulatory status of each specific nonnutritive sweetener varies by country.
- Regulatory organizations establish an acceptable daily intake (ADI) which is the amount of sweetener thought to be safe to consume every day for lifetime. The sweetener is approved if the estimated intake is lower than the ADI.
- Nonnutritive sweeteners are present in a wide variety of foods and beverages including diet soda, other carbonated and noncarbonated soft drinks, dairy products, condiments, canned fruit, frozen desserts, chewing gum, baked goods, and cereals as well as in sweetener packets.
- Approximately 30–35% of the general adult population consumes nonnutritive sweetener-containing items on a given day.
- Nonnutritive sweeteners and other sweet-tasting substances are sensed via heterodimeric G-protein-coupled taste receptors.

- Sweet-taste receptors are located on taste buds of the tongue and in the oral cavity, and also on specific cells in the small intestine, pancreas, biliary tract, and lungs.
- *In vitro* studies have demonstrated that nonnutritive sweeteners can induce secretion of gastrointestinal hormones, including insulin, GLP-1, and GIP, yet these results have not been reliably replicated *in vivo*.
- Epidemiologic studies suggest that nonnutritive sweetener use is associated with weight gain, metabolic syndrome, vascular dysfunction, preterm delivery, renal problems, and lymphoma. However, the contribution of nonnutritive sweeteners relative to other dietary and environmental factors is not clear.
- Randomized controlled trials evaluating nonnutritive sweeteners for weight control suggest that nonnutritive sweeteners are weight-neutral or may result in modest weight reduction.
- Nonnutritive sweeteners are differentiated from caloric sugars by the brain, yet how this may influence food choice and calorie intake remains to be elucidated.
- The metabolism of nonnutritive sweeteners, including their potential effects on nutrient and drug absorption, requires further investigation.
- Potential effects of nonnutritive sweeteners on taste preferences in children have not been studied.
- Most studies of nonnutritive sweeteners on glycemia control and satiety have examined acute effects (less than one day); the long-term effects require further study.

INTRODUCTION

Nonnutritive sweeteners (NNSs) are sweet-tasting compounds that do not substantially contribute to energy intake when ingested [1,2]. NNSs are also referred to as artificial sweeteners, low-calorie sweeteners, noncaloric sweeteners, and high-intensity sweeteners. The first NNS was discovered accidentally in the late nineteenth century. After working with coal and neglecting to wash his hands, a chemist ate lunch and tasted sweetness on his bread. He later traced the sweetness to a specific compound in his laboratory, known today as saccharin [3]. By the 1980s, a second generation of NNSs, including cyclamates, acesulfame potassium, and aspartame emerged, followed by sucralose and neotame, and most recently by products based on extracts of the stevia and monk fruit plants. With obesity rates increasing rapidly since the 1980s, dieting and diet programs have become increasingly popular, creating an important market for NNS.

NNSs have much higher sweetness intensity than sucrose, ranging from 32 times that of 5% sucrose (for cyclamate) to 11,000 times (for neotame) [4]. This allows NNSs to be used in very low concentrations in foods and beverages. The relative sweetness of sweeteners is typically assessed using psychophysical techniques, in which trained observers subjectively assess the sweetness intensity of different solutions of sweeteners compared to a set of standard sucrose solutions at varying concentrations [5]. Using these techniques, a number of parameters may be calculated, including the lowest concentration at which the sweet taste is identified (sweetness recognition threshold), the concentration of the sweetener that achieves half-maximal sweetness response (analogous to the Michaelis–Menton constant KM50), and the overall sweetness relative to sucrose by weight (Table 7.1).

REGULATION AND CONSUMPTION OF NONNUTRITIVE SWEETENERS (NNS)

How Are NNSs Regulated?

Which specific NNSs are approved and how each NNS is regulated differs by country (see Table 7.1). In the USA, six NNSs have been approved by the Food and Drug Administration (FDA) for use in the general population: acesulfame potassium, aspartame, neotame, saccharin, sucralose, and stevia. In 1958, Congress had passed the Food Additives Amendment to the Food, Drug, and

TABLE 7.1
Approval Status, Chemical Structure, and Relative Sweetness of NNSs

Sweetener	Structure	ADI (mg/kg/day) USA EU JECFA FSANZ	Sweetness (Compared to 5% Sucrose)	Mean Concentration in Carbonated Soft Drinks (mmol/L)
Sucrose	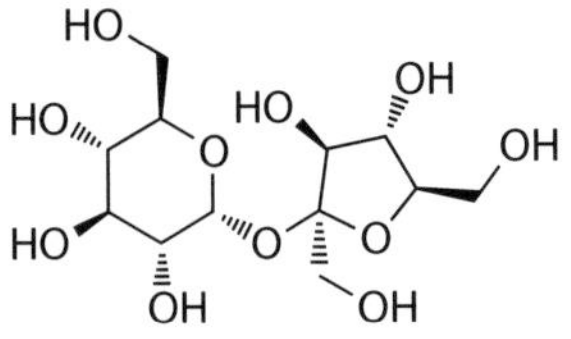	NA	1	329
Acesulfame potassium	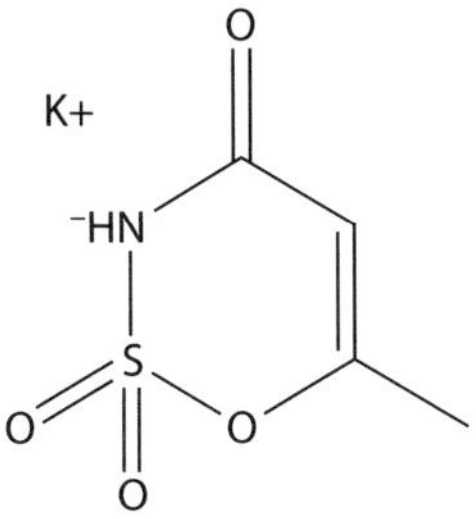	15 9 15 15	140	0.44
Advantame	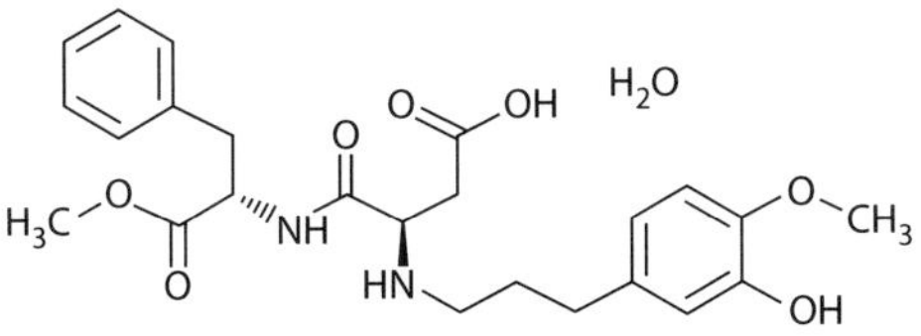	NA NA NA 5	20,000	0.015
Alitame	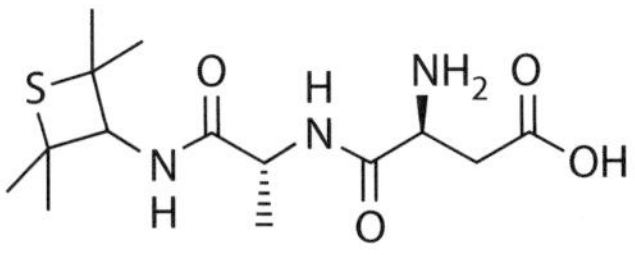	NA NA 1 1	2000	0.13
Aspartame	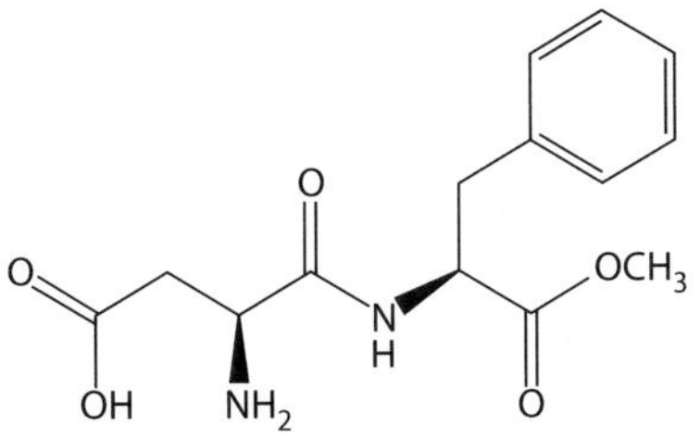	50 40 40 40	200	0.16
Cyclamate	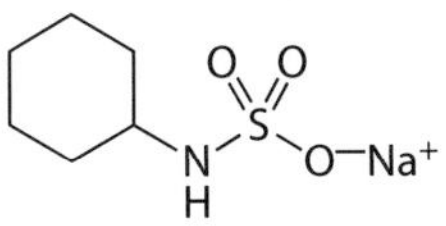	NA 7 11 11	32	0.86

continued

TABLE 7.1 (continued)
Approval Status, Chemical Structure, and Relative Sweetness of NNSs

Sweetener	Structure	ADI (mg/kg/day) USA EU JECFA FSANZ	Sweetness (Compared to 5% Sucrose)	Mean Concentration in Carbonated Soft Drinks (mmol/L)
Luo Han Guo	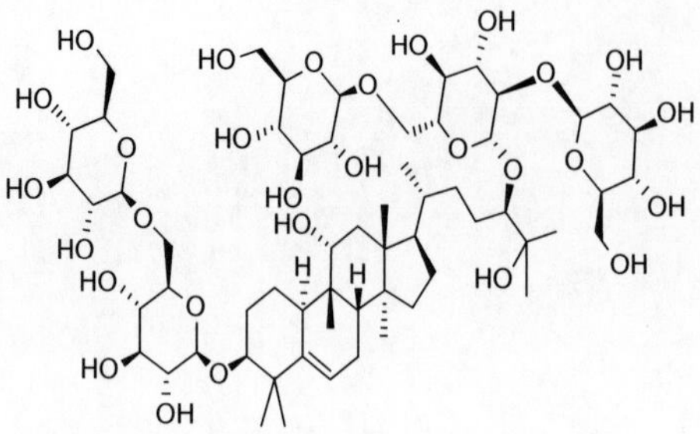	No ADI[a] NA[a] NA[a] NA[a]	150	Not tested
Neotame	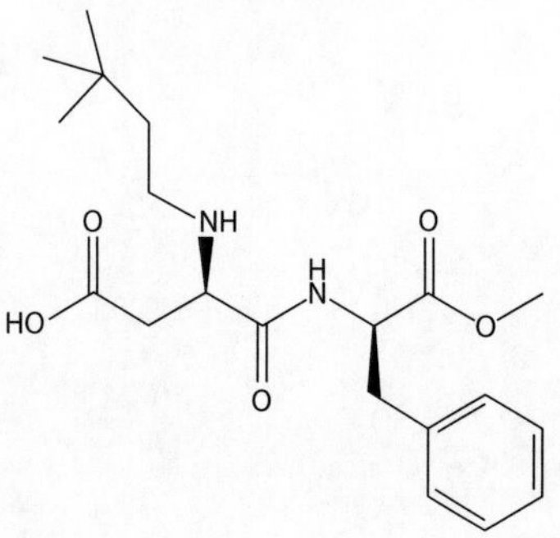	2 2 2 2	11,000	Not tested
Saccharin	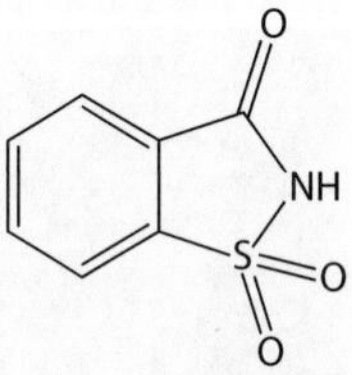	5 5 5 5	450	0.15
Steviol glycosides	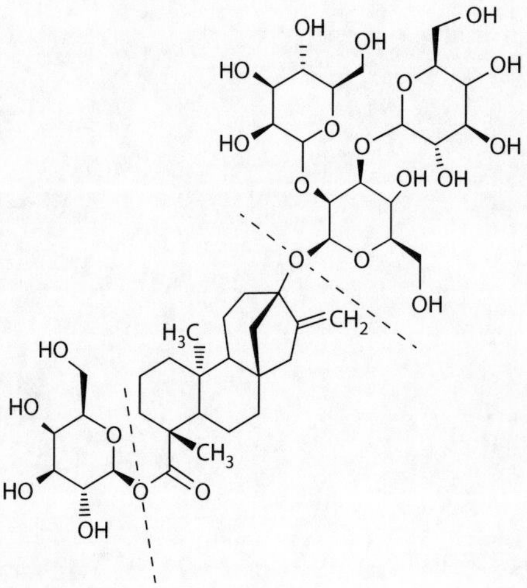	No ADI[b] No ADI[b] 4 4	250	Not tested

continued

TABLE 7.1 (continued)
Approval Status, Chemical Structure, and Relative Sweetness of NNSs

Sweetener	Structure	ADI (mg/kg/day) USA EU JECFA FSANZ	Sweetness (Compared to 5% Sucrose)	Mean Concentration in Carbonated Soft Drinks (mmol/L)
Sucralose	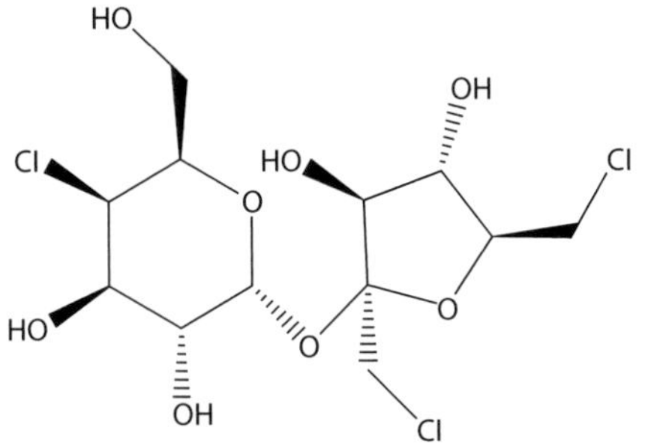	5 15 15 15	60	0.14

Note: Advantame was approved for use as a general purpose sweetener by the United States Food and Drug Administration in May 2014, subsequent to the writing of this chapter.

[a] Monk fruit extracts (Luo Han Guo) are not approved as food additives in the USA and have been designated GRAS as dietary supplements. Monk fruit extracts are also not yet approved for use as NNSs in Europe or Australia/New Zealand, but can be used as a flavor modifier.

[b] Extracts of the Stevia Rebaudiana Bertoni plant are approved for use as dietary supplements by the US FDA and as novel food ingredients in the European Union.

Cosmetic Act, requiring the FDA to approve food additives, such as artificial sweeteners. However, this legislation does not apply to products that are "generally recognized as safe (GRAS)" and thus do not require FDA approval. An example is luo han guo (monk fruit extract) which is a zero-calorie sweetener marketed alone and in combination with sucralose [6,7]. The difference between products that are labeled as food additives and others labeled as GRAS is not necessarily obvious. The primary distinguishing factor for being labeled as GRAS versus as a food additive is the level of common knowledge about the use and/or safety of the product in question (and not whether a product is plant-derived versus chemically synthesized) [8]. Cyclamate, which had been on the US market since the 1950s, was banned by the US FDA in 1969 due to concerns about bladder cancer, liver failure, and other negative health effects, but remains available in more than 50 other countries [9]. Alitame is a dipeptide compound similar to aspartame approved in Australia, New Zealand, Mexico, and China [10], and advantame is another dipeptide approved for use in Australia and New Zealand [11]. Petitions for these sweeteners have been submitted to the US FDA for approval (or re-approval, in the case of cyclamate).

The processes by which regulatory organizations including the FDA [12], the Bureau of Chemical Safety (Canada), the Scientific Committee on Food of the European Commission (Europe) [13], Food Standards Australia New Zealand (Australia and New Zealand) [14], and the Joint Expert Committee on Food Additives (JECFA) [15] (worldwide) regulate and approve the use of NNSs are similar, in that an acceptable daily intake (ADI) is established based on available toxicological data [16–18]. The ADI is the amount of a substance that people can consume on a daily basis during their whole life without any appreciable risk to health and is determined by dividing the lowest dose shown to cause toxicity in animal studies by a safety factor of 100. In order for an ADI to be established and an NNS approved for use, the manufacturer must submit a petition containing detailed information about the additive, its proposed use, the results of safety tests, and information on the sweetener's effectiveness for its intended use [16–18]. Identity and purity specifications are also developed [16] to ensure that the materials ingested are the same materials that were evaluated in toxicological testing and subsequently approved for general use. The ADI is then compared to estimates of consumption of the specific sweetener in the population and the sweetener is approved only if the ADI exceeds the estimated levels of actual intake [13,18,19]. In addition to the ADI, some regulatory organizations such as the Canadian Bureau of Health [20] and Food Standards Australia New Zealand also have detailed specifications for the amounts of each NNS that can be used in specific types of commercially prepared foods and beverages (shown in Table 7.1). In contrast, the FDA does not regulate the quantities of NNSs that can be added to different categories of manufactured foods and beverages (i.e., carbonated soft drinks or processed foods), with the exception of saccharin, for which stipulations for use in specific types of products exist. There are additional regulations for the use of tabletop sweeteners, which are regulated universally in accordance with good manufacturing practices, meaning that the lowest possible level of a food additive necessary for a specific function (sweetening) is to be used.

What Types of Foods and Beverages Are Sweetened with NNSs?

The availability of NNSs in commercially prepared foods and beverages has increased dramatically and thousands of new products containing NNSs have been released in the last decade [21]. The most commonly consumed NNS worldwide is sucralose, which recently surpassed aspartame to hold the majority of the market share [22]. NNSs are consumed by more than 200 million people around the world and are found in more than 6000 products [23]. Common types of items sweetened with NNSs include diet soda and other carbonated and noncarbonated soft drinks, powdered drink mixes, yogurts, puddings and fillings, condiments, canned fruit, frozen desserts, chewing gum, confections, gelatins, baked goods, breads, cereals, snack foods, frozen entrees, and tabletop sweeteners. Some pharmaceuticals (e.g., vitamins, sugar-free cough drops, and toothpaste) also contain NNSs.

Different NNSs are suitable for use in different types of products because each NNS has a different taste profile and dissimilar chemical and physical properties. For example, sucralose is highly stable and does not degrade at high temperatures [24], making it ideal for use in baked goods, whereas aspartame will degrade when heated [25]. Other sweeteners such as acesulfame potassium and saccharin also have bitter taste properties; as a result, acesulfame potassium is usually found blended with other NNSs, most commonly aspartame or sucralose [26]. Taste profiles of NNSs are also influenced by other food and beverage components including carbonation, pH, and the presence of other food ingredients such as gelling agents, starches, and fats [27].

How Common Is NNS consumption?

Consumption of NNSs occurs worldwide, yet up-to-date consumption data are scarce and are readily available only in the USA [28] and in several European countries [29–31]. Data from the Calorie Control Council showed that 85% of the US population reported ever using an NNS in 2007 [32], while a study evaluating daily NNS consumption using dietary recall data demonstrated that approximately 34% of adults and 15% of children in the USA reported use of NNSs on a given day [28]. European studies have provided similar estimates, with 36% of the general population reporting consumption of NNSs in Germany on a given day [30].

How Do Consumers Identify Foods and Beverages with NNSs?

Given that advances in food technology have enabled combinations of NNSs to closely resemble the taste of sugar, many food and beverage companies have turned to NNSs as a means of lowering the sugar and calorie content of their products. Food claims including "sugar-free," "no sugar added," "no added sugar," "reduced sugar," "light," "weight control," "carb smart," "low-carbohydrate," "low-joule," and "energy-reduced," often accompany products containing NNSs to increase their appeal to health- or weight-conscious consumers.

While the number of products sweetened with NNSs has increased [33], regulations requiring manufacturers to indicate the presence and quantity of NNSs in their products vary by country. In the USA, for example, the specific NNS (i.e., aspartame) must be listed on the ingredients label on the back of the package, yet information about the amount (milligrams) or concentration of each NNS in the product is not required. Since many consumers do not recognize NNSs by their generic names (e.g., acesulfame potassium), NNS-containing products are likely to be purchased and consumed without awareness of the presence of NNSs. In contrast, Canadian food and drug regulations require a statement on the principal display panel that the food "contains (name of the sweetener)" or is "sweetened with (name of the sweetener)" and also requires a listing of the sweetener content in milligrams per standard serving [34].

BIOLOGICAL EFFECTS OF NNSs

How Are NNSs Recognized by the Body?

All sweet compounds have the ability to bind to sweet-taste receptors, although they bind to different ligand binding domains of the receptor [35,36]. Sweet-tasting substances vary widely in chemical structure and include caloric sugars (e.g., sucrose, glucose, and fructose), sweet proteins such as thaumatin and monellin, sugar alcohols, and NNSs. Some of these chemicals bear structural homology to sucrose, while others do not. Important species differences exist in the perception of sweet tastes. For example, rodents do not perceive aspartame as sweet, and cats do not perceive sweet tastes at all [37].

Sweet tastes are sensed via heterodimeric G-protein-coupled taste receptors consisting of a T1R2 and T1R3 subunit. These receptors are located on taste receptor cells within taste buds of the tongue, and elsewhere in the oropharynx. When sweet-tasting compounds bind to sweet-taste receptors, associated G-proteins, such as α-gustducin, are activated, resulting in increased phospholipase Cβ2. This in turn leads to increases in second messengers inositol trisphosphate and diacylglycerol, resulting in activation of the taste-transduction channel, TRPM5 (transient receptor potential cation channel subfamily M member 5, also known as long transient receptor potential channel 5). Activation of this ion channel causes increased intracellular calcium and neurotransmitter release [38]. In cells of the oropharynx that express sweet-taste receptors, this neurotransmitter release conveys signals via projections to neurons in the brain, permitting conscious awareness of sweetness.

Where Are Sweet-Taste Receptors Located?

In recent years, sweet-taste receptors have been identified outside of the oral cavity using immunohistochemical stains for the receptor subunits or their associated G-proteins. Components of the sweet-taste signaling system have been identified in enteroendocrine L and K cells in the intestinal mucosa [39], pancreatic β-cells [40], preadipocytes [41], the biliary tract [42], and the lungs [43]. Stimulation of sweet-taste receptors outside of the oral cavity does not convey a conscious perception of sweetness; instead, these receptors appear to function as part of a nutrient-sensing system.

Among the extra-oral sweet-taste receptors, the role of enteroendocrine cell receptors has been best characterized. The functional importance of these receptors was studied in humans using an inhibitor of sweet-taste receptors, lactisole, which interferes with receptor signaling by binding to the transmembrane domain of the T1R3 subunit [44]. In healthy adults, secretion of hormones made by enteroendocrine L cells in response to an intragastric glucose infusion was decreased by the addition of lactisole, which resulted in approximately 25–50% lower glucagon-like peptide 1 (GLP-1), and approximately 15–30% lower peptide YY (PYY) concentrations [45,46]. In contrast, lactisole did not alter secretion of the hormone cholecystokinin (CCK), which is made by enteroendocrine I cells that do not express sweet-taste receptors. These data support a model in which hormone secretion from L-cells is partly, but not entirely, mediated via binding of ligands to sweet-taste receptors on those cells.

Do NNSs Have Effects via Extra-Oral Taste Receptors?

Since nutritive sweeteners (NSs) and NNSs bind to oral sweet-taste receptors, resulting in the perception of sweetness, one can hypothesize that NNS activation of extra-oral sweet-taste receptors may lead to signal transduction in the tissues where these receptors are expressed. Indeed, *in vitro* studies have demonstrated that GLP-1 [47,48] and glucose-dependent insulinotropic peptide (GIP) [48] secretion can be induced by the NNS sucralose and that this effect is mediated via sweet-taste receptors. Similarly, insulin secretion can be induced *in vitro* by exposure of pancreatic beta-cells to sucralose [40], saccharin [40,49], and acesulfame potassium [40], an effect also mediated by sweet-taste receptor signaling. If these *in vitro* data are applicable to whole organisms, it would suggest that NNSs could alter hormone secretion, potentially impacting glycemia and appetite. Other *in vitro* studies, however, have failed to demonstrate a GLP-1 or GIP response to NNSs [50,51].

Studies in humans and animals have shown that the NNSs sucralose, acesulfame potassium, stevia, and D-tryptophan (in animals) in the absence of glucose do not stimulate GLP-1, PYY, ghrelin, or GIP secretion [39,45,52–54]. Two human studies have suggested that NNSs might alter gut hormone secretion when given in conjunction with caloric sugars. Ingestion of sucralose and acesulfame potassium containing diet cola (versus a carbonated water control) increased glucose-stimulated total GLP-1 secretion in adolescents and young adults who were healthy or had type 1 diabetes [55,56]. However, the clinical significance of this finding was unclear, as no differences in glucose or insulin were observed. Another study [57] of overweight, African-American women demonstrated higher glucose and insulin responses after consumption of sucralose (versus a water control) prior to an oral glucose load, but did not show differences in active GLP-1 or GIP [57]. A third study showed no effect of intragastric sucralose in saline (versus a saline control) on either GLP-1 or blood glucose; insulin was not measured [58]. Taken together, these data support the notion that NNSs do not exert metabolic activity when administered alone but may have synergistic effects when administered in combination with NSs; however, the data supporting the synergistic effects of NNSs with NSs are conflicting and require confirmation [59]. Increases in the rate of intestinal glucose absorption [60] have also been demonstrated in response to NNSs in animal studies, but a single human study to date has not confirmed this effect [58]. Thus, at the current time, there is no good evidence that NNSs significantly alter glucose homeostasis via interactions with sweet-taste receptors *in vivo*.

HEALTH EFFECTS OF NNSs

Is There a Relationship between NNS Consumption and Body Weight?

From a theoretical perspective, replacing NSs with NNSs should cause a net reduction in caloric intake and hence result in weight loss or slowed weight gain. However, individuals using NNSs for weight control may consciously or unconsciously compensate for the reduced calorie intake. For example, they may replace a sugar-sweetened soda with a diet soda, but then allow themselves an extra cookie. In fact, several epidemiologic studies have shown NNS use to be associated with adverse health outcomes including weight gain [61–63], metabolic syndrome [64,65], and vascular dysfunction [66,67], leading to the hypothesis that dieters may *over*compensate for these "missing calories" from foods and drinks sweetened with NNSs, potentially resulting in sustained increases in caloric intake. Meanwhile, a minority of epidemiologic studies have shown no association or a negative association between NNS consumption and body weight [68–72].

What Are Plausible Explanations for the Observed Association between NNSs and Body Weight in Epidemiologic Studies?

In addition to caloric compensation, another explanation for the observed association between NNS consumption and body weight is that individuals who are already overweight or who have been gaining weight might consume NNSs as a strategy to reduce calorie intake, a phenomenon referred to as reverse causality [73]. However, several other explanations have been proposed to explain how NNS consumption could lead to changes in appetite and food intake, and, ultimately, promote weight gain and related complications. One explanation supported by rodent data is that NNS consumption may lead to a disconnect between sweetness and calories [74,75]. This could cause animals to associate sweetness with low caloric content, resulting in overeating and weight gain [76]. As detailed in the "How are NNSs Recognized by the Body?" section, another proposed explanation is that NNSs may alter gut peptide secretion through interactions with sweet-taste receptors present on intestinal enteroendocrine and pancreatic islet cells, potentially altering glycemia and satiety [77]. Finally, it has been suggested that consumption of NNSs may lead to alterations in preferences for sweet taste, thereby adversely affecting dietary patterns [78,79]. This is supported by cross-sectional data, such as those in the Nurses' Health Study, which have demonstrated that consumption of diet drinks is associated with poorer dietary patterns involving high intake of sugar-sweetened drinks, refined grains, and processed meat, and a lower intake of vegetables [80]. Positive correlations between consumption of carbonated soft drinks (regular and diet) and less healthy dietary patterns have been shown in numerous other cohorts [81–85]. However, contrasting data suggesting an association between NNS use and neutral [86] or even healthier [87] dietary patterns exist as well. While these proposed explanations have limited support in rodent studies, human data are lacking and additional experimental studies are required to determine whether NNSs play any causal role in weight change in humans.

What Have Intervention Trials Determined about NNSs and Body Weight?

A number of randomized controlled trials examining the effects of NNSs on body weight have been performed to help resolve the conundrum of observed associations between consumption of NNSs and weight gain in epidemiologic studies. In adults, short-term (3–10 weeks) randomized controlled trials of supplementation with sugar versus NNSs showed reduced calorie intake with NNSs, but minimal effects on body weight [88,89]. A long-term study randomizing adults to consume or abstain from NNSs showed no difference in weight loss, but reduced weight regain among the NNS consumers [90]. Similarly, an observational study showed that individuals who successfully maintained weight loss consumed more NNSs than those who experienced weight regain; however, weight loss maintainers used numerous other dietary strategies in addition to NNS use [91].

Among children, short-term (12–25 weeks) randomized controlled trials using NNSs showed no or minimal differences in weight or body mass index (BMI) z-scores between those randomized to NNSs versus not [1,92,93]. Two long-term (1–2 years) randomized controlled trials in children showed minimal (1–2 kg) but statistically lower body weight and/or weight gain in the groups randomized to NNSs [94,95]. In one of these studies, children were blinded to whether or not their drinks contained NNSs versus NSs [95]. The lower weight gain in the NNS group suggests that, when NNS is given covertly (i.e., without conscious awareness), children do not completely compensate for the "missing calories" from drinks with NNSs, leading to overall reduced caloric intake and slower weight gain. However, this study lacked a control arm (e.g., providing water), thus it remains unclear whether the children exposed to NNSs gained more weight than expected had no supplemental sweet drink been provided. In summary, randomized controlled trials of NNSs for weight control suggest that NNSs are weight-neutral or result in weight reduction that is not clinically significant in the management of obesity.

Is the Consumption of NNSs Associated with Other Adverse Health Effects?

In addition to the relationship between NNS consumption and body weight, observational studies have described associations between NNS and a variety of negative health effects. Two Scandinavian natural history studies reported that consumption of NNS-containing beverages by pregnant woman was associated with preterm delivery. It was suggested that metabolites of aspartame, acesulfame potassium, saccharin, and cyclamate may have played a role [96,97]. In the Nurses' Health Study it was found that women who consumed two or more servings per day of diet soda were at a 2-fold increased risk for clinically relevant worsening of renal function [98]. The authors pointed out that limitations of their analysis included the inability to pinpoint consumption to specific sweeteners or other ingredients in diet soda. Based on analyses from the Health Professionals Follow-Up Study, it was recently reported that men who consumed more than one daily serving of diet soda had an increased risk of developing non-Hodgkin lymphoma and multiple myeloma in comparison with men who did not consume diet soda [99]. However, the same findings were not observed in women enrolled in the Nurses' Health Study. Further reports have concluded that there may be a link between stroke and diet soft drink consumption [100], though the association was only marginally significant and was no longer significant after adjustment for BMI and diabetes status. While the results of these epidemiologic studies are thought-provoking, the contribution of NNSs relative to additional dietary and life-style factors remains unknown. Few studies have distinguished among the various NNSs, each of which has different chemical properties. This reinforces the need to improve dietary assessment of NNS consumption and to reduce the number of confounders to enable future studies to pinpoint specific compounds requiring further analysis.

Do NNSs Activate Reward Pathways in the Brain?

Reward is defined as a positive stimulus that reinforces a behavior and increases the probability of performing that behavior [101]. In fact, studies show that reward pathways activated in response to the consumption of palatable foods and beverages are similar to those involved in the brain response to alcohol and other drugs of abuse. Food- and drug-induced reward responses are largely controlled by the neurotransmitter dopamine and involve several brain regions including the ventral tegmental area, the hypothalamus, medial forebrain bundle, and the prefrontal cortex [102]. Analogous to the development of tolerance in drug users, recent research has shown that reward responses to sweet taste may differ according to whether or not an individual habitually consumes NNSs [103,104].

In several studies using functional magnetic resonance imaging, it was found that NNSs only partially replicate brain responses elicited by NSs. In two human studies, NSs (e.g., glucose or sucrose) activated reward circuits to a greater extent than NNSs (e.g., sucralose and aspartame) [105, 106]. Similar results have been demonstrated in rodent experiments, during which animals without functional sweet-taste receptors released more dopamine when given solutions of sucrose compared to sucralose, supporting the necessity of a caloric stimulus in fully activating reward circuits [107]. Thus, it appears that NNSs are differentiated from NSs in the human brain, yet whether or not this distinction influences food choices remains to be elucidated.

UNANSWERED QUESTIONS AND FUTURE DIRECTIONS

The growing presence of NNSs in commercially available foods and beverages, as well as in the soil [108] and in the water supply [109], raises questions about their role in human health. Important areas which require further study include how NNSs may influence the intestinal microbiome and gut function and to which compartments NNSs and their metabolites are localized following ingestion [110–112]. Additional questions relating specifically to the role of NNSs in weight management include whether NNSs influence the development of taste preferences in young children, how NNSs may impact glucose homeostasis and satiety hormone response following prolonged exposure, and the ways in which NNSs may impact the central reward system. It is imperative that additional clinical and laboratory research be conducted to address these questions, as public health campaigns to reduce the consumption of added sugars are likely to result in continued increases in the consumption of NNSs.

REFERENCES

1. Brown RJ, de Banate MA, Rother KI. Artificial sweeteners: A systematic review of metabolic effects in youth. *Int J Pediatr Obes*. 2010;5(4):305–12. Epub 2010/01/19.
2. Gardner C, Wylie-Rosett J, Gidding SS, Steffen LM, Johnson RK, Reader D et al. Nonnutritive sweeteners: Current use and health perspectives. A scientific statement from the American Heart Association and the American Diabetes Association. *Circulation*. 2012;126(4):509–19.
3. Bartoshuk LM. Artificial sweeteners: Outwitting the wisdom of the body? *Observer*. 2009; 22(8).
4. Schiffman S, Sattely-Miller E, Ihab B. Sensory properties of neotame: Comparison with other sweeteners. *Sweetness and Sweeteners*. Washington DC: American Chemical Society; 2008. p. 511–29.
5. DuBois Grant E, Walters DE, Schiffman Susan S, Warwick Zoe S, Booth Barbara J, Pecore Suzanne D et al. Concentration? Response relationships of sweeteners. *Sweeteners*. Washington DC: American Chemical Society; 1991. p. 261–76.
6. BioVittoria. Biovittoria: The Monk Fruit Company. 2013; Available from: http://www.biovittoria.com/.
7. Niutang. 2013; Available from: http://www.niutang.com/food-ingredients/sweeteners/monk-fruit/.
8. Neltner TG, Alger HM, O'Reilly JT, Krimsky S, Bero LA, Maffini MV. Conflicts of interest in approvals of additives to food determined to be generally recognized as safe: Out of balance. *JAMA Intern Med.* 2013;173(22):2032–6.
9. Calorie Control Council. Worldwide Approval Status of Cyclamate. Atlanta, GA: Calorie Control Council; 2009.
10. Calorie Control Council. Alitame. 2013; Available from: http://www.caloriecontrol.org/sweeteners-and-lite/sugar-substitutes/other-sweeteners/alitame.
11. AJINOMOTO. Advantame. 2013; Available from: http://www.advantame.com/.
12. Food Additives Permitted for Direct Addition to Food for Human Consumption, 21 CFF Part 172, 1999.
13. European Commission Scientific Committee on Food. Opinion of the Scientific Committee on Food: Update on the Safety of Aspartame. 2002.
14. Australian Government. Australia New Zealand Food Standards Code-Standard 1.3.1-Food Additives. 2013.
15. Online Editon: Combined Comendium of Food Additive Specifications, 2013.
16. World Health Organization. Food Safety-About the Joint Fao/Who Expert Committee on Food Additives (Jecfa). 2013.
17. United States Food and Drug Administration. Guidance for Industry and Other Stakeholders: Toxicological Principles for the Safety Assessment of Food Ingredients. In: Department of Health and Human Services, editor. 2000.
18. Health Canada. Food Additives. 2005.
19. United States Food and Drug Administration. Guidance for Industry: Estimating Dietary Intake of Substances in Food. In: United States Department of Health and Human Services, editor. 2006.
20. Health Canada. Lists of permitted food additives. 2013; Available from: http://www.hc-sc.gc.ca/fn-an/securit/addit/list/9-sweetener-edulcorant-eng.php.
21. Yang Q. Gain weight by "going diet?" Artificial sweeteners and the neurobiology of sugar cravings: Neuroscience 2010. *Yale J Biol Med*. 2010;83(2):101–8.
22. BCC Research. Global markets for sugars and sweeteners in processed foods and beverages. 2013.
23. Calorie Control Council. Aspartame Information Center: Consumer Products. 2013.
24. Knight I. The development and applications of sucralose, a new high-intensity sweetener. *Can J Physiol Pharmacol*. 1994;72(4):435–9.
25. Boehm MF, Bada JL. Racemization of aspartic acid and phenylalanine in the sweetener aspartame at 100 degrees C. *Proc Natl Acad Sci USA*. 1984;81(16):5263–6.
26. Calorie Control Council. The facts about acesulfame-potassium. 2010; Available from: http://www.acesulfamek.org/.
27. Binns NM. Sucralose—All sweetness and light. *Nutr Bull*. 2003;28:53–8.
28. Sylvetsky AC, Welsh JA, Brown RJ, Vos MB. Low-calorie sweetener consumption is increasing in the United States. *Am J Clin Nutr*. 2012;96(3):640–6.

29. Leth T, Fabricius N, Fagt S. Estimated intake of intense sweeteners from nonalcoholic beverages in Denmark. *Food Addit Contam*. 2007;24(3):227–35.
30. Bar A, Biermann C. Intake of intense sweeteners in Germany. *Z Ernahrungswiss*. 1992;31(1):25–39.
31. Ilback NG, Alzin M, Jahrl S, Enghardt-Barbieri H, Busk L. Estimated intake of the artificial sweeteners acesulfame-K, aspartame, cyclamate and saccharin in a group of Swedish diabetics. *Food Addit Contam*. 2003;20(2):99–114.
32. Bloomgarden ZT. Nonnutritive sweeteners, fructose, and other aspects of diet. *Diabetes Care*. 2011;34(5):e46–51.
33. Piernas C, Ng SW, Popkin B. Trends in purchases and intake of foods and beverages containing caloric and low-calorie sweeteners over the last decade in the United States. *Pediatr Obes*. 2013;8(4):294–306. Epub 2013/03/27.
34. Canadian Food Inspection Agency. Chapter 9: Supplementary Information on Specific Products. 2011.
35. Xu H, Staszewski L, Tang H, Adler E, Zoller M, Li X. Different functional roles of T1r subunits in the heteromeric taste receptors. *Proc Natl Acad Sci USA*. 2004;101(39):14258–63.
36. Jiang P, Ji Q, Liu Z, Snyder LA, Benard LM, Margolskee RF et al. The cysteine-rich region of T1r3 determines responses to intensely sweet proteins. *J Biol Chem*. 2004;279(43):45068–75. Epub 2004/08/10.
37. Nelson G, Hoon MA, Chandrashekar J, Zhang Y, Ryba NJ, Zuker CS. Mammalian sweet taste receptors. *Cell*. 2001;106(3):381–90.
38. Chandrashekar J, Hoon MA, Ryba NJ, Zuker CS. The receptors and cells for mammalian taste. *Nature*. 2006;444(7117):288–94. Epub 2006/11/17.
39. Fujita Y, Wideman RD, Speck M, Asadi A, King DS, Webber TD et al. Incretin release from gut is acutely enhanced by sugar but not by sweeteners in vivo. *Am J Physiol Endocrinol Metab*. 2009;296(3):E473–9.
40. Nakagawa Y, Nagasawa M, Yamada S, Hara A, Mogami H, Nikolaev VO et al. Sweet taste receptor expressed in pancreatic beta-cells activates the calcium and cyclic amp signaling systems and stimulates insulin secretion. *PLoS One*. 2009;4(4):e5106. Epub 2009/04/09.
41. Masubuchi Y, Nakagawa Y, Ma J, Sasaki T, Kitamura T, Yamamoto Y et al. A novel regulatory function of sweet taste-sensing receptor in adipogenic differentiation of 3t3-L1 cells. *PLoS One*. 2013;8(1):e54500.
42. Toyono T, Seta Y, Kataoka S, Toyoshima K. Ccaat/enhancer-binding protein beta regulates expression of human T1r3 taste receptor gene in the bile duct carcinoma cell line, Hucct1. *Biochim Biophys Acta*. 2007;1769(11–12):641–8. Epub 2007/10/12.
43. Finger TE, Kinnamon SC. Taste isn't just for taste buds anymore. F1000. *Biol Rep*. 2011;3:20. Epub 2011/09/24.
44. Jiang P, Cui M, Zhao B, Liu Z, Snyder LA, Benard LM et al. Lactisole interacts with the transmembrane domains of human T1r3 to inhibit sweet taste. *J Biol Chem*. 2005;280(15):15238–46. Epub 2005/01/26.
45. Steinert RE, Gerspach AC, Gutmann H, Asarian L, Drewe J, Beglinger C. The functional involvement of gut-expressed sweet taste receptors in glucose-stimulated secretion of glucagon-like peptide-1 (Glp-1) and peptide Yy (Pyy). *Clin Nutr*. 2011;30(4):524–32. Epub 2011/02/18.
46. Gerspach AC, Steinert RE, Schonenberger L, Graber-Maier A, Beglinger C. The role of the gut sweet taste receptor in regulating Glp-1, Pyy, and Cck release in humans. *Am J Physiol Endocrinol Metab*. 2011;301(2):E317–25. Epub 2011/05/05.
47. Jang HJ, Kokrashvili Z, Theodorakis MJ, Carlson OD, Kim BJ, Zhou J et al. Gut-expressed gustducin and taste receptors regulate secretion of glucagon-like peptide-1. *Proc Natl Acad Sci USA*. 2007;104(38):15069–74.
48. Margolskee RF, Dyer J, Kokrashvili Z, Salmon KS, Ilegems E, Daly K et al. T1r3 and gustducin in gut sense sugars to regulate expression of Na + -glucose cotransporter 1. *Proc Natl Acad Sci USA*. 2007;104(38):15075–80.
49. Corkey BE. Banting Lecture 2011: Hyperinsulinemia: Cause or consequence? *Diabetes*. 2012;61(1):4–13. Epub 2011/12/22.
50. Reimann F, Habib AM, Tolhurst G, Parker HE, Rogers GJ, Gribble FM. Glucose sensing in L cells: A primary cell study. *Cell Metab*. 2008;8(6):532–9. Epub 2008/12/02.
51. Parker HE, Habib AM, Rogers GJ, Gribble FM, Reimann F. Nutrient-dependent secretion of glucose-dependent insulinotropic polypeptide from primary murine K cells. *Diabetologia*. 2009;52(2):289–98. Epub 2008/12/17.
52. Ma J, Bellon M, Wishart JM, Young R, Blackshaw LA, Jones KL et al. Effect of the artificial sweetener, sucralose, on gastric emptying and incretin hormone release in healthy subjects. *Am J Physiol Gastrointest Liver Physiol*. 2009;296(4):G735–9. Epub 2009/02/18.

53. Ford HE, Peters V, Martin NM, Sleeth ML, Ghatei MA, Frost GS et al. Effects of oral ingestion of sucralose on gut hormone response and appetite in healthy normal-weight subjects. *Eur J Clin Nutr.* 2011;65(4):508–13. Epub 2011/01/20.
54. Brown AW, Bohan Brown MM, Onken KL, Beitz DC. Short-term consumption of sucralose, a non-nutritive sweetener, is similar to water with regard to select markers of hunger signaling and short-term glucose homeostasis in women. *Nutr Res.* 2011;31(12):882–8. Epub 2011/12/14.
55. Brown RJ, Walter M, Rother KI. Ingestion of diet soda before a glucose load augments glucagon-like peptide-1 secretion. *Diabetes Care.* 2009;32(12):2184–6. Epub 2009/10/08.
56. Brown RJ, Walter M, Rother KI. Effects of diet soda on gut hormones in youths with diabetes. *Diabetes care.* May 2012; 35(5):959–964.
57. Pepino MY, Tiemann CD, Patterson BW, Wice BM, Klein S. Sucralose affects glycemic and hormonal responses to an oral glucose load. *Diabetes Care.* 2013;36(9):2530–5. Epub 2013/05/02.
58. Ma J, Chang J, Checklin HL, Young RL, Jones KL, Horowitz M et al. Effect of the artificial sweetener, sucralose, on small intestinal glucose absorption in healthy human subjects. *Br J Nutr.* 2010;104(6):803–6. Epub 2010/04/28.
59. Brown RJ, Rother KI. Non-nutritive sweeteners and their role in the gastrointestinal tract. *J Clin Endocrinol Metab.* 2012;97(8):2597–605.
60. Mace OJ, Affleck J, Patel N, Kellett GL. Sweet taste receptors in rat small intestine stimulate glucose absorption through apical Glut2. *J Physiol.* 2007;582(Pt 1):379–92.
61. Stellman SD, Garfinkel L. Artificial sweetener use and one-year weight change among women. *Prev Med.* 1986;15(2):195–202.
62. Fowler SP, Williams K, Resendez RG, Hunt KJ, Hazuda HP, Sterns MP. Fueling the obesity epidemic? Artificially sweetened beverage use and long-term weight gain. *Obesity (Silver Spring).* 2008;16(8):1894–900.
63. Colditz GA, Willett WC, Stampfer MJ, London SJ, Segal MR, Speizer FE. Patterns of weight change and their relation to diet in a cohort of healthy women. *Am J Clin Nutr.* 1990;51(6):1100–5.
64. Nettleton JA, Lutsey PL, Wang Y, Lima JA, Michos ED, Jacobs Jr DR. Diet soda intake and risk of incident metabolic syndrome and type 2 diabetes in the multi-ethnic study of atherosclerosis. *Diabetes Care.* 2009;32(4):688–94.
65. Lutsey PL, Steffen LM, Stevens J. Dietary intake and the development of the metabolic syndrome: The atherosclerosis risk in communities study. *Circulation.* 2008;117(6):754–61.
66. Gardener H, Rundek T, Markert M, Wright CB, Elkind MS, Sacco RL. Diet soft drink consumption is associated with an increased risk of vascular events in the Northern Manhattan Study. *J Gen Intern Med.* 2012;27(9):1120–6. Epub 2012/01/28.
67. Dhingra R, Sullivan L, Jacques PF, Wang TJ, Fox CS, Meigs JB et al. Soft drink consumption and risk of developing cardiometabolic risk factors and the metabolic syndrome in middle-aged adults in the community. *Circulation.* 2007;116(5):480–8.
68. Kral TV, Stunkard AJ, Berkowitz RI, Stallings VA, Moore RH, Faith MS. Beverage consumption patterns of children born at different risk of obesity. *Obesity (Silver Spring).* 2008;16(8):1802–8. Epub 2008/06/07.
69. Serra-Majem L, Ribas L, Ingles C, Fuentes M, Lloveras G, Salleras L. Cyclamate consumption in Catalonia, Spain (1992): Relationship with the body mass index. *Food Addit Contam.* 1996;13(6):695–703.
70. Striegel-Moore RH, Thompson D, Affenito SG, Franko DL, Obarzanek E, Barton BA et al. Correlates of beverage intake in adolescent girls: The National Heart, Lung, and Blood Institute Growth and Health Study. *J Pediatr.* 2006;148(2):183–7.
71. Newby PK, Peterson KE, Berkey CS, Leppert J, Willett WC, Colditz GA. Beverage consumption is not associated with changes in weight and body mass index among low-income preschool children in North Dakota. *J Am Diet Assoc.* 2004;104(7):1086–94.
72. Anderson GH, Foreyt J, Sigman-Grant M, Allison DB. The use of low-calorie sweeteners by adults: Impact on weight management. *J Nutr.* 2012;142(6):1163S–9S.
73. Pepino MY, Bourne C. Non-nutritive sweeteners, energy balance, and glucose homeostasis. *Curr Opin Clin Nutr Metab Care.* 2011;14(4):391–5.
74. Swithers SE, Martin AA, Davidson TL. High-intensity sweeteners and energy balance. *Physiol Behav.* 2010;100(1):55–62. Epub 2010/01/12.
75. Swithers SE. Artificial sweeteners produce the counterintuitive effect of inducing metabolic derangements. *Trends Endocrinol Metab.* 2013;24(9):431–41.
76. Swithers SE, Laboy AF, Clark K, Cooper S, Davidson TL. Experience with the high-intensity sweetener saccharin impairs glucose homeostasis and Glp-1 release in rats. *Behav Brain Res.* 2012;233(1):1–14.

77. Egan JM, Margolskee RF. Taste cells of the gut and gastrointestinal chemosensation. *Mol Interv.* 2008;8(2):78–81. Epub 2008/04/12.
78. Birch LL, Anzman-Frasca S. Learning to prefer the familiar in obesogenic environments. *Nestle Nutr Workshop Ser Pediatr Program.* 2011;68:187–96; discussion 96–9. Epub 2011/11/03.
79. Sartor F, Donaldson LF, Markland DA, Loveday H, Jackson MJ, Kubis HP. Taste perception and implicit attitude toward sweet related to body mass index and soft drink supplementation. *Appetite.* 2011;57(1):237–46.
80. Schulze MB, Hoffmann K, Manson JE, Willett WC, Meigs JB, Weikert C et al. Dietary pattern, inflammation, and incidence of type 2 diabetes in women. *Am J Clin Nutr.* 2005;82(3):675–84; quiz 714–5.
81. Marshall TA, Eichenberger Gilmore JM, Broffitt B, Stumbo PJ, Levy SM. Diet quality in young children is influenced by beverage consumption. *J Am Coll Nutr.* 2005;24(1):65–75.
82. Leung CW, Ding EL, Catalano PJ, Villamor E, Rimm EB, Willett WC. Dietary intake and dietary quality of low-income adults in the supplemental nutrition assistance program. *Am J Clin Nutr.* 2012;96(5):977–88.
83. Ranjit N, Evans MH, Byrd-Williams C, Evans AE, Hoelscher DM. Dietary and activity correlates of sugar-sweetened beverage consumption among adolescents. *Pediatrics.* 2010;126(4):e754–61.
84. Mullie P, Aerenhouts D, Clarys P. Demographic, socioeconomic and nutritional determinants of daily versus non-daily sugar-sweetened and artificially sweetened beverage consumption. *Eur J Clin Nutr.* 2012;66(2):150–5.
85. Fiorito LM, Marini M, Mitchell DC, Smiciklas-Wright H, Birch LL. Girls' early sweetened carbonated beverage intake predicts different patterns of beverage and nutrient intake across childhood and adolescence. *J Am Diet Assoc.* 2010;110(4):543–50.
86. Piernas C, Tate DF, Wang X, Popkin BM. Does diet-beverage intake affect dietary consumption patterns? Results from the Choose Healthy Options Consciously Everyday (Choice) Randomized Clinical Trial. *Am J Clin Nutr.* 2013;97(3):604–11.
87. Binkley J, Golub A. Comparison of grocery purchase patterns of diet soda buyers to those of regular soda buyers. *Appetite.* 2007;49(3):561–71.
88. Tordoff MG, Alleva AM. Effect of drinking soda sweetened with aspartame or high-fructose corn syrup on food intake and body weight. *Am J Clin Nutr.* 1990;51(6):963–9.
89. Raben A, Vasilaras TH, Moller AC, Astrup A. Sucrose compared with artificial sweeteners: Different effects on ad libitum food intake and body weight after 10 wk of supplementation in overweight subjects. *Am J Clin Nutr.* 2002;76(4):721–9.
90. Blackburn GL, Kanders BS, Lavin PT, Keller SD, Whatley J. The effect of aspartame as part of a multidisciplinary weight-control program on short- and long-term control of body weight. *Am J Clin Nutr.* 1997;65(2):409–18.
91. Phelan S, Lang W, Jordan D, Wing RR. Use of artificial sweeteners and fat-modified foods in weight loss maintainers and always-normal weight individuals. *Int J Obes (Lond).* 2009;33(10):1183–90.
92. Williams CL, Strobino BA, Brotanek J. Weight control among obese adolescents: A pilot study. *Int J Food Sci Nutr.* 2007;58(3):217–30.
93. Ebbeling CB, Feldman HA, Osganian SK, Chomitz VR, Ellenbogen SJ, Ludwig DS. Effects of decreasing sugar-sweetened beverage consumption on body weight in adolescents: A randomized, controlled pilot study. *Pediatrics.* 2006;117(3):673–80. Epub 2006/03/03.
94. Ebbeling CB, Feldman HA, Chomitz VR, Antonelli TA, Gortmaker SL, Osganian SK et al. A randomized trial of sugar-sweetened beverages and adolescent body weight. *N Engl J Med.* 2012;367(15):1407–16.
95. de Ruyter JC, Olthof MR, Seidell JC, Katan MB. A trial of sugar-free or sugar-sweetened beverages and body weight in children. *N Engl J Med.* 2012;367(15):1397–406. Epub 2012/09/25.
96. Englund-Ogge L, Brantsaeter AL, Haugen M, Sengpiel V, Khatibi A, Myhre R et al. Association between intake of artificially sweetened and sugar-sweetened beverages and preterm delivery: A large prospective cohort study. *Am J Clin Nutr.* 2012;96(3):552–9. Epub 2012/08/03.
97. Halldorsson TI, Strom M, Petersen SB, Olsen SF. Intake of artificially sweetened soft drinks and risk of preterm delivery: A prospective cohort study in 59,334 Danish pregnant women. *Am J Clin Nutr.* 2010;92(3):626–33.
98. Lin J, Curhan GC. Associations of sugar and artificially sweetened soda with albuminuria and kidney function decline in women. *Clin J Am Soc Nephrol.* 2011;6(1):160–6.
99. Schernhammer ES, Bertrand KA, Birmann BM, Sampson L, Willett WC, Feskanich D. Consumption of artificial sweetener- and sugar-containing soda and risk of lymphoma and leukemia in men and women. *Am J Clin Nutr.* 2012;96(6):1419–28.
100. Fung TT, Malik V, Rexrode KM, Manson JE, Willett WC, Hu FB. Sweetened beverage consumption and risk of coronary heart disease in women. *Am J Clin Nutr.* 2009;89(4):1037–42.

101. McClure SM, York MK, Montague PR. The neural substrates of reward processing in humans: The modern role of fMRI. *Neuroscientist.* 2004;10(3):260–8.
102. Wise RA. Neurobiology of addiction. *Curr Opin Neurobiol.* 1996;6(2):243–51.
103. Green E, Murphy C. Altered processing of sweet taste in the brain of diet soda drinkers. *Physiol Behav.* 2012;107(4):560–7.
104. Rudenga KJ, Small DM. Amygdala response to sucrose consumption is inversely related to artificial sweetener use. *Appetite.* 2012;58(2):504–7.
105. Frank GK, Oberndorfer TA, Simmons AN, Paulus MP, Fudge JL, Yang TT et al. Sucrose activates human taste pathways differently from artificial sweetener. *Neuroimage.* 2008;39(4):1559–69.
106. Smeets PA, Weijzen P, de Graaf C, Viergever MA. Consumption of caloric and non-caloric versions of a soft drink differentially affects brain activation during tasting. *Neuroimage.* 2011;54(2):1367–74. Epub 2010/09/02.
107. de Araujo IE, Oliveira-Maia AJ, Sotnikova TD, Gainetdinov RR, Caron MG, Nicolelis MA et al. Food reward in the absence of taste receptor signaling. *Neuron.* 2008;57(6):930–41. Epub 2008/03/28.
108. Scheurer M, Brauch HJ, Lange FT. Analysis and occurrence of seven artificial sweeteners in German waste water and surface water and in soil aquifer treatment (Sat). *Anal Bioanal Chem.* 2009;394(6):1585–94.
109. Lange FT, Scheurer M, Brauch HJ. Artificial sweeteners—A recently recognized class of emerging environmental contaminants: A review. *Anal Bioanal Chem.* 2012;403(9):2503–18.
110. Abou-Donia MB, El-Masry EM, Abdel-Rahman AA, McLendon RE, Schiffman SS. Splenda alters gut microflora and increases intestinal P-glycoprotein and cytochrome P-450 in male rats. *J Toxicol Environ Health A.* 2008;71(21):1415–29.
111. Schiffman SS, Abou-Donia MB. Sucralose revisited: Rebuttal of two papers about splenda safety. *Regul Toxicol Pharmacol.* 2012;63(3):505–8; author reply 9–13.
112. Schiffman SS. Rationale for further medical and health research on high-potency sweeteners. *Chem Senses.* 2012;37(8):671–9.

8 Nutrition Economics Related to Consumption of Dietary Sugars

Adam Drewnowski

CONTENTS

KEY POINTS

- Diet-related chronic diseases, including obesity and diabetes, follow a social gradient. Higher rates are observed in poor neighborhoods and among lower-income groups.
- One of the mediating factors may be diet quality. Diet quality is related to food prices and diet costs. Lower-cost diets can be energy-rich but nutrient-poor.
- Based on observed eating habits in countries including the USA and France, the recommended healthier diets cost approximately $1.50 more per 2000 kcal.
- In France, each additional 100 g of fats and sweets reduced diet cost by 0.05–0.40 Euros per day.
- Lower-income groups consume lower-cost diets. Such groups may also differ in other unobserved ways from higher-income groups.
- The consumption of added sugars in the USA was inversely linked to education and incomes. The effect of education was estimated at 4 tsp/day or 64 kcal/day.
- It is difficult to separate the effect on health of a single food or dietary ingredient from the broader effects of chronic poverty, poor housing, or unemployment.
- The continued focus on single nutrients may be misplaced: it is time to address food patterns in their totality.
- Food patterns reflect socio-demographics, culture, and social norms.
- Food patterns may be context-specific, reflecting the local built environment. New measures of socioeconomic status now include neighborhood residential property values and supermarket choice.

- Lower diet costs may be a better predictor of adverse health outcomes than any one food or nutrient.

INTRODUCTION

Diet-related chronic diseases are known to follow a socioeconomic gradient [1–3]. In more affluent societies, groups with lower education and incomes suffer from higher rates of obesity, type 2 diabetes (T2D), and cardiovascular disease (CVD). While all groups consume similar amounts of dietary energy, lower-income groups have both cheaper and lower-quality diets. Although sugar-rich diets cost less per calorie, the recommended higher-quality diets generally cost more [4]. Unacknowledged disparities in diet quality and diet cost may be at the root of the observed socioeconomic disparities in health [1,5].

Whether dietary sugar or dietary fat is the principal cause of the global obesity epidemic is a contentious issue. In the past years, dietary fat was said to be the principal cause of obesity and weight gain [6]. With attention shifting to dietary sugars, studies have explored temporal parallels between rising obesity rates and the rising consumption of added sugars, including both sucrose and high-fructose corn syrup (HFCS) [7,8]. The consumption of HFCS-sweetened beverages, in particular, was linked to T2D, CVD risk, and long-term weight gain [9]. The links between dietary sugars and health outcomes are reviewed more specifically in other chapters in this book.

What diets high in added sugars and added fats have in common is the lower per calorie diet cost [10]. The inclusion of the cost variable in dietary studies may help explain why obesity and other diet-related diseases are concentrated among the lower socioeconomic status (SES) groups [1]. To date, relatively few epidemiologic studies have focused on the role of cheap added sugars in relation to body weights and health [10–14]. Rather, the impact of dietary sugars on health continues to be viewed through the prism of physiology and metabolism. Yet the main contribution of added sugars to overeating and weight gain may be through their greater affordability, real or perceived, to lower-income groups [10]. Differences in food prices and diet costs may help explain, if only in part, the observed impact of socioeconomic variables on body weights and health [1].

First, lower-cost diets are more likely to be energy-rich but nutrient-poor [4,15]. Based on existing food prices and eating habits, diets high in added sugars cost less, whereas the recommended nutrient-rich diets cost more [4]. Second, there is general agreement that the recommended diets containing vegetables, whole fruit, whole grains, nuts, and seafood are associated with better health outcomes [16,17]. Such diets are not only more expensive, but are also consumed by higher-income groups [18,19]. By contrast, lower-cost, lower-quality diets tend to be consumed by the poor [14,20].

Despite best attempts, studies in nutritional epidemiology have not been successful in separating a given food or dietary ingredient from the person consuming it. As studies in social sciences have shown, food consumption patterns represent a key component of social and cultural identity [21]. Higher consumption of added sugars has been associated both with lower diet cost per calorie [4] and with lower education and incomes [22]. In other words, added sugars consumption in the USA appears to be inversely associated with social class.

The intrusion of social class into epidemiologic studies has further implications for clinicians and for public health policy. Consumers of healthier and therefore more expensive diets are likely to be wealthier, better educated, insured, and may have more opportunities to purchase better foods or engage in physical activity than do the poor [5]. Different levels of nutrient exposure, adjusted for energy, may be associated further with unobserved differences in neighborhood wealth, social capital, and social context. As discussed below, such socio-demographic factors are either missing from epidemiologic studies altogether or, even when available, are treated as covariates rather than as important variables in their own right [23]. Based on existing studies on consumer profiles and their diet quality in relation to diet cost, chronic disease prevention appears to be an economic issue [24].

CURRENT KNOWLEDGE

The present review of current knowledge covers studies in nutrition economics on the relation between the various dietary sugars (including sucrose and HFCS), prevailing food prices, and estimated diet costs. Studies continue to link the consumption of low-cost foods with weight gain, whereas the consumption of more expensive foods tends to be associated with weight loss [16]. Yet the likely influence of food prices on dietary choices is rarely acknowledged in mainstream studies on diets and health [5].

The mechanisms by which SES influences dietary choices are difficult to isolate and quantify. Food choices are subject to a myriad of influences at the individual, group, and societal levels and there are many reasons why lower-income groups select cheaper energy-dense foods [25]. While limited economic resources are one barrier, attitudes and nutrition knowledge have also been implicated in food selection [26]. The present emphasis will be on the relatively understudied economics of food choice. Discussing the role of dietary sugars in nutrition economics is the specific purpose of this review.

Much of the evidence that SES factors affect diet quality has come from studies of household food expenditures. However, studies on household food expenditures have not collected any data on health outcomes, whereas studies on diets and disease risk have not concerned themselves with food prices and diet costs. Further, although food expenditures are typically collected at the household level, epidemiologic studies on diet quality, body weights, and health require that data be collected at the individual level. Reconciling these diverse approaches to the study of dietary choices has been a conceptual and methodological challenge.

Linking food consumption databases to food price data has allowed for novel analyses of individual-level diet quality in relation to cost [12,14]. At this time, retail food prices have been attached to dietary data collected using food records, dietary histories, and food frequency questionnaires [18]. In such studies, retail food prices per 100 g edible portion were merged with the food composition database to estimate diet costs in a manner analogous to that used to estimate energy and nutrient intakes. Such studies, conducted for the most part outside the USA, have allowed for new insights into the relation between food, health, and incomes.

DIETARY SUGARS AND ENERGY COSTS

One critical distinction in the economics of sugar consumption is between added sugars (sucrose and HFCS) and other natural sugars from milk, vegetables, and fruits. It is the added sugars that provide dietary energy at an exceptionally low cost, whereas fruits and vegetables do not. Further, import tariffs on foreign sugar keep retail prices of refined sugar in the USA at approximately three times the world price [27]. For this reason, HFCS is significantly cheaper. In the USA, HFCS has become the principal caloric sweetener in processed foods and beverages.

For the past 100 years, the usual way of comparing the relative cost of different foods was to compare prices per calorie. Comparisons based on food weight or serving size are not meaningful. As noted by Atwater in 1894 [28], some foods are 90% water, which provides bulk and weight but no calories and no nutrients. Based on FDA regulations, a "serving" of food can provide anywhere from 1 to 500 kcal. As early as 1902, commonly eaten foods were grouped by the USDA according to their energy costs [29,30]. Among "cheap" foods, providing >1900 cal for 10 cents were sugars, cereals, starches, lard, dried beans and peas, cheap cuts of meat, salt pork and bacon, potatoes, and sweet potatoes. Lean meats and fish, chicken, eggs, green vegetables, and most fresh fruit were described by the USDA as "expensive" foods that provided <800 cal for 10 cents. Then as now, sugar calories were cheaper than fresh produce [29,30].

Using contemporary food prices from France that were merged with the national nutrient composition data, Darmon et al. [18,24] confirmed that added sugars provided lower-cost calories than did fresh produce. As later confirmed in multiple studies, fats, grains, sugar, beans, and potatoes had substantially lower energy costs than did meats, fish, lettuce, or fresh fruit [29–31].

Recent analyses of the nutrient value of US foods in relation to their cost [29,30], made use of the USDA Food and Nutrient Database for Dietary Studies 1.0 (FNDDS) [32]. Used to analyze the What We Eat in America food intake data, the FNDDS database contains some 6940 foods from all food groups [32]. Those foods were first grouped into milk and milk products; meat, poultry, and fish; eggs; dry beans, legumes, nuts and seeds; grain products; fruits; vegetables; fats, oils, and salad dressings; and sugars, sweets, and beverages. The nutrient composition data were then merged with national food prices released by the USDA Center for Nutrition Policy and Promotion (CNPP) [33,34]. One national price, corrected for preparation and waste and expressed per gram of edible portion, was provided for each food that was listed as consumed by National Health and Nutrition Examination Survey (NHANES) participants.

Food price analyses by major food group showed that energy cost ($/100 kcal) was lowest for grains, fats, eggs, and milk. Energy cost for vegetables was higher than that for every other food group except for fruit. Mean energy cost for vegetables was more than five times that of grains and fats and more than double the cost of sugars, sweets, and beverages [29].

Although an expensive sources of calories, vegetables provide several key nutrients at low cost [24,31]. Measuring food prices per gram, rather than per calorie, is one way to make healthy vegetables appear less expensive. However, a better measure of affordability would be to take the nutrient content of vegetables into account. Recent studies on the nutritive value of US foods in relation to cost therefore compared relative prices per nutrient by food group [35]. Potatoes were the lowest cost source of potassium, while fruits were the lowest cost sources of vitamin C. Milk and dairy products were the lowest cost sources of dietary calcium, whereas lowest cost fiber was provided by beans. With some exceptions made for fortified products, foods and beverages containing high levels of added sugars were poor (and expensive) sources of key nutrients.

ADDED SUGARS AND DIET COSTS

The merging of nutrient composition data with local or national food prices has allowed researchers to estimate energy intakes as well as the quality and cost of individual diets. Linking diet quality to diet cost is the first step in estimating the impact of different quality diets on weights and health.

One early study estimated diet costs of 837 adults in the Val-de-Marne database, whose diets had been assessed using a dietary history method [18]. French national retail prices in Euros per kg were obtained for 57 foods in the nutrient database. Individual diet costs were estimated by multiplying the weight of each food by its unit cost and summing over all foods and beverages consumed by each person. Dietary energy density was calculated by dividing total dietary energy by the edible weight of foods and caloric beverages. Energy-dense diets high in refined grains, fats, and sweets were associated with lower diet costs, whereas diets high in vegetables and fruit were associated with higher diet costs [18].

Consuming a high-sugar diet was a way to save on daily diet costs [13]. Depending on energy intakes, each additional 100 g of fats and sweets was associated with a 0.05- to 0.40-Euro drop per day in diet costs. In contrast, depending on energy intakes, each additional 100 g of fruits and vegetables was associated with a 0.18–0.29-Euro per day increase in diet costs (equivalent to $0.25–0.40/day).

The preliminary conclusion was that as incomes drop and food budgets shrink, food purchases may shift toward refined grains and added sugars and fats. Although higher food spending does not guarantee a better diet, reducing food spending below a certain minimum virtually ensures that the resulting diet will be high in energy but low in essential nutrients. Such studies were consistent with the notion of hidden hunger, that is, vitamin and mineral deficiencies found in developed countries among lower-income groups.

The Val-de-Marne data were subsequently confirmed using data from the nationally representative study of individual food consumption patterns in France (INCA). That study was based on 7-day food records completed by over 1500 adult respondents and dietary intake data were merged with food prices for over 600 foods [36–38]. US-based studies have also confirmed that diets high in cereals, fats, and sweets were associated with lower per calorie diet costs [39]. Similar results have now been obtained from Spain [11], Japan [40], Australia [41], and the Netherlands [42].

A recent review of the literature, followed by meta-analysis placed the cost differential between healthy and unhealthy diets at approximately $1.50 per person per day [43]. Such a differential translates into a difference of $42/week or $2200 over the course of a year for a family of 4. By comparison, the current food assistance allotment, said to be adequate for a nutritious diet at low cost is in the range of $127–146/week for a family of 4. For lower-income groups, adopting a higher quality diet might be associated with a >30% increase in daily diet costs.

On the national basis, an increase of $1.50 per day translates into $109 billion per year, assuming a population of 200 million adults. Although those figures may be less than the cost of health care for diet-related chronic disease, they are not trivial and cannot be dismissed lightly.

SES, DIET QUALITY, AND HEALTH

Observational studies have linked higher intakes of sugars, including both sucrose and HFCS with a higher risk of heart disease, obesity, and diabetes as reviewed in other chapters. Insufficient intake of higher cost foods was also linked to adverse health outcomes. In most such studies, participants were divided into quintiles of nutrient exposure, adjusted for energy using the method of residuals [44]. Exposures were adjusted for SES using proxy indicators such as smoking and physical activity, since data on education and incomes were rarely available. Higher chronic disease risk was also linked in a dose-dependent manner to lower intakes of dietary fibers, folates, carotenoids, vitamins A, C, and E, calcium, and potassium. Each of these nutrients was directly related to diet costs [4].

The relation between nutrient content of the diet and diet cost was examined for adult participants in the Seattle Obesity Study [4]. Dietary intake data were based on a food frequency questionnaire instrument, whereas prices for FFQ foods were obtained from area supermarkets. Participants were divided into quintiles of nutrient intakes, adjusted for energy using the method of residuals. Analyses confirmed that higher intakes of added sugars and saturated and trans fats were associated with lower per calorie diet costs. Lower-cost diets were also associated with lower intakes of dietary fiber and of vitamins A, C, D, E, and B12, beta carotene, folates, iron, calcium, potassium, and magnesium. As expected, persons with the lower-cost, lower-quality diets were more likely to be from lower SES groups.

Nutrient content is one measure of diet quality; composite scores are another. Among composite measures of diet quality are the Healthy Eating Index 2005 and its alternatives [45]. These are designed to reflect compliance with the US dietary recommendations and guidelines and are often based on foods as well as nutrients. The consumption of total or added sugars detracts from the quality of the total diet. For example, the chief sources of "empty calories" in the US diet are said to be SoFAAS (solid fats, alcoholic beverages and added sugars). The SoFAAs subscore is a negative component of the Healthy Eating Index (HEI) 2005, reducing overall diet quality.

Applying these measures to a representative sample of the US population showed that higher HEI scores were linked with higher-cost diets and with higher SES. Monetary costs of diets consumed by 2001–2002 NHANES participants were estimated using the national food prices database. Mean daily diet costs, energy-adjusted diet costs, and values of the HEI-2005 were estimated for each respondent. Analyses showed that higher HEI-2005 scores for both men and women were associated with higher energy-adjusted diet costs. Higher diet cost was strongly associated with consuming more servings of fruit and vegetables and with fewer calories from SoFAAs. Women in the highest quintile of diet costs had a mean HEI-2005 score of 69.6 compared with 52.5 for women in the lowest-cost quintile. According to the USDA, scores in the range of 51–80 indicate a diet in need of improvement, whereas scores >80 denote a "good" diet. Clearly, the lowest cost diets were also in the need of most improvement.

Based on analyses of federal US data using USDA diet quality metrics, there can be no doubt that healthier diets cost more and are preferentially consumed by higher SES groups. In other words, much like health status, diet quality in the USA is a function of social class. Some of these disparities may be explained by diet cost [46].

SUGAR AND SOCIAL CLASS

That food consumption patterns vary by social class has been known for a long time. Writing in 1936, John Boyd Orr [47] observed that the diets of lower-income groups were based around cheap sources of energy and therefore cheap satisfiers of hunger. By contrast, the consumption of vegetables, fruit, and meat was associated with higher incomes. In his view, the five-fold increase in sugar consumption observed over the previous 100 years (1834–1934) had been very likely caused by the great fall in sugar price. Sugar consumption in the UK in 1934 was estimated at 94 lb. per capita per annum.

Then, as of now, sugar consumption was higher among lower-income groups. In 1937, George Orwell [48] noted that the British miners subsisted on white bread and margarine, corned beef, sugar, and potatoes—calling it an appalling diet. The miner's family was reported to spend 10 pence a week on green vegetables and nothing on fruit but one shilling and nine pence on sugar and a shilling on tea.

The US Bureau of Labor Statistics has estimated that the bottom quintile of the US population by income spent no more than $5.80 per person per day for all foods purchased at retail and eaten at home. Current estimates suggest that the average household spends about 10% of income on foods at home and away from home, although that percentage is substantially higher among lower-income groups, consistent with Engel's Law. Food spending can determine diet quality, given that most people do not want to deviate from the cultural norms.

ECONOMICS OF DIETARY SUGARS CONSUMPTION

Studies in nutrition economics have allowed us to examine consumption patterns across SES strata. In economic terms, the type of product the demand for which declines as incomes rise is called an inferior good. In the USA, sugar and sweetened beverages appear to meet that definition. Epidemiologic studies have shown that the consumption of added sugars was inversely linked to incomes [22]. Likewise, the consumption of sugar sweetened beverages (SSBs) was more common among lower-income groups.

Conversely, for the so-called normal goods, an increase in income causes a growth in demand. In observational studies based on NHANES data, consumption of diet beverages, bottled water, skim milk, and whole fruit increased together with incomes. Economists have also identified a category of luxury goods, the demand for which rises disproportionately with income. Based on the sharp SES gradient, fresh fruits and vegetables excluding potatoes appeared to be luxury goods in the UK in 1934 [47]. More contemporary analyses suggest that they may be still [5].

Our energy density model, introduced in 2004 [1], proposed that attempting to reduce diet costs would lead to diets that were higher in added sugars and fats and lower in vegetables and fruit. Such diets would have higher energy density and would provide more calories per unit cost. Given that energy-dense foods also tend to be more palatable and have less satiating power, there was potential for unintended overconsumption [49]. One consequence of reduced food expenditures would be a surfeit of empty calories. In other words, it was possible to spend less and eat more.

Evidence for this notion was initially provided by diet optimization studies using a linear programming model [50]. The goal was to predict food choices that could be made by people trying to reduce their food budgets without a major departure from their usual eating habits [51]. The USDA used a similar linear programming model to create the Thrifty Food Plan, a nutritious diet at low cost [52]. To ensure these diets were consistent with habitual food consumption patterns, consumption constraints minimized departure from the average French diet and imposed limits on portion size and the allowed amount of energy from food groups.

Imposing the cost constraint in the absence of nutrition considerations led to modeled food patterns that were energy-dense and contained more added sugars, sweets, and added fats and were lacking in fruit and vegetables, meat, and dairy products [53]. The nutritional quality of modeled diets was markedly reduced. The composition of the modeled food patterns reproduced the food intakes observed among the lower SES groups in France.

The energy density model and the results of linear programming were recently confirmed by empirical studies conducted by the Institute for Fiscal Studies in the UK [54]. The study dealt with the combined impact on diet quality of stagnating wages, rising unemployment, and an increase in food prices relative to other goods since the Great Recession of 2008. Data analyses showed that between 2005 and 2012, households reduced the amount of calories by 3.6% but reduced food expenditures by 8.5%. By buying and substituting cheaper foods, households spent 5.2% less per calorie. The reduction in diet quality was driven by a trend away from fruit and vegetables and their substitution by processed fats and sweets. Most affected were households with young children and single-parent households.

OBESITY AND POVERTY

In most US-based research, measures of SES have been restricted to only two variables: education and income. More recent studies based on geographic information system (GIS) approaches suggest multiple new variables for a better assessment of social class that are linked to residential context and the built environment. In particular, residential property values may become a useful wealth metric for use in health studies [55].

In Seattle-King County, obesity rates at the census tract level were best predicted by education and residential property values. At the individual level, property values were linked to higher HEI 2005 scores and to lower body mass index values in women. Women in the bottom quartile of property values were 3.4 times more likely to be obese than women in the top quartile. No association between property values and obesity was observed for men [3]. Such studies have permitted the mapping of obesity and diabetes at the census tract level, pointing to a geographic concentration in lower income areas [56].

Incidentally, those studies failed to observe any effects of access to healthy foods when formulated as proximity to the nearest store. Only one in seven respondents reported shopping at the nearest supermarket. Obesity risk was not associated with distance to the nearest supermarket or with living in a food desert. By contrast, the type of supermarket, by price, was found to be inversely and significantly associated with obesity rates, even after adjusting for individual-level socio-demographic and lifestyle variables, and proximity measures. Attitudes toward a healthy diet were also predictive of better diet quality.

OPEN QUESTIONS

Confounding by Diet Cost

Studies on the impact of dietary factors on weight gain and health have attempted to isolate the contribution of specific beverages and foods [16]. In general, changes in consumption of starches, refined grains, and processed foods were more likely to contribute to weight gain. Conversely, additional consumption of fruits, vegetables, nuts, and whole grains was associated with less weight gain. The consumption of 100% juice was associated with less weight gain that the consumption of sweetened beverages. Interestingly, since diets and incomes appear to be linked, changes in dietary patterns may have been secondary to changes in household resources and food budgets.

The observed differences were said to relate to varying portion sizes, patterns of eating, effects on satiety, or substitution for other beverages or foods. For example, 100% juices may have been consumed in smaller servings than SSBs or in different patterns. Another possibility is that these foods were consumed by different groups that differed from each other in various unobserved ways.

What SSBs, starches, and refined grains and processed foods may have in common is their low per calorie cost. What many epidemiologic studies seem to show is that more expensive foods consumed by wealthier people are associated with better health outcomes. In many cases, the controlling for SES has been problematic at best.

Confounding by Social Norms

The confounding by cultural attitudes deserves a mention. Throughout history, sugar has been the means of providing inexpensive calories to lower-income groups. As such, sugar and sweets have acquired a place in global food culture. Attempts to reduce consumption of dietary sugars to improve diet quality will need to address aspects of culture, economics, and behavior.

One argument is that not all healthy foods cost more. Some nutrient-rich foods can be obtained at very low cost [38]. For example, a recent article on value metrics identified potatoes and beans as providing most nutrients per penny [35]. However, food choices are a part of social identity, and the ability to adhere to a socially acceptable diet is one of the necessities of life. The custom of the country—to borrow a phrase from Adam Smith—may place some foods outside the accepted social norms [38].

Public health interventions need to come to terms with the fact that some healthy foods may be rejected by the consumer. All too often, the low cost of powdered milk, ground pork, organ meats, beans, lentils, carrots, and cabbage is cited as proof that lower-income groups in the USA have full access to inexpensive yet nourishing foods. Home-cooked lentil soup and inexpensive rice and beans have been proposed as suitable staple diets for the US poor. Indeed, nuts, seeds, legumes, cereals, potatoes, and cabbage offer good nutrition at an affordable cost [30]. The search for affordable, nutrient-rich foods is being aided further by the new techniques of nutrient profiling [51] and by the new metrics of nutrients per energy and nutrients per unit cost [35].

What Really Matters—Sugar or Its Price?

The rates of obesity and type II diabetes in the USA are largely driven by SES. The geographic concentration of chronic disease in lower SES neighborhoods is readily apparent in small-area GIS studies. Higher rates are observed in the more disadvantaged neighborhoods and among groups with lower education and income. The impact of SES on weights and health may be mediated, in part, by diet quality. In general, lower-quality diets are associated with higher disease risk, whereas the recommended higher-quality diets are associated with lower disease risk. However, based on food prices and existing eating habits in the USA, lower-quality diets are also associated with lower per calorie diet costs. By contrast, the recommended higher-quality diets are more costly and more likely to be purchased by higher SES groups. Lower-income groups selecting cheaper diets are more likely to be obese and have associated health problems.

The importance of economic factors when it comes to sugar consumption is listed in Table 8.1. The relative prices per kilocalorie for a number of sugar-containing beverages, from generic cola to 100% fruit juices and meal replacement products, are also shown. Previous studies have associated the low-cost sugars with obesity and weight gain, whereas the higher-cost juices and meal replacement shakes have been associated with weight maintenance or weight loss. Although beverage prices per 100 kcal varied by an order of magnitude, their sugar content per 100 g was much the same. In other words, the same sugars, differently priced, have been associated in epidemiologic and in clinical studies with both weight gain and weight loss.

The point is that these beverages, containing added or natural sugars, may be selected by consumers at different levels of SES. Added sugars, including sucrose and HFCS, have been associated with lower SES, lower diet quality, lower diet costs, and higher disease risks. However, it now appears that the relevant obesogenic factor is not the foods' sugar content of foods but its low price.

TABLE 8.1
Price of Sweetened Beverages and Their Sugar Content (AJCN 2007)[a]

Sugar Content	Sugar g/100	Cost $/MJ
Tampico Tropical Punch[b]	10.8	0.25
Safeway Select Cola[c]	12.1	0.32
Reduced-fat Chocolate Milk[d]	12.3	0.38
A&W Root Beer[e]	12.9	0.40
Coca-Cola Classic[f]	11.3	0.44
Sunny D Tangy Original (5% juice)[g]	11.3	0.44
Hi-C Blast Fruit Pow (10% juice)[f]	2.7	0.66
Safeway White Grape Juice (100%)[c]	15.8	0.77
Welch's Grape Juice (100% juice)[h]	16.7	0.82
Ocean Spray Cranberry Juice Cocktail (27% juice)[i]	13.8	0.89
Minute Maid Orange Juice (100% conc)[f]	10.0	0.94
Tropicana Orange Juice (100% pure squeezed)[j]	9.2	1.08
V8 Fusion Fruit and Vegetable Juice[k]	11.2	1.49
Slim Fast Optima French Vanilla (low sugar)[l]	4.8	1.59
Slim Fast French Vanilla Classic (original formula)[l]	10.8	1.59
Odwalla Orange Juice (100% juice squeezed)[f]	10.0	2.92

[a] All prices were obtained from www.safeway.com (accessed 23 March 2006).
[b] Heartland Farms, City of Industry, CA, USA.
[c] Safeway, Inc., Pleasanton, CA, USA.
[d] Darigold Dairies, Seattle, WA, USA.
[e] Dr. Pepper/SevenUp, Inc., Plano, TX, USA.
[f] Coca-Cola Company, Atlanta, GA, USA.
[g] Sunny Delight Beverages, Cincinnati, OH, USA.
[h] Welch Foods, Inc., Concord, MA, USA.
[i] Ocean Spray Cranberries, Inc., Lakeville-Middleboro, MA, USA.
[j] PepsiCo, Inc., Purchase, NY, USA.
[k] Campbell's, Camden, NJ, USA.
[l] Unilever, Vlaardingen, the Netherlands.

Epidemiologic studies have not fully disentangled the potential impact of multiple SES variables, food prices, and diet costs on body weights and health. High dietary energy density and low per calorie diet cost may be better predictors of disease risk than is any one single nutrient, beverage, or food. Future studies should address overall food patterns and their social, economic, and cultural aspects in relation to health.

REFERENCES

1. Drewnowski A, Specter SE. Poverty and obesity: The role of energy density and energy costs. *Am J Clin Nutr*. 2004;79(1):6–16.
2. Loucks EB, Magnusson KT, Cook S, Rehkopf DH, Ford ES, Berkman LF. Socioeconomic position and the metabolic syndrome in early, middle, and late life: Evidence from NHANES 1999–2002. *Ann Epidemiol*. 2007;17(10):782–90.
3. Rehm CD, Moudon AV, Hurvitz PM, Drewnowski A. Residential property values are associated with obesity among women in King County, WA, USA. *Soc Sci Med*. 2012;75(3):491–5.
4. Aggarwal A, Monsivais P, Drewnowski A. Nutrient intakes linked to better health outcomes are associated with higher diet costs in the US. *PLoS One*. 2012;7(5):e37533.

5. Darmon N, Drewnowski A. Does social class predict diet quality? *Am J Clin Nutr*. 2008;87(5):1107–17.
6. Bray GA, Popkin BM. Dietary fat intake does affect obesity! *Am J Clin Nutr*. 1998;68(6):1157–73.
7. Bray GA, Nielsen SJ, Popkin BM. Consumption of high-fructose corn syrup in beverages may play a role in the epidemic of obesity. *Am J Clin Nutr*. 2004;79(4):537–43.
8. Gross LS, Li L, Ford ES, Liu S. Increased consumption of refined carbohydrates and the epidemic of type 2 diabetes in the United States: An ecologic assessment. *Am J Clin Nutr*. 2004;79(5):774–9.
9. Malik VS, Popkin BM, Bray GA, Despres JP, Hu FB. Sugar-sweetened beverages, obesity, type 2 diabetes mellitus, and cardiovascular disease risk. *Circulation*. 2010;121(11):1356–64.
10. Drewnowski A. The real contribution of added sugars and fats to obesity. *Epidemiol Rev*. 2007;29:160–71.
11. Schroder H, Marrugat J, Covas MI. High monetary costs of dietary patterns associated with lower body mass index: A population-based study. *Int J Obes (Lond)*. 2006;30(10):1574–9.
12. Drewnowski A, Darmon N. The economics of obesity: Dietary energy density and energy cost. *Am J Clin Nutr*. 2005;82(1 Suppl):265s–73s.
13. Drewnowski A, Darmon N, Briend A. Replacing fats and sweets with vegetables and fruits—A question of cost. *Am J Public Health*. 2004;94(9):1555–9.
14. Drewnowski A, Darmon N. Food choices and diet costs: An economic analysis. *J Nutr*. 2005;135(4):900–4.
15. Andrieu E, Darmon N, Drewnowski A. Low-cost diets: More energy, fewer nutrients. *Eur J Clin Nutr*. 2006;60(3):434–6.
16. Mozaffarian D, Hao T, Rimm EB, Willett WC, Hu FB. Changes in diet and lifestyle and long-term weight gain in women and men. *N Engl J Med*. 2011;364(25):2392–404.
17. United States. Dietary Guidelines for Americans 2010, 7th ed. Washington, DC: U.S. Department of Agriculture and U.S. Department of Health and Human Services; 2010.
18. Darmon N, Briend A, Drewnowski A. Energy-dense diets are associated with lower diet costs: A community study of French adults. *Public Health Nutr*. 2004;7(1):21–7.
19. Rehm CD, Monsivais P, Drewnowski A. The quality and monetary value of diets consumed by adults in the United States. *Am J Clin Nutr*. 2011;94(5):1333–9.
20. Mendoza JA, Drewnowski A, Christakis DA. Dietary energy density is associated with obesity and the metabolic syndrome in U.S. adults. *Diabetes Care*. 2007;30(4):974–9.
21. Rozin P, Fischler C, Imada S, Sarubin A, Wrzesniewski A. Attitudes to food and the role of food in life in the USA, Japan, Flemish Belgium and France: Possible implications for the diet-health debate. *Appetite*. 1999;33(2):163–80.
22. Thompson FE, McNeel TS, Dowling EC, Midthune D, Morrissette M, Zeruto CA. Interrelationships of added sugars intake, socioeconomic status, and race/ethnicity in adults in the United States: National Health Interview Survey, 2005. *J Am Diet Assoc*. 2009;109(8):1376–83.
23. Braveman PA, Cubbin C, Egerter S, Chideya S, Marchi KS, Metzler M et al. Socioeconomic status in health research: One size does not fit all. *JAMA*. 2005;294(22):2879–88.
24. Darmon N, Darmon M, Maillot M, Drewnowski A. A nutrient density standard for vegetables and fruits: Nutrients per calorie and nutrients per unit cost. *J Am Diet Assoc*. 2005;105(12):1881–7.
25. Maillot M, Darmon N, Drewnowski A. Are the lowest-cost healthful food plans culturally and socially acceptable? *Public Health Nutr*. 2010;13(8):1178–85.
26. Aggarwal A, Monsivais P, Cook AJ, Drewnowski A. Positive attitude toward healthy eating predicts higher diet quality at all cost levels of supermarkets. *J Acad Nutr Diet*. 2014;114(2):266–72.
27. US Department of Agriculture, Economic Research Service. Sugar and sweeteners yearbook tables [Internet]. Washington, DC: US Department of Agriculture, Economic Research Service; Available from: http://www.ers.usda.gov/data-products/sugar-and-sweeteners-yearbook-tables.aspx#25442 (accessed on 21 March 2014).
28. Atwater W. Food: Nutritive value and cost. Washington, DC: US Department of Agriculture Farmers Bulletin #23; 1894. Available from: US Government Printing Office.
29. Drewnowski A. The cost of US foods as related to their nutritive value. *Am J Clin Nutr*. 2010;92(5):1181–8.
30. Drewnowski A. The Nutrient Rich Foods Index helps to identify healthy, affordable foods. *Am J Clin Nutr*. 2010;91(4):1095s–101s.
31. Drewnowski A. New metrics of affordable nutrition: Which vegetables provide most nutrients for least cost? *J Acad Nutr Diet*. 2013;113(9):1182–7.
32. USDA Food and Nutrient Database for Dietary Studies, 1.0 [monograph on the Internet]. Beltsville, MD: Agricultural Research Service, Food Surveys Research Group; 2004. Available from: http://www.ars.usda.gov/services/docs.htm?docid=12082 (accessed on 8 June 2007).
33. Bowman SA. A methodology to price foods consumed: Development of a food price database. *Family Econ Nutr Rev*. 1997;10(1):26.

34. Carlson A, Lino M, Juan W, Marcoe K, Bente L, Hiza H et al. Development of the CNPP prices database. Alexandria, VA: US Department of Agriculture, Center for Nutrition Policy and Promotion; May 2008. Available from: http://www.cnpp.usda.gov/Publications/FoodPlans/MiscPubs/PricesDatabaseReport.pdf.
35. Drewnowski A, Rehm CD. Vegetable cost metrics show that potatoes and beans provide most nutrients per penny. *PLoS One*. 2013;8(5):e63277.
36. Drewnowski A, Monsivais P, Maillot M, Darmon N. Low-energy-density diets are associated with higher diet quality and higher diet costs in French adults. *J Am Diet Assoc*. 2007;107(6):1028–32.
37. Maillot M, Darmon N, Vieux F, Drewnowski A. Low energy density and high nutritional quality are each associated with higher diet costs in French adults. *Am J Clin Nutr*. 2007;86(3):690–6.
38. Maillot M, Darmon N, Darmon M, Lafay L, Drewnowski A. Nutrient-dense food groups have high energy costs: An econometric approach to nutrient profiling. *J Nutr*. 2007;137(7):1815–20.
39. Townsend MS, Aaron GJ, Monsivais P, Keim NL, Drewnowski A. Less-energy-dense diets of low-income women in California are associated with higher energy-adjusted diet costs. *Am J Clin Nutr*. 2009;89(4):1220–6.
40. Murakami K, Sasaki S, Takahashi Y, Uenishi K. Monetary cost of dietary energy is negatively associated with BMI and waist circumference, but not with other metabolic risk factors, in young Japanese women. *Public Health Nutr*. 2009;12(8):1092–8.
41. Brimblecombe JK, O'Dea K. The role of energy cost in food choices for an aboriginal population in northern Australia. *Med J Aust*. 2009;190(10):549–51.
42. Waterlander WE, de Haas WE, van Amstel I, Schuit AJ, Twisk JW, Visser M et al. Energy density, energy costs and income—How are they related? *Public Health Nutr*. 2010;13(10):1599–608.
43. Rao M, Afshin A, Singh G, Mozaffarian D. Do healthier foods and diet patterns cost more than less healthy options? A systematic review and meta-analysis. *BMJ Open*. 2013;3(12):e004277.
44. Willett W. Nutritional Epidemiology. New York: Oxford University Press; 1998.
45. Chiuve SE, Fung TT, Rimm EB, Hu FB, McCullough ML, Wang M et al. Alternative dietary indices both strongly predict risk of chronic disease. *J Nutr*. 2012;142(6):1009–18.
46. Monsivais P, Aggarwal A, Drewnowski A. Are socio-economic disparities in diet quality explained by diet cost? *J Epidemiol Commun Health*. 2012;66(6):530–5.
47. Boyd Orr J. Food, Health and Income: Report on a Survey of Adequacy of Diet in Relation to Income. London: MacMillan; 1936.
48. Orwell G. The Road to Wigan Pier. London: Victor Gollancz Publisher; 1937.
49. Ledikwe JH, Blanck HM, Kettel Khan L, Serdula MK, Seymour JD, Tohill BC et al. Dietary energy density is associated with energy intake and weight status in US adults. *Am J Clin Nutr*. 2006;83(6):1362–8.
50. Darmon N, Ferguson EL, Briend A. A cost constraint alone has adverse effects on food selection and nutrient density: An analysis of human diets by linear programming. *J Nutr*. 2002;132(12):3764–71.
51. Maillot M, Ferguson EL, Drewnowski A, Darmon N. Nutrient profiling can help identify foods of good nutritional quality for their price: A validation study with linear programming. *J Nutr*. 2008;138(6):1107–13.
52. Wilde PE, Llobrera J. Using the thrifty food plan to assess the cost of a nutritious diet. *J Consumer Affairs*. 2009;43(2):274–304.
53. Darmon N, Ferguson E, Briend A. Do economic constraints encourage the selection of energy dense diets? *Appetite*. 2003;41(3):315–22.
54. Griffith R, O'Connell M, Smith K. Food expenditure and nutritional quality over the Great Recession [Internet]. UK: The Institute for Fiscal Studies. Available from: http://www.ifs.org.uk/bns/bn143.pdf (accessed on 29 November 2913).
55. Moudon AV, Cook AJ, Ulmer J, Hurvitz PM, Drewnowski A. A neighborhood wealth metric for use in health studies. *Am J Prev Med*. 2011;41(1):88–97.
56. Drewnowski A, Rehm CD, Arterburn D. The geographic distribution of obesity by census tract among 59 767 insured adults in King County, WA. *Int J Obes (Lond)*. 2014;38(6):833–9.

9 Sugar Consumption in the Food and Beverage Supply across the Globe

Barry M. Popkin

CONTENTS

KEY POINTS

- Added sugars are found in 75% of all the consumer packaged foods and beverages sold in the USA, suggestive of the large number of ways added sugar is used in our entire supply of processed foods and beverages globally.
- Fruit juice concentrate is the new "healthy," "natural" added sugar increasingly used in foods and beverages.
- In the USA and a few other high-income countries, noncaloric or diet sweeteners are increasingly being used to replace added sugars in beverages and foods. This is linked with a decline in total calories from added sugars in the USA and UK.
- While the bottom 40% of US individuals aged 2 and older consume 120 kcal/day or less, the top two quintiles average 326 and 662 kcal/day of added sugar.
- Outside of the high-income countries, low- and middle-income country (LMIC) dietary intake and other data suggest major increases in added sugar intake, particularly from caloric sugar-sweetened beverages.
- Mexico and Brazil are two of the largest consumers of caloric beverages and use added sugar in a wide variety of processed beverages.

INTRODUCTION

Sugars are found in our food supply either as a natural component of the food or as an added sugar of various types. Sugars are added to food not only for their impact on taste, but also because it is economical and has many properties, such as a preservative to prevent growth of many organisms and keep perishable foods from spoiling (e.g., jams, candied fruit peels) as well as to improve texture of cooked products. Added sugars provide only empty calories with no nutrient value, are highly refined, and also serve to sweeten foods and beverages and enhance desirability. As a beverage, a vast literature has shown how our bodies do not compensate for beverage calories, and sugary beverage intake is linked with many cardiometabolic problems [1–5] as reviewed in other chapters. Surprisingly, much less is understood about the sweetening of our food supply than one would imagine. Partly this relates to the impossibility of measuring the specific type and amount of the different added sugars versus naturally occurring sugars directly in any food or beverage. Partly this relates to the vast number of different sugars used in the food supply.

The sweetening of the US and global food supply has been occurring for a long time [6]. Outside the USA, some of the very first research in the world funded to systematically increase the productivity of sugar plantations was in the Caribbean area and Indonesia. Cane-breeding research began in the 1880s in Barbados at the Dodds Botanical Station and in Java at the East Java Research Station. The USA was not far behind. The Sugar Station, founded in 1885, is the oldest of the Louisiana Agricultural Experiment Station and one of the firsts in the USA.

John Yudkin, more than any scholar, deserves credit for pushing forward our modern understanding of the role of dietary sugars and refined carbohydrates in our diet [7,8]. Yudkin's work did not receive full credit until more recently. As early as the 1950s, he displayed a stronger linkage between English sugar consumption and coronary heart disease than the saturated fats from animal foods but his work was largely ignored by major scholars and dietary policy groups [8,9].

The other critical issue to understand about the role of sugars in our food supply is the enormous early and continued research undertaken to keep sugars economical [10]. Our history over the last five to six centuries has often revolved around sugar but here we will focus not on this history but on our current food supply and what we know from various data sources about the role of sugars in our food supply. In the next section, we use food ingredient data for the 600,000 consumer packaged foods in the US food supply to provide some sense of sugar use. We follow this with some global data on long-term shifts in total sugar use and some of our work on total added sugar use in the USA. This is followed by a discussion of some of the patterns and trends of calorically sweetened beverages across the globe.

MODERN FOOD SUPPLY: THE US EXAMPLE FROM THE CONSUMER PACKAGED FOOD AND BEVERAGE SECTOR

Little is known about the use of sweeteners in foods and beverages sold and consumed in the USA. As noted, there is no direct measurement of sweetener content of foods and beverages. Since added sugars cannot be chemically distinguished from intrinsic (naturally occurring) sugars, the primary food-composition databases in the USA do not contain composition information for either intrinsic or added sugars [11]. There are two supplementary sources of added sugars information available from the US Department of Agriculture (USDA). The USDA Database for the Added Sugars Content of Selected Foods, Release 1 (2006) [12] provides data for the added sugars content of 2038 commonly consumed foods, excluding brand name foods. A second source, the MyPyramid Equivalents Database (MPED), provides data on added sugars content of foods reported in Continuing Survey of Food Intakes of Individuals 1994–1996 and 1998, and the National Health and Nutrition Examination Survey 2001–2002 and 2003–2004 [13] and more recently a new released updated version for the 2005–2010 period [14,15]. An updated interim data set has been used to estimate added sugar for the 2005–2010 period [16]. The government uses their own recipe files and linear programming algorithms to estimate the amount of added sugar in each product comparable to that used by the University of Minnesota's nutrient data system [17,18].

In one study, we utilized details of the ingredients in each packaged food and beverage to estimate the foods that contain added sugars [11]. Elsewhere we review these databases which when combined provide nutrition facts panel and full ingredients lists [19]. Essentially we matched the nutrition facts label NFP data with the 2005–2009 Homescan data on household purchases at the barcode (universal package code or UPC) level in order to create a more complete measure of the nutritional content of UPCs reported purchased. This was successful for more than 98% of the volume and dollar sales of foods reported purchased in Homescan.

There are a vast array of sugars used in our food supply, many of which will surprise most public health and nutrition scholars [11]. In Table 9.1, we provide a list of all these sugars. We included fruit juice concentrate as it is used in a great number of foods and beverages.

Essentially we searched the full set of ingredients for each food and beverage with a unique set of ingredients to estimate the proportion of the unique food products with various combinations of sugars, NCS (noncaloric sweetener, really low calorie sweeteners or diet sweeteners). We are defining unique food products as those with unique formulations (e.g., a 1.5-l bottle of Coca-Cola Classic will be nutritionally equivalent to a 12 fl. oz. can of Coca-Cola Classic and a 20 fl. Oz. bottle of Coca-Cola Classic, so even though they will have different barcodes, they only count as one food product). We searched not only for sugars, but also low calorie sweeteners (NCS or diet sweeteners).

TABLE 9.1
CSs Used in the US Food Supply

Caloric Sweeteners	Search Terms Used
Fruit juice concentrate (FJC)[a]	Juice concentrate/conc., concentrated/conc. juice, concentrated/conc. fruit juice, concentrated/conc juice sweetener (where included were apple, pear, grapefruit, orange, peach, plum, mango, lemon, lime, apricot, nectarine, prune, grape, pineapple, blueberry, strawberry, raspberry, blackberry, boysenberry, lingonberry, gooseberry, elderberry, mulberry, currant, cherry, pomegranate, cranberry, kiwi, melon, lychee, mangosteen, coconut, mixed)
Cane sugar	Cane sugar, cane juice, cane syrup, turbinado, golden syrup, treacle, caramel, Sucanat
Beet sugar	Beet sugar, sugar beet
Sucrose	Sucrose, table sugar
Corn syrup	Corn syrup, maltodextrin, TruSweet, C Sweet, Versatose, Clintose, Benchmate, Corn Sweet
HFCS	High-fructose corn syrup
Agave-based sweeteners	Agave nectar, agave syrup, agave sap, agave juice
Honey	Honey, nectar, Honi-Bake, Honi-Flake, Sweet'N'Neat
Molasses	Molasses
Maple	Maple
Sorghum/malt/maltose	Sorghum, malt, maltose, mizuame
Rice syrup	Rice syrup, rice sugar, Sweet Dream
Fructose	Fructose
Lactose	Lactose
Inverted sugars	Invert sugar, inverted sugar, sugar invert, Nulomoline, sucrovert, invertase
Sugar alcohol	Sorbitol, glucitol, erythritol, xylitol, mannitol, lactitol, maltitol, glycerol, hydrogenated starch hydrolysates, isomalt, isoglucose, lycasin, tastes like honey, Maltidex
Low-calorie sweeteners	luo han guo, luo han kuo, tagatose, trehalose, brazzein, Cweet, pentadin, Oubli, mabinlin, monellin, thaumatin, curculin, lumbah, miraculin, monatin, inulin, osladin, licorice, glycyrrhizin, fructooligosaccharide, oligofructose, oligofructan
Other CSs	Syrup, gomme, starch sweetener

[a] Juices from concentrate or reconstituted fruit juice are not considered FJC or CS.

TABLE 9.2
Percentage of Uniquely Formulated Consumer Packaged Food Products Purchased During 2005–2009 by Sweetener Category for Select Food Groups

Select Food or Beverage Group	Number of Unique Products	% Among all Unique Products	% Unique Products Within Food Group[a] Containing			
			No Sweetener	CS (Including FJC) Only	NCS Only	Both CS and NCS
Baby food, formula	993	1.2	47.5	52.5	0.0	0.0
Cakes, cookies, pies	5592	6.5	0.7	95.3	0.1	4.0
Fruit, fresh, frozen, canned, or dried	1722	2.0	36.6	59.9	2.7	0.7
Granola, protein, or energy bars	2526	3.0	3.0	78.2	0.0	18.8
Ready-to-eat cereals	1378	1.6	3.6	94.0	0.3	2.1
Salad dressings and dips	3305	3.9	26.9	71.0	1.5	0.7
Savory snacks	5734	6.7	28.8	69.9	0.7	0.6
Sweet breads and pastries	1440	1.7	17.3	79.3	0.5	2.9
Sweet snacks	6710	7.9	0.6	84.6	0.6	14.1
Yogurt	1152	1.3	6.4	60.8	6.8	26.0
Sports and energy drinks	506	0.6	1.2	63.4	6.9	28.5
Sugar sweetened beverage	2513	2.7	1.5	83.6	1.0	13.9
Diet sweetened beverage[b]	974	1.4	9.9	17.2	14.6	58.3
Milk and milk/yogurt/soy drinks	1483	1.7	32.4	56.6	2.4	8.6
100% Fruit juice	1404	1.6	33.6	66.0	0.0	0.4
Vegetable juice	230	0.3	22.2	69.1	0.4	8.3
Water, plain, or flavored	799	0.9	36.4	21.7	22.3	19.7
All food and beverage groups	85,451	100	25.4	67.9	1.0	5.6

Source: Nielsen Homescan 2005–2009, Gladson Nutrition Database 2007 and 2010.
Note: CS = Caloric sweetener; FJC = Fruit juice czoncentrate; NCS = Noncaloric sweetener.
[a] The % of unique products within this food group (e.g., yogurt) with various types of sweeteners.
[b] Not strictly products that contain zero calories, rather items that are marketed as "nonregular" or less calories than the regular version.

We determined the total calories and volume (or gram weight) of each product using the Homescan purchase and NFP data. We then calculated the proportion of total calories and total volume purchased by Americans that contain any sugars, and any NCS for each food group and all food groups.

From the commercial databases described above, we identified 85,451 unique processed and packaged food and beverage products that were not raw or single ingredient foods [11] (see Table 9.2). Among these, 75% contain some sweetener (68% with sugar only, 1% with NCS only, 6% with both sugar and NCS).

It is useful to see the ranking of use of these sugars in the USA. In Table 9.3, the top five sweetener types included in ingredient lists within each food group are ranked. We found that between 2005 and 2009, across all unique food products, corn syrup is the most commonly listed sweetener, followed by sorghum, cane, HFCS, and FJC. Corn syrup is the most common sweetener used in baby food/formula, salad dressings and dips, sweet snacks, milk and milk/yogurt/soy drinks. HFCS is the most common for cakes/cookies/pies, fruit products, yogurt and sugar sweetened beverages and FJC came up top for fruit juice and vegetable juice. The NCSs, acesulfame potassium, aspartame, and sucralose were the three most common sweeteners found in diet sweetened beverages, and both acesulfame potassium and sucralose were also highly ranked among water products. Unfortunately, since each unique food product's formulation is proprietary information, it is not

TABLE 9.3
Most Common Sweeteners Used in Unique Consumer Packaged Food Products Purchased During 2005–2009 for Select Food Groups

Select Food or Beverage Group	Most Common	Second Most Common	Third Most Common	Fourth Most Common	Fifth Most Common
Baby food, formula	Corn syrup	FJC	Lactose	Sorghum	Cane
Cakes, cookies, pies	HFCS	Sorghum	Corn syrup	Cane	Molasses
Fruit, fresh, frozen, canned, or dried	HFCS	Cane	FJC	Corn syrup	Sucralose
Granola, protein, or energy bars	Sorghum	Cane	Corn syrup	Honey	Alcohol
Ready-to-eat cereals	Sorghum	Cane	Honey	Corn syrup	Molasses
Salad dressings and dips	Corn syrup	FJC	Cane	Sorghum	HFCS
Savory snacks	Sorghum	Corn syrup	Cane	HFCS	Lactose
Sweet breads and pastries	Sorghum	Corn syrup	Cane	HFCS	Honey
Sweet snacks	Corn syrup	Sugar alcohol	Sorghum	Lactose	Honey
Yogurt	HFCS	Fructose	Aspartame	Sucralose	FJC
Sports and energy drinks	Cane	Sucrose	HFCS	Sucralose	Corn syrup
Sugar sweetened beverage	HFCS	FJC	Cane	Corn syrup	Fructose
Diet sweetened beverage[a]	Acesulfame potassium	Aspartame	Sucralose	Cane	FJC
Milk and milk/yogurt/soy drinks	Corn syrup	Cane	HFCS	Sucralose	Sorghum
100% fruit juice	FJC	HFCS	Cane	Fructose	Sorghum
Vegetable juice	FJC	HFCS	Sucralose	Cane	Fructose
Water, plain, or flavored	Sucralose	Acesulfame potassium	Fructose	Cane	Sugar alcohol
All food and beverage groups	Corn syrup	Sorghum	Cane	HFCS	FJC

Source: Nielsen Homescan 2005–2009, Gladson Nutrition Database 2007 and 2010.
[a] NS = Nutritive sweetener; FJC = Fruit juice concentrate not reconstituted; NNS = Nonnutritive sweetener.

possible to determine exactly how much of each sweetener is used, and therefore these rankings are based on frequency of occurrence, rather than volume.

Elsewhere we have explored this topic in more depth but these highlights ultimately show that 77% of all foods and beverages purchased in 2005–2009 from US stores selling packaged foods and beverages contained added sugars [11,20]. We are unable to estimate the amount of these added sugars at this time.

Furthermore, we explored the types of common caloric sweeteners (CSs). Surprisingly, the sweetener in the USA used in the most foods and beverages was not sugarcane or HFCS but rather corn syrup followed by sorghum (a common grass globally which is one source of lower cost sugar used in many foods).

GLOBAL TRENDS—SWEETENING OF THE GLOBAL DIET

At the global level, the only data available are very crude approximations of the amount of CSs available for consumption. These are from food disappearance (called also food balance) data from the Food and Agricultural Organization of the United Nations. These represent approximations from each country across the globe of the amount of added sugar available for human food consumption [6]. They exclude fruit juice concentrate as an added sweetener. These data presented in Table 9.4 show marked increases in selected regions (e.g., Southeast Asia) and much less change in others (e.g., Americas). The largest increase occurred in the regions where the modern food supply

TABLE 9.4
Global Trends on Caloric Sugars Available for Consumption (kcal/capita/day): Food Balance Trends 1961–2009

Regions Not Mutually Exclusive	1961	1970	1980	1990	2000	2009	kcal/day Change 1961–2009
Africa	101	118	155	141	148	153	52
Eastern Africa	63	87	91	79	100	102	39
Northern Africa	167	183	271	278	278	281	114
Southern Africa	361	364	380	344	301	285	–76
Western Africa	38	46	86	61	82	101	63
Americas	421	456	489	487	486	473	52
Caribbean	356	384	424	389	438	367	11
Central America	250	346	437	480	458	468	218
South America	363	377	457	414	376	387	24
Northern America	512	561	546	576	626	585	73
Asia							
Central Asia					162	159	NA
Southeastern Asia	96	118	136	143	184	170	74
Southern Asia	176	194	187	186	203	205	29
Western Asia	107	201	281	303	303	305	198
Oceania	523	518	498	455	414	410	–113
Europe							
Northern Europe	492	481	424	411	381	371	–121
Southern Europe	211	284	320	303	294	275	64
Western Europe	339	395	390	378	419	442	103
World	192	222	236	234	228	224	32

Source: FAOSTAT, accessed April 8, 2013.

is increasing rapidly, particularly caloric beverage intake such as Central America, North Africa, and Western Asia (essentially what we term the Middle East). It must be recognized that these data are very crude approximations and do not account for all sweeteners with calories. Moreover, as we show below with US trends, these trends might not mirror the trends based on dietary intake data. Furthermore, the critical issue from a health perspective is not just consuming excess sugar but whether this is from a beverage or a food product.

US ADDED SUGAR CONSUMPTION FROM NATIONAL DIETARY INTAKE ESTIMATES

The only country for which we have strong estimates of added sugars in the food supply is the USA. Because Brazil also use the same food composition for its last national survey, we can also report on some Brazilian results. The United States Department of Agriculture has developed methods for estimation of the amount of added sugars in the food supply [21,22]. These methods rely on linear programming algorithms used by both USDA and the University of Minnesota Nutrition Coordinating Center [17,18] and data on total sugar intake and other components of each food to estimate the added sugar in each food in the USDA food composition. MPED version 1.0 was used for NFCS1965. NFCS 1977–1978, CSFII 1989–1901, CSFII 1994–1998; MPED version 2.0 was used for WWEIA, NHANES 2003–2004; and MPED version 2.0 addendum was used for WWEIA, NHANES 2005–2006, 2007–2008, and 2009–2010 [16,23,24].

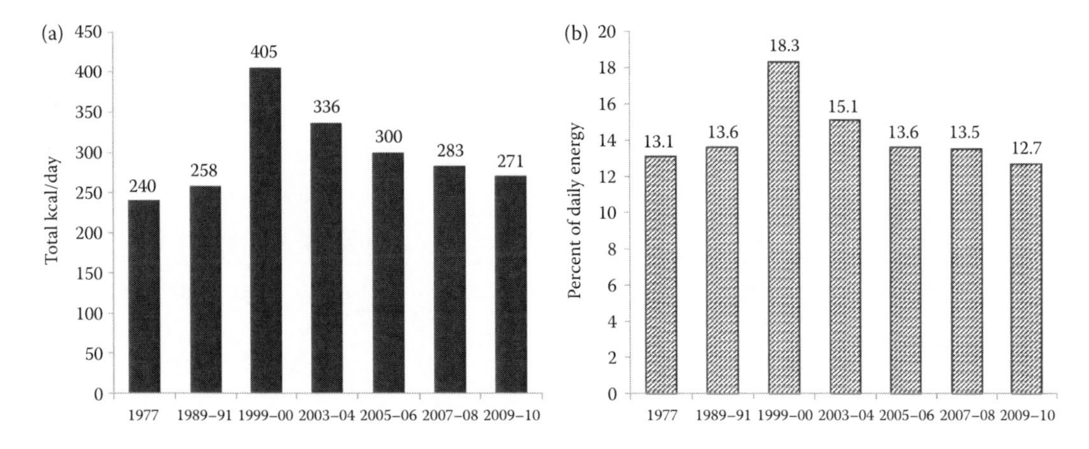

FIGURE 9.1 US nationally representative added sugar trends, 1977–2010, ages 2 and older. (a) Total kcal per day from added sugars, (b) percent of daily energy from added sugars.

Dietary intake data from each survey period were linked to a food composition database developed by the USDA with nutrient values corresponding to the diets of individuals at the time of processing. Prior to 2003–2004, the only surveys to use this same food composition database were the USDA nationally representative surveys. For WWEIA, NHANES 2003–2004, 2005–2006, 2007–2008, and 2009–2010, data were used from the USDA's Food and Nutrient Database for Dietary Studies (FNDDS) which is used to code, process, and analyze the data assessed in the course of the WWEIA survey [25–29]. Each nutrient database was derived from the USDA Nutrient Data Base for Standard Reference (SR), versions 11, 18, 20, and 22 [30].

Figure 9.1 provides estimates of consumption of added sugars from these dietary intake nationally representative surveys that use the same USDA food composition table. We see that the large increase in added sugars that began in the 1970s and peaked in 1999–2000 started to decline for the USA in the past decade [31]. This coincided with a marked reduction in added sugar from beverages, in particular [32]. We see how the percentage of kcal/day from added sugar in the USA peaked at 18.3% in 1999–2000 and has declined subsequently.

Figure 9.2 provides data on the total distribution by quintile of added sugar consumers in the USA. For those consuming CS beverages, the reduction occurred in all quintiles. Smaller declines occurred among the third and fourth quintiles of 70 and 100 kcal/day from peak intake in 1999–2000 but these are major meaningful decreases. There were also equally meaningful declines in added sugar from foods but in absolute and relative terms they are much smaller. Figure 9.2 highlights the marked increase among the top quintile of added sugar users of 396 kcal/day between 1977 and 1999–2000 and then the precipitous decline of 294 kcal/day between that peak and 2009–2010. This is mainly linked with a decline in sugar-sweetened beverage intake (data not shown).

In Brazil, a nationally representative dietary intake survey found that added sugar in 2008–2009 represents 13% of total calories with about half coming from food (mainly sweets and desserts) and half from an array of beverages [33]. This is essentially at about the same level as the USA.

GLOBAL TRENDS ON BEVERAGES—THE LEADING SOURCE OF ADDED SUGAR INCREASES GLOBALLY

There are surprisingly few diet surveys across LMICs, and only a few higher-income countries (US, UK, Japan, South Korea) have annual or episodic dietary intake surveys. In the last several years, Brazil conducted its first national dietary intake survey and Mexico has collected detailed dietary intake data in its national nutrition surveys in 1999 and 2011–2012. We have also utilized

Total	Q1	Q2	Q3	Q4	Q5	
1977	32	114	195	299	560	
1989-91	29	113	206	324	616	+396kcal
1999-2000	62	194	321	491	956	
2003-2004	57	160	270	416	775	
2005-2006	46	136	233	369	715	−294kcal
2007-2008	43	129	217	339	686	
2009-2010	41	120	205	326	662	

Source: Duffey & Popkin(2008) AJCN 88 (suppl):1722S
* Underestimate,due to omission fruit juice concentrate

FIGURE 9.2 Shifts in added sugar by Quintile of Consumption among US individuals aged 2 and older.

in some of our research sales data on caloric beverages from Euromonitor by company to provide some sense of the dynamics of sugary beverage use. The major limitation with all of this work is the continued introduction of hundreds of new versions of caloric beverages—be they energy drinks, sugars, vitamin waters, sports drinks, or any number of other new variants. As we have shown in other research [20], the commercial sector changes are often not accurately captured by the food composition tables used in national surveys and because these beverages are often consumed in ad hoc ways throughout the day, they are often missed in both surveys using recall methods or scanning of the foods.

Here we report on a limited set of studies across LMICs along with data from selected European studies we conducted.

EUROPE

Our only consumption data was on adolescents aged 12.5–17.5 years selected using a multistage random cluster sampling procedure from the 10 selected European cities [34]. Mean beverage consumption was 1611 ml/day in boys and 1316 ml/day in girls. Energy intake from beverages was about 470 and 370 cal/day in European boys and girls, respectively, with sugar-sweetened beverages (defined as carbonated and noncarbonated beverages, including soft drinks, fruit drinks, and powders/concentrates with any type of CS) contributing to daily energy intake more than other groups of beverages. Boys and older adolescents consumed the most amount of per capita total energy from beverages. Among all age and gender subgroups, sugar-sweetened beverages, sweetened milk (including chocolate milk and flavored yogurt drinks all with added sugar), low-fat milk, and fruit juice provided the highest amount of per capita energy. Water was consumed by the largest percent of adolescents followed by sugar-sweetened beverages, fruit juice, and sweetened milk. Among consumers, water provided the greatest fluid intake and sweetened milk accounted for the largest amount of energy intake followed by sugar-sweetened beverages. Patterns of energy intake from each beverage varied between countries.

Trends in a European country—the UK: This is the only country we were able to obtain consistently measured nationally representative beverage intake data for [34]. In 2008/2009, beverages accounted for 21, 14, and 18% of daily energy intake for children aged 1.5–18 years, 4–18 years, and adults (19–64 years), respectively. Since the 1990s, the most important shifts are a reduction in consumption of high-fat dairy products (−13 kcal/day) and an increased consumption of fruit juices (+9 kcal/day) and sweetened milk (+10 kcal/day) among preschoolers, children, and adolescents.

Among adults between 1986–1987 and 2008–2009, consumption of high-fat milk beverages (−6 kcal/day) and sweetened tea and coffee (−94 kcal/day) fell, but reduced-fat milk (+14 kcal/day), alcohol (particularly beer) (+49 kcal/day), and fruit juice (+7 kcal/day) rose. The beverage consumption patterns of these UK adolescents mirrored that of the European countries noted above.

Trends in Mexico and Brazil: As the two largest countries in Central and South America, these countries represent some of the major new targets for sales of caloric beverages. Elsewhere we have shown that kcal/ounce of beverages sold in the USA by Coca-Cola and Pepsi Cola have been declining as they push in the USA and UK for enhanced sales of noncalorically sweetened beverages and waters [35]. In contrast, we showed that in China and Brazil, among many LMICs, they have pushed for increased sales of caloric beverages of a wide array from classic sugar-sweetened beverages to flavored waters and energy drinks.

Mexico is a remarkable case study of the dynamics of this sector and its efforts to reach into LMICs. By 1996, Mexicans consumed more than 20% of their daily energy intake from caloric beverages [36,37]. In an unpublished work, Stern et al. [38] examined daily intake for nationally representative data in 2011–2012. They found high levels of caloric beverage intake among adolescents and adults. In both cases, about 50% of males and females aged 12–18 and 19–59 consumed sodas and among those consuming sodas (excluding sports and energy drinks and many other added sugar beverages), adults 20–59 consumed 215 kcal/day and adolescents consumed 194 kcal/day. The figures for female consumers aged 20–49 of sodas only in 1999 and 2012 were 149 and 187 kcal/day, respectively.

In Brazil, based on a national representative survey from those aged 10 and older, we found that the overall contribution of beverages to total daily energy intake was 17.1%, which decreased slightly with age ($\beta = -0.005\%$; $p < 0.01$; data not shown) [39]. The beverage groups that contributed most to total daily energy intake in the full sample were the calorie coffee beverages (6.4%), fruit/vegetable juices (4.7%), and calorie milk/soymilk beverages (2.9%) (Table 9.2). Calorie coffee beverages provided the greatest level of calories overall (111 kcal/day). Individuals from 10 to 18 (58 kcal/day) and from 19 to 39 years old (55 kcal/day) consumed higher proportion of energy from sugar sweetened soft drinks than individuals over this age (34 kcal/day for those 40–59 and 19 kcal/day for those >60 years old).

SUMMARY

There are several patterns and trends that emerge from this chapter. First, it is clear that added sugars/sweeteners are found in far more products than would be expected. That approximately 75% of all foods and beverages have some type of added sugar in the US food supply suggests that added sugar may be increasingly being used in our diet although we do not have historical data from earlier periods to act as a comparison. A recent book by an established journalist on this topic provides important insights into this behavior [40]. One important element for readers seeking natural or organic products is the increasing use of fruit juice concentrate as an added sugar.

Second, aside from Europe and Oceana, few regions seem to be seeing a decline in added sugar available for consumption. Rather, it is the opposite, particularly for Central America and North Africa. This is based on the food disappearance data as studies on individual dietary intake exist only for Mexico, Brazil, and the UAE [41] among these regions.

Third, when we have data like we have for the USA and Brazil on added sugar intake in our diet, we find levels that can vary from 12.7 to 18%. However, it is important to note that these US estimates exclude fruit juice concentrate.

Fourth are the global beverage trends. The USA, and I expect also Western Europe, are reducing their intake of added sugar, particularly from beverages as they shift to noncaloric sweetened beverages or unsweetened beverages (e.g., water, tea, coffee). The opposite is true in LMICs where we have documentation. These include Mexico, which is one of the major consumers of added sugar, and this has had a profound effect on consumption of calorically sweetened beverages across all age groups.

ACKNOWLEDGMENTS

We thank the Carolina Population Center (5 R24 HD050924) and UNC for financial support. We also thank Ms. Frances L. Dancy for administrative assistance and Mr. Tom Swasey for graphics support and for research assistance. This author has participated as co-investigator in a grant funded by Nestlé's Water USA and as a consultant to the Mexican National Institute of Public Health and in a second one funded by Danome Water. Otherwise, he does not have any conflict of interests of any type with respect to this manuscript.

CONFLICTS OF INTEREST

Barry Popkin does not and has never been consulted for the beverage industry or, for that matter, for any company. He has been involved with two separate grants to the University of North Carolina at Chapel Hill (as a co-investigator) and to the Mexican National Institute of Public Health (as a collaborator and mentor) on the issue of beverage intake and health. He was a co-investigator on a grant for which Deborah Tate was the principal investigator who received funds from Nestlé's Water. In addition, he has taken remuneration for costs to speak on beverage intake patterns and trends at the British Nutrition Society annual meeting from Danone Research. In 2004, prior to an AJCN publication in 2006, George Bray, Walter Willett, Balz Frey, and Lawrence Armstrong took funding from Unilever to support travel and the venue for a daylong meeting in New York City to create a US beverage guidance review. He has never been involved in any company that manufactures or markets any sweetener-caloric or low caloric.

REFERENCES

1. Mattes RD. Dietary compensation by humans for supplemental energy provided as ethanol or carbohydrate in fluids. *Physiol Behav*. 1996;59(1):179–87.
2. DiMeglio DP, Mattes RD. Liquid versus solid carbohydrate: Effects on food intake and body weight. *Int J Obes Relat Metab Disord*. 2000;24(6):794–800.
3. Mourao DM, Bressan J, Campbell WW, Mattes RD. Effects of food form on appetite and energy intake in lean and obese young adults. *Int J Obes (London)*. 2007;31(11):1688–95.
4. Malik VS, Popkin BM, Bray GA, Despres JP, Willett WC, Hu FB. Sugar-sweetened beverages and risk of metabolic syndrome and type 2 diabetes: A meta-analysis. *Diabetes Care*. 2010;33(11):2477–83.
5. Malik VS, Schulze MB, Hu FB. Intake of sugar-sweetened beverages and weight gain: A systematic review. *Am J Clin Nutr*. 2006;84(2):274–88.
6. Popkin BM, Nielsen SJ. The sweetening of the world's diet. *Obes Res*. 2003;11(11):1325–32.
7. Yudkin J. Dietary fat and dietary sugar in relation to ischemic heart-disease and diabetes. *Lancet*. 1964;2:4.
8. Yudkin J. Sweet and Dangerous: The New Facts About the Sugar You Eat As a Cause of Heart Disease, Diabetes, and Other Killers. London: Bantam Books; 1972.
9. Trowell HC, Burkett DP. Western Diseases: Their Emergence and Prevention. Cambridge, MA: Harvard University Press; 1981.
10. Popkin BM. The World is Fat—The Fads, Trends, Policies, and Products that are Fattening the Human Race. New York: Avery-Penguin Group; 2008.
11. Ng SW, Slining MM, Popkin BM. Use of caloric and noncaloric sweeteners in US consumer packaged foods, 2005–2009. *J Acad Nutr Diet*. 2012;112(11):1828–34.e6.
12. U.S. Department of Agriculture. USDA Database for the Added Sugars Content of Selected Foods, Release 1. Beltsville, MD: USDA; 2006. Available from: http://www.ars.usda.gov/services/docs.htm?docid=12107.
13. U.S. Department of Agriculture. MyPyramid Equivalents Database. Beltsville, MD: USDA; 2012. Available from: http://www.ars.usda.gov/Services/docs.htm?docid=17558 (accessed 31 January 2012).
14. USDA. Discretionary calories: What are "added sugars". Washington, DC: USDA; 2011. Available from: http://www.mypyramid.gov/pyramid/discretionary_calories_sugars.html.
15. USDA. Food Patterns Equivalents Database. In: Agricultural Research Service Food Surveys Division, editor. Beltsville, MD: USDA; 2013.

16. Koegel KL, Kuczynski KJ. Center for Nutrition Policy and Promotion Addendum to the MyPyramid Equivalents Database 2.0; 2011. Available from: Center for Nutrition Policy and Promotion Addendum to the MyPyramid Equivalents Database 2.0 [Online].
17. Westrich BJ, Altmann MA, Potthoff SJ. Minnesota's nutrition coordinating center uses mathematical optimization to estimate food nutrient values. *Interfaces*. 1998;28(5):86–99.
18. Westrich BJ, Buzzard IM, Gatewood LC, McGovern PG. Accuracy and efficiency of estimating nutrient values in commercial food products using mathematical optimization. *J Food Composition Analysis*. 1994;7(4):223–39.
19. Ng SW, Popkin BM. Monitoring foods and nutrients sold and consumed in the US: Dynamics and challenges. *J Acad Nutr Diet*. 2012;112(1):41–5.e4.
20. Piernas C, Ng SW, Popkin BM. Trends in purchases and intake of foods and beverages containing caloric and low-calorie sweeteners over the last decade in the United States. *Pediatr Obes*. 2013;8(4):294–306.
21. Slining MM, Popkin BM. Trends in intakes and sources of solid fats and added sugars among U.S. children and adolescents: 1994–2010. *Pediatr Obes*. 2013;8:307–24.
22. Duffey KJ, Popkin BM. High-fructose corn syrup: Is this what's for dinner? *Am J Clin Nutr*. 2008;88(6):1722S–32S.
23. Friday JE, Bowman SA. MyPyramid Equivalents Database for USDA Survey Food Codes, 1994–2002 Version 1.0; 2006. Available from: http://www.barc.usda.gov/bhnrc/fsrg.
24. Bowman SA, Friday JE, Moshfegh AJ. My Pyramid Equvalents Database, 2.0 for USDA Survey Foods, 2003–2004. Food Surveys Research Group 2008. Available from: http://www.ars.usda.gov/Services/docs.htm?docid=17558.
25. Ahuja J, Montville J, Omolewa-Tomobi G, Heendeniya KY, Martin CL, Steinfeldt LC et al. USDA Food and Nutrient Database for Dietary Studies, 5.0. In: Department of Agriculture ARS, Food Surveys Research Group, editor. Beltsville, MD: USDA; 2012.
26. Food Surveys Research Group. USDA Food and Nutrient Database for Dietary Studies, 4.1. In: Agricultural Research Service, editor. Beltsville, MD: USDA; 2010.
27. Food Surveys Research Group. USDA Food and Nutrient Database for Dietary Studies, 3.0. In: Agricultural Research Service, editor. Beltsville, MD: USDA; 2008.
28. Food Surveys Research Group. USDA Food and Nutrient Database for Dietary Studies, 2.0. In: Agricultural Research Service, editor. Beltsville, MD: USDA; 2006.
29. Food Surveys Research Group. USDA Food and Nutrient Database for Dietary Studies, 5.0. In: Agricultural Research Service, editor. Beltsville, MD: USDA; 2012.
30. USDA. Food and Nutrient Database for Dietary Studies, 2.0. In: Department of Agriculture ARS, Food Survey Research Group, editor. 2006.
31. Ng SW, Slining MM, Popkin BM. A turning point for US diets? Recessionary effects or behavioral shifts in foods purchased and consumed. University of North Carolina, 2013.
32. Kit BK, Fakhouri TH, Park S, Nielsen SJ, Ogden CL. Trends in sugar-sweetened beverage consumption among youth and adults in the United States: 1999–2010. *Am J Clin Nutr*. 2013;98(1):180–8.
33. Pereira RA, Duffey KJ, Sichieri R, Popkin BM. Sources of excessive saturated fat, trans fat and sugar consumption in Brazil: An analysis of the first Brazilian Nationwide Individual Dietary Survey. *Public Health Nutr*. 2014;1(1):113–21.
34. Duffey KJ, Huybrechts I, Mouratidou T, Libuda L, Kersting M, Devriendt K et al. Beverage consumption among European adolescents in the HELENA Study. *Eur J Clin Nutr*. 2011;66:244–52.
35. Kleiman S, Ng SW, Popkin BM. Drinking to our health: Can beverage companies cut calories while maintaining profits? *Obes Rev*. 2012;13(3):258–74.
36. Barquera S, Campirano F, Bonvecchio A, Hernández L, Rivera JA, Popkin BM. Caloric beverage consumption patterns in Mexican children. *Nutr J*. 2010;9:47–56.
37. Barquera S, Hernandez-Barrera L, Tolentino ML, Espinosa J, Ng SW, Rivera JA et al. Energy intake from beverages is increasing among Mexican adolescents and adults. *J Nutr*. 2008;138(12):2454–61.
38. Stern D, Duffey K, Barquera S, Rivera-Dommarco JA, Popkin BM. Sugar sweetened beverage sales and consumption trends in Mexico: 1999–2012. Unpublished Manuscript; 2013.
39. Pereira RA, Souza AM, Duffey KJ, Sichieri R, Popkin BM. Beverages sales and consumption in Brazil. Unpublished Manuscript; 2013.
40. Moss M. Salt Sugar Fat: How the Food Giants Hooked Us. New York: Random House; 2013.
41. Ng SW, Zaghloul S, Ali H, Harrison G, Yeatts K, El Sadig M et al. Nutrition transition in the United Arab Emirates. *Eur J Clin Nutr*. 2011;65(12):1328–37.

10 Dietary Intake and Availability of Fructose and Sweeteners in the USA

Bernadette P. Marriott

CONTENTS

KEY POINTS

- Estimated mean total fructose intake, as a percentage of total energy, was higher in 2004 (9.1%) than in 1978 (8.1%), with significant increases in some age groups occurring. Compared with 1978, overall average energy intake in the USA also was higher in 2004 (2004: 2148 ± 12.8 kcal/day; 1978: 1817 ± 11.0 kcal/day).
- Estimated mean total fructose intake expressed as a percentage of carbohydrate intake was less in 2004 (17.1%) compared to 1978 (18.6%), which reflected the estimated 41% higher intake of carbohydrates in 2004 in the USA compared to 1978.
- With the exception of 1–3-year-olds, the estimated intake of *naturally occurring* fructose was 3–7 g/day less in 2004 than in 1978.
- Overall, 13% of the population had added sugars intake >25%; mean added sugars intake: 83.1 g-eq/day. More non-Hispanic Black individuals (15.1%), those with a poverty-income ratio below the poverty line (17.5%), and underweight individuals (15.4%) consumed the highest level of added sugars intake (>25% of total energy from added sugars).
- Between 1999–2000 and 2007–2008, the absolute intake of added sugars decreased significantly by 23.4% from a mean of 100.1 to 76.7 g/day. The mean percentage of total energy from added sugars decreased significantly from 18.1% (in 1999–2000) to 14.6% (in 2007–2008). The total energy intake also decreased from 2145 kcal/day (in 1999–2000) to 2069 kcal/day (in 2007–2008), a mean decrease of 76 kcal/day or 4%.

- In 1985, 1999, and 2010, while the *total average per capita calories available* in the US food supply continued to increase (2270, 2508, and 2546 kcal), the per capita availability of energy from sugar and added sweeteners increased and then decreased: 1985: 352 kcal (16%); 1999: 429 kcal (17%); 2010: 379 kcal (15%), and energy available from added fats and oils and dairy fats steadily increased: 1985: 427 kcal (19%); 1999: 444 kcal (18%); 2010: 588 kcal (23%).
- Between 1978 and 2004, fructose intake increased, while availability of fructose in the food supply as a percent of total sweetener increased until 2000 and then remained constant through 2005. Current data indicate that overall intake and availability of added sweeteners in the USA is decreasing.

INTRODUCTION

Sugar production is one of the world's oldest industries and was first described in northern India around 500 BC [1]. Sugar began being produced in large quantities at lower prices during the seventeenth century and became more accessible to the general population. By the nineteenth century, sugar was considered an indispensable part of the diet and was linked with industrialization and to economic and societal changes [2]. In 1913, the USA was reported to have consumed nearly 82 pounds per capita of the world's production of approximately 16 million tons of sucrose sugar [3]. Currently, the USA, as a marketplace, consumes more sweeteners than any other country in the world and is also one of the largest producers and importers of sugar [4].

The purpose of this chapter is to provide an overview of dietary intake of caloric sweeteners and their consumption in the USA. There is no laboratory analysis method that can distinguish between sugars that naturally occur in foods and sugars that are added [5]. Thus, in attempting to describe dietary sugar intake, three major challenges arise: (1) for sweeteners, both intrinsic to food and added, dietary intake research has tended to focus on specific sweeteners such as sucrose, high-fructose corn syrup (HFCS), fructose, glucose, and the ever widening array of new sweeteners on the global market such as agave nectar, stevia, etc. or sweeteners grouped in different ways resulting in data that are difficult to compare; (2) as described in Chapter 17 and by others, [5] national dietary guidelines differ both in amount of recommended sugar intake levels and focus of the recommendation, whether on free sugars, added sugars, etc. and (3) of most concern, data on intake are generated by a number of diverse dietary assessment techniques.

In this chapter, an overview of national *intake* data on fructose and added sugars in the USA is provided. Many studies have also cited data on sweetener "availability" in the market, henceforth termed "consumption data." Therefore, this chapter will also include fructose and added sweetener *availability* information. Throughout, the focus will be on *added* fructose, sugar, and sweeteners and not on the food sources such as beverages, bakery products, or confectionary. For the individual intake data collected as part of national surveys, the terms "decreased" or "increased" may be used to describe the changes over time. These terms are being used in a relational context only as it is important to remember that the data in these interview-based surveys are cross-sectional not longitudinal and thus each sample contains data on different individuals not repeated samples from the same individuals.

INDIVIDUAL DIETARY ASSESSMENT

Methods for dietary intake estimation in national health surveillance studies and large clinical trials vary among multi-pass 24-h recall methods [6], single or multiple day food frequency questionnaires (FFQs) [7–9], and food diaries [10–12]. In the USA, the current "gold standard" is the United States Department of Agriculture's (USDA's) validated 24-h individual, *interviewer-based*, food and beverage recall, the Automated Multi-Pass Method (AMPM) [13]. Two AMPM interview-based dietary assessments, the first conducted by in-person interview and the second interview typically by telephone, are used by the US Center for Disease Control and Prevention (CDC) as the dietary assessment approach in its continuing nationally stratified health surveillance of the US population, the National Health and Nutrition Examination Survey (NHANES). NHANES also incorporates an FFQ, which obtains information about the approximate frequency food and beverage intake by interview over a set time period, such as the last 30 days, last week, etc. FFQs may or may not include collection of data on portion sizes. The NHANES FFQ uses a look-back time period of 12 months with specific questions that address seasonal intake of foods such as fruits and vegetables. The NHANES FFQ does not include portion size (see http://appliedresearch.cancer.gov/diet/usualintakes/ffq.html). Usual dietary intake can be estimated using two AM/PM assessments and the National Cancer Institute (NCI) method of long-term average estimation with or without the FFQ as a covariate [14]. Dietary intake assessment methods vary greatly in the USA and often use FFQs of variable look-back durations, and food diaries, as well as single and multiple 24-h recalls (see, e.g., the NCI web site for a discussion of recommended, validated methods: http://appliedresearch.cancer.gov/resource/collection.html).

Food Consumption or Availability

In addition to national surveillance intake information compiled through individual dietary assessment, data on per capita food *available* for intake (historically in the USA termed "disappearance data") are collected throughout the world and compiled by the Food and Agriculture Organization (FAO) of the United Nations (http://faostat3.fao.org/faostat-gateway/go/to/home/E). The FAO presents these data as food balance sheets (FBSs), which are calculated from the food produced within and imported into a country minus the food exported (net of imports), fed to animals, or otherwise not available for human consumption, and then divided by the population size. FBSs thus can provide comprehensive information about a country's food supply during a specified time period and are a measure of the total food *available* for human consumption per capita. FBSs are an approximation of the average availability of foods per person and do not represent the actual food intake because they are *not* compilations of what individuals in the region reported eating/drinking. FBSs and other food availability data are typically presented in the literature as food *consumed* by a country or region and thus termed *food consumption* data [15].

In some countries such as the USA, the food availability data are systematically corrected for loss due to wastage at specific points from production to plate, such as food spoilage in the supply chain, at home, plate waste, etc. The USDA has compiled and provided food availability data since the 1860s. The USDA Economic Research Service (ERS) currently generates three per capita and total data sets: food availability, loss-adjusted food availability, and an estimate of nutrient availability; these data sets enable researchers to estimate the nutrient availability of the US food supply and compare the nutrient availability for the US population to national nutrition recommendations [4]. By definition and method of compilation therefore, even loss-adjusted food availability estimates and FBSs overestimate actual food intake in a country. However, because FBSs are available *for every country in the world* through the FAO for a wide variety of food items, they provide an additional method to compare international trends in food use that can reflect changes in dietary patterns worldwide [16].

In the USA, food availability data are constructed by the ERS for hundreds of basic commodities, not processed foods, and compiled as follows:

> Available commodity supply (production + imports + beginning stocks) − Measurable nonfood use (farm inputs + exports + ending stocks, etc.) = Total annual food supply of a commodity.

The ERS has included annual US total and per capita availability of caloric sweeteners since 1941. These dry-weight availability estimates include refined cane and beet sugar, corn sweeteners, honey, and edible syrups [4]. Through the annual FBSs, the FAO provides per capita sugar and sweetener availability estimates from all the countries in the world [17].

INDIVIDUAL DIETARY ASSESSMENT OF INTAKE

INTAKE OF FRUCTOSE IN THE USA

In 1993, Park and Yetley [18] reported estimates of fructose intake in the US diet based on dietary recall data for 30,770 individuals collected during the nationally representative 1977–1978 Nationwide Food Consumption Survey (NFCS). The NFCS compiled up to 3 days of dietary records for each participant with at least one 24-h interviewer-based recall and 1 or 2 days of participant self-administered food records. These authors estimated fructose intake by applying conversion factors to measures of added and naturally occurring (NO) sugar. The conversion factors were based on the landmark Glinsmann et al.'s report of the Sugars Task Force from the mid-1980s [19]. Conversion factors comprised the fructose percentage of added sugar for the food group, based on sugar deliveries to an industry sector such as bakery. Basically, the conversion factors were calculated by multiplying the total amount of each type of sweetener (glucose, dextrose, HFCS-42, HFCS-55) by the sugar content of the sweetener (e.g., sucrose is 100% sugar; HFCS contains 98% sugar), which enabled the derivation of total sugar deliveries. While the conversion factors were equivalent to the percent of total sugar deliveries from each source, sucrose, HFCS, and other corn sweeteners, an additional conversion factor was calculated by multiplying the amount of sugars in HFCS by the fructose content of HFCS (42 or 55% fructose), and included estimates of free and bound (one-half the conversion factor for sucrose) fructose (see Reference 18 for detail). In 1978, the overall estimated mean total fructose intake as a percentage of energy was 8.1%.

In 2009, we published data on estimated national fructose *intake* based on 1999–2004 NHANES [20]. While acknowledging that methodological changes in the intervening years were limitations to our comparison [20], we estimated usual intake of fructose following the then most current approach using C-side analysis of two NHANES 24-h recalls [21–23]. We also used the same conversion factor approach as Park and Yetley [18].

We found that estimated fructose gram intake was higher in all gender and age groups in 2004 compared to 1978 (see Table 10.1). In terms of estimated grams of fructose intake, young men in age groups 15–18 years and 19–22 years had the highest mean intake of total fructose at 75 g/day. Women aged 19–22 years similarly consumed the highest mean total fructose: 61 g/day. These 2004 figures represented 33 and 30 g/day higher intake for 19–22-year-old men and women, respectively, compared with 1978. The 95th percentile intake for these groups was men: 121, 134 g/day and women: 116 g/day. As discussed by White [24], a number of studies have reported adverse health effects through intake experiments. These experimental studies have provided as much as a three-fold above these 95th percentile US intake levels [25]. It is important to note that the increase in total fructose intake between the two time periods is due to an increase in *added fructose* not *naturally occurring fructose intake.* For all age and gender groups represented in Table 10.1, with the exception of 1–3-year olds, the estimated intake of naturally occurring fructose was 3–7 g/day less in 2004 than in 1978.

We found that the overall estimated total fructose intake as a percentage of total energy was 9.1% (range 7.4–11.6%) in 2004 and thus higher than the 8.1% of total energy reported in 1978. Compared with the 1978 data of Park and Yetley, overall average energy intake in the USA also was higher in 2004 (1978: 1817 ± 11.0 kcal/day; 2004: 2148 ± 12.8 kcal/day). Similarly, we found that the overall estimated mean total fructose intake expressed as a percentage of carbohydrate was less in 2004 (17.1%) compared to 1978 (18.6%), which reflected the estimated general 41% higher intake of carbohydrates in 2004 in the USA compared to 1978 (see Table 10.2).

TABLE 10.1
Mean Fructose Intake (g/day ± SEM): NFCS (1977–1978) and NHANES (1999–2004)

Sex/Age Group	Sample Size 1999–2004 (1977–1978)	Added Fructose 1977–1978	Added Fructose 1999–2004	Naturally Occurring Fructose 1977–1978	Naturally Occurring Fructose 1999–2004	Total Fructose 1977–1978	Total Fructose 1999–2004
Both sexes							
1–3 years	2087 (1716)	18 ± 0.5	22 ± 0.9	12 ± 0.4	12 ± 0.5	29 ± 0.6	34 ± 1.0
4–6 years	1458 (1947)	24 ± 0.5	34 ± 1.3	12 ± 0.3	9 ± 0.5	36 ± 0.6	43 ± 1.3
7–10 years	2001 (2788)	28 ± 0.5	44 ± 2.1	14 ± 0.3	7 ± 0.5	42 ± 0.6	51 ± 2.1
Males							
11–14 years	1504 (1592)	34 ± 0.6	53 ± 2.5	14 ± 0.4	7 ± 0.5	49 ± 0.7	60 ± 2.3
15–18 years	1704 (1510)	39 ± 0.8	68 ± 2.4	15 ± 0.4	8 ± 0.8	54 ± 0.9	75 ± 2.7
19–22 years	746 (738)	34 ± 1.1	67 ± 4.5	14 ± 0.5	8 ± 1.1	47 ± 1.2	75 ± 4.2
23–50 years	2925 (3792)	28 ± 0.5	54 ± 1.7	14 ± 0.3	8 ± 0.6	43 ± 0.5	63 ± 1.8
51+ years	3076 (2677)	21 ± 0.4	32 ± 1.3	16 ± 0.4	9 ± 0.4	36 ± 0.6	41 ± 1.5
Females							
11–14 years	1639 (1591)	29 ± 0.6	43 ± 1.9	13 ± 0.3	7 ± 0.4	42 ± 0.7	50 ± 2.0
15–18 years	1485 (1596)	29 ± 0.6	48 ± 2.2	12 ± 0.3	7 ± 0.4	40 ± 0.7	55 ± 2.3
19–22 years	609 (922)	24 ± 0.7	54 ± 3.3	11 ± 0.4	7 ± 0.8	35 ± 0.7	61 ± 3.4
23–50 years	2769 (5220)	20 ± 0.4	39 ± 1.4	12 ± 0.3	7 ± 0.4	32 ± 0.4	45 ± 1.2
51+ years	3167 (4113)	16 ± 0.3	24 ± 0.9	14 ± 0.3	8 ± 0.3	29 ± 0.5	32 ± 0.8

Source: Adapted from Park YK, Yetley EA. *Am J Clin Nutr.* 1993;58(suppl):737S–47S; Marriott BP, Cole N, Lee E. *J Nutr.* 2009;139(6):1228S–35S.

Added Sugar Intake in the USA

In 2010, we looked more broadly at assessment of usual intake of added sugar in the USA, based on NHANES 2003–2006 data [26]. One purpose of the study was to update and expand the earlier results published as Appendix Table J in the Institute of Medicine (IOM) Dietary Reference Intake (DRI) report on macronutrients in 2002 [27]. The IOM macronutrient report recommended a maximal intake level of 25% or less of energy from added sugars for both adults and children. It is important to note that this recommendation was not presented as a tolerable upper intake level or UL. The IOM Committee made the 25% maximal intake recommendation in part due to concern about the potential for low micronutrient intake of persons whose diet exceeded 25% of energy from added sugars. The recommendation was based on the existing literature and also estimated median intakes of selected micronutrients at 5% increments of added sugars intake included in Appendix Table J of the Committee report. The data in Table J were based on NHANES III data, which was collected between 1988 and 1994 (http://www.cdc.gov/nchs/nhanes/nh3rrm.htm).

Outside the USA, international recommendations vary greatly with regard to added sugar intake. Majority of countries address sugar consumption and provide qualitative recommendations such as to "limit" or "reduce sugar consumption" (Argentina, Germany), or "reduce sugar intake and choose foods low in sugar" (Mexico) [5]. Other counties specifically address added sugars quantitatively, recommend a maximum of 10% (Finland, Iceland, Norway or 15% (Italy) of energy from added sugars [5].

TABLE 10.2
Estimated Mean and 90th and 95th Percentile Usual Fructose Intake as Percentage of Energy Intake of the US Population (≥1-Year Old) by DRI Gender and Age Groups (NHANES, 1999–2004)[a–c]

Gender/Age Group	Sample Size, n[d]	Energy Intake (kcal/Day)[e]	Mean			90th Percentile			95th Percentile		
			Added	Naturally Occurring	Total[f]	Added	Naturally Occurring	Total[g]	Added	Naturally Occurring	Total[g]
			% of Energy Intake			% of Energy Intake			% of Energy Intake		
Both sexes											
1–3 years	2087	1509 ± 25.5	5.8 ± 0.20	3.2 ± 0.14	9.0 ± 0.21	9.5 ± 0.32	5.7 ± 0.24	12.5 ± 0.31	10.8 ± 0.38	6.8 ± 0.35	13.7 ± 0.36
4–8 years	2473	1892 ± 34.0	7.9 ± 0.22	1.8 ± 0.11	9.7 ± 0.19	10.9 ± 0.26	3.3 ± 0.18	12.6 ± 0.23	11.9 ± 0.29	3.9 ± 0.22	13.6 ± 0.26
Males											
9–13 years	1600	2289 ± 60.0	8.8 ± 0.25	1.2 ± 0.07	10.0 ± 0.25	11.8 ± 0.30	2.2 ± 0.11	13.0 ± 0.29	12.8 ± 0.33	2.6 ± 0.12	14.0 ± 0.32
14–18 years	2103	2735 ± 64.6	9.9 ± 0.38	1.2 ± 0.08	11.0 ± 0.35	13.9 ± 0.58	2.2 ± 0.16	14.6 ± 0.53	15.3 ± 0.70	2.8 ± 0.19	15.8 ± 0.64
19–30 years	1555	2890 ± 62.6	8.9 ± 0.36	1.1 ± 0.11	10.0 ± 0.32	13.5 ± 0.52	2.2 ± 0.24	14.9 ± 0.48	15.1 ± 0.69	2.8 ± 0.30	16.6 ± 0.56
31–50 years	2115	2775 ± 36.9	7.5 ± 0.21	1.3 ± 0.09	8.8 ± 0.22	12.2 ± 0.41	2.5 ± 0.17	13.3 ± 0.36	14.0 ± 0.51	3.1 ± 0.19	15.0 ± 0.45
51–70 years	1889	2289 ± 44.4	5.8 ± 0.21	1.7 ± 0.07	7.4 ± 0.22	10.2 ± 0.38	3.1 ± 0.14	11.7 ± 0.36	11.9 ± 0.47	3.8 ± 0.18	13.3 ± 0.45
71+ years	1187	1878 ± 32.4	5.4 ± 0.18	2.1 ± 0.09	7.5 ± 0.17	8.7 ± 0.33	3.6 ± 0.15	10.6 ± 0.28	9.8 ± 0.42	4.2 ± 0.18	11.7 ± 0.35

Females											
9–13 years	1673	1954 ± 36.8	8.7 ± 0.33	1.5 ± 0.09	10.2 ± 0.33	11.7 ± 0.39	2.6 ± 0.14	12.5 ± 0.39	12.7 ± 0.42	3.0 ± 0.15	13.3 ± 0.41
14–18 years	1939	1968 ± 39.9	9.6 ± 0.33	1.4 ± 0.10	11.0 ± 0.34	13.3 ± 0.49	2.8 ± 0.22	14.9 ± 0.48	14.5 ± 0.54	3.4 ± 0.25	16.2 ± 0.56
19–30 years	1305	2033 ± 42.4	9.5 ± 0.37	1.3 ± 0.10	10.8 ± 0.38	15.1 ± 0.62	2.6 ± 0.21	16.1 ± 0.60	17.2 ± 0.80	3.2 ± 0.28	18.0 ± 0.76
31–50 years	2073	1910 ± 27.9	7.5 ± 0.30	1.6 ± 0.09	9.1 ± 0.27	12.8 ± 0.49	3.0 ± 0.20	14.0 ± 0.43	14.8 ± 0.61	3.6 ± 0.25	15.8 ± 0.54
51–70 years	1938	1689 ± 33.8	5.8 ± 0.23	2.1 ± 0.11	7.9 ± 0.22	10.1 ± 0.40	3.9 ± 0.23	12.2 ± 0.38	11.8 ± 0.45	4.6 ± 0.34	13.8 ± 0.46
71+ years	1228	1480 ± 28.0	5.6 ± 0.22	2.4 ± 0.11	8.0 ± 0.20	8.8 ± 0.34	4.3 ± 0.19	11.1 ± 0.27	9.9 ± 0.42	5.1 ± 0.24	12.2 ± 0.32
Total	25,165	2148 ± 12.8	7.5 ± 0.16	1.6 ± 0.03	9.1 ± 0.13	11.7 ± 0.41	3.2 ± 0.19	13.2 ± 0.38	13.1 ± 0.50	3.8 ± 0.23	14.5 ± 0.46

Source: From Marriott BP, Cole N, Lee E. *J Nutr.* 2009;139(6):1228S–35S. With permission.

[a] Values are means ± SE.

[b] The DRI gender/age groups as described in the DRI volumes [3] with the exception that we did not include children less than 1 year of age and pregnant and lactating women.

[c] NHANES 1999–2004 self-reported 24-h recall data from two recalls combined. Usual intake was estimated using *C-SIDE: Software for Intake Distribution Estimation* (14).

[d] Unweighted sample size.

[e] 1 kcal = 4186.8 J.

[f] Sums of added and naturally occurring fructose may not agree with totals presented due to rounding.

[g] Data for the 90th and 95th percentile and SE for each gender/age group are presented for added, naturally occurring, and total fructose, respectively; therefore, the 90th and 95th percentile of added and naturally occurring fructose in each column will not sum to equal the total.

For our study, we used the USDA definition of added sugars:

> "... all sugars used as ingredients in processed and prepared foods such as breads, cakes, soft drinks, jams, chocolates, and ice cream, and sugars eaten separately or added to foods at the table .... Added sugars do not include naturally occurring sugars such as lactose in milk or fructose in fruit, unless the sugar is added to the food item". [28]

We used the USDA MyPyramid Equivalents Database (MPED) 2.0 [28] as developed for 2003–2004 NHANES and we calculated the added sugars content in each individual food as reported in the two NHANES 24-h recalls. For this analysis, we used two 24-h recalls from the NHANES data to estimate usual intake. Since the NCI had recently released their new usual intake analysis macros, we were able to use this software and also incorporate NHANES FFQ data, where appropriate, to further refine our estimates [14,16]. Specifically, we incorporated total energy as a covariate in our added sugars intake models to control for differences in usual intake that might be driven by variation in total energy intake. This allowed for the control of total energy intake for each individual, which is significant because individuals who ingest more total calories could have a higher intake of specific nutrients than individuals who ingest less total energy. By controlling for total energy in the analysis, appropriate comparisons of the nutrient data could be made across subgroups whose average energy intake may have differed. Previous assessment of the use of FFQ data as covariate in models had demonstrated that this method could often improve the power to detect relationships between dietary intake and other variables [29]. The final analytic sample included 15,189 children and adults aged 4 years or older [30]. We calculated the percent of the total daily energy intake from added sugars and placed each individual into one of eight added sugars categories from 0 to >35%, calculated usual dietary intakes of nutrients based on the NCI method [16] for each individual, and compared the intake to DRIs.

We found that overall 13% of the population had added sugars intake >25% and the mean added sugars intake was 83.1 g-eq/day. While specific nutrient intake was less, with each 5% increase in added sugars intake above 5–10%, and higher added sugar intake was associated with higher proportions of individuals with nutrient intakes below the estimated average requirement (EAR), the overall high calorie and low quality of the US diet remained the predominant issue.

Specifically, our analysis revealed that more than 87% of the US population had estimated intakes of added sugars from >0 to ≤25% of total energy intake (see Table 10.3). Approximately 13% had added sugar intake >25% of total energy and of these, 6.6% were in the >25% to ≤30% category, while approximately 3% were in each of the >30 to ≤35% and the >35% of total energy from added sugar categories. The mean daily total energy intake was 2063–2138 kcal and controlling for total energy intake, this yielded an estimated range of 45–92 mean gram-equivalents (g-eq) of added sugars intake daily. Males and females were evenly distributed in the total sample and also across the added sugar categories.

The largest proportion of individuals in all of the life-stage groups ingested >5 to ≤20% of total energy from added sugars. More adolescents obtained >15 to ≤20% of total energy from added sugars than any other life-stage group (males and females 9–13 years: 31.2 and 27.8%, respectively, and 14–18 years: 27.8 and 25.7%, respectively). In addition, a considerable number of males (22.7%) and females (17.5%) 14–18 years ingested >20 to ≤25% of their total energy from added sugars.

As reported in other studies [31,32], the majority of older adults (≥51 years: ≈72–84%) in the USA obtained ≤15% of their total energy from added sugars. Compared to the overall population (12.5%), more non-Hispanic Black individuals (15.1%), those with a poverty-income ratio below the poverty line (17.5%), and underweight individuals (15.4%) had the highest level of added sugars intake (>25% of total energy from added sugars). Thompson et al. [32] also found an inverse relationship of added sugar intake with family income when analyzing intake data from the 2005 US National Health Interview Survey.

TABLE 10.3

Sample Size, Weighted Population Estimates, Percentage, Estimated Daily Energy Intake, Estimated Daily Intake of Added Sugars, Dietary Reference Intake (DRI) Life Stage Groups,[a] and Selected Demographic Characteristics by Range of Percent of Estimated Daily Intake from Added Sugars, National Health and Nutrition Examination Survey (NHANES) 2003–2006

		Categories of Individuals Based on Percent of Energy Intake from Added Sugar[b]							
Characteristic[c]	Full Sample[c]	$0 \le x \le 5\%$	$5 < x \le 10\%$	$10 < x \le 15\%$	$15 < x \le 20\%$	$20 < x \le 25\%$	$25 < x \le 30\%$	$30 < x \le 35\%$	>35%
N	15,190	1387	2877	3666	3311	2055	1078	432	384
Weighted *N*	287,845,042	33,743,743	60,083,772	68,584,551	55,570,985	33,778,579	18,911,454	8,754,407	8,417,551
Percent	100.0	11.7	20.9	23.8	19.3	11.7	6.6	3.0	2.9
Estimated total daily energy intake, kcal: median (SE)	2118 (13.1)	2028 (17.4)	2063 (15.4)	2104 (12.9)	2138 (14.1)	2177 (15.2)	2221 (19.7)	2261 (22.49)	2298 (28.3)
Estimated daily added sugar intake, with total energy intake as a covariate in the analysis gram equivalents: mean (SE)[d]	82.9 (0.06)	24.9 (0.06)	44.9 (0.07)	66.9 (0.07)	91.5 (0.08)	127.1 (0.13)	160.3 (0.21)	197.6 (0.40)	232.8 (0.50)
Mean age: years (SE)[e]	38.6 (0.5)	47.2 (0.9)	44.5 (0.8)	38.4 (0.7)	34.8 (0.7)	32.2 (0.6)	30.9 (0.8)	32.6 (1.1)	33.9 (1.2)
Gender:% (SE)									
Male	49.4 (0.6)	11.1 (0.8)	20.5 (0.9)	23.6 (0.9)	20.1 (0.8)	12.6 (0.7)	6.8 (0.4)	3.0 (0.4)	2.4 (0.3)
Female	50.6 (0.6)	12.0 (1.0)	22.6 (0.9)	24.5 (0.8)	18.8 (0.6)	10.7 (0.6)	6.2 (0.5)	2.6 (0.3)	2.6 (0.4)
DRI group:% (SE)									
Children aged 4–8	7.5 (0.3)	3.3 (0.7)	15.4 (1.4)	31.4 (2.0)	24.8 (1.7)	15.1 (1.3)	7.5 (1.4)	1.9 (0.5)	0.7 (0.7)
Males 9–13 years	4.1 (0.2)	2.3 (0.7)	10.1 (1.5)	24.8 (2.0)	31.2 (2.8)	17.2 (2.5)	9.7 (2.0)	2.9 (1.0)	1.8 (0.4)
Females 9–13 years	3.8 (0.2)	4.3 (1.2)	16.0 (1.8)	25.4 (2.3)	27.8 (2.3)	15.1 (1.7)	8.6 (1.0)	1.6 (0.7)	1.2 (0.8)
Males 14–18 years	4.1 (0.3)	2.7 (0.6)	10.6 (1.6)	19.2 (2.1)	27.8 (2.3)	22.7 (2.3)	9.4 (1.5)	4.3 (0.7)	3.3 (1.1)
Females 14–18 years	3.8 (0.3)	3.4 (0.8)	13.1 (1.7)	20.0 (1.7)	25.7 (1.8)	17.5 (1.8)	12.6 (1.7)	3.7 (1.0)	4.0 (1.0)
Males 19–30 years	8.1 (0.5)	10.1 (1.5)	15.9 (1.7)	22.7 (2.1)	18.4 (1.7)	14.9 (1.5)	8.6 (1.3)	5.3 (1.2)	4.2 (1.1)
Females 19–30 years	7.2 (0.4)	9.8 (1.7)	16.2 (2.2)	22.9 (1.8)	19.3 (2.0)	12.5 (1.5)	9.4 (1.7)	5.0 (1.0)	4.9 (0.6)
Males 31–50 years	15.0 (0.5)	13.4 (1.5)	21.7 (1.3)	23.2 (1.6)	18.6 (1.2)	11.1 (1.3)	6.7 (0.7)	2.4 (0.5)	2.9 (0.7)
Females 31–50 years	15.1 (0.5)	14.3 (1.6)	23.4 (1.7)	23.4 (1.8)	15.6 (1.5)	11.4 (1.2)	5.5 (0.7)	3.1 (0.6)	3.4 (0.3)

continued

TABLE 10.3 (continued)
Sample Size, Weighted Population Estimates, Percentage, Estimated Daily Energy Intake, Estimated Daily Intake of Added Sugars, Dietary Reference Intake (DRI) Life Stage Groups,[a] and Selected Demographic Characteristics by Range of Percent of Estimated Daily Intake from Added Sugars, National Health and Nutrition Examination Survey (NHANES) 2003–2006

			Categories of Individuals Based on Percent of Energy Intake from Added Sugar[b]													
Characteristic[c]	Full Sample[c]		$0 \le x \le 5\%$		$5 < x \le 10\%$		$10 < x \le 15\%$		$15 < x \le 20\%$		$20 < x \le 25\%$		$25 < x \le 30\%$		$30 < x \le 35\%$		>35%	
Males 51–70 years	10.7	(0.5)	17.0	(1.4)	28.6	(1.7)	22.8	(1.7)	16.4	(1.6)	7.7	(1.1)	4.2	(1.1)	2.4	(0.6)	1.0	(0.3)
Females 51–70 years	12.3	(0.6)	18.0	(1.6)	30.2	(1.7)	24.0	(1.8)	15.2	(1.2)	5.8	(1.0)	3.9	(0.7)	1.4	(0.4)	1.5	(0.5)
Males >70 years	3.5	(0.3)	15.7	(1.7)	31.2	(2.3)	26.1	(1.6)	16.4	(1.5)	6.4	(0.8)	2.2	(0.7)	1.1	(0.5)	0.9	(0.5)
Females >70 years	4.6	(0.3)	12.6	(1.6)	28.3	(2.2)	27.9	(2.0)	19.2	(2.1)	7.7	(1.2)	2.2	(0.7)	0.8	(0.4)	1.3	(0.6)
Race/ethnicity:% (SE)																		
Non-Hispanic White	71.6	(2.3)	12.6	(0.8)	22.3	(0.9)	23.7	(0.9)	18.6	(0.7)	11.1	(0.6)	6.3	(0.5)	2.9	(0.4)	2.4	(0.3)
Non-Hispanic Black	11.8	(1.4)	7.2	(0.9)	15.3	(1.2)	24.5	(0.8)	23.2	(0.9)	14.7	(0.8)	8.7	(0.6)	3.2	(0.4)	3.2	(0.6)
Hispanic[f]	11.3	(1.3)	8.3	(0.9)	21.0	(1.4)	27.4	(1.5)	20.8	(1.0)	13.5	(1.1)	5.6	(0.6)	2.2	(0.4)	1.2	(0.4)
Other race/ethnicity[f]	5.3	(0.6)	15.4	(2.5)	26.6	(3.2)	19.6	(2.3)	19.6	(2.4)	7.8	(1.2)	5.1	(1.3)	1.5	(0.5)	4.4	(1.7)
Poverty-income ratio (PIR):% (SE)																		
Below poverty line	13.4	(0.8)	6.8	(0.9)	17.4	(1.6)	23.5	(1.3)	21.1	(1.0)	13.7	(0.8)	8.9	(1.1)	4.7	(0.9)	3.9	(0.6)
At/above poverty line	37.5	(1.3)	9.7	(0.9)	21.0	(0.8)	23.4	(0.9)	20.8	(0.8)	12.3	(0.7)	6.7	(0.5)	2.8	(0.5)	3.3	(0.5)
Above 3× poverty line	49.1	(1.7)	14.4	(0.9)	23.2	(1.1)	24.6	(0.9)	18.0	(0.9)	10.5	(0.5)	5.6	(0.5)	2.2	(0.3)	1.4	(0.2)
Mean body mass index (BMI)	26.6	(0.2)	28.9	(0.4)	27.4	(0.2)	26.1	(0.3)	25.5	(0.2)	25.6	(0.3)	26.1	(0.3)	25.5	(0.5)	28.1	(0.7)
BMI weight categories: % (SE)[g]																		
Underweight	1.6	(0.1)	11.5	(2.9)	23.2	(3.4)	17.1	(3.5)	20.8	(2.8)	12.1	(2.6)	7.1	(2.2)	3.5	(1.6)	4.8	(1.8)
Normal weight	39.3	(1.0)	8.6	(0.7)	19.7	(1.0)	25.5	(1.2)	21.3	(0.9)	12.5	(0.6)	6.8	(0.5)	3.4	(0.5)	2.2	(0.4)

Overweight	29.5	(0.7)	12.8	(0.9)	22.5	(0.9)	24.3	(1.1)	18.2	(1.0)	11.1	(0.6)	6.5	(0.6)	2.7	(0.4)	2.0	(0.5)
Obese	29.6	(1.0)	14.5	(1.1)	22.9	(1.3)	22.1	(0.7)	18.2	(0.9)	11.0	(0.8)	6.0	(0.5)	2.0	(0.3)	3.2	(0.5)

Source: From Marriott BP, Cole N, Lee E. *J Nutr.* 2009;139(6):1228S–35S. With permission.

[a] Dietary Reference Intake Life Stage groups (Institute of Medicine [27]).

[b] Our analyses employed 2 days of 24-h dietary recall data from the National Health and Nutrition Examination Survey (NHANES), What We Eat in America 2003–2006. We restricted our sample to children and adults as defined by the DRIs as aged 4 years or older. Our sample was further restricted to individuals with reliable recall status, excluding fasters, pregnant women, and lactating women. The final analytic sample included 29,099 days of recall data from 15,189 individual respondents. For 2539 individuals in the sample, only one 24-h recall was reported.

[c] Percentages for characteristics are indicated in this table as follows: in the full sample column, the percent for each level of the characteristic totals to 100%; for rows of levels within a characteristic, each specific row totals to 100%. For example, while the full sample was comprised of 49.5% male, of the total 100% of these males 23.6% ingested >10 but ≤15% of their energy from added sugar.

[d] One Gram-equivalent (g-eq) equals an amount of added sugar comparable to 1 g sucrose in carbohydrate content. Added sugar gram-equivalents were calculated based on 2-day mean intake from MyPyramid Equivalents Database servings.

[e] NHANES top-codes age at 85 years, therefore the mean age estimate is biased slightly downwards.

[f] Hispanic includes Mexican-Americans and Other Hispanics. Other race ethnicity includes (1) individuals whose reported racial or ethnic identity was not Mexican-American, Other Hispanic, Non-Hispanic White, or Non-Hispanic Black and (2) multiracial persons.

[g] BMI (kg/m^2) for this study was calculated from the measured height and weight collected in the NHANES exam unit. Respondents aged 21 or older were classified as underweight if BMI was less than 18.5, normal weight if BMI was 18.5 or above but below 25, overweight if BMI was 25 or above but below 30, and obese if BMI was 30 or above. Respondents aged 20 or younger were classified by their BMI age/sex percentile ranking relative to 2000 CDC Growth Reference values: underweight if BMI was below the 5th percentile, normal weight if BMI was at or above the 5th percentile but below the 85th percentile, overweight if BMI was at or above the 85th percentile but below the 95th percentile, and obese if BMI was at or above the 95th percentile.

Based on calculated BMIs, 1.6% of the respondents were underweight, 39.3% were normal weight, 29.5% were overweight, and 29.6% were obese. The highest percentage of individuals who were overweight or obese consumed >5 to ≤15% of their energy from added sugars. With each 5% increase in added sugars category above 15% added sugars intake, there was a lower prevalence of overweight and obese individuals, with the exception of >35% added sugars where the prevalence increased to 3.2% for the obese individuals. A greater percentage of underweight and normal weight individuals reported higher levels of added sugars intake than individuals classified as overweight or obese. Details of estimated nutrient intake estimates by added sugar intake category for the 13 adult and child DRI life stage groups can be found in the original paper [26].

Since our analysis, several reports have addressed intake of added sugars in the USA using NHANES data [33–35]. Although somewhat different methods for data analyses were used [36], similar gram/day findings support the contention of Welsh et al. [33] that added sugar intake in the USA is decreasing, although it remains much higher than in the 1980s [33].

Welsh et al. [33] analyzed trends in added sugar intakes in the USA from 1999 to 2008 by using dietary recall data from NHANES in five sequential 2-year cycles and obtained the added sugar content of the reported foods from the MyPyramid Equivalents Database. Their sample included individuals ≥2 years of age with a combined sample size of 42,316. Between 1999–2000 and 2007–2008, the absolute intake of added sugars decreased significantly by 23.4% from a mean of 100.1 to 76.7 g/day. Added sugars consumption was significantly higher in males than in females, but when this was adjusted for total energy intake, there was no statistical difference by sex, which is consistent with our study. The mean percentage of total energy from added sugars decreased significantly from 18.1% (in 1999–2000) to 14.6% (in 2007–2008). The total energy intake also decreased from 2145 kcal/day (in 1999–2000) to 2069 kcal/day (in 2007–2008), a mean decrease of 76 kcal/day or 4%.

This decreasing trend of added sugars intake was observed across all age, race/ethnicity, and income groups, consistent with other studies [16,26,37], with the exception of those studies that were restricted to children and adolescents [33]. Non-Hispanic Blacks ingested the greatest percentage of total calories from added sugars; however, this decreased from 20.5% (1999–2000) to 16.1% (2007–2008). Hispanics evidenced the lowest amounts of added sugar intake with their intake decreasing from 15.9% (1999–2000) to 13.4% (2007–2008) of energy. Added sugar intake decreased with increasing family income, with subjects in the lowest quartile of income having the highest intake of added sugars and those in the highest income quartile having the lowest intake of added sugars. Mean intake decreased in both groups by 15–16%. Added sugars intake decreased in the middle-income quartiles by 22–23%.

The National Center for Health Statistics, CDC, reported the intake of added sugars by adults (≥20 years) in the USA from 2005 to 2010 [35]. Men obtained more energy from added sugars per day than women, but this was a nonsignificant difference when considered as a percentage of total calories ingested per day. The percentage of total calories from added sugars significantly decreased with increasing age from 20 to over 60 years. With respect to race ethnicity, non-Hispanic Black men ingested a significantly larger percentage of total energy from added sugars than non-Hispanic White and Mexican-American men. Non-Hispanic Black women also obtained a significantly larger percentage of their total energy from added sugars than Non-Hispanic White and Mexican-American women. No significant difference was observed between Non-Hispanic White and Mexican-American men or women. These results are consistent with those reported by Welsh et al. [33] in which non-Hispanic Blacks ≥2 years evidenced a mean percentage of total energy from added sugar that decreased from 20.5% in 1999–2000 to 16.1% in 2007–2008. Also, added sugars intake as a percentage of total energy decreased linearly with increasing income for adult men and women in the USA. These results are consistent with our study and that of Welsh et al. [33].

Wang et al. [31] used generalized linear mixed regressions to describe trends in added-sugar intake and BMI by gender and age groups and by weight status in data from the Minnesota Heart Survey

(1980–1982 to 2007–2009). These authors found that energy intake from added sugar increased by 54% in women between 1980–1982 and 2000–2002, but declined somewhat in 2007–2009; men followed the same pattern ($P < 0.001$). Added sugar intake was lower among women than men and higher among younger than older adults. BMI in women paralleled added-sugar intake, but men's BMI increased overall. Percentage of energy intake from added sugar was similar among BMI groups.

Added Sugar Intake among Children and Adolescents in the USA

The CDC reported intake of added sugars among children and adolescents (2–19 years) in the US based on NHANES 2005–2008 [34]. This CDC analysis showed that American children and adolescents derived approximately 16% of their total calories from added sugar in 2005–2008 and boys exhibited a significantly higher intake of calories (362 kcal) than girls (282 kcal). Energy intake from added sugar significantly increased linearly with age in both boys and girls (boys and girls, respectively: 218 and 196 kcal for 2–5-year-olds; 345 and 293 kcal for 6–11-year-olds; 442 and 314 kcal for 12–19-year-olds). Non-Hispanic White boys and girls obtained a significantly larger percent of calories from added sugar than their Mexican-American counterparts boys: 17.2%, 14.8%; girls: 16.1%, 14.0%) and non-Hispanic Black girls ingested significantly more than Mexican-American girls (15.9%, 14.0%). There was no significant difference in added sugar intake among children and adolescents based on family income.

Recently, Slining and Popkin [38] analyzed trends in the intake and sources of solid fats and added sugar among US children and adolescents (2–18 years) from 1994 to 2010, only the added sugar intake will be described here. This study assessed individual dietary intake data from the Continuing Survey of Food Intakes by Individuals Surveys (1994–1996) and NHANES, What We Eat in America (2003–2004, 2005–2006, 2007–2008, and 2009–2010).

As shown in Table 10.4, the mean estimated average daily energy intake of 2–18-year-olds decreased from 2115 kcal/day (2003–2004) to 1914 kcal/day (2009–2010), except for the specific intake of 12–18-year-olds, non-Hispanic Blacks, and children from middle-income families, which did not change significantly. The mean added sugars intake as a percentage of total energy also decreased from 18% in 1994–1998 to 14% in 2009–2010. In addition, the mean daily intake of energy from added sugars decreased from 371 to 278 kcal/day during the same time frame. For most of the age, race/ethnicity, and income groups, added sugars intakes were significantly lower during 2005–2008 compared to 1994–2004. However, only 6–11-year-olds showed a decrease in added sugars intake from 2007–2008 to 2009–2010.

TRENDS IN THE AVAILABILITY (COUNTRY CONSUMPTION) OF FRUCTOSE AND SWEETENERS

Sweetener availability or "consumption" *into the market* is recognized as not representative of individual intake. However, these data provide an important framework for understanding food and nutrient availability. Loss-adjusted food availability data also can be used to assess whether or not a country is producing enough food and nutrients to meet national dietary recommendations. These data can demonstrate the production and movement of sugar into the food supply and its distribution thus forming a background for understanding dietary intake information.

Availability of Fructose and Sweeteners in the USA

Earlier studies showed that per capita availability of sweeteners from 1960 to 1992 were relatively stable at 155 ± 2.9 g/day [18,29]. Marriott et al. [20] showed that after 1993 per capita, total sweetener availability in the US market (g/day dry weight) increased to 187.9 g/day in 1999 and then decreased to 175.6 g/day in 2003 where it remained relatively constant at 176 g/day through 2005. As shown in Table 10.5, while sucrose was the main sweetener in 1970 (85% of sweeteners dry

TABLE 10.4
Mean Percentage of Total Energy from Added Sugars and Added Fats, and Total Energy Intake of US Children and Adolescents (2–18 years), 1994–2010[a]

	1994–1998	2003–2004	2005–2006	2007–2008	2009–2010
All					
Total energy (kcal)	2016 ± 26	2115 ± 22	2035 ± 33	1906 ± 26 [b–d]	1914 ± 27 [c]
% energy from added sugars	18	17	16[b]	15[b,c]	14[b–d]
% energy from solid fat	21	20	20	20[b]	19[b,d]
2–5 Years					
Total energy (kcal)	1587 ± 13	1721 ± 25[b]	1566 ± 23[c]	1510 ± 25[c]	1543 ± 26[c]
% energy from added sugars	15	14	14[b]	13[b]	12[b–d]
% energy from solid fat	21	21	19[b]	20[c]	20
6–11 Years					
Total energy (kcal)	1934 ± 22	2120 ± 49	1981 ± 37	1931 ± 27[c]	1865 ± 20[c]
% energy from added sugars	18	17	16[b]	16[b]	14[b,c,e]
% energy from solid fat	21	20	21	20[b]	19[b,d]
12–18 Years					
Total energy (kcal)	2352 ± 49	2317 ± 48	2315 ± 51	2106 ± 44[a–d]	2157 ± 58
% energy from added sugars	19	19	17[b]	16[b]	15[b,c]
% energy from solid fat	20	19[b]	20	19	18[b]
Male					
Total energy (kcal)	2242 ± 34	2295 ± 42	2258 ± 50	2065 ± 36[b,c]	2066 ± 39[c]
% energy from added sugars	18	18	16	16	14
% energy from solid fat	21	20	20	19	19
Female					
Total energy (kcal)	1777 ± 26	1924 ± 26[b]	1798 ± 21[c]	1747 ± 33[c]	1761 ± 28[c]
% energy from added sugars	18	17	16[b]	15[b,c]	14[b,c]
% energy from solid fat	20	20	20	20	19[c]
Non-Hispanic White					
Total energy (kcal)	2059 ± 32	2133 ± 32	2101 ± 41	1956 ± 41[c]	1921 ± 36[b–d]
% energy from added sugars	18	18	16[b]	16[b]	15[b,c]
% energy from solid fat	21	20	20	20	19[b,c]
Non-Hispanic Black					
Total energy (kcal)	1975 ± 41	2093 ± 48	1941 ± 40	1847 ± 44[c]	1937 ± 57
% energy from added sugars	17	17	16	15[b,c]	14[b,c]
% energy from solid fat	22	20[b]	20[b]	19[b]	19[b,d]
Mexican Americans					
Total energy (kcal)	1846 ± 75	2131 ± 45[b]	1930 ± 33[c]	1810 ± 39[c]	1849 ± 40[b]
% energy from added sugars	16	16	14	14[b,c]	13[b,c]
% energy from solid fat	20	20	19	19	18[b]

[a] Adapted from Slining and Popkin [38].
[b] Significantly different from 1994–1998, $p < 0.05$.
[c] Significantly different from 2003–2004, $p < 0.05$.
[d] Significantly different from 2005–2006, $p < 0.05$.
[e] Significantly different from 2007–2008, $p < 0.05$.

TABLE 10.5
Percent (%) of Sucrose, HFCS, and Other Sweetener Availability Relative to Total Sweeteners, USA, 1970–2005

Year	Sucrose	HFCS	Other[a]
1970	85	0.5	14
1975	78	4	17
1980	73	12	15
1985	50	36	14
1990	49	37	14
1995	45	40	15
2000	44	42	14
2005	44	42	14

Source: Adapted from Marriott BP, Cole N, Lee E. *J Nutr*. 2009;139(6):1228S–35S; USDA Economic Research Service.

[a] Honey, edible syrups, crystalline fructose, and fructose only syrups.

weight basis with HFCS = 0.5%) by 15 years later in 1985, sucrose had dropped to 50%, and 36% of sweeteners in the US food supply were HFCS. In 2000, shortly after the 1999 peak in sweetener availability in the USA, the ratio of percent sucrose to percent HFCS was 44:42. Since 1999, while the total sweetener availability has declined, the percentage ratio of sucrose to HFCS availability has remained constant.

Since 1993, while change in the overall per capita availability of sweeteners has been small (1%), the composition has evidenced a larger change (6%): total sweetener availability increased by 2.2 g/day, sucrose availability decreased by 0.9 g/day, HFCS availability increased by 4.0 g/day, and other sweeteners decreased by 1.0 g/day [20].

The US 2013 *Sugar and Sweeteners Outlook* [39] from the USDA Economic Research Service (ERS) presented a comparison of the average daily per capita calories from the US food availability data, adjusted for spoilage, in 1985, 1999, and 2010. At these three time points while the *total average per capita calories available* in the US continued to increase (2270, 2508, and 2546 kcal), the per capita availability of energy from sugar and added sweeteners increased as indicated above in 1999 and then decreased: 1985: 352 kcal (16%); 1999: 429 kcal (17%); 2010: 379 kcal (15%), while energy available from added fats and oils and dairy fats have steadily increased: 1985: 427 kcal (19%); 1999: 444 kcal (18%); 2010: 588 kcal (23%). These historical trends in US availability of sucrose and HFCS from 1910 to 2010 have been previously reviewed by White [24,28] who showed that HFCS consumption into the marketplace peaked in 1999 and since that time has declined steadily. The most recent USDA data illustrate that current availability of added sugar and sweeteners to levels comparable to 1992 (see Figure 10.1).

Nonetheless, global analysis based on the FAO FBS shows that the North American region while declining in overall intake continues to remain the area of the world with the highest level of sweetener availability (consumption into the market) (Food and Agriculture Organization; United Nations data available at http://faostat3.fao.org/home/index.html).

CONCLUSION

Our analysis indicated that added fructose intake in the USA increased significantly between 1978 and 2004 on a gram/day basis and as a percent of energy intake but that HFCS *availability* had plateaued relative to other sweeteners as of 2005. Assessment of dietary intake data from nationally

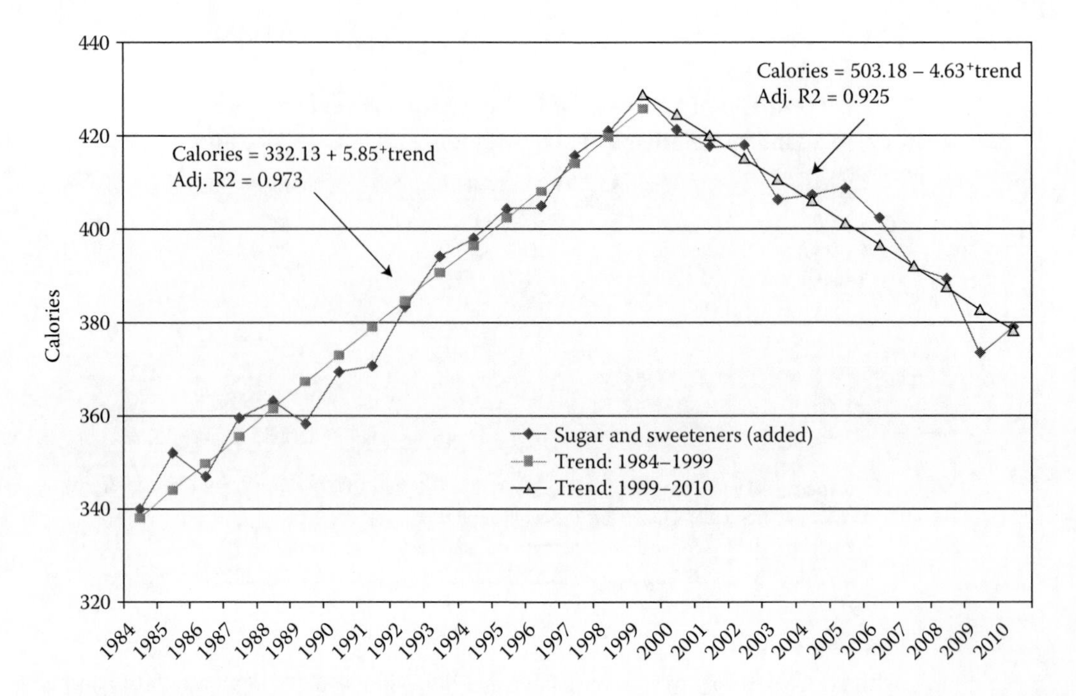

FIGURE 10.1 **(See color insert.)** Average daily per capita calories from added sugar and sweeteners availability, adjusted for spoilage and other waste.

representative surveys in the USA show that added sugar intake as a percent of energy has declined and that this trend appears to be currently continuing [35]. The most recent USDA data indicated that per capita availability of energy from added sweeteners and sugar has decreased to 15% of energy which is below the 1985 levels for *availability*. In contrast, the per capita availability of energy from fats, oils, and dairy fat in the US market in the US diet is on the increase [39]. Between 1978 and 2004 fructose intake increased, while availability of fructose in the food supply as a percent of total sweetener increased until 2000 and then remained constant through 2005. No newer data are available on fructose intake to determine the current pattern of added fructose intake relative to the decline in added sugar intake and availability.

The rise in available food energy globally has been accompanied by changes in the composition of the diet and this process has been characterized as having followed a two-stage transition pattern [15]. In stage 1: "the expansion effect," the main change is an increase in energy supplies with extra calories being contributed by cheaper foods of vegetable origin. In stage 2, "the substitution effect," food intake patterns change without a change in total energy. This stage shift is evidenced mainly as a change in use of carbohydrate-rich staples (e.g., cereals, tubers) to vegetable oils, animal products (meat and dairy), and sugar. The stage 2 transition is viewed as country-specific and dependent upon culture and religious traditions. This theory views that as the main drivers of food use, such as income, urbanization, trade liberalization, retailing and marketing, and consumer attitudes [15] shape the global intake of sweeteners, we can expect that the global nutrition transition will continue. This transition will be reflected in sugar availability and intake and linked to individual economic status of each country. Thus, the place of sugar in the overall diet will continue to transition and evolve as it has since 500 BC [1]. However, with growth in understanding the health impacts of added sweeteners and other food components, public health information, and policies have the potential to shape this transition and lead to more healthful food intake in the USA and globally.

ACKNOWLEDGMENTS

The author appreciates the contributions of Christopher Fink, MS, and Terri Krakower, Ph.D., for data and table development, and Samantha Wise in formatting and preparation of the final manuscript.

REFERENCES

1. Kiple KF, Ornelas K. The Cambridge World History of Food, 2 vols. Cambridge, UK: Cambridge University Press; 2000.
2. Mintz SW. Sweetness and Power: The Place of Sugar in Modern History. New York: Viking Penguin, Inc.; 1985. 274 pp.
3. Reiling J. 100 Years ago: Sugar as food. *JAMA*. 2013;310(7):752.
4. ERS U. Sugars & Sweeteners. USDA Economic Research Service, 2013 Contract No.: 8/24/2013.
5. Hess J, Latulippe M, Ayob K, Slavin S. The confusing world of dietary sugars: Definitions, intakes, food sources and international dietary recommendations. *Food Function*. 2012;3:477–86.
6. Colucci AC, Cesar CL, Marchioni DM, Fisberg RM. Factors associated with added sugars intake among adolescents living in Sao Paulo, Brazil. *J Am Coll Nutr*. 2012;31(4):259–67.
7. Fidler Mis N, Kobe H, Stimec M. Dietary intake of macro- and micronutrients in Slovenian adolescents: Comparison with reference values. *Ann Nutr Metab*. 2012;61(4):305–13.
8. MacIntyre UE, Venter CS, Kruger A, Serfontein M. Measuring micronutrient intakes at different levels of sugar consumption in a population in transition: The Transition and Health during Urbanisation in South Africa (THUSA) study. *South Afr J Clin Nutr*. 2012;25(3):122–30.
9. Husoy T, Mangschou B, Fotland TO, Kolset SO, Notvik Jakobsen H, Tommerberg I et al. Reducing added sugar intake in Norway by replacing sugar sweetened beverages with beverages containing intense sweeteners—A risk benefit assessment. *Food Chem Toxicol*. 2008;46(9):3099–105.
10. Pereira RA, Duffey KJ, Sichieri R, Popkin BM. Sources of excessive saturated fat, trans fat and sugar consumption in Brazil: An analysis of the first Brazilian nationwide individual dietary survey. *Public Health Nutr*. 2014;17(1):113–21.
11. Herbst A, Diethelm K, Cheng G, Alexy U, Icks A, Buyken AE. Direction of associations between added sugar intake in early childhood and body mass index at age 7 years may depend on intake levels. *J Nutr*. 2011;141(7):1348–54.
12. Elmadfa I, Meyer A, Nowak V, Hasenegger V, Putz P, Verstraeten R et al. European nutrition and health report 2009. *Ann Nutr Metab*. 2009;55(Suppl 2):1–40.
13. Moshfegh AJ, Rhodes DG, Baer DJ, Murayi T, Clemens JC, Rumpler WV et al. The US Department of Agriculture Automated Multiple-Pass Method reduces bias in the collection of energy intakes. *Am J Clin Nutr*. 2008;88(2):324–32.
14. Tooze J, Midthune D, Dodd K, Freedman L, Krebs-Smith SM, Subar A et al. A new statistical method for estimating the usual intake of episodically consumed foods with application to their distribution. *J Am Dietetic Assoc*. 2006;106:1575–87.
15. Kearney J. Food consumption trends and drivers. *Philos Trans R Soc Lond B Biol Sci*. 2010;365(1554):2793–807.
16. Wells HF, Buzby JC. ERS food availability data look at consumption in three ways. *Amber Waves*. 2007;5(3):40–1.
17. FAO. FAOSTAT 2013. Available from: http://faostat3.fao.org/faostat-gateway/go/to/home/E.
18. Park YK, Yetley EA. Intake and food sources of fructose in the United States. *Am J Clin Nutr*. 1993;58(suppl):737S–47S.
19. Glinsmann WH, Irausquin H, Park YK. Evaluation of health aspects of sugars contained in carbohydrate sweeteners: Report of Sugars Task Force. *J Nutr*. 1986;116(11S):S1–S216.
20. Marriott BP, Cole N, Lee E. National estimates of dietary fructose intake increased from 1977 to 2004 in the United States. *J Nutr*. 2009;139(6):1228S–35S.
21. Carriquiry AL. Estimation of usual intake distributions of nutrients and foods. *J Nutr*. 2003; 133(2):601S–8S.
22. Carriquiry AL, Camano-Garcia G. Evaluation of dietary intake data using the tolerable upper intake levels. *J Nutr*. 2006;136:507S-13S.
23. Dwyer J, Picciano MF, Raiten DJ. Estimation of usual intakes: What we eat in America-NHANES. *J Nutr*. 2003;133(2):609S–23S.

24. White JS. Challenging the fructose hypothesis: New perspectives on fructose consumption and metabolism. *Adv Nutr*. 2013;4(2):246–56.
25. Collino M. High dietary fructose intake: Sweet or bitter life? *World J Diabetes*. 2011;2(6):77–81.
26. Marriott B, Olsho L, Hadden L, Connor P. Intake of added sugars and selected nuritents in the United States, National Health and Nutrition Examination Survey (NHANES). *Crit Rev Food Sci Nutr*. 2010;50:228–58.
27. Medicine Io. Dietary Reference Intakes for Energy, Carbohydrate, Fiber, Fat, Fatty Acids, Cholesterol, Protein, and Amino Acids. Washington, DC: National Academy Press; 2002.
28. Bowman SA, Friday JE, Moshfegh AJ. MyPyramid Equivalents Database, 2.0 for USDA Survey Foods, 2003–2004: Documentation and User Guide. Food Surveys Research Group, Beltsville Human Nutrition Research Center, Agricultural Research Service, US Department of Agriculture; 2008. Available from: http://www ars usda gov/ba/bhnrc/fsrg (accessed August 2009).
29. Subar A, Dodd K, Guenther PM, Kipnis V, Midthune D, McDowell MM et al. The food proponsity questionnaire: Concept, development, and validation for use as a covariate in a model to estimate ususal food intake. *J Am Dietetic Assoc*. 2006;106:1556–63.
30. Moshfegh A, Goldman J, Cleveland L. What we eat in America, NHANES 2001–2002: Usual nutrient intakes from food compared to dietary reference intakes. Washington, DC: USDA, Agricultural Research Service; 2005.
31. Wang H, Steffen LM, Zhou X, Harnack L, Luepker RV. Consistency between increasing trends in added-sugar intake and body mass index among adults: The Minnesota Heart Survey, 1980–1982 to 2007–2009. *Am J Public Health*. 2013;103(3):501–7.
32. Thompson FE, McNeel TS, Dowling EC, Midthune D, Morrissette M, Zeruto CA. Interrelationships of added sugars intake, socioeconomic status, and race/ethnicity in adults in the United States: National Health Interview Survey, 2005. *J Am Diet Assoc*. 2009;109(8):1376–83.
33. Welsh JA, Sharma AJ, Grellinger L, Vos MB. Consumption of added sugars is decreasing in the United States. *Am J Clin Nutr*. 2011;94(3):726–34.
34. Ervin RB, Kit BK, Carroll MD, Ogden CL. Consumption of added sugar among U.S. children and adolescents, 2005–2008. *NCHS Data Brief*. 2012(87):1–8.
35. Ervin RB, Ogden CL. Consumption of added sugars among U.S. adults, 2005–2010. *NCHS Data Brief*. 2013(122):1–8.
36. Marriott B, Olsho L, Hadden L, Connor P. Intake of added sugars in the United States: What is the measure? *AJCN*. 2011;94(6):1652–3.
37. EFSA. General principles for the collection of national food consumption data in the view of a pan-European dietary survey. *EFSA J*. 2009;7:1435–86.
38. Slining MM, Popkin BM. Trends in intakes and sources of solid fats and added sugars among U.S. children and adolescents: 1994–2010. *Pediatr Obes*. 2013;8(4):307–24.
39. Haley S. Sugar and Sweeteners Outlook—Jan 2013. wwwersusdagov Electronic Outlook Report from the Economic Research Service. 2013; SSS-M-293 (17 January 2013).

11 Metabolism of Hexoses

Yeo Shi Hui, Lim Wen Bin, and Mary Chong Foong Fong

CONTENTS

KEY POINTS

- Digestible carbohydrates consist mainly of complex carbohydrate (starch), disaccharides (sucrose, lactose), and simple sugars (glucose and fructose).
- In the gut, starch is hydrolyzed to glucose, sucrose to glucose and fructose, and lactose to glucose and galactose; dietary carbohydrates are finally absorbed in the hepatic portal blood as simple carbohydrates (glucose, fructose, and galactose).
- Glucose plays a central role in energy production and can be used as an energy substrate by all cells of the organism. Complex regulatory mechanisms such as hormonal and allosteric regulations are present to ensure glucose homeostasis. Glucose metabolism is largely determined by the nutritional state and level of physical activity.

- Fructose and galactose, unlike glucose, cannot be directly used as energy substrates by many cells of the organism; it needs first to be converted into glucose, lactate, and fatty acids in splanchnic organs for fructose, into glucose in the liver for galactose.
- Fructose ingestion elicits modest increases in glycemia, as its initial steps for metabolism are not regulated by insulin.
- Sugar alcohols (sorbitol, galacticol) are endogenously produced from glucose and galactose under the action of the enzyme aldose reductase.

INTRODUCTION

Dietary carbohydrates are mainly absorbed in the form of three monosaccharides: glucose, fructose, and galactose. These monosaccharides are delivered first into the portal bloodstream to be used as energy substrates in other organs and tissues. Glucose constitutes the largest portion of the digestion products of dietary carbohydrate and is widely used as the main source of fuel for body cells. Fructose is consumed mainly with glucose as part of the disaccharide sucrose, while galactose is usually consumed with glucose as part of lactose, found mainly in milk products. Glucose is the prime energy substrate of the organism and can be used by all cell types, while fructose and galactose will eventually be converted into glucose (or other energy substrates, such as lactate or fatty acids) in the liver. Some cells, such as brain and red blood cells, rely exclusively on glucose as an energy fuel under normal conditions [1–3].

In this chapter, the metabolism of sugar alcohols will also be briefly described. Sugar alcohols are alcohols which occur naturally, although they are more often industrially prepared by hydrogenation of sugars. They are widely used in the food industry as thickeners and sweeteners. Among the various sugar alcohols available, we focus on the two commonly used, namely sorbitol and xylitol. The metabolic pathways used for energy production from glucose, fructose, galactose, and sugar alcohols are closely interrelated, as shown in Figure 11.1.

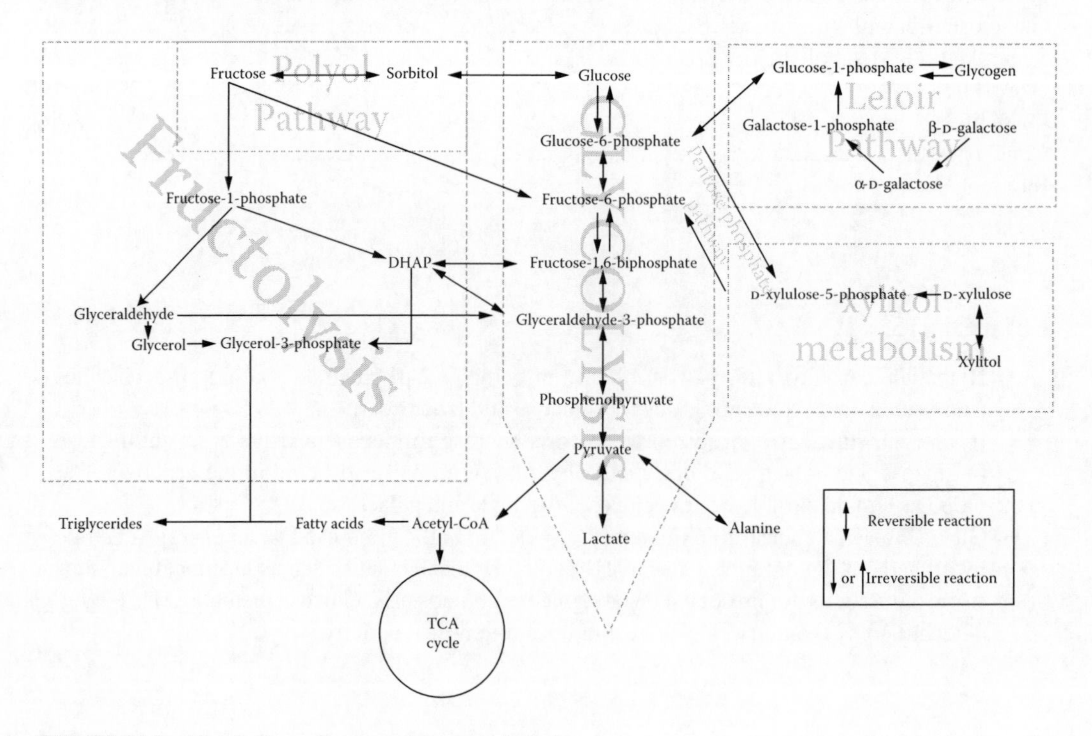

FIGURE 11.1 Metabolism of sugars and sugar alcohols.

GLUCOSE METABOLISM

Fasting blood glucose is maintained within relatively tight limits through complex regulatory mechanisms. Normal fasting blood glucose concentration is approximately 1 g/L. Given that glucose in the blood is nearly equilibrated with glucose concentration in extracellular fluid, this corresponds, for a 70-kg healthy male, to approximately 15 g of glucose, which can readily be used by all cells of the organism for energy production. Exogenous dietary carbohydrates, glycogen stored in the liver, and de novo synthesis of glucose from nonglucose precursors (lactate, glycerol, amino acids) in the liver and kidney contribute to blood glucose in a closely regulated way. Our intake of dietary carbohydrates is roughly partitioned into starch (large polymers of glucose linked by alpha-1,4 and alpha-1,6 glycoside bonds; 60% of carbohydrate intake), sucrose (made up of one molecule of glucose linked to one molecule of fructose; 30% of carbohydrate intake), and lactose (made up of one molecule of glucose linked to one molecule of galactose; 10% of carbohydrate intake). Seventy to eighty percent of our dietary carbohydrates are, therefore, ultimately absorbed from the gut as glucose, and only 20–30% is absorbed as fructose and galactose [3–6].

Blood glucose is first transported into cells and converted into glucose-6-phosphate, a branch point for several pathways for carbohydrate disposal. This is determined largely by the nutritional state and energy needs of the organism. In the fed state, glucose uptake is stimulated in insulin-sensitive tissues, and glucose-6-phosphate is preferentially degraded by glycolysis to pyruvate and acetyl-CoA, which are subsequently oxidized to produce the energy needed by the cells. When excess glucose is present, the amount of glucose taken up by cells and not needed to cover the cells' adenosine triphosphate (ATP) needs is stored, mainly as glycogen (in muscles and liver) and as triglycerides (as glycerol backbone of triglycerides in adipose tissue). Under special conditions associated with a demand of nicotinamide adenine dinucleotide phosphate (reduced) (NADPH) for biosynthetic processes (i.e., de novo lipogenesis in lactating mammary gland, or reduction of oxidized glutathione in inflammatory tissues), some glucose is also used to fuel the pentose phosphate pathway (PPP). Some of the glucose transported into cells is degraded down to pyruvate in the glycolytic pathway and released in the extracellular space as lactate and pyruvate, which are secondarily reconverted into glucose in the liver (Cori- and glucose-alanine cycles). These cycles are known to be activated during exercise. Finally, glucose may be metabolized to lactate and released into the extracellular space, to be subsequently taken up by other cells as an oxidative fuel. This is known to occur in astrocytes, which produce lactate as a metabolic fuel to adjacent neurons, and in muscle to convey lactate to oxidative muscle fibers [7,8]. Figure 11.2 shows the various aforementioned pathways in glucose metabolism, which are further described below.

GLUCOSE METABOLISM IN THE FED STATE

Oxidative Glucose Metabolism

Glycolysis, also known as the Emben-Meyerhof-Parnas pathway, occurs in the cytosol of all cells and is a key pathway by which energy is released from the glucose. The isomerization of glucose-6-phosphate to fructose-6-phosphate marks the initiation of glycolysis. Fructose-6-phosphate is next catalyzed by phosphofructokinase-1 to fructose-1,6-biphosphate, which is then cleaved into two 3-carbon molecules, glyceraldehyde-3-phosphate and dihydroxyacetone phosphate. In the final step of glycolysis, two molecules of pyruvate are formed by pyruvate kinase.

Under aerobic conditions, pyruvate will be transported into the mitochondria of the cell, where it is converted into acetyl-CoA by pyruvate dehydrogenase and then enters the tricarboxylic acid (TCA) cycle. TCA cycle is a common pathway for the final oxidative degradation of acetyl-CoA (or, other amino acid metabolites) produced from carbohydrates, fat, and amino acid metabolism. It is an aerobic 5-step degradation pathway in which acetyl-coA is broken down to carbon dioxide and water, which is associated with the release of large amounts of energy [in the form of ATP,

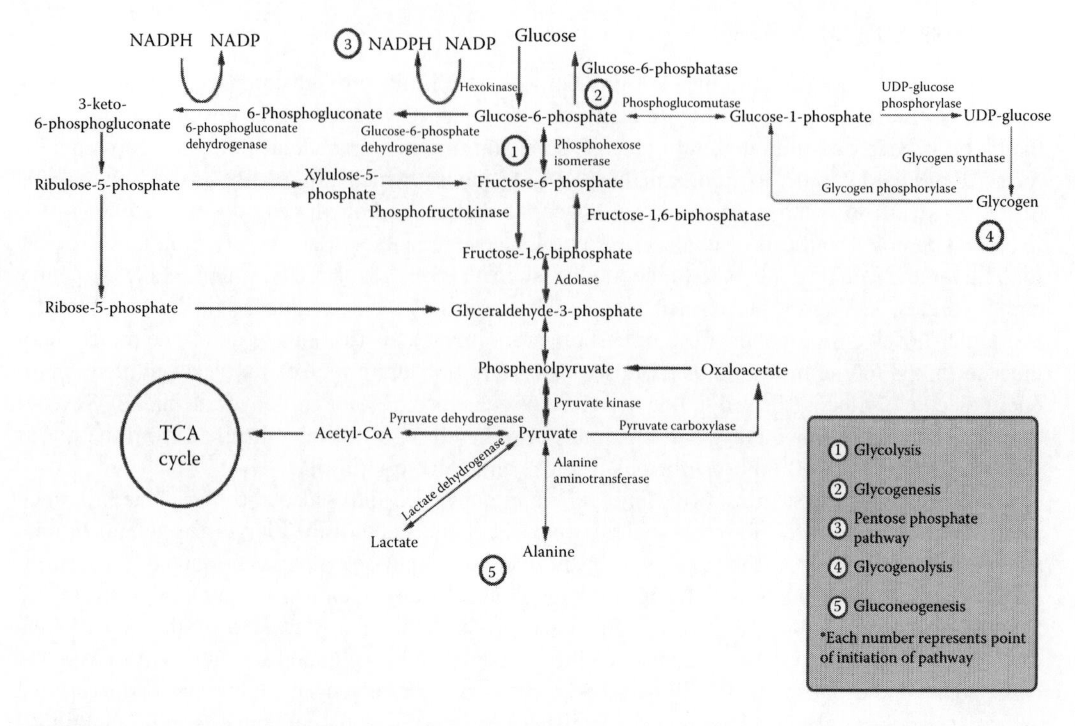

FIGURE 11.2 Glucose metabolism.

guanosine triphosphate, nicotinamide adenine dinucleotide (reduced) (NADH), and flavin adenine dinucleotide (reduced form) (FADH)] and key metabolites (ketogutarate, citrate, oxaloacetate) for synthesis of other compounds.

Under hypoxic conditions (e.g., severe exercise), excessive pyruvate is reduced to produce lactate. This allows for the glycolytic degradation of glucose in hypoxic cells, and the production while at the same time providing lactate for energy production in nonhypoxic cells [2–4,7,9].

Nonoxidative Glucose Metabolism

When glucose-6-phosphate production exceeds the energy need of the cell, its excess is preferentially stored as glycogen. This pathway is initiated when glucose-6-phosphate is isomerized to glucose-1-phosphate, which is then used for the synthesis of UDP-glucose. UDP-glucose is added to the glycogen backbone by glycogen synthase which creates the alpha-1,4 linkages, and branching enzymes which create the alpha-1,6 linkages in glycogen. Although many cell types can synthesize small amounts of glycogen, only the liver and skeletal muscles can build up large glycogen stores. The capacity to store glucose as intracellular glycogen is, however, quantitatively limited. Once the maximal capacity for glycogen storage is attained, some cell types, such as liver cells, can also convert excess glucose into fat. During this process, referred to as de novo lipogenesis, acetyl-CoA derived from pyruvate is used for either fatty acid or cholesterol synthesis.

Pentose Phosphate Pathway

The PPP, also called the hexose monophosphate shunt, is an alternative metabolic pathway for glucose. It is initiated when glucose-6-phosphate is oxidized by glucose-6-phosphate dehydrogenase to form 6-phosphogluconate and NADPH. Subsequently, 6-phophogluconate will be converted into ribulose-5-phosphate in a reaction catalyzed by 6-phosphogluconate dehydrogenase, to produce more NADPH. The PPP is present in most tissues and is the source of pentoses needed for the synthesis of nucleotides and nucleic acid. It is therefore highly active in tissues which have a high rate of cellular replication; NADPH is also a source of reducing power to counteract oxidative stress. In the liver and adipose tissue, the activity of glucose-6-phosphate dehydrogenase is stimulated by excess carbohydrate availability. Although the ensuing amount of glucose metabolized in the PPPs remains quantitatively small, it is essential for producing the NADPH, which is required for de novo lipogenesis [1–3,9,10].

SHORT-TERM FASTING AND STARVATION

Glycogenolysis

In fasted or starved conditions, glycogen is broken down to yield glucose, a process known as glycogenolysis. In the liver, glycogen is broken down to glucose, which is released into bloodstream for other tissues in need of glucose. After hydrolysis of the linkages in glycogen, glucose-1-phosphate is converted into glucose-6-phosphate and then into glucose by glucose-6-phosphatase. The presence of glucose-6-phosphatase allows the liver to release glucose into the bloodstream and hence to maintain glycemia during fasting. This glucose-producing ability, conferred by the presence of glucose-6-phosphatase, is being shared only by the kidney and the gut [11]. The role of the latter in the control of glycemia remains debated however [12,13].

In the muscle, glycogenolysis follows a different route as the muscle lacks the enzyme glucose 6-phosphatase and hence cannot release glucose into the blood. Instead, it releases glucose-6-phosphate which will enter glycolysis and the TCA cycle to produce energy needed for muscle contraction.

Gluconeogenesis

During fasting or starvation, lactate, glycerol, or amino acids are used to synthesize glucose in the liver and the kidneys via a process known as gluconeogenesis. Lactate and amino acids are first converted into pyruvate. From this point, gluconeogenesis is essentially a "revert glycolysis," since many glycolytic enzyme catalyze reversible reactions. There are, however, three irreversible reactions in glycolysis which require the presence of specific gluconeogenic enzymes. One of these irreversible steps is the conversion of phosphoenolpyruvate into pyruvate for gluconeogenesis; this reverse reaction involves an initial carboxylation of pyruvate to oxaloacetate by pyruvate carboxykinase, followed by oxaloacetate decarboxylation to phosphoenolpyruvate by phosphoenolpyruvate carboxykinase. The next irreversible glycolytic step involves the synthesis of fructose-6-phosphate from fructose-1,6-biphosphate by fructose biphosphate phosphatase. Finally, the last irreversible step involves glucose-6-phosphate conversion into glucose, which requires the action of glucose-6-phosphatase. When glycerol is converted into glucose, the initial step is the synthesis of glycerol-3-phosphate, catalyzed by the enzyme glycerokinase: glycerol-3-phosphate.

The liver is the main gluconeogenic organ during short-term fasting. During prolonged fasting and starvation, however, the kidney becomes a major contributor to overall glucose production. Gluconeogenesis in the kidney uses glutamine as a major substrate. Conversion of glutamine into glucose is associated with urine acidification due to renal excretion of NH_4^+. Renal gluconeogenesis therefore has a dual role in starvation since it contributes to glucose homeostasis at the same time as it counteracts the metabolic acidosis associated to starvation-induced ketogenesis [2,3,5,9,10,12,13].

GLUCOSE CYCLING ASSOCIATED WITH EXERCISE

During exercise, an increased amount of glucose is required and glycogen stores will be degraded by glycogenolysis to generate energy. However, during periods of intense exercise, oxygen is limited in muscle cells, and excessive pyruvate will be reduced to produce either lactate or/and alanine.

Lactate released from the muscle is taken by the liver where it is converted back to glucose via gluconeogenesis, a process known as the Cori cycle. Similarly, alanine formed from pyruvate transamination will be transported to the liver and reconverted back to glucose for energy generation, a process known as the glucose–alanine cycle [14].

REGULATION OF GLUCOSE METABOLISM

Due to the central role played by glucose in energy production and also due to the fact that cells within the central nervous system rely almost exclusively on blood glucose for their energy production, the organism has evolved complex regulatory mechanisms to ensure constant blood glucose concentration. Glucose homeostasis is mainly maintained through hormonal regulations and biochemical allosteric mechanisms.

HORMONAL REGULATION

Blood glucose control and energy homeostasis are mainly regulated by peptide hormones released from the pancreatic endocrine islets and from gut endocrine cells. The secretion of most peptide hormones is rapidly altered by changes in blood glucose concentration, but as their half-life in the blood is short, any increase in their blood concentration is usually limited in time. They interact with specific receptors present in the membrane of cells and exert very rapid actions, mainly activating or inhibiting key metabolic enzymes through phosphorylation or dephosphorylation, and to a lesser extent by altering the expression of genes coding for key metabolic enzymes. We will focus only on the most relevant hormones in this chapter, and the reader can refer to standard textbooks of physiology for a more comprehensive description of endocrine factors involved in energy homeostasis [11,15,16].

Insulin: Insulin is an anabolic hormone produced and released by the beta-cells of the pancreatic islets in response to hyperglycemia, which occurs normally in the postprandial state. Insulin stimulates glucose disposal by facilitating the uptake of glucose into insulin-sensitive cells (skeletal muscles, adipose tissue, and many other cell types) through a translocation of glucose transporters (GLUT-4). In muscle cells, it promotes glucose oxidation by activating glycolytic enzymes and by stimulating the decarboxylation of pyruvate and the entry of glucose-derived acetyl-CoA into the TCA cycle; it also stimulates glycogen synthesis by activating glycogen synthase. In adipose tissue, it stimulates the production of glycerol-3-phosphate from glucose, thus furnishing the glycerol backbone for triglyceride synthesis. Glucose metabolism in the liver is mainly regulated through allosteric mechanisms (see below) and hence the role of insulin in the control of glucose metabolism in the liver is relatively small compared to skeletal muscles and adipose tissue. Insulin, however, plays a major role by regulating the expression of glucokinase, the key enzyme catalyzing glucose-6-phophate production in the liver and by activating key enzymes required for de novo lipogenesis. This occurs through alteration of gene transcription and hence is more determined by insulin concentrations prevalent over the previous hours to days rather than an acute effect of insulin.

Glucagon: Glucagon is a catabolic hormone produced by the alpha cells of pancreas in response to hypoglycemia, sympathetic nervous system activation, and stress. Its secretion is physiologically increased in the fasting state and during exercise. It is involved in maintaining normal blood glucose and has opposing effects to insulin. It acts mainly on the liver, where it enhances glycogenolysis by activating glycogen phosphorylase and key gluconeogenic processes.

Other hormones involved in postprandial stimulation of glucose disposal: Besides the key hormone insulin, other hormones that contribute to stimulate glucose disposal include amylin, gut hormones, and insulin-like growth factor 1 (IGF1). Amylin is produced by pancreatic beta cells. It primarily inhibits postprandial glucagon secretion and slows down gastric emptying. Gut hormones, also known as incretins, include glucose-dependent insulinotropic peptide (GIP) and glucagon-like peptide-1 (GLP-1). Both GLP-1 and G1P enhance glucose-induced insulin production and secretion after ingestion of carbohydrate-rich meal, while GLP-1 additionally inhibits the secretion of glucagon and slows down gastric emptying. Blood IGF1 is mainly secreted in the liver under the control of growth hormone and exerts anabolic effects similar to insulin.

Other hormones that contribute to the stimulation of glucose production: Apart from glucagon, the stress-related hormones epinephrine and cortisol also contribute in the release of glucose into the bloodstream. Epinephrine promotes glycogenolysis in both liver and muscles and stimulates hepatic glyconeogenesis, while cortisol mainly stimulates gluconeogenesis in liver.

ALLOSTERIC REGULATION

Besides hormones regulation, allosteric effectors also play an important role in the regulation of carbohydrate metabolism. An allosteric effector is a solute compound which can activate or inhibit key enzymes. These allosteric regulations are often reflective of the cellular metabolic state. Allosteric effectors can be intermediary metabolites or high-energy molecules such as adenosine diphosphate, adenosine monophosphate (AMP), and ATP. An example of allosteric regulation by a metabolite is the inhibition of hexokinase by increased intracellular glucose-6-phosphate (a metabolite of glycolysis), which subsequently prevents further phosphorylation of glucose. The activation of pyruvate kinase by high AMP concentration during energy shortage and its inhibition by high intracellular concentrations of ATP and acetyl-Co when the cells are energy-repleted are examples of regulation by high-energy compounds. The presence of high concentration of ATP and acetyl-coA during times when cellular needs are met inhibits the action of pyruvate kinase [2,3,9,11,15–17].

ORGAN-SPECIFIC GLUCOSE METABOLISM

The metabolism of glucose is markedly different in the liver, the skeletal muscle fibers, and adipose tissue, and varies according to the nutritional status. This reflects the coordinated role of these key tissues in glucose homeostasis. The liver mainly acts as the key organ responsible for maintaining blood glucose concentrations; for this purpose, it switches from a glucose-utilizing organ in fed conditions, when exogenous glucose is mainly used to restore hepatic glycogen stores, to a glucose-producing organ in interprandial conditions. Skeletal muscle is quantitatively the most important energy-consuming tissue of the organism and relies to a large extent on glucose during high-intensity exercise; it has evolved as a tissue capable of relying mainly on fatty acids for energy production in the interprandial period and on glucose during postprandial periods. Due to its high mass and large capacity for metabolizing glucose, it plays a prominent role in the disposal of exogenous glucose in the postprandial state. Finally, adipose tissue is mainly involved in the storage of exogenous fat as triglyceride in postprandial conditions and in its release as fatty acids during interprandial periods. Triglyceride synthesis in adipocytes is insulin-dependent and requires the glycolytic degradation of glucose to glycerol-3-phosphate to form the glycerol backbone of triglycerides.

FRUCTOSE METABOLISM

Substantial amounts of fructose can be absorbed from fruits, honey, and caloric sweeteners (sucrose, high fructose corn syrup) in the diet. Both fructose and glucose have the same chemical formula: $C_6H_{12}O_6$; their chemical structure, however, differs by the presence of an aldose group in glucose versus a ketone group in fructose. Due to this difference, the affinity of hexokinase for fructose is markedly lower than that for glucose, and only a very minor portion of dietary fructose is directly converted into fructose-6-phosphate [18].

The majority of fructose is metabolized by a specific set of enzymes present in the gut, the liver, and the kidney. Fructose absorbed from the gut first reaches the liver, where it is converted into fructose-1-phophate by the enzyme fructokinase. Fructose-1-phosphate is then split into two 3-carbon molecules, namely glyceraldehyde and dihydroxyacetone phosphate (DHAP) by

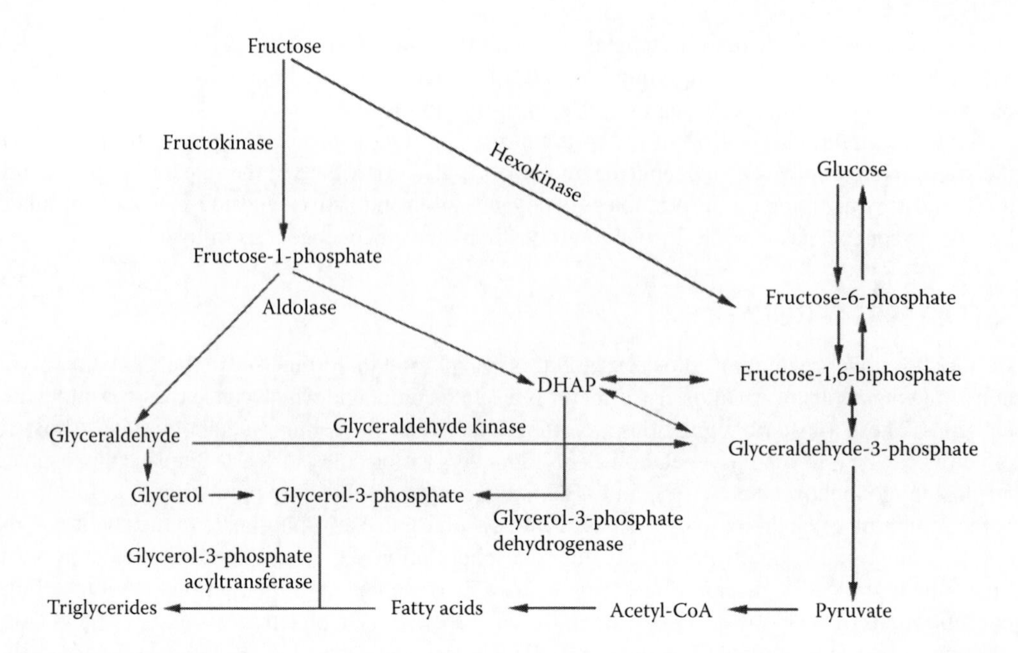

FIGURE 11.3 Fructose metabolism.

aldolase B. Glyceraldehyde is further converted into glyceraldehyde-3-phosphate by triokase, and DHAP and glyceraldehyde-3-P can then enter various metabolic pathways, that is, glycolysis, glycogenesis, gluconeogenesis, and lipogenesis to form "classical" energy substrates such as glucose, glycogen, lactate, and fatty acids. Small amounts of these carbon-3 compounds are also directly oxidized to carbon dioxide in the liver [19,20] (Figure 11.3).

Fructokinase has a very high affinity for fructose and is not inhibited by its product fructose-1-6-diphsphate. Aldolase B rapidly removes fructose-1-phosphate to cleave it into trioses-phosphate. Fructokinase and aldolase B therefore catalyze reactions similar to the generation of trioses-phosphate from glucose by phosphofructokinase and aldolase in the glycolytic pathway. The rate of trioses-phosphate formation in glycolysis is, however, regulated by cellular energy needs through a feedback inhibition of phosphofructokinase by increased ATP and citrate concentrations. No such inhibition is observed for fructokinase activity, and the rate of trioses-phosphate formation is therefore proportional to the rate of fructose entry into the cell. When dietary fructose intake is high, the rate of fructose appearance in the portal blood and of hepatic fructose uptakes results in the intrahepatic production of trioses-phosphate in excess of cellular energy needs. Nonoxidized trioses-phosphate is therefore converted into lactate and released into the bloodstream as energy fuel for extrahepatic cells, or converted into glucose, which is either released into the blood or stored as hepatic glycogen. Part of the pyruvate formed from fructose can also enter the mitochondria to form acetyl-CoA, which is then re-transported into the cytosol to serve as a substrate for de novo lipogenesis. The end product of this pathway, palmitic acid, can secondarily be elongated to stearic acid, and desaturated to some extent by stearoyl-CoA desaturase to yield oleic acid. Fatty acids issued from de novo lipogenesis are ultimately incorporated into triglycerides and either stored as intrahepatic fat or secreted with very-low-density lipoproteins.

Mutations of key enzymes for fructose metabolism give rise to inherited metabolic diseases. Genetic deficiency of fructokinase causes essential fructosuria; this is a benign condition, in which ingestion of fructose containing foods is associated with urinary excretion of free fructose. Genetic deficiency of aldolase B causes hereditary fructose intolerance. In affected subjects, ingested fructose is taken up by liver cells, where it is rapidly metabolized into fructose-1-phosphate; lack of aldolase B prevents further oxidative metabolism of fructose-1-phosphate. Since fructokinase is not inhibited by fructose-1-phosphate, the reaction continues as long as fructose is present in the portal blood and is associated with a large ATP consumption and an acute cellular ATP and inorganic phosphate depletion. This occurs in tissues where fructokinase and aldolase B are both expressed, that is, the gut, the liver, and the kidney. In the liver, this acute cellular energy crisis is associated with episodes of severe hypoglycemia; in the kidney, it is associated with proximal renal tubule dysfunction, causing aminoaciduria and renal acidosis. These acute reactions to fructose exposure can be life-threatening, but the condition is essentially benign in the absence of fructose intake. Treatment consists of withdrawing all fructose (and sorbitol)-containing foods from the diet.

EFFECTS OF FRUCTOSE ON BLOOD GLUCOSE

The initial steps for fructose metabolism are not regulated by insulin and hence are not impaired in patients with diabetes mellitus. Furthermore, although a major portion of fructose carbons is converted into glucose, fructose ingestion elicits only modest increases in glycemia. This is explained by autoregulatory mechanisms which prevent an increase in net hepatic glucose output in conditions when gluconeogenesis is acutely increased. Due to these properties, it has been proposed that fructose may be a suitable sweetener for diabetic patients, and several studies have indeed reported that replacing sucrose with fructose in the diet of diabetic patients decreases postprandial glycemia and glycated hemoglobin levels [18,21].

EFFECTS OF FRUCTOSE ON LIPID METABOLISM

While fructose appears to exert beneficial effects on blood glucose when it replaces relatively small amounts of dietary sucrose, its consumption has also been associated with adverse effects on blood lipid concentrations. When ingested together with a lipid-containing meal, it causes a substantial increase in postprandial blood triglycerides. This effect may be explained by the fact that fructose does not stimulate insulin secretion and hence that insulin-induced activation of lipoprotein lipase and postprandial lipid clearance is lower with fructose than with glucose-containing meals. It has also been suggested that fructose may directly impair blood triglyceride clearance, through mechanisms remain to be further clarified. In addition, a fructose-induced stimulation of de novo lipogenesis, although it is generally thought to be quantitatively small, may contribute to the development of both fasting and postprandial hypertriglyceridemia.

With the chronic consumption of a high-fructose diet, the pattern of fructose metabolism becomes substantially altered. Enhanced activities of fructose-1-6-biphosphastase, glycogen synthase, and glucose-6-phosphatase increase the liver's ability to channel fructose carbons into gluconeogenesis and hepatic glycogen synthesis. Increased activity of lipogenic enzymes in the liver stimulate long-chain fatty acid synthesis, leading to hypertriglyceridemia [18].

GALACTOSE METABOLISM

Galactose is an epimer of glucose present in our diet essentially as a constituent of lactose in dairy products. Its consumption is highly variable and closely linked to consumption of dairy products. In addition, a large proportion of the adult population world-wide is deficient in lactate, the brush border enzyme responsible for the hydrolysis of lactose into glucose and galactose in the gut, and hence has virtually no galactose intake. Like fructose, galactose is not metabolized by hexokinase and requires the presence of specific enzymes. It is predominantly metabolized in the liver via the Leloir pathway (Figure 11.4). β-D-galactose, the main form of galactose in foods, is first epimerized by galactose mutarotase to α-D-galactose and then phosphorylated to galactose-1-phosphate by galactokinase. Galactose-1-phosphate uridyltransferase catalyzes the transfer of a uridine monophosphate group from uridine diphosphate (UDP)-glucose to galactose-1-phosphate, thereby generating glucose-1-phosphate and UDP-galactose. This cycle is then completed by conversion

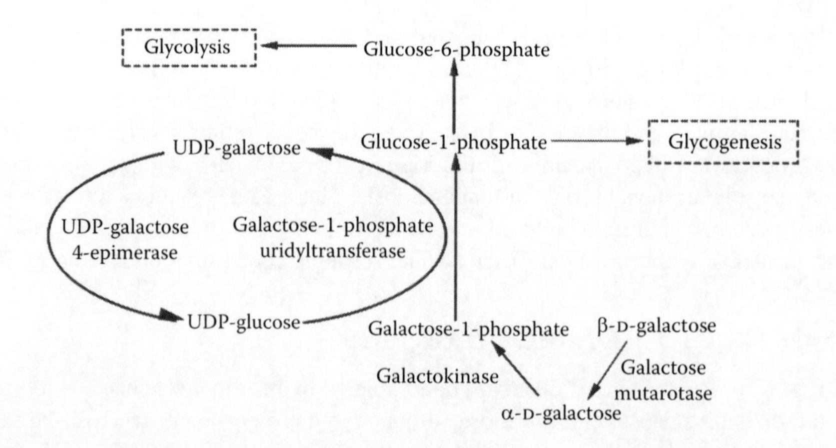

FIGURE 11.4 Leloir pathway for galactose metabolism.

of UDP-galactose back to UDP-glucose by UDP-galactose epimerase. The key product, glucose-1-phosphate, can be a substrate for glycogenesis or can be converted into glucose-6-phosphate to enter the glycolysis pathway [21,22].

In humans, defects in the genes encoding for galactokinase, uridyl transferase, or epimerase can give rise to an inherited metabolic diseases referred to as galactosemia. The most common form is due to the deficiency of galactose-1-phosphate uridyltransferase (GALT); the clinical diagnosis rests on increased galactose-1-phosphate concentration and low GALT activity in isolated red blood cells. Disorders in galactose metabolism can result in life-threatening complications in children, including feeding problems, failure to thrive, hepatocellular damage, bleeding, and sepsis. Treatment consists essentially in withdrawing galactose-containing foods in the diet. Even with adequate treatment, galactosemic children remain at increased risk for developmental delay, speech problems, and abnormalities of motor function [22].

SUGAR ALCOHOL METABOLISM

Sorbitol

Sorbitol is present in the human body as an intermediate product in the polyol pathway, which converts glucose into fructose. The function of this pathway, active in many organs, including the nervous system, the placenta, and endothelial cells, remains incompletely understood. Flux through this pathway is stimulated by hyperglycemia, which is thought to contribute to the development of the microvascular and nervous complications of diabetes. Sorbitol is present in our diet as a calorie-reduced sweetener and can only be metabolized intracellularly after conversion to fructose or glucose. Most studies suggest that sorbitol in humans is primarily converted into fructose, and only a small portion is metabolized directly to glucose, due to higher concentrations of glucose than fructose in cells. As seen in Figure 11.5, sorbitol is converted into fructose by nicotinamide adenine dinucleotide (NAD)-dependent polyol dehydrogenase or sorbitol dehydrogenase. Due to the low affinity of the NAD-dependent polyol dehydrogenase for a number of polyols, sorbitols, and other sugar alcohols can accumulate in lens, sciatic nerve, and renal papilla in certain diseased states such

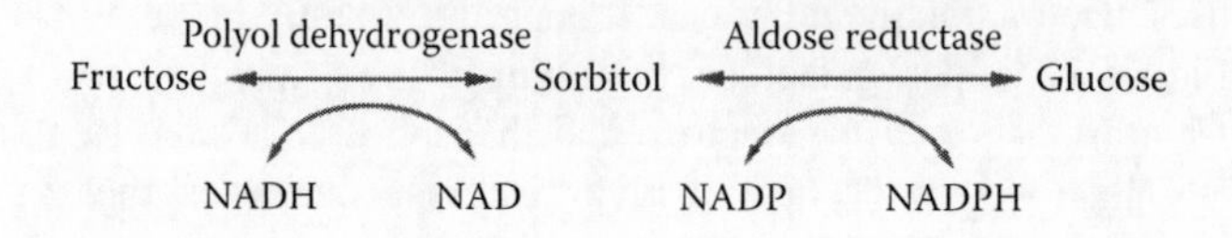

FIGURE 11.5 Polyol pathway for sorbitol metabolism.

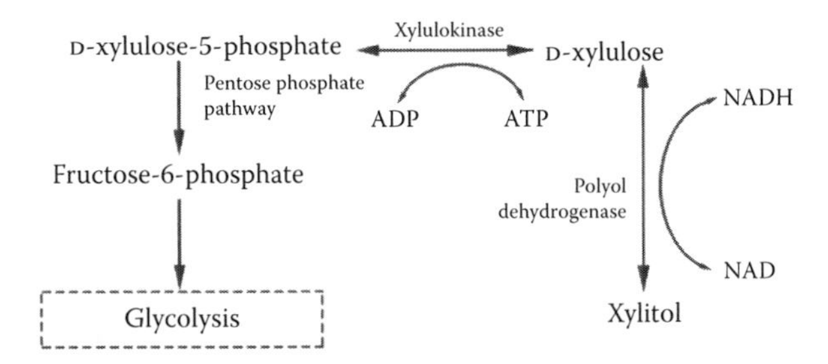

FIGURE 11.6 Xylitol metabolism.

as diabetes mellitus and consequently lead to toxicity. Both sorbitol and fructose can accumulate in the human lens in diabetics, causing osmotic damage, which has been suggested to be involved in the pathogenesis of diabetic cataract. Of importance, administration of sorbitol to patients with hereditary fructose intolerance will trigger acute metabolic crisis as does fructose [19,20].

Xylitol

Xylitol is another sugar alcohol commonly used by the food industries as a calorie-reduced sweetener. While xylitol can enter almost all cells of an organism, the liver cells are especially permeable. Enzymes for metabolizing xylitol are present in the kidney and testes, but the liver cells contain the most considerable amount and are thus the most important site of xylitol metabolism.

Xylitol has two possible pathways of metabolism in the liver. It can be oxidized to L-xylulose by a specific NADP-linked polyol dehydrogenase or to D-xylulose by a nonspecific NAD-linked polyol dehyrogenase, although the latter pathway is normally preferred. D-Xylulose is rapidly phosphorylated by xylulokinase to D-xylulose-5-phosphate, which can be converted into fructose-6-phosphate by the reactions of the PPP. Fructose-6-phosphate, an intermediate of glycolysis and gluconeogenesis, can be metabolized either to glucose and glycogen or to pyruvate and lactate (Figure 11.6).

Xylitol-induced dose-dependent abnormalities can occur in certain situations. Due to limited gut absorption capacity, ingestion of large doses of xylitol can cause osmotic diarrhea. Excessive xylitol intake can result in an imbalance of NADH/NAD ratio in the liver cytosol and in a depletion of hepatic ATP and inorganic phosphate can lead to hyperuricemia and occasionally lactic acidosis [19,20].

CONCLUSIONS

While most investigations to study sugar metabolism are carried out in laboratory animals, particularly rats, there has been increasing noteworthy contributions by studies conducted in humans using state-of-the-art techniques such as stable isotopes and nuclear magnetic resonance spectroscopy. While there is growing interest in the area of glucose metabolism in the brain, the capacity of individual tissues to utilize and metabolize nonglucose carbohydrates and their level of human tolerance and safety, particularly in the longer term, remains to be truly established.

REFERENCES

1. Appleton A, Bergen OV. *Carbohydrate Metabolism. Metabolism and Nutrition*, 4th edition. London: Elsevier Health Sciences; 2013. p. 23–44.
2. Dashty M. A quick look at biochemistry: Carbohydrate metabolism. *Clinical Biochemistry*. 2013;46(15):1339–52.
3. McKee T, McKee JR. *Carbohydrate Metabolism. Biochemistry the Molecular Basis of Life*, 5th edition. UK: Oxford University Press; 2013.

4. Alpers DH. Carbohydrates—Digestion, absorption, and metabolism. In: Caballero B, editor. *Encyclopedia of Food Sciences and Nutrition*, 2nd edition. Oxford: Academic Press; 2003. p. 881–7.
5. Sibley E. Carbohydrate digestion and absorption. In: Johnson LR, editor. *Encyclopedia of Gastroenterology*. New York: Elsevier; 2004. p. 275–8.
6. Gray GM. Carbohydrate absorption and malabsorption. In: Green M, Greene HL, editors. *The Role of the Gastrointestinal Tract in Nutrient Delivery*. Orlando: Academic Press; 1984. p. 133–44.
7. Brooks GA. Cell–cell and intracellular lactate shuttles. *J Physiol*. 2009;587(Pt 23):5591–600. Epub 2009/10/07.
8. Pellerin L, Magistretti PJ. Glial energy metabolism: Overview. In: Squire LR, editor. *Encyclopedia of Neuroscience*. Oxford: Academic Press; 2009. p. 783–8.
9. Stylianopoulos CL. Carbohydrates: Regulation of metabolism. In: Caballero B, editor. *Encyclopedia of Human Nutrition*, 2nd edition. Oxford: Elsevier; 2005. p. 309–15.
10. Leverv XM. Integration of metabolism 1: Energy. In: Lanham SA, MacDonald IA, Roche HM, editors. *Nutrition and Metabolism*, 2nd edition. UK: Wiley-Blackwell; 2011. p. 35–48.
11. Feher J. The endocrine pancreas and control of blood glucose. In: Feher J, editor. *Quantitative Human Physiology*. Boston: Academic Press; 2012. p. 799–809.
12. Marsenic O. Glucose control by the kidney: An emerging target in diabetes. *Am J Kidney Diseases*. 2009;53(5):875–83.
13. Mitrakou A. Kidney: Its impact on glucose homeostasis and hormonal regulation. *Diabetes Res Clin Practice*. 2011;93(Suppl 1):S66–S72.
14. Egan B, Zierath Juleen R. Exercise metabolism and the molecular regulation of skeletal muscle adaptation. *Cell Metabolism*. 2013;17(2):162–84.
15. Goodman HM. Hormonal regulation of fuel metabolism. In: Goodman HM, editor. *Basic Medical Endocrinology*, 4th edition. San Diego: Academic Press; 2009. p. 151–74.
16. Yeo R, Sawdon M. Hormonal control of metabolism: Regulation of plasma glucose. *Anaesth Intensive Care Med*. 2013;14(7):296–300.
17. Macdonald I. Carbohydrates: Metabolism of sugars. In: Caballero B, editor. *Encyclopedia of Food Sciences and Nutrition*, 2nd edition. Oxford: Academic Press; 2003. p. 889–91.
18. Mayes PA. Intermediary metabolism of fructose. *Am J Clin Nutr*. 1993;58(5 Suppl):754S–65S. Epub 1993/11/01.
19. Sestoft L. An evaluation of biochemical aspects of intravenous fructose, sorbitol and xylitol administration in man. *Acta Anaesthesiol Scand Suppl*. 1985;82:19–29. Epub 1985/01/01.
20. Wang YM, van Eys J. Nutritional significance of fructose and sugar alcohols. *Annu Rev Nutr*. 1981;1:437–75. Epub 1981/01/01.
21. Coss-Bu JA, Sunehag AL, Haymond MW. Contribution of galactose and fructose to glucose homeostasis. *Metabolism*. 2009;58(8):1050–8. Epub 2009/06/02.
22. Holden HM, Rayment I, Thoden JB. Structure and function of enzymes of the Leloir pathway for galactose metabolism. *J Biol Chem*. 2003;278(45):43885–8. Epub 2003/08/19.

12 Sugars and Metabolic Disorders in Animal Models Including Primates

Michael Pagliassotti, Kimberly Cox-York, and Tiffany Weir

CONTENTS

KEY POINTS

- Glucose extraction by the liver is ~30%, whereas fructose extraction is ~60–80%.
- High amounts of fructose induce metabolic impairments in rodents and nonhuman primates.
- Sex and strain influence susceptibility to sucrose and fructose.
- The gut microbiome and intestinal barrier contribute to fructose-induced metabolic impairments.
- Hyperuricemia may link fructose to metabolic impairments.
- Fructose has direct effects on the liver and hepatocytes.

INTRODUCTION

Metabolic disorders, including dyslipidemia, metabolic syndrome, obesity, and type 2 diabetes, are major public health problems. Thus, large research efforts are in place to understand the etiology, prevention, and treatment of these disorders. Although the causes of obesity and type 2 diabetes are complex, lifestyle changes can prevent or delay their onset. For example, the Diabetes and Prevention Program demonstrated that changes in diet and physical activity reduced the development of type 2 diabetes by 58% [1].

Diet composition plays an important role in the development of metabolic disorders [2]. The most researched adverse consequence related to diet composition relates to the role of excess calories, in the form of fat and simple sugars in the development of comorbidities associated with obesity [3–5].

However, these macronutrients can also have potent effects on glucose and lipid metabolism, insulin action, and the inflammatory response that are independent of calorie content and fat mass [6–11]. More recently, dietary fat and simple sugars have been implicated in the development of metabolic disorders via effects on the composition of the intestinal microbiota [12,13]. Thus, diet composition has the potential to influence the development and exacerbation of metabolic disorders directly and indirectly through effects on fat mass, fat distribution, and intestinal bacteria.

Along with a shift in total energy consumption over the past few decades, there has been a shift in the type of nutrients in the American diet. It has recently been estimated that the annual per capita intake of fructose is ~17 kg [14]. Major sources of fructose include sucrose, high-fructose corn syrup, fruit juice concentrate, fruits, and honey. In this chapter, we will discuss evidence related to the ability of sucrose and fructose to produce metabolic impairments in animal models that have relevance to human disease. There are a large number of review articles related to this topic [15–19]. We will begin by summarizing the acute and chronic effects of sucrose and fructose in animal models and nonhuman primates and then discuss putative tissue/organ targets and potential mechanisms of action.

ACUTE EFFECTS OF SUCROSE AND FRUCTOSE

The liver occupies a central role in the maintenance of blood glucose homeostasis due to its ability to both release glucose into and remove glucose from the circulation. In the postabsorptive state, glucose arising from glucose-6-phosphate, derived from glycogenolysis and gluconeogenesis, is released into the circulation. Following ingestion of a meal containing complex carbohydrates or glucose, the liver becomes a net consuming organ, accounting for ~30% of the total dietary carbohydrate/glucose disposal [20]. In contrast, fructose extraction by the liver can approach 60–80% and the presence of even small quantities of fructose in the portal vein increase glucose uptake by activating glucokinase translocation [21,22]. Thus, when complex carbohydrates or glucose are replaced by sucrose or fructose, the contribution of the liver to the disposal of dietary carbohydrate will be increased. The liver engages the pentose phosphate pathway, de novo lipogenesis, and glycolysis to deal with this increased carbohydrate load [23,24], resulting in a vastly different intrahepatic and/or circulating environment, characterized by increased pentose phosphate and lipid intermediates, triglycerides, and lactate. Hence, the magnitude of carbohydrate metabolism in the liver can be dramatically altered by the presence of sucrose or fructose in the diet.

OVERVIEW OF CHRONIC EFFECTS OF SUCROSE AND FRUCTOSE

The majority of animal studies that have examined the effects of diets enriched in sucrose or fructose have been conducted in rodents and the sucrose/fructose has generally, but not always, been supplied in the drinking water. Most of these studies have reported adaptations that include dyslipidemia, hypertension, hyperuricemia, insulin resistance, and adipose tissue fat accumulation [6,19, 25–31] (Figure 12.1). There are a small proportion of animal studies that have not observed some or all of these adaptations [32–34].

In a recent long-term study, rhesus monkeys were fed a grain-based standard primate diet (30% of energy from protein, 11% from fat, 59% from carbohydrate) that was supplemented with ~75 g of fructose as a fruit-flavored beverage over a 12-month period [35]. The intent of this study was to develop a "nonhuman primate model of diet-induced insulin resistance and dyslipidemia (and not to compare the metabolic effects of fructose vs. glucose in the animals)". It was reported that over the course of the 12-month study, every monkey ($n = 29$) developed components of the metabolic syndrome (increased adiposity, insulin resistance, and/or dyslipidemia). Four monkeys developed diabetes, based on a fasting glucose of ≥126 mg/dl. Together with the rodent-based studies, these results indicate that a relatively high amount of fructose (~30% of energy), provided in the form of a beverage, induces metabolic impairments.

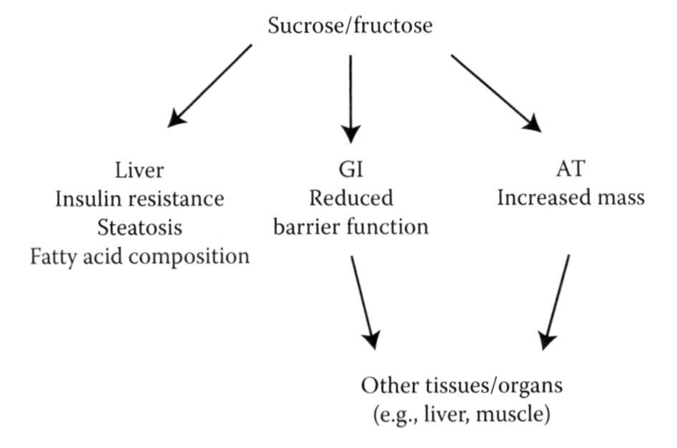

FIGURE 12.1 Schematic diagram of sucrose/fructose-mediated effects in rodents and nonhuman primates. Sucrose and fructose may have direct effects on the liver, gastrointestinal tract (GI), and adipose tissue (AT). Adaptations in GI and AT may influence other tissues and organ systems.

FACTORS THAT CAN INFLUENCE SUCROSE- AND FRUCTOSE-INDUCED METABOLIC IMPAIRMENTS

A primary criticism of animal models has been the amount of sucrose or fructose introduced into the diet. In most cases, animal studies have used a strategy in which the carbohydrate content of the diet has been replaced or supplemented through the water with sucrose or fructose at levels that approximate 32–69 or 34–88% of total calories, respectively [6,25–28,31,36–40]. The extent to which such studies relate to the development of human disease must therefore be considered cautiously. It should be noted, however, that a relatively low sucrose diet (18% of energy as sucrose) over a period of ≥16 weeks has been shown to induce insulin resistance and dyslipidemia in rats [41] (Figure 12.2).

Female Wistar rats, unlike their male counterparts, do not develop insulin resistance nor accumulate plasma or liver triglycerides in response to a high-sucrose diet provided for up to 8 weeks [42]. Other studies have reported that the development of hypertension was delayed and that there was protection against sucrose-induced oxidative stress in female rats [43,44]. CD36 is an integral membrane glycoprotein found on the surface of a variety of cells and plays an important role in fatty

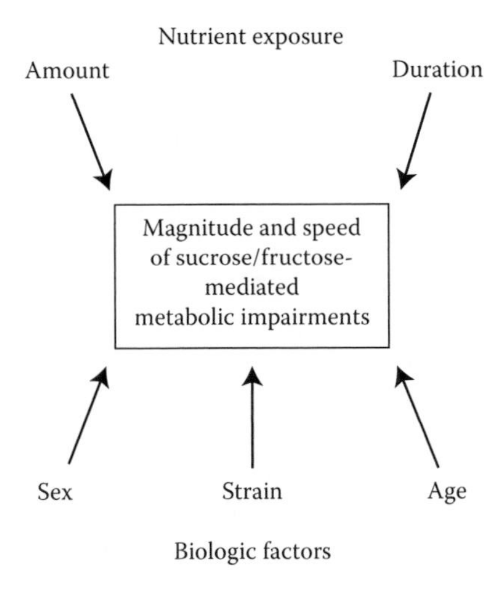

FIGURE 12.2 The magnitude and speed of adaptations to sucrose/fructose will be influenced by the amount and duration of nutrient exposure and biologic factors, such as sex, strain, and age.

acid transport [45]. Increased expression of CD36 mRNA was observed in the liver of female compared to male rats, and CD36 null mice were more susceptible to fructose-induced insulin resistance compared to their wild-type counterparts [45,46]. Thus, there appear to be sex-based differences in susceptibility to sucrose- and fructose-induced metabolic impairments that may involve CD36 and have been attributed to the antioxidant effects of estrogen [43] (Figure 12.2).

Susceptibility to the negative effects of a high-fructose diet in mice appears also to be dependent on strain. In one study, mice were provided a high-carbohydrate diet (58% carbohydrate with no fructose) or a high-fructose diet (66% fructose) for 8 weeks. Relative to the high-carbohydrate diet, the fructose diet induced postprandial hyperinsulinemia, hypertriglyceridemia, and visceral fat accumulation in CBA/JN, C3H/He, and BALB/c mice; however, these responses were either blunted or absent in DBA/2N, DBA/JN, and C57BL/6N mice [47] (Figure 12.2).

TISSUE/ORGAN TARGETS

In 1980, Kelly et al. [48] reported that a high-sucrose diet (73% sucrose) increased mesenteric lymph triglyceride output and speculated that the intestine participated in sucrose-induced hypertriglyceridemia in rats. This theory was supported by a study by Bergheim et al. [49] in 2008, who demonstrated that antibiotics provided protection against fructose-induced (fructose in the drinking water) hepatic lipid accumulation in mice. It was hypothesized that high rates of fructose consumption increased intestinal translocation of endotoxin [49]. These authors have postulated a working model that involves fructose-mediated bacterial overgrowth, increased intestinal permeability, increased portal vein endotoxin, activation of hepatic Kupffer cells, and Kupffer cell-derived tumor necrosis factor-α-mediated hepatocyte insulin resistance and triglyceride accumulation [50–53]. In addition, fructose-fed mice treated with pro- and pre-biotics, restoring the homeostasis of the gut microbiota, were protected from fructose-induced liver damage [54,55].The gut microbiota and intestinal barrier, therefore, appears to be involved in fructose-mediated (likely also sucrose-mediated) metabolic impairments (Figure 12.1).

Although metabolic impairments associated with high sucrose or fructose feeding have been observed in the absence of significant adipose tissue accumulation [6,56], several studies have reported that these nutrients can promote increased adiposity [38,57–59]. Glucocorticoids can promote visceral obesity and metabolic complications [60]. 11β-Hydroxysteroid dehydrogenase type 1 (11β-HSD1) plays a central role in the regulation of tissue-specific intracellular glucocorticoid levels [61]. Increased 11β-HSD1 mRNA and protein in the liver, and mRNA in adipose tissue, was observed in rats within 24 h of ingestion of 16% fructose solution [62]. These differences were not, however, observed in rats exposed to a 16% sucrose solution, likely due to the lower amount of fructose present in the sucrose group. The molecular mechanisms that link fructose to 11β-HSD1 in liver and adipose tissue may have implications for the regulation of lipid accumulation in these tissues. Incubation of murine 3T3-L1 cells with fructose increased adipogenesis and adipocyte-related gene expression [63]. Interestingly, GLUT5, the key fructose transporter, was also shown to be expressed in early-stage adipocyte differentiation, but not in mature adipocytes. Moreover, epididymal adipose tissue was reduced in GLUT5 –/– mice compared to their wild-type counterparts [63]. Thus, fructose transport/metabolism in adipocytes may be an important determinant of adipose tissue morphology and function (Figure 12.1).

The liver and hepatocytes are primary targets of sucrose- and fructose-mediated adaptations, such as hepatic insulin resistance and steatosis [19,64]. Several studies have demonstrated that sucrose- and fructose-mediated hepatic steatosis and insulin resistance occur rapidly and often precede adaptations in muscle and/or adipose tissue [6,19,25,26]. To examine the direct effects of fructose on the liver, we performed hyperglycemic, hyperinsulinemic pancreatic clamps for 3 or 6 h in the presence or absence of low (portal vein fructose concentration of <0.3 mmol/L) or high (portal vein fructose concentration >1 mmol/L) intraportal fructose infusions [65]. Selective delivery of fructose activated stress signaling pathways and reduced insulin signaling. Several studies have demonstrated that fructose delivery and metabolism in hepatocytes also activates stress signaling pathways and reduces insulin signaling [66,67]. In summary, fructose has direct effects on the liver and hepatocytes that can be elicited independent of the gastrointestinal tract and adipose tissue (Figure 12.1).

ROLE OF FRUCTOKINASE IN METABOLIC IMPAIRMENTS

Fructose metabolism and extraction by the liver are high (relative to glucose) due to both the extensive amount of fructokinase (ketohexokinase) in the liver and to the subsequent metabolism of fructose-1-phosphate at the triose phosphate level, which bypasses control exerted by phosphofructokinase [21,68]. Recent studies have provided new information pertaining to fructokinase and its role in fructose-induced metabolic impairments [69–71]. Fructokinase exists in two alternatively spliced isoforms, fructokinase A and C, that differ in exon 3 [72]. Fructokinase C is characterized by a high affinity for fructose (low K_m) and is expressed primarily in the liver, kidney, and intestines [73]. Mice lacking both isoforms were protected from fructose (30% fructose in the drinking water)-induced increases in body fat, hyperinsulinemia, and lipid accumulation in the liver [69]. In contrast, fructose-mediated effects were exacerbated in mice lacking fructokinase A. The protective effects of fructokinase A may be mediated by its low affinity (high K_m) for fructose. Future studies that modulate fructokinase in a tissue-specific manner are needed to elucidate the relative importance of fructose metabolism in different tissues/organs to sucrose- and fructose-mediated metabolic impairments.

HEPATIC STEATOSIS

It is well established that sucrose- and fructose-enriched diets produce hepatic steatosis in animal models [19,25,26,37]. In addition, these diets produce a change in the fatty acid composition of membrane phospholipids and triglycerides. A high-sucrose diet (68% of energy from sucrose) increased the degree of saturation of sinusoidal membrane phospholipids and liver triglyceride fatty acids after 1 and 5 weeks [74]. These changes were associated with reduced sinusoidal membrane fluidity [74]. More recently, it was demonstrated that high-sucrose diet-mediated increases in the saturated fatty acid content of microsomal membrane phospholipids and triglycerides were associated with the presence of endoplasmic reticulum (ER) stress and increased caspase activity in the liver [75]. These studies suggest that the deleterious effects of hepatic steatosis may involve the composition of lipids delivered to and stored within the liver.

A recent study examined the effects of diet-induced hepatic steatosis on liver regeneration. Male Sprague-Dawley rats were fed a high fructose (H-fruc; 66% fructose), high fat (H-fat; 54% fat), or control chow diet for 4 weeks [76]. Although hepatic steatosis, based on hepatic triglyceride content and oil red O staining, was less severe in H-fruc compared to H-fat liver, regeneration after 70% partial hepatectomy was reduced in H-fruc compared to H-fat. It is unclear whether differences in fatty acid composition were involved in the differential regenerative capacity following partial hepatectomy [75].

URIC ACID

Uric acid has been linked to pro- and anti-oxidant activity, inflammation, and regulation of nitric oxide bioavailability [77]. Fructose metabolism can raise plasma uric acid concentrations [78]. Uric acid dose-dependently inhibited the vasodilatory response of aortic artery rings to acetylcholine, indicating that uric acid may be involved in fructose-mediated metabolic impairments, particularly those involving the endothelium. The inclusion of allopurinol (a xanthine oxidase inhibitor) in the drinking water lowered plasma uric acid and prevented or reversed many of the metabolic impairments (hyperinsulinemia, systolic hypertension, hypertriglyceridemia, weight gain) associated with consumption of a high-fructose diet in rats [31]. It should be mentioned that although hypertension in response to high-sucrose or -fructose diets has been observed in several studies, this is not a universal finding [79–83].

FRUCTOSE AND THE PROTEOME

Morand et al. [84] examined the effects of a high-fructose diet (60% fructose) compared to a chow diet on hepatic ER-associated protein in hamsters. After 2 weeks of high-fructose diet feeding, 34 differentially expressed proteins were identified. Hepatic ER proteins that were >2-fold upregulated included α-glucosidase, P-glycoprotein, fibrinogen, protein disulfide isomerase, glucose-regulated protein-94, and apolipoprotein E. Hepatic ER proteins that were reduced >2-fold included ER60, ERp46, ERp29, glutamate dehydrogenase, and TAP1. More recently, hamsters were fed a regular rodent chow or high-fructose (60% fructose) diet for 8 weeks [85]. Fructose-fed hamsters were characterized by hyperinsulinemia, hyperlipidemia, and hepatic steatosis. Matrix-assisted laser desportion/ionization (MALDI)-based proteomics analysis of livers resulted in the identification of 33 protein spots with a >2-fold change in expression. Proteins that were induced in fructose-fed livers included fatty acid-binding protein, protein disulfide isomerase, apolipoprotein A-1, peroxiredoxin 2, glutathione *S*-transferase, and leucyl aminopeptidase. Proteins that were reduced in fructose-fed livers included carbamoyl-phosphate synthase 1,10-formyltetrahydrofolate dehydrogenase, ferritin heavy chain, and heat shock protein-70. While chronic high-fructose feeding provokes a number of proteomic changes in the liver, the extent to which these changes mediate or result from metabolic impairments is presently unknown.

SUMMARY

Fructose is pervasive in the western diet, and evidence from numerous animal studies support its role in the growing obesity epidemic. In addition to influencing obesity, excessive fructose consumption can result in hepatic steatosis, dyslipidemia, hypertension, and insulin resistance in rodents and primates. Fructose can act on host systems via direct effects on the liver or indirectly through alterations in intestinal microbiota or through alterations in adipose tissue morphology and function (Figure 12.1). Fructose-induced metabolic impairments appear to be linked to the ratio of fructokinase A and C, but models exploring tissue- and isoform-specific expression of fructokinase are needed to clarify this mechanism. New "omics" technologies offer the opportunity to further explore the role of the gastrointestinal tract and its associated microorganisms as well as provide insights into host-specific polymorphisms in fructose metabolism and to identify novel gene and protein targets that are altered by fructose consumption. Further research is also needed to clarify whether the mode of consumption (food versus beverage) alters the nature or magnitude of metabolic impairments associated with sucrose and fructose consumption.

REFERENCES

1. Albright AL, Gregg EW. Preventing type 2 diabetes in communities across the U.S.: The National Diabetes Prevention Program. *Am J Prev Med*. 2013;44(4 Suppl 4):S346–51. Epub 2013/03/27.
2. Hamman RF. Genetic and environmental determinants of non-insulin dependent diabetes mellitus (Niddm). *Diabetes/Metabolism Rev*. 1992;8(4):287–338.
3. Bray GA, Nielsen SJ, Popkin BM. Consumption of high-fructose corn syrup in beverages may play a role in the epidemic of obesity. *Am J Clin Nutr*. 2004;79:537–43.
4. Bray GA, Popkin BM. Dietary fat intake does affect obesity! *Am J Clin Nutr*. 1998;68:1157–73.
5. Doucet E, Almeras N, White MD, Despres JP, Bouchard C, Tremblay A. Dietary fat composition and human adiposity. *Eur J Clin Nutr*. 1998;52(1):2–6.

6. Pagliassotti MJ, Prach PA, Koppenhafer TA, Pan DA. Changes in insulin action, triglycerides, and lipid composition during sucrose feeding in rats. *Am J Physiol.* 1996;271(5 Pt 2):R1319–26. Epub 1996/11/01.
7. Dirlewanger M, Schneiter P, Jequier E, Tappy L. Effects of fructose on hepatic glucose metabolism in humans. *Am J Physiol Endocrinol Metab.* 2000;279:E907–E11.
8. Wei Y, Pagliassotti MJ. Hepatospecific effects of fructose on C-Jun Nh2-terminal kinase: Implications for hepatic insuliin resistance. *Am J Physiol Endocrinol Metab.* 2004;287:E926–E33.
9. Bergman RN, Ader M. Free fatty acids and pathogenesis of type 2 diabetes mellitus. *Trends Endocrinol Metab.* 2000;11(9):351–6.
10. Buettner R, Parhofer KG, Woenckhaus M, Wrede CE, Kunz-Schughart LA, Scholmerich J et al. Defining high-fat-diet rat models: Metabolic and molecular effects of different fat types. *J Mol Endocrinol.* 2006;36(3):485–501.
11. Wellen KE, Hotamisligil GS. Inflammation, stress, and diabetes. *J Clin Invest.* 2005;115:1111–9.
12. Cheng J, Palva AM, de Vos WM, Satokari R. Contribution of the intestinal microbiota to human health: From birth to 100 years of age. *Curr Top Microbiol Immunol.* 2013;358:323–46. Epub 2011/11/19.
13. Payne AN, Chassard C, Lacroix C. Gut microbial adaptation to dietary consumption of fructose, artificial sweeteners and sugar alcohols: Implications for host–microbe interactions contributing to obesity. *Obes Rev.* 2012;13(9):799–809. Epub 2012/06/13.
14. Marriott BP, Cole N, Lee E. National estimates of dietary fructose intake increased from 1977 to 2004 in the United States. *J Nutr.* 2009;139:1228S–35S.
15. Elliott SS, Keim NL, Stern JS, Teff K, Havel PJ. Fructose, weight gain, and the insulin resistance syndrome. *Am J Clin Nutr.* 2002;76:911–22.
16. Hallfrisch J. Metabolic effects of dietary fructose. *FASEB J.* 1990;4:2652–60.
17. Tappy L, Le KA. Metabolic effects of fructose and the worldwide increase in obesity. *Physiol Rev.* 2010;90(1):23–46. Epub 2010/01/21.
18. Rippe JM, Angelopoulos TJ. Sucrose, high-fructose corn syrup, and fructose, their metabolism and potential health effects: What do we really know? *Adv Nutr.* 2013;4(2):236–45. Epub 2013/03/16.
19. Bizeau ME, Pagliassotti MJ. Hepatic adaptations to sucrose and fructose. *Metabolism.* 2005;54(9):1189–201. Epub 2005/08/30.
20. Cherrington AD. Control of glucose uptake and release by the liver in vivo. *Diabetes.* 1999;48:1198–214.
21. Mayes PA. Intermediary metabolism of fructose. *Am J Clin Nutr.* 1993;58:754S–65S.
22. Shiota M, Galassetti P, Monohan P, Neal D, Cherrington AD. Small amounts of fructose markedly augment het hepatic glucose uptake in the conscious dog. *Diabetes.* 1998;47:867–73.
23. Wei Y, Bizeau ME, Pagliassotti MJ. An acute increase in fructose concentration increases hepatic glucose-6-phosphatase Mrna via mechanisms that are independent of glycogen synthase kinase-3 in rats. *J Nutr.* 2004;134(3):545–51.
24. Carmona A, Nishina PM, Avery EH, Freedland RA. Time course changes in glycogen accretion, 6-phosphogluconate, fructose-2,6-bisphosphate, and lipogenesis upon refeeding a high sucrose diet to starved rats. *Int J Biochem.* 1991;23(4):455–60.
25. Storlien LH, Kraegen EW, Jenkins AB, Chisholm DJ. Effects of sucrose vs. starch diets on in vivo insulin action, thermogenesis, and obesity in rats. *Am J Clin Nutr.* 1988;47:420–7.
26. Thorburn AW, Storlien LH, Jenkins AB, Khouri S, Kraegen EW. Fructose-induced in vivo insulin resistance and elevated plasma triglyceride levels in rats. *Am J Clin Nutr.* 1989;49:1155–63.
27. Collison KS, Saleh SM, Bakheet RH, Al-Rabiah RK, Inglis AL, Makhoul NJ et al. Diabetes of the liver: The link between nonalcoholic fatty liver disease and Hfcs-55. *Obesity (Silver Spring).* 2009;17(11):2003–13.
28. Kelley GL, Allan G, Azhar S. High dietary fructose induces a hepatic stress response resulting in cholesterol and lipid dysregulation. *Endocrinology.* 2004;145(2):548–55.
29. Nagai Y, Nishio Y, Nakamura T, Maegawa H, Kikkawa R, Kashiwagi A. Amelioration of high fructose-induced metabolic derangements by activation of PPARalpha. *Am J Physiol Endocrinol Metab.* 2002;282(5):E1180–90. Epub 2002/04/06.
30. Johnson RJ, Segal MS, Sautin Y, Nakagawa T, Feig DI, Kang DH et al. Potential role of sugar (fructose) in the epidemic of hypertension, obesity and the metabolic syndrome, diabetes, kidney disease, and cardiovascular disease. *Am J Clin Nutr.* 2007;86(4):899–906. Epub 2007/10/09.
31. Nakagawa T, Hu H, Zharikov S, Tuttle KR, Short RA, Glushakova O et al. A causal role for uric acid in fructose-induced metabolic syndrome. *Am J Physiol Renal Physiol.* 2006;290(3):F625–31. Epub 2005/10/20.
32. Vallerand AL, Lupien J, Bukowiecki LJ. Synergistic improvement of glucose tolerance by sucrose feeding and exercise training. *Am J Physiol Endocrinol Metab.* 1986;250:E607–14.

33. Maegawa H, Kobayashi M, Ishibashi O, Takata Y, Shigeta Y. Effect of diet change on insulin action: Difference between muscle and adipocytes. *Am J Physiol Endocrinol Metab.* 1986;251:E616–23.
34. Stark AH, Timar B, Madar Z. Adaptation of Sprague-Dawley rats to long-term feeding of high fat or high fructose diets. *Eur J Nutr.* 2000;39:229–34.
35. Bremer AA, Stanhope KL, Graham JL, Cummings BP, Wang W, Saville BR et al. Fructose-fed rhesus monkeys: A nonhuman primate model of insulin resistance, metabolic syndrome, and type 2 diabetes. *Clin Transl Sci.* 2011;4(4):243–52. Epub 2011/09/03.
36. Bezerra RMN, Ueno M, Silva MS, Tavares DQ, Carvalho CRO, Saad MF. A high fructose diet affects the early steps of insulin action in muscle and liver of rats. *J Nutr.* 2000;130:1531–5.
37. Gutman RA, Basilico MZ, Bernal CA, Chicco A, Lombardo YB. Long-term hypertriglyceridemia and glucose intolerance in rats fed chronically an isocaloric sucrose-rich diet. *Metabolism.* 1987;36(11):1013–20.
38. Soria A, D'Alessandro ME, Lombardo YB. Duration of feeding on a sucrose-rich diet determines metabolic and morphological changes in rat adipocytes. *J Appl Physiol.* 2001;91:2109–16.
39. Wright DW, Hansen RI, Mondon CE, Reaven GM. Sucrose-induced insulin resistance in the rat: Modulation by exercise and diet. *Am J Clin Nutr.* 1983;38:879–83.
40. Thresher JS, Podolin DA, Wei Y, Mazzeo RS, Pagliassotti MJ. Comparison of the effects of sucrose and fructose on insulin action and glucose tolerance. *Am J Physiol Regul Integr Comp Physiol.* 2000;279(4):R1334–40. Epub 2000/09/27.
41. Pagliassotti MJ, Prach PA. Quantity of sucrose alters the tissue pattern and time course of insulin resistance in young rats. *Am J Physiol.* 1995;269(3 Pt 2):R641–6. Epub 1995/09/01.
42. Horton TJ, Gayles EC, Prach PA, Koppenhafer TA, Pagliassotti MJ. Female rats do not develop sucrose-induced insulin resistance. *Am J Physiol.* 1997;272(5 Pt 2):R1571–6. Epub 1997/05/01.
43. Busserolles J, Mazur A, Gueux E, Rock E, Rayssiguier Y. Metabolic syndrome in the rat: Females are protected against the pro-oxidant effect of a high sucrose diet. *Exp Biol Med (Maywood).* 2002;227(9):837–42.
44. Roberts CK, Vaziri ND, Barnard RJ. Protective effects of estrogen on gender specific development of diet-induced hypertension. *J Appl Physiol.* 2001;91:2005–9.
45. Hajri T, Abumrad NA. Fatty acid transport across membranes: Relevance to nutrition and metabolic pathology. *Ann Rev Nutr.* 2002;22:383–415.
46. Stahlberg N, Rico-Bautista E, Fisher RM, Wu X, Cheung L, Flores-Morales A et al. Female-predominant expression of fatty acid translocase/Cd36 in rat and human liver. *Endocrinology.* 2004;145:1972–9.
47. Nagata R, Nishio Y, Sekine O, Nagai Y, Maeno Y, Ugi S et al. Single nucleotide polymorphism (–468 G to a) at the promoter region of Srebp-1c associates with genetic defect of fructose-induced hepatic lipogenesis. *J Biol Chem.* 2004;279:29031–42.
48. Kelly TJ, Holt PR, Wu AL. Effect of sucrose on intestinal very low-density lipoprotein production. *Am J Clin Nutr.* 1980;33(5):1033–40. Epub 1980/05/01.
49. Bergheim I, Weber S, Vos M, Kramer S, Volynets V, Kaserouni S et al. Antibiotics protect against fructose-induced hepatic lipid accumulation in mice: Role of endotoxin. *J Hepatol.* 2008;48:983–92.
50. Spruss A, Bergheim I. Dietary fructose and intestinal barrier: Potential risk factor in the pathogenesis of nonalcoholic fatty liver disease. *J Nutr Biochem.* 2009;20(9):657–62.
51. Kanuri G, Spruss A, Wagnerberger S, Bischoff SC, Bergheim I. Role of tumor necrosis factor alpha (Tnfalpha) in the onset of fructose-induced nonalcoholic fatty liver disease in mice. *J Nutr Biochem.* 2011;22(6):527–34. Epub 2010/08/31.
52. Spruss A, Kanuri G, Wagnerberger S, Haub S, Bischoff SC, Bergheim I. Toll-like receptor 4 is involved in the development of fructose-induced hepatic steatosis in mice. *Hepatology.* 2009;50(4):1094–104. Epub 2009/07/29.
53. Spruss A, Kanuri G, Uebel K, Bischoff SC, Bergheim I. Role of the inducible nitric oxide synthase in the onset of fructose-induced steatosis in mice. *Antioxid Redox Signal.* 2011;14(11):2121–35. Epub 2010/11/19.
54. Busserolles J, Gueux E, Rock E, Demigne C, Mazur A, Rayssiguier Y. Oligofructose protects against the hypertriglyceridemic and pro-oxidative effects of a high fructose diet in rats. *J Nutr.* 2003;133(6):1903–8. Epub 2003/05/29.
55. Suganthi R, Rajamani S, Ravichandran MK, Anuradha CV. Effect of food seasoning spices mixture on biomarkers of oxidative stress in tissues of fructose-fed insulin-resistant rats. *J Med Food.* 2007;10(1):149–53. Epub 2007/05/03.
56. Pagliassotti MJ, Shahrokhi KA, Moscarello M. Involvement of liver and skeletal muscle in sucrose-induced insulin resistance: Dose–response studies. *Am J Physiol.* 1994;266(5 Pt 2):R1637–44. Epub 1994/05/01.
57. Toida S, Takahashi M, Shimizu H, Sato N, Shimomura Y, Kobayashi I. Effect of high sucrose feeding on fat accumulation in the male wistar rat. *Obes Res.* 1996;4(6):561–8.

58. Jurgens H, Haass W, Castaneda TR, Schurmann A, Koebnick C, Dombrowski F et al. Consuming fructose-sweetened beverages increases body adiposity in mice. *Obes Res*. 2005;13(7):1146–56. Epub 2005/08/04.
59. Alzamendi A, Giovambattista A, Raschia A, Madrid V, Gaillard RC, Rebolledo O et al. Fructose-rich diet-induced abdominal adipose tissue endocrine dysfunction in normal male rats. *Endocrine*. 2009;35(2):227–32. Epub 2009/01/24.
60. Bjorntorp P. The regulation of adipose tissue distribution in humans. *Int J Obes Relat Metab Disord*. 1996;20(4):291–302. Epub 1996/04/01.
61. London E, Castonguay TW. Diet and the role of 11beta-hydroxysteroid dehydrogenase-1 on obesity. *J Nutr Biochem*. 2009;20(7):485–93. Epub 2009/05/16.
62. London E, Castonguay TW. High fructose diets increase 11beta-hydroxysteroid dehydrogenase type 1 in liver and visceral adipose in rats within 24-h exposure. *Obesity (Silver Spring)*. 2011;19(5):925–32. Epub 2010/12/04.
63. Du L, Heaney AP. Regulation of adipose differentiation by fructose and Glut5. *Mol Endocrinol*. 2012;26(10):1773–82. Epub 2012/07/26.
64. Wei Y, Wang D, Topczewski F, Pagliassotti MJ. Fructose-mediated stress signaling in the liver: Implications for hepatic insulin resistance. *J Nutr Biochem*. 2007;18(1):1–9.
65. Wei Y, Pagliassotti MJ. Hepatospecific effects of fructose on C-Jun Nh2-terminal kinase: Implications for hepatic insulin resistance. *Am J Physiol Endocrinol Metab*. 2004;287(5):E926–33. Epub 2004/06/17.
66. Wei Y, Wang D, Pagliassotti MJ. Fructose selectively modulates C-Jun N-terminal kinase activity and insulin signaling in rat primary hepatocytes. *J Nutr*. 2005;135(7):1642–6.
67. Wei Y, Wang D, Moran G, Estrada A, Pagliassotti MJ. Fructose-induced stress signaling in the liver involves methylglyoxal. *Nutr Metab (Lond)*. 2013;10(1):32. Epub 2013/04/10.
68. Heinz F, Lamprecht W, Kirsch J. Enzymes of fructose metabolism in human liver. *J Clin Invest*. 1968;47:1826–32.
69. Ishimoto T, Lanaspa MA, Le MT, Garcia GE, Diggle CP, Maclean PS et al. Opposing effects of fructokinase C and A isoforms on fructose-induced metabolic syndrome in mice. *Proc Natl Acad Sci USA*. 2012;109(11):4320–5. Epub 2012/03/01.
70. Diggle CP, Shires M, Leitch D, Brooke D, Carr IM, Markham AF et al. Ketohexokinase: Expression and localization of the principal fructose-metabolizing enzyme. *J Histochem Cytochem*. 2009;57(8):763–74. Epub 2009/04/15.
71. Diggle CP, Shires M, McRae C, Crellin D, Fisher J, Carr IM et al. Both isoforms of ketohexokinase are dispensable for normal growth and development. *Physiol Genomics*. 2010;42A(4):235–43. Epub 2010/09/16.
72. Hayward BE, Bonthron DT. Structure and alternative splicing of the ketohexokinase gene. *Eur J Biochem*. 1998;257(1):85–91. Epub 1998/11/03.
73. Asipu A, Hayward BE, O'Reilly J, Bonthron DT. Properties of normal and mutant recombinant human ketohexokinases and implications for the pathogenesis of essential fructosuria. *Diabetes*. 2003;52(9):2426–32. Epub 2003/08/28.
74. Podolin DA, Sutherland E, Iwahashi M, Simon FR, Pagliassotti MJ. A high-sucrose diet alters the lipid composition and fluidity of liver sinusoidal membranes. *Horm Metab Res*. 1998;30(4):195–9.
75. Wang D, Wei Y, Pagliassotti MJ. Saturated fatty acids promote endoplasmic reticulum stress and liver injury in rats with hepatic steatosis. *Endocrinology*. 2006;147:943–51.
76. Tanoue S, Uto H, Kumamoto R, Arima S, Hashimoto S, Nasu Y et al. Liver regeneration after partial hepatectomy in rat is more impaired in a steatotic liver induced by dietary fructose compared to dietary fat. *Biochem Biophys Res Commun*. 2011;407(1):163–8. Epub 2011/03/05.
77. Johnson RJ, Sautin YY, Oliver WJ, Roncal C, Mu W, Gabriela Sanchez-Lozada L et al. Lessons from comparative physiology: Could uric acid represent a physiologic alarm signal gone awry in western society? *J Comp Physiol B*. 2009;179(1):67–76. Epub 2008/07/24.
78. Stirpe F, Della Corte E, Bonetti E, Abbondanza A, Abbati A, De Stefano F. Fructose-induced hyperuricaemia. *Lancet*. 1970;2(7686):1310–1. Epub 1970/12/19.
79. Pagliassotti MJ, Gayles EC, Podolin DA, Wei Y, Morin CL. Developmental stage modifies diet-induced peripheral insulin resistance in rats. *Am J Physiol Regul Integr Comp Physiol*. 2000;278(1):R66–73. Epub 2000/01/25.
80. Ackerman Z, Oron-Herman M, Grozovski M, Rosenthal T, Pappo O, Link G et al. Fructose-induced fatty liver disease: Hepatic effects of blood pressure and plasma triglyceride reduction. *Hypertension*. 2005;45(5):1012–8.
81. Hulman S, Falkner B. The effect of excess dietary sucrose on growth, blood pressure, and metabolism in developing Sprague-Dawley rats. *Pediatr Res*. 1994;36:95–101.

82. Santure M, Pitre M, Marette A, Deshaies Y, Lemieux C, Lariviere R et al. Induction of insulin resistance by high-sucrose feeding does not raise mean arterial blood pressure but impairs haemodynamic responses to insulin in rats. *Br J Pharm*. 2001;137:185–96.
83. van der Schaaf MR, Joles JA, van Tol A, Koomans HA. Long-term fructose versus corn starch feeding in the spontaneously hypertensive rat. *Clin Sci*. 1995;88:719–25.
84. Morand JP, Macri J, Adeli K. Proteomic profiling of hepatic endoplasmic reticulum-associated proteins in an animal model of insulin resistance and metabolic dyslipidemia. *J Biol Chem*. 2005;280(18):17626–33. Epub 2005/03/12.
85. Zhang L, Perdomo G, Kim DH, Qu S, Ringquist S, Trucco M et al. Proteomic analysis of fructose-induced fatty liver in hamsters. *Metabolism*. 2008;57(8):1115–24. Epub 2008/07/22.

13 Contributions of Sugars to Metabolic Disorders in Human Models

Kim-Anne Lê and Luc Tappy

CONTENTS

KEY POINTS

- Sugar ingestion results in the absorption of glucose and fructose in the gut, while starch ingestion results in the exclusive absorption of glucose. Whatever specific metabolic effects of sugar are therefore likely to be due to its fructose component.
- Glucose absorbed from the gut elicits satiety signals and is metabolized by means of tightly regulated metabolic pathways under the control of insulin. In contrast, fructose is entirely and almost immediately metabolized in splanchnic organs by essentially unregulated metabolic pathways. In the liver, it is converted into glucose, lactate, and fatty acid as a first step, and these substrates are subsequently used by extra-splanchnic cells as energy substrates.
- Epidemiological studies show an association between sugar intake and obesity, but the obesogenic role of sugar remains unclear. Since sugar does not significantly decrease energy expenditure, any causal effect in the development of obesity should involve an excess food intake, following sugar ingestion.

- The material reviewed in this chapter includes many human studies having used very high amounts of sugar or pure fructose to workout possible pathogenic mechanisms. Such studies do not imply that sugars have the same effects when ingested at doses encountered in usual diets.
- A high sugar intake causes an increase in fasting and postprandial blood triglycerides and an increase in intrahepatic fat. Stimulation of de novo lipogenesis, mainly in the liver, but also possibly in the gut, and alterations of extrahepatic clearance of triglycerides are responsible for this effect.
- A high sugar intake decreases insulin-mediated suppression of glucose production, which may contribute to an increased postprandial glycemic response. In the short-term, however, it does not impair muscle insulin resistance.
- Increased de novo lipogenesis and hepatic glucose production may be normal adaptive responses elicited by the presence of fructose in the diet rather than pathogenic events. Future research should focus on identification of maladaptive responses to fructose as a cause of metabolic diseases.

INTRODUCTION

Sugars have always been present in the human diet from time immemorial, but were consumed only in small amounts with fruits, berries, and honey. Consumption of sugar extracted from sugarcane started only after the crusade, but remained quantitatively small due to its low availability and high price. In these times, it was used in minute amounts and is mentioned amongst spices in medieval cookbooks. The use of sugar really increased in the colonial era, when it became available in large amounts at an affordable price. Its consumption has gradually increased since then, as it became introduced in "solid" food items such as pastries, jams, marmelades, and preservatives, on the one hand, and was used extensively to sweeten the new beverages brought from colonies such as tea, coffee, and chocolates. Since then, sugar consumption has increased continuously throughout the world. It is important to take note that, since the early days of its consumption, a substantial portion of sugar is consumed together with beverages: initially with hot beverages, and more recently with sodas, fruit juices, and energy drinks. As a consequence, the consumption of "liquid" calories in comparison with more traditional, solid foods has increased and constitutes now a substantial portion of our diet [1].

Fruits, vegetables, and honey contain fructose, glucose, and sucrose (i.e., one molecule of glucose linked to one molecule of fructose) in various amounts, together with dietary fibers, minerals, vitamins, polyphenols, and various other nutritional compounds. Sugar refined from sugarcane or beet contains almost only sucrose, without free glucose or fructose, and with virtually no other macro- or micronutrients. High-fructose corn syrup (HFCS), prepared from corn starch through industrial procedures, has substituted for sucrose in many beverages and industrial food products; it contains free fructose and free glucose in various proportions, together with a small amount of oligosaccharides [2].

Both sugar and starch are carbohydrates. Starch digestion in the gut yields glucose molecules which are subsequently absorbed into the hepatic portal circulation. Sucrose is hydrolyzed into glucose and fructose by intestinal disaccharidases present in the brush-border of enterocytes and is subsequently absorbed as free glucose and fructose. Free glucose and fructose ingested with fruits or HFCS are directly absorbed by the enterocytes to be released into the portal vein. The consumption of natural, sweet foods therefore includes both glucose and fructose which are ingested together. Since sugar differs from starch by yielding fructose in addition to glucose in the intestinal lumen, it is logical to assume that the differences between the effects of sugar and starch on health-related variables are essentially mediated by fructose. It is, however, well recognized that even starchy foods devoid of fructose can differentially affect health outcomes according to their glycemic index, indicating that other factors, such as the rate of hexose absorption, the glycemic response, or postprandial insulin concentrations are also important factors [3].

WHY DO WE SUSPECT THAT SUGARS ARE ASSOCIATED WITH ADVERSE HEALTH OUTCOMES?

There is no naturally occurring food providing only fructose in our diet. However, in the 1980s, there was a huge interest in the use of pure fructose as a sweetener for subjects with diabetes mellitus, since this sugar can be metabolized to some extent independent of insulin secretion and elicits much smaller glycemic responses than sucrose. Many small-scale clinical trials were performed to assess the effects of substituting pure fructose for sucrose in healthy individuals and in subjects with diabetes mellitus. These trials indeed documented that pure fructose reduced blood glucose, decreased insulin requirements, and, in patients with diabetes, lowered the blood-glycated hemoglobin concentrations [4]. Some trials, however, observed that fructose also increased fasting and postprandial triglyceride concentrations, raising the suspicion that it may increase cardiovascular risk and, in the long-term, produce more deleterious than beneficial effects [5]. The hypothesis that fructose may have adverse metabolic effects in the long-term was further strengthened by the observations that animals put on a high-sucrose or -fructose diet developed many features of the metabolic syndrome, such as obesity, insulin resistance and impaired glucose homeostasis, dyslipidemia, hepatic steatosis, and even high blood pressure [6]. Since then, numerous experiments, having mainly used rodents, documented that fructose and fructose-containing caloric sweeteners such as sucrose and HFCS may indeed cause diabetes mellitus.

The initial hypothesis that fructose may have deleterious effects on health was supported by in vitro and in vivo animal data showing that it caused cellular oxidative stress and insulin resistance. It was further strengthened by many epidemiological studies showing that the consumption of either total sugar, fructose, or sweetened beverages was associated with obesity and with metabolic diseases.

In addition, ecological observations are also supporting a possible role of sugar in obesity and metabolic diseases: sugar consumption has increased progressively in Europe and North America from about 2 kg per person per year in the 1750s to about 50 kg per person per year in the 1970s, and close to 70 kg per person per year in the 2000s. Recent increases have also been reported in South America, Oceania, and Asia. Although there is some debate whether it still increases, has stabilized, or has slightly decreased over the past 10 years, there is no doubt that we have presently the highest consumption of sugar in human history. The prevalence of obesity and of noncommunicable diseases such as diabetes and cardiovascular diseases has increased dramatically since the 1970s, and some observers have suggested that it paralleled sugar consumption [7]. This hypothesis appears plausible, since sugar constitutes an important source of energy; it also implies that some kind of threshold was reached in the 1970s, above which sugar consumption started exerting deleterious health effects. This is consistent with recent ecological studies showing a high prevalence of diabetes mellitus in countries where there is a high intake of added sugars [8,9].

In the USA, HFCS has become increasingly available since the 1970s and has gradually replaced about 30% of dietary sugar. Large-scale HFCS consumption in the USA was really concomitant with the increase in obesity prevalence, arising the suspicion that, more than sugar, HFCS may be causally involved. This hypothesis appeared furthermore plausible based on the fact that HFCS 55, the most common form of HFCS used for the preparation of sweetened beverages, contains on a weight:weight basis somewhat more fructose than sucrose [10].

IN WHAT WAYS DOES THE METABOLISM OF FRUCTOSE DIFFER FROM THAT OF GLUCOSE?

Glucose is the universal energy substrate for our organism. It can be transported virtually into every cell of our organism due to the presence of facilitative glucose transporter proteins, called glucose transporters (GLUTs), which facilitate the diffusion of extracellular glucose into the cell according to its concentration gradient. It exists several types of glucose transporters with various kinetic characteristics. As a consequence, glucose uptake varies according to the type of GLUT transporter present at the cell surface of a cell. GLUT1 and GLUT3 are permanently present at the surface of the cell. They have a low K_m for fructose (1–3 mmol/L) and hence they transport glucose at half the maximal rate even when blood glucose is lower than normal (3.9–5.2 mmol/L). Cells expressing GLUT1 and/or GLUT3, such as neurons, glial cells, red blood cells, and placental cells, have a fairly constant cellular glucose uptake, which shows little variations according to the nutritional status or to changes in blood glucose and insulin concentrations. Insulin-sensitive cells such as skeletal muscles or adipose cells express GLUT4 transporters. When insulin is low, GLUT4 transporters are located in the membrane of intracellular vesicles, where they have no access to extracellular glucose and hence are quiescent. After ingestion of a meal, insulin triggers their translocation toward the cell membrane, thus increasing cellular glucose uptake. GLUT2 transporters have a very low affinity for glucose (K_m of about 12–20 mmol/L); due to this low affinity, glucose uptake of GLUT2-expressing cells will vary mainly according to extracellular glucose concentration. GLUT2 transporters are expressing cells involved with glucose-sensing, such as pancreatic A and B cells, liver cells, and some hypothalamic cells [11].

Once inside the cells, glucose is rapidly converted into glucose-6-phosphate by hexokinases, then to fructose-1,6-diphosphate by the enzyme phosphofructokinase. Fructose-1,6-diphosphate is further degraded along the glycolytic pathway, generating pyruvate which will mainly be further degraded into acetyl-CoA and be degraded to CO_2 and H_2O in the tricarboxylic acid cycle, fueling the mitochondrial synthesis of adenosine triphosphate (ATP). Inhibition of phosphofructokinase by increased cellular ATP and citrate concentration ensures that glygolytic degradation of glucose does not exceed cellular energy needs.

Glucose can be used as an energy substrate in all tissues and organs of the human body, since all cells of the organism express at least one type of GLUT protein, one type of hexokinase, and phosphofructokinase. In brain cells, due to the presence of GLUT1 and GLUT3, glucose uptake and oxidation is nearly continuous and produces a continuous supply of ATP. Brain cells use glucose almost exclusively as a metabolic substrate in physiological condition and do not synthesize the enzymes required for lipid oxidation. Most other cells in the organism synthesize the enzymes for fatty acid oxidation and will rely on either glucose or fatty acid for energy production according to the nutritional state; in muscle cells, the increase in blood glucose and insulin concentrations which occurs after a meal activates the translocation of GLUT4 to the cell surface, thus increasing glucose transport, and simultaneously activates glycolysis while inhibiting fat oxidation. In liver cells, the postprandial increase in portal blood glucose enhances hepatocytes' glucose uptake; furthermore, hepatocytes express an isoform of hexokinase, glucokinase, which has also a high K_m for glucose, and glucose metabolism is therefore enhanced as the sole consequence of portal hyperglycemia [12]. Phosphofructokinase is, however, inhibited by ATP and citrate in the liver as in muscles and hence glucose metabolism is adjusted to cell energy needs (see Chapter 11).

Although fructose has the same chemical formula as glucose ($C_6H_{12}O_6$) and has the same energy content (enthalpy for degradation = 686 kcal/mol), these two hexoses have a different molecular structure: fructose displays a ketone group on its second carbon, while glucose displays an aldehyde group on its first carbon. Due to its different conformation, fructose is not efficiently transported by GLUT1, GLUT3, or GLUT4, but is transported by a specific fructose transporter, GLUT5, expressed in enterocytes, renal cells, and to a lesser extent in adipocytes, skeletal and heart muscles, and various other cell types [13]. In the liver, fructose is transported by GLUT2, but with a lesser affinity than glucose. As for glucose, hepatic fructose uptake requires that portal blood fructose concentration is substantially increased.

Once inside the hepatocyte, fructose follows a different metabolic pathway than glucose, however. Hepatocytes express three key enzymes specific for fructose metabolism. The first of these enzymes, fructokinase, converts fructose to fructose-1-phosphate; the second, aldolase B, cleaves fructose-1-phosphate into glyceraldehyde and dihydroxyacetone phosphate; the third, triokinase, phosphorylates glyceraldehyde to glyceraldehyde phosphate, which can be secondarily converted into dihydroxyacetone phosphate. Dihydroxyacetone phosphate is a normal glycolytic intermediate which is further catabolized to pyruvate, while glyceraldehyde is further phosphorylated to glyceraldehyde-3-phosphate before joining glycolysis. Fructokinase has a very high affinity for fructose, and both fructokinase and adolase B have high maximal velocity. In addition, these enzymes do not require to be activated by insulin and are not inhibited by ATP or citrate as phosphofructokinase. As a consequence, all the fructose entering the hepatocyte is rapidly converted into glycolytic intermediates irrespective of the energy need of hepatocytes. The degradation of pyruvate in the Krebs cycle is, however, dependent on the amount of adenosine diphosphate to be regenerated to ATP and therefore matches cellular energy expenditure. The trioses-phosphate generated in excess is largely cleared by being either metabolized to lactate or to glucose and these two substrates are released into the hepatic vein to be made available as energy substrate by other cells of the organism. Part of the glucose synthesized from fructose in the hepatocyte can also be used to replenish hepatic glycogen stores. Trioses-phosphate can also be converted into acetyl-CoA to be used for the de novo synthesis of fatty acid. This pathway can be fueled by acetyl-CoA issued from fructose, glucose, or amino acid, but fructose appears to be more lipogenic than other energy substrate, most likely due to the unregulated production of intrahepatic trioses [14].

Fructokinase and aldolase B are expressed in enterocytes, hepatocytes, and renal cells. In hepatocytes, the presence of these enzymes, together with enzymes for gluconeogenesis and de novo lipogenesis, allows for the conversion of fructose to glucose, lactate, and fatty acids, which are substrates which can be readily used by most cells in the body. In enterocytes, their role remains speculative. Glucose is transported from the gut lumen into the enterocytes by means of a sodium glucose cotransporter, SGLT1; glucose transport through this process is driven by the positive sodium gradient between the gut lumen and the inside of the enterocyte, maintained through the constant extrusion of sodium by Na-K ATPase at the basolateral pole of the enterocyte. In contrast, fructose is transported from the gut lumen into the enterocyte through a facilitative fructose carrier, GLUT5; this transport requires higher intraluminal fructose concentration than free fructose concentration within the enterocyte [13]. Fructose metabolism to lactate and glucose may therefore be instrumental for intestinal fructose absorption. The role of fructose-metabolizing enzymes in the kidney remains a puzzle. When fructose is administered intravenously, arterial blood fructose can increase to 2–3 mmol/L, and a substantial amount of fructose is metabolized to glucose and/or lactate metabolism in the kidney [15]. After oral fructose administration, splanchnic fructose uptake is nearly complete, and only a small portion reaches the arterial circulation, causing only a small transient increase in arterial blood fructose in the 0.1–0.5 mmol/L range. Given the low affinity of hexokinases for fructose, it is very unlikely that this triggers any significant fructose metabolism in muscles, adipose tissue, or brain cells, and it is therefore possible that the presence of fructose-metabolizing enzymes in the kidney are responsible for the metabolism of fructose having escaped splanchnic metabolism.

SUGAR-INDUCED METABOLIC ALTERATIONS IN ANIMAL MODELS AND PROPOSED MECHANISMS

Many studies in animal models (see Chapter 12) indicate that animal fed diets containing large amount of fructose (whether as pure fructose or as sucrose or HFCS) lead to increased body fat stores and development of dyslipidemia, ectopic lipid deposition in the liver and skeletal muscles, and insulin resistance and/or diabetes mellitus [6]. These effects could largely be attributed to the fructose component of the diet. In some studies, high-fructose diet also causes high blood pressure [16]. These effects are largely documented in rodents, but have been reported in primates as well [17].

The mechanisms underlying these effects are complex and not yet understood. In most studies, the presence of sugars in drinking solutions or to solid food is associated with an increased energy consumption, which accounts for body weight gain and excess body fat deposition. An increased palatability of sugar-enriched diets and/or disruption of the mechanisms regulating food intake

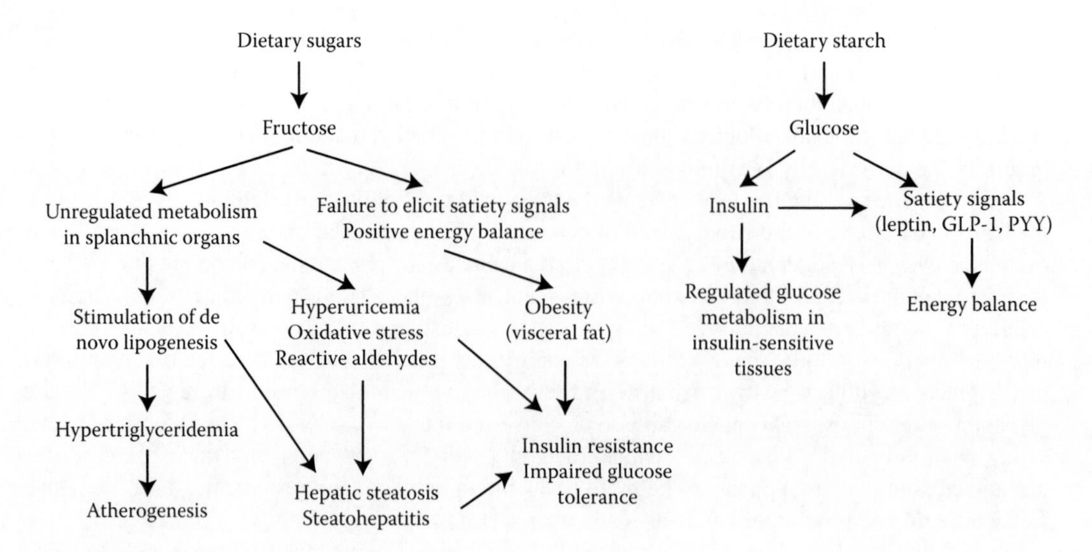

FIGURE 13.1 Major factors identified as possible links between sugars and metabolic disease in animal models.

may therefore be involved. Rats fed a high-fructose diet together with a modest energy restriction, however, still gained body fat mass, suggesting that fructose may specifically enhance body fat accretion [18]. Whatever the mechanisms, changes in body fat mass may be central in sugar-induced metabolic dysfunction.

In addition to metabolic changes secondary to increased body fat, several factors have been proposed to mediate adverse metabolic effects of fructose. Fructose-induced de novo lipogenesis in the liver may lead to hepatic steatosis, increased very-low-density lipoprotein (VLDL)-triglyceride (TG) secretion, ectopic lipid deposition, and insulin resistance secondary to lipotoxicity in the liver and skeletal muscles [19]. Fructose-induced hyperuricemia may cause endothelial dysfunction, which may contribute to increased blood pressure, on the one hand, and play a role in muscle insulin resistance by inhibiting insulin-induced muscle vasodilation [20]. In liver cells, exposure to large amounts of fructose can cause an oxidative stress and trigger endoplasmic reticulum stress responses [21]; its hepatic metabolism can further generate reactive carbohydrate metabolites, such as methylglyoxal, which can secondarily alterate hepatic metabolism [22]; these effects are likely to be limited to the liver, however, since the concentration of fructose observed in the systemic circulation is too low to predict direct extrahepatic effects. Dietary fructose may also trigger hepatic and systemic inflammation by altering gut microbiota, increasing gut permeability, and enhancing the absorption of microbial products such as bacterial lipopolysaccharides into the portal vein [23]. All these proposed mechanisms, summarized in Figure 13.1, are animal-based hypothetical mechanisms which certainly raise concerns regarding the safety of sugar in the human diet. Whether they are indeed operative in humans, and at which level of exposure to sugar, has however not been clearly demonstrated. The following sections will therefore review our present understanding of the effects of dietary sugar in human subjects.

EPIDEMIOLOGICAL DATA LINKING CONSUMPTION OF DIETARY SUGARS AND HUMAN OBESITY

Epidemiological data generally report an association between consumption of sugars and obesity as reviewed in more detail in Chapters 16 and 17. Cross-sectional studies show strong associations between consumption of sucrose, fructose, or sugar-sweetened beverages and body weight [24]. Prospective studies indicate that sugar consumption is associated with weight gain over time, but also point to effects of other nutritional factors, such as energy dense foods, or low consumption of whole grains, fruits, and vegetables [25]. These data are generally consistent with the hypothesis that dietary sugars can be involved in body weight gain, but cannot reliably assess a causal roe of sugars in this process.

There has been recently some confusion regarding the mechanisms involved in the development of obesity, and the concept of obesity as an excess energy intake in regard to energy expenditure has been challenged [26]. During the development of obesity, however, body mass and body fat stores increase, and the total amount of energy stored within the body therefore increases. In other words, somebody who would gain 20 kg body fat over any time lapse will have increased body energy content by 160,000 kcal. The pathogenesis of obesity therefore implies a positive energy balance, which may be secondary to either decreased energy expenditure or increased food intake, or both together.

EFFECTS OF SUGARS ON ENERGY EXPENDITURE

Given the fact that the build-up of body fat results in an imbalance between energy expenditure and energy intake, it may be hypothesized that sugars, and more specifically fructose, may cause obesity by decreasing energy expenditure. There is presently no evidence for such a mechanism. Several studies have documented that acute ingestion of fructose elicits a larger thermic effect than isocaloric glucose. This is mainly accounted for by a lower energy efficiency of fructose compared to glucose, due to energy loss when fructose is converted into glucose or fat in splanchnic tissues. One study reported that long-term fructose decreased basal metabolic rate (but not postprandial energy expenditure) [27], but most other studies observed no significant changes in resting or postprandial energy expenditure [28].

EFFECTS OF SUGARS ON ENERGY INTAKE

In the absence of patent alterations in energy expenditure, the development of obesity has to be accounted for by an energy intake exceeding energy requirements. The effects of dietary sugars on satiety and on brain centers involved in food intake control are reviewed in more detail in Chapters 14 and 15, and we will only mention briefly some relevant aspects here.

The hypothesis that sugars, more than any other dietary nutrients, specifically cause obesity by increasing energy intake implies that sugars disrupt the complex homeostatic mechanism regulating food intake and body weight. This indirectly implies that, when sugars are consumed before or added to a mixed meal, the amount of energy consumed from other nutrients in the meal is not adequately reduced, and the total energy consumed is increased. This may be due to protein, complex carbohydrate, and fat eliciting satiety signals to match food intake to the energy requirements, but sugar failing to elicit such signals. Studies having assessed the effects of sucrose or fructose on spontaneous food intake in humans have failed to clearly document that sugars present in solid foods or in beverages are actually not adequately compensated by a reduction of energy intake from other nutrients [29]. Experimental evaluation of food intake in human subjects is technically difficult and has many sources of errors, however. In addition, there is evidence that body weight control is achieved by matching energy intake to energy expenditure over periods of several days rather than at each meal.

The mechanisms regulating food intake are multiple, highly complex, and yet not fully understood. In fasting conditions, low blood glucose and insulin, and a high secretion of ghrelin from gastric endocrine cells, all contribute to stimulate food intake. In contrast, after ingestion of a meal, high blood glucose, amino acids, lactate, and insulin all exert direct effects on hypothalamic and brain stem centers to reduce food intake. In addition, gut peptides such as GLP1 and PYY contribute to inhibit food intake. On top of these acute metabolic signals providing information on minute-to minute nutrients availability, blood leptin concentration provides information on the level of adipose tissue stores: when adipose stores are low, hypoleptinemia further stimulates food intake, while at the opposite, excess body fat mass causes hyperleptinemia, which should suppress food intake [30]. The latter mechanisms appears, however, little efficient, since most obese subjects maintain excessive body fat stores in spite of hyperleptinemia.

It has been reported that fructose ingestion fails to stimulate several of the above-mentioned satiety factors. In healthy or overweight subjects, ingestion of a test meal together with a drink sweetened with pure glucose elicited significant postprandial increases in blood glucose, insulin, GLP1, and leptin concentrations, together with a suppression in ghrelin concentration. All these responses were significantly blunted when the same meal was ingested together with a fructose drink. When meals were ingested with sucrose, glucose:fructose mixtures, or HFCS-sweetened drinks, glucose, insulin, and leptin responses were higher, and ghrelin concentrations were intermediate between those observed with pure fructose or glucose [31,32]. In addition, it was observed, using brain imaging in healthy humans, that consumption of fructose compared with glucose resulted in a distinct pattern of regional cerebral blood flow consistent with fructose-containing sugar being less satiating than glucose [33]. This may, however, be related to lower insulin concentrations after fructose ingestion.

ROLE OF SUGARS IN THE DEVELOPMENT OF DYSLIPIDEMIA

It has been recognized for several decades that diets containing sucrose or fructose can increase blood triglyceride concentration and lower HDL-cholesterol concentrations, as reviewed in more detail in Chapter 19. The increase in blood triglyceride is essentially accounted for by an increase in VLDL triglycerides [34]. Furthermore, dietary fructose is associated with the production of small, dense LDL particles, which may be secondary to an increased modeling of VLDL-TG by cholesteryl-esther transfer protein and hepatic lipase [35]. All these alterations of blood lipid have been associated with an enhanced atherogenic risk.

Interestingly, consumption of a high-fructose diet is associated with two distinct alterations of blood lipoprotein metabolism. On the one hand, consuming a high-fructose diet is associated with increased fasting VLDL-triglyceride and apoB concentrations, which are mainly secondary to an enhanced VLDL secretion by the liver. A marked stimulation of hepatic de novo lipogenesis is observed shortly after starting on a high-fructose diet and may contribute to stimulate hepatic VLDL secretion [36,37]. On the other hand, there is an increased postprandial blood triglyceride response after ingestion of mixed meal together with added fructose or sucrose than after ingestion of the same meal with equivalent amounts of glucose [32]. This postprandial VLDL-TG response involves both a stimulation of hepatic VLDL secretion and a decreased extrahepatic VLDL-TG clearance; the latter may be explained by adipose lipoprotein lipase being stimulated by hyperinsulinemia when meals are consumed with glucose, but less so when they are consumed with fructose [38].

The amount of daily fructose needed to enhance blood triglyceride concentrations is still debated. Based on meta-analyses having assessed the data of a large number of small-scale fructose studies, it was concluded that fasting blood triglyceride concentrations were increased with 100 g fructose consumed every day, whereas postprandial concentrations were already increased with 50 g fructose/day [39]. Given that the average daily sugar consumption in the USA is about 100 g/day, corresponding to 50 g fructose/day, these effects may be relevant for half the population. The absolute increase in blood triglyceride observed with very large doses of fructose as part of short-term hypercaloric feeding is relatively small, however (about 50% increase for fasting blood triglyceride [40], and about 50–130% for postprandial triglyceride), and its real impact on atherogenesis remains to be established [32].

EFFECTS OF DIETARY SUGARS ON GLUCOSE HOMEOSTASIS

Ingestion of pure fructose is associated with a much lower blood glucose and insulin response than ingestion of an isocaloric amount of glucose. This is observed not only in healthy, lean subjects, but also in obese subjects and patients with type 2 diabetes. As a consequence of this lower glycemic response, 24-h blood glucose profile and glycated hemoglobin concentration decreased when sucrose is partially replaced with fructose in the diet of type 2 diabetic subjects [41].

In spite of this improved blood glucose profile, insulin resistance may develop upon exposure to high amounts of sugar in the diet, mainly related to fructose impairing insulin's actions. This rests mainly on the observations that animals on a high-fructose diet are prone to develop insulin resistance and diabetes mellitus [6].

The effects of fructose on insulin sensitivity in humans are, however, more contrasted. When insulin sensitivity was directly measured with the euglycemic-hyperinsulinemic clamp method, i.v. fructose administration did not decrease whole body insulin-mediated glucose disposal, indicating that it did not impair extrahepatic glucose transport [42]. Fructose, however, increased hepatic glucose production, most likely due to intrahepatic fructose conversion into glucose and release of the newly formed glucose into the systemic circulation [43]. This was unexpected because gluconeogenesis and hepatic glucose output are normally inhibited by insulin. It suggests that the high availability of trioses-phosphate as gluconeogenesis precursors overcame insulin inhibition, resulting in some degree of hepatic insulin resistance [44].

Although a single administration of fructose did not cause extrahepatic insulin resistance, it has been hypothesized that fructose consumption over several days to several weeks may impair insulin's actions in skeletal muscles. One putative mechanism was that fructose-induced hypertriglyceridemia would secondarily increase fat deposition in skeletal muscle fibers and cause muscle lipotoxicity. This was, however, not observed. Several studies measured the effects of a high-fructose diet on insulin sensitivity with hyperinsulinemic-euglycemic clamps in healthy subjects. Although the amount of fructose in the diet was quite large in some of these studies, there was no decrease in whole body insulin-mediated glucose disposal [42,43,45,46]. There was also no, or only, minimal accumulation of fat in skeletal muscles. In contrast, several studies observed a mild impairment of hepatic insulin sensitivity, without any substantial increase in fasting glucose concentrations, however [43,46].

It has also been proposed that fructose may adversely affect insulin's actions in subjects with preexisting insulin resistance. Although one study observed that a 6-day high-fructose diet decreased insulin sensitivity in nondiabetic offsprings of patients with type 2 diabetes [47], another similar study failed to observe any such fructose-induced insulin resistance [45]. Furthermore, substituting fructose for sucrose in patients with type 2 diabetes mellitus did not alter insulin resistance [48].

Collectively, studies which have directly measured insulin sensitivity generally observed some impairment of hepatic insulin sensitivity, but no extrahepatic insulin resistance in response to a high-fructose diet. These observations were obtained in small groups of subjects, however, and generally involved hypercaloric feeding with very large amounts of pure fructose; similar studies using more physiological high-sucrose diet are unfortunately not available. It also remains possible that insulin resistance may require much longer exposure to dietary fructose and/or be dependent on fructose-induced alterations of body composition.

DE NOVO LIPOGENESIS AND ECTOPIC LIPID DEPOSITION IN LIVER CELLS AS KEY MECHANISMS LINKING FRUCTOSE AND METABOLIC RISK FACTORS

Nonalcoholic fatty liver disease (NAFLD) is a highly prevalent condition among obese subjects. It can evolve from hepatic steatosis to nonalcoholic steatohepatitis, hepatic fibrosis, and eventually to nonalcoholic cirrhosis. The accumulation of fat in the liver is highly associated with insulin resistance. Intrahepatic fat has even been shown to be a better predictor of insulin resistance than visceral fat volume [49].

Although nonesterified fatty acid make the major contribution to intrahepatic fat in NAFLD [50], fatty acids synthetized from dietary sugar can also represent up to about 30% of intrahepatic lipids

[51]. Genetic factors appear to be involved as well: at similar excess body fat mass, obese Hispanics have a higher prevalence of NAFLD than Caucasians [52]. A common polymorphism of PNPLA3, a lipase expressed in hepatic and extrahepatic tissues, which may act both as a lipolytic and lipogenic enzyme [53], is associated with increased hepatic fat content [54]. In mice, overexpression of PNPLA3 increases de novo lipogenesis and deposition of newly formed lipids in the liver [55]. In a multi-ethnic US adolescent population, dietary sugar intake is associated with intrahepatic fat only in subjects expressing the PNPLA3 variant [56]. The presence of the PNPLA3 polymorphism conferring an increase hepatic fat content is not associated with insulin resistance, however. It has been recently reported that the fatty acid composition of intrahepatic fat secondary to obesity differed from that of lipids synthesized by Hyysalo et al. [57], providing a possible explanation for this discrepancy.

There are several reasons to suspect that intake of dietary sugars may play a role in the development of NAFLD. Rodents rapidly develop hepatic steatosis when put on a high-fructose diet [6]. In healthy humans, intrahepatic fat content can be increased two-fold after only a few days on a high-fructose, hypercaloric diet [58,59].

This increase in hepatic fat content is quantitatively modest, but the effects of longer time fructose administration remain unknown. Animal experiments indicate that fructose produces an oxidative stress on liver cells, which may in the long run trigger the development of hepatic inflammation and fibrosis. In addition, fructose metabolism leads to the intrahepatic synthesis of methyglyoxal, which may also promote tissue fibrosis [22]. Therefore, a high-fructose intake may play a role in the development of hepatic inflammation and in the progression of hepatic steatosis to nonalcoholic steatohepatitis.

URIC ACID AS A MEDIATOR OF FRUCTOSE'S ADVERSE EFFECTS

Hyperuricemia is observed in high-fructose-fed rodents and it is generally attributed to an increase in uric acid production [60]. A high-fructose intake has also been reported to cause hypertension in some rat models [61]. It has further been reported that fructose-induced hyperuricemia may impair endothelium-mediated vasodilation, thus contributing to the development, not only of hypertension, but also of muscle insulin resistance [60]. In humans, however, the role of uric acid as a mediator of fructose's adverse effects has yet received little attention. One study reported that consumption of a fructose-supplemented diet increased both blood pressure and uric acid concentration; in this study, prevention of hyperuricemia by the administration of an uricosuric agent prevented the rise in blood pressure, but not the development of other metabolic disturbances induced by fructose [62].

GENDER DIFFERENCES FOR FRUCTOSE'S METABOLIC EFFECTS

Several observations indicate that the effects of a high-fructose intake vary according to gender. The metabolic consequences of a high-fructose diet are markedly attenuated in females compared to male rats. Oophorectomy, however, abolishes these differences, suggesting that female sex hormones may attenuate fructose's effects [63]. Short-term fructose overfeeding increases fasting plasma triglyceride to a lesser extent in normal weight premenopausal women than in men [64]. A short-term high-fructose diet also fails to decrease hepatic insulin sensitivity in premenopausal women [64]. Furthermore, a high-fructose diet, when administered over a 10-week period, increases visceral fat mass and enhances the blood glucose responses to a glucose load only in men [65].

GENERAL CONCLUSIONS AND FUTURE PERSPECTIVES

Starchy foods, yielding directly glucose when digested, represent the largest source of dietary carbohydrates in nature. Many frugivorous animals also feed on fruits and honey containing fructose, glucose, and sucrose in substantial amounts. Although fruit availability is seasonal in most parts of the world, this source of energy has long been appreciated, as attested by the widespread presence of fructose-metabolizing enzymes in vertebrates. Expressing specific enzymes in all cell types for the sole purpose of metabolizing one seasonal substrate was certainly not advantageous; it made more sense to concentrate them in a limited number of organs which would convert fructose into substrates that could be used by all cell types, that is, glucose, lactate, and fatty acids.

Specific enzymes for fructose metabolism are fructokinase, aldolase B, and triokinase; together, they convert fructose into trioses-phosphate, which can be converted into glucose, lactate, or fatty acids. Contrary to glycolytic enzymes, they do not need to be activated by insulin and are not inhibited by intracellular metabolites or ATP and hence metabolize fructose at a very high rate [66]. They are mainly expressed in the gut mucosa, the liver, and the kidney [67]. Interestingly, these are also the only organs in the body which synthesize quantitative amounts of glucose-6-phosphatase, the enzyme enabling to release glucose into the blood. The functional role of fructose-metabolizing enzymes is somewhat different in each of these organs, however. In the gut, fructose is absorbed by the facilitative transporter GLUT5, and this process requires the presence of a concentration gradient between the intestinal lumen and the enterocytes; the main role for fructose-metabolizing enzymes in the gut may therefore be to maintain a low intracellular fructose concentration to facilitate fructose absorption. In the liver, they are responsible for the near-complete extraction of fructose released from the gut and its immediate conversion into trioses-phosphate. Trioses-phosphate are primarily converted into glucose and lactate and released in the blood to serve as energy substrates in extrahepatic cells; one part also ends up to replenish hepatic glycogen; finally, some fructose can be converted into fat which is either stored as intrahepatic fat or secreted with VLDLs [68]. Whatever fructose escapes hepatic uptake is metabolized in the kidney, whereas in the liver, it is converted into lactate and glucose [69].

This two-step metabolism allows for the efficient use of an energy-rich substrate inconstantly present in our diet. It comes, however, with some energetic cost, since the synthesis of glucose and fat are energy-requiring processes, in which, respectively, 5–10 and 30% of the energy content of fructose is lost as heat [70]. Although energetically suboptimal, hepatic de novo fat synthesis is clearly advantageous under special conditions. Black bears take advantage of the high availability of fruits and berries in late summer and fall to build up their body fat stores before hibernating. Humming birds support the high energy cost of their hovering flight by metabolizing the sugar present in the nectar of flowers, while at the same time storing fat required for their migration [71]. For most birds, hepatic fat synthesis is indeed the major pathway for storing body fat.

In humans, switching from a low- to a high-fructose diet comes together with substantial changes regarding how nutrients are distributed within the body. In this context, an increase in glucose production, a rise in blood triglycerides, or a stimulation of hepatic de novo lipogenesis are all normal, adaptive changes, which cannot be considered as early markers of metabolic dysfunction. The fate of fructose carbons depend on key regulatory steps illustrated in Figure 13.2. Intrahepatic conversion of fructose into trioses-phosphate is directly related to the rate of intestinal fructose absorption; synthesis and release of lactate and glucose are likely to be the prime pathways to be activated, since they involve little energy loss; the rate of glucose and lactate release is, however, limited, by glucoregulatory mechanisms for glucose, and by unknown mechanisms, possibly related to lactate transport or pH regulation, for lactate; fructose can also be stored as hepatic glycogen, although in limited amounts. When all these pathways are saturated, trioses-phosphate are converted into lipids, but their release into the blood is limited by the rate of VLDL assembly, and some fat is temporarily stored within liver cells. Knowing these bottlenecks for trioses-phosphate disposal, one may predict how fructose's effects will vary according to prevalent conditions. First, in individuals with a high energy turnover, utilization of fructose-derived glucose and lactate will be enhanced. Second, a high energy turnover will also increase hepatic glycogen breakdown and therefore will allow conversion of more fructose into glycogen at the next meal. Exercise, the major factor increasing energy turnover, plays therefore a key role in preventing fructose conversion into fat [72]. Third, with ingestion of large fructose loads, maximal rates for fructose disposal as lactate and glucose/

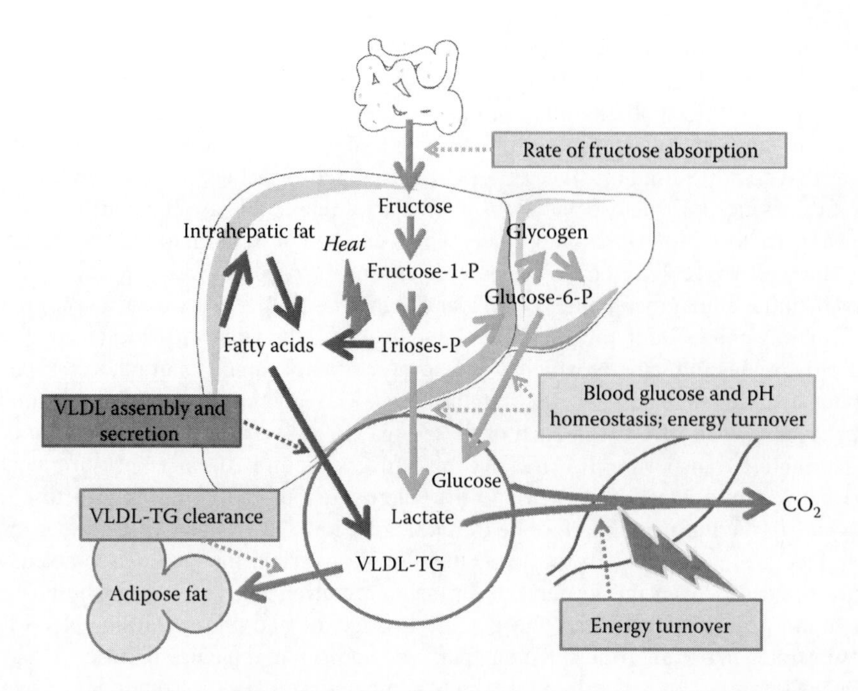

FIGURE 13.2 Key regulatory steps for fructose metabolism and possible links to diseases. Fructose carbons are initially processed in the liver, and end up as blood glucose, lactate and VLDL-TG, hepatic glycogen, and hepatic or adipose fat, before being ultimately oxidized to CO_2 in any cells of the body. Bottlenecks for fructose carbon disposal are: (1) in the liver: glucose and lactate production and VLDL-TG secretion; (2) from the blood: glucose and lactate utilization and VLDL-TG clearance. Increased glucose production, hepatic de novo lipogenesis, and VLDL-TG concentrations are normal adaptive responses to very-high-fructose diet, but inappropriate disposal of intra- or extrahepatic fructose carbon disposal may be at the origin of long-term metabolic dysfunctions.

glycogen and for VLDL secretion are likely to be exceeded, and intrahepatic fat synthesis will increase. Therefore, not only the amount of fructose ingested daily, but also its pattern of intake may determine its metabolic effects. Finally, there may be interindividual variations in trioses-phosphate disposal according to genetic factors, gender, or environmental variables, which may have consequences on body fat distribution or on exposure of the liver to stress. Such mechanisms have been documented in chickens, in which body fat gain in chicken inversely related to the hepatic secretion of lipoproteins [73]. The issues to be addressed in future studies are therefore not whether fructose stimulates de novo lipogenesis or increases intrahepatic fat, but whether these adaptive responses may be abnormal in subjects at risk of developing metabolic or cardiovascular diseases.

ACKNOWLEDGMENTS

The various studies done in Luc Tappy's laboratory have been supported by SNF grants 320030-135782 and 320030-138428 from the Swiss National Foundation for Science.

CONFLICTS OF INTEREST

Kim-Anne Lê is employed by Nestec Ltd, which is a subsidiary of Nestlé Ltd and provides professional assistance, research, and consulting services for food, dietary, dietetic, and pharmaceutical products of interest to Nestlé Ltd. Luc Tappy's research has been mainly supported by grants from the Swiss National Science Foundation and has included research projects funded by Nestlé SA, Vevey, Switzerland, and by Ajinomoto Co., Inc., Japan.

REFERENCES

1. Mintz SN. *Sweetness and Power: The Place of Sugar in Modern History*; 1985. Penguin Books, New York. ISBN 978-0-14-009233-2.
2. Hanover LM, White JS. Manufacturing, composition, and applications of fructose. *Am J Clin Nutr*. 1993;58(5 Suppl):724S–32S.
3. Ludwig DS. The glycemic index: Physiological mechanisms relating to obesity, diabetes, and cardiovascular disease. *JAMA*. 2002;287(18):2414–23.
4. Bantle JP. Clinical aspects of sucrose and fructose metabolism. *Diabetes Care*. 1989;12(1):56–61.
5. Bray GA. Fructose: Pure, white, and deadly? Fructose, by any other name, is a health hazard. *J Diabetes Sci Technol*. 2010;4(4):1003–7.
6. Bizeau ME, Pagliassotti MJ. Hepatic adaptations to sucrose and fructose. *Metabolism*. 2005;54(9):1189–201.
7. Johnson RJ, Segal MS, Sautin Y, Nakagawa T, Feig DI, Kang DH et al. Potential role of sugar (fructose) in the epidemic of hypertension, obesity and the metabolic syndrome, diabetes, kidney disease, and cardiovascular disease. *Am J Clin Nutr*. 2007;86(4):899–906.
8. Basu S, Yoffe P, Hills N, Lustig RH. The relationship of sugar to population-level diabetes prevalence: An econometric analysis of repeated cross-sectional data. *PLoS One*. 2013;8(2):e57873.
9. Goran MI, Ulijaszek SJ, Ventura EE. High fructose corn syrup and diabetes prevalence: A global perspective. *Glob Public Health*. 2013;8(1):55–64.
10. Bray GA, Nielsen SJ, Popkin BM. Consumption of high-fructose corn syrup in beverages may play a role in the epidemic of obesity. *Am J Clin Nutr*. 2004;79(4):537–43.
11. Thorens B, Mueckler M. Glucose transporters in the 21st Century. *Am J Physiol Endocrinol Metab*. 2010;298(2):E141–5.
12. Postic C, Shiota M, Magnuson MA. Cell-specific roles of glucokinase in glucose homeostasis. *Recent Progr Hormone Res*. 2001;56:195–217.
13. Douard V, Ferraris RP. Regulation of the fructose transporter GLUT5 in health and disease. *Am J Physiol Endocrinol Metab*. 2008;295(2):E227–37.
14. Mayes PA. Intermediary metabolism of fructose. *Am J Clin Nutr*. 1993;58(5 Suppl):754S–65S.
15. Ahlborg G, Bjorkman O. Splanchnic and muscle fructose metabolism during and after exercise. *J Appl Physiol*. 1990;69(4):1244–51.
16. Hwang IS, Ho H, Hoffman BB, Reaven GM. Fructose-induced insulin resistance and hypertension in rats. *Hypertension*. 1987;10:512–6.
17. Bremer AA, Stanhope KL, Graham JL, Cummings BP, Wang W, Saville BR et al. Fructose-fed rhesus monkeys: A nonhuman primate model of insulin resistance, metabolic syndrome, and type 2 diabetes. *Clin Transl Sci*. 2011;4(4):243–52.
18. Sanchez-Lozada LG, Mu W, Roncal C, Sautin YY, Abdelmalek M, Reungjui S et al. Comparison of free fructose and glucose to sucrose in the ability to cause fatty liver. *Eur J Nutr*. 2010;49(1):1–9.
19. Stanhope KL, Havel PJ. Fructose consumption: Potential mechanisms for its effects to increase visceral adiposity and induce dyslipidemia and insulin resistance. *Curr Opin Lipidol*. 2008;19(1):16–24.
20. Nakagawa T, Hu H, Zharikov S, Tuttle KR, Short RA, Glushakova O et al. A causal role for uric acid in fructose-induced metabolic syndrome. *Am J Physiol (Renal Physiol)*. 2006;290(3):F625–31.
21. Zhang C, Chen X, Zhu RM, Zhang Y, Yu T, Wang H et al. Endoplasmic reticulum stress is involved in hepatic SREBP-1c activation and lipid accumulation in fructose-fed mice. *Toxicol Lett*. 2012;212(3):229–40.
22. Lee O, Bruce WR, Dong Q, Bruce J, Mehta R, O'Brien PJ. Fructose and carbonyl metabolites as endogenous toxins. *Chem Biol Interact*. 2009;178(1–3):332–9.
23. Bergheim I, Weber S, Vos M, Kramer S, Volynets V, Kaserouni S et al. Antibiotics protect against fructose-induced hepatic lipid accumulation in mice: Role of endotoxin. *J Hepatol*. 2008;48(6):983–92.
24. Malik VS, Popkin BM, Bray GA, Despres JP, Hu FB. Sugar-sweetened beverages, obesity, type 2 diabetes mellitus, and cardiovascular disease risk. *Circulation*. 2010;121(11):1356–64.
25. Mozaffarian D, Hao T, Rimm EB, Willett WC, Hu FB. Changes in diet and lifestyle and long-term weight gain in women and men. *New Engl J Med*. 2011;364(25):2392–404.
26. Taubes G. Treat obesity as physiology, not physics. *Nature*. 2012;492(7428):155.
27. Cox CL, Stanhope KL, Schwarz JM, Graham JL, Hatcher B, Griffen SC et al. Consumption of fructose-sweetened beverages for 10 weeks reduces net fat oxidation and energy expenditure in overweight/obese men and women. *Eur J Clin Nutr*. 2012;66(2):201–8.
28. Tappy L, Egli L, Lecoultre V, Schneider P. Effects of fructose-containing caloric sweeteners on resting energy expenditure and energy efficiency: A review of human trials. *Nutr Metab*. 2013;10(1):54.

29. Rodin J. Comparative effects of fructose, aspartame, glucose, and water preloads on calorie and macronutrient intake. *Am J Clin Nutr*. 1990;51(3):428–35.
30. Cummings DE, Overduin J. Gastrointestinal regulation of food intake. *J Clin Invest*. 2007;117(1):13–23.
31. Teff KL, Elliott SS, Tschöp M, Kieffer TJ, Rader D, Heiman M et al. Dietary fructose reduces circulating insulin and leptin, attenuates postprandial suppression of ghrelin, and increases triglycerides in women. *J Clin Endocrinol Metab*. 2004;89:2963–72.
32. Stanhope KL, Griffen SC, Bair BR, Swarbrick MM, Keim NL, Havel PJ. Twenty-four-hour endocrine and metabolic profiles following consumption of high-fructose corn syrup-, sucrose-, fructose-, and glucose-sweetened beverages with meals. *Am J Clin Nutr*. 2008;87(5):1194–203.
33. Page KA, Chan O, Arora J, Belfort-Deaguiar R, Dzuira J, Roehmholdt B et al. Effects of fructose vs glucose on regional cerebral blood flow in brain regions involved with appetite and reward pathways. *JAMA*. 2013;309(1):63–70.
34. Fried SK, Rao SP. Sugars, hypertriglyceridemia, and cardiovascular disease. *Am J Clin Nutr*. 2003;78(4):873S–80S.
35. Gerber PA, Berneis K. Regulation of low-density lipoprotein subfractions by carbohydrates. *Curr Opin Clin Nutr Metab Care*. 2012;15(4):381–5.
36. Theytaz F, Noguchi Y, Egli L, Campos V, Buehler T, Hodson L et al. Effects of supplementation with essential amino acids on intrahepatic lipid concentrations during fructose overfeeding in humans. *Am J Clin Nutr*. 2012;98:1008–16.
37. Egli L, Lecoultre V, Theytaz F, Campos V, Hodson L, Schneiter P et al. Exercise prevents fructose-induced hypertriglyceridemia in healthy young subjects. *Diabetes*. 2013;62(7):2259–65.
38. Chong MF, Fielding BA, Frayn KN. Mechanisms for the acute effect of fructose on postprandial lipemia. *Am J Clin Nutr*. 2007;85(6):1511–20. PubMed PMID: 17556686.
39. Livesey G, Taylor R. Fructose consumption and consequences for glycation, plasma triacylglycerol, and body weight: Meta-analyses and meta-regression models of intervention studies. *Am J Clin Nutr*. 2008;88(5):1419–37.
40. Lecoultre V, Carrel G, Egli L, Binnert C, Boss A, Macmillan EL et al. Coffee consumption attenuates short-term fructose-induced liver insulin resistance in healthy men. *Am J Clin Nutr*. 2014;99(2):268–75.
41. Sievenpiper JL, Vuksan V, Wong EY, Mendelson RA, Bruce-Thompson C. Effect of meal dilution on the postprandial glycemic response: Implications for glycemic testing. *Diabetes Care*. 1998;21(5):711–6.
42. Le KA, Faeh D, Stettler R, Ith M, Kreis R, Vermathen P et al. A 4-wk high-fructose diet alters lipid metabolism without affecting insulin sensitivity or ectopic lipids in healthy humans. *Am J Clin Nutr*. 2006;84(6):1374–9.
43. Faeh D, Minehira K, Schwarz JM, Periasamy R, Park S, Tappy L. Effect of fructose overfeeding and fish oil administration on hepatic de novo lipogenesis and insulin sensitivity in healthy men. *Diabetes*. 2005;54(7):1907–13.
44. Schwarz JM, Acheson KJ, Tappy L, Piolino V, Muller MJ, Felber JP et al. Thermogenesis and fructose metabolism in humans. *Am J Physiol*. 1992;262(5 Pt 1):E591–8.
45. Le KA, Ith M, Kreis R, Faeh D, Bortolotti M, Tran C et al. Fructose overconsumption causes dyslipidemia and ectopic lipid deposition in healthy subjects with and without a family history of type 2 diabetes. *Am J Clin Nutr*. 2009;89(6):1760–5.
46. Aeberli I, Hochuli M, Gerber PA, Sze L, Murer SB, Tappy L et al. Moderate amounts of fructose consumption impair insulin sensitivity in healthy young men: A randomized controlled trial. *Diabetes Care*. 2013;36(1):150–6.
47. Hokayem M, Blond E, Vidal H, Lambert K, Meugnier E, Feillet-Coudray C et al. Grape polyphenols prevent fructose-induced oxidative stress and insulin resistance in first-degree relatives of type 2 diabetic patients. *Diabetes Care*. 2013;36(6):1454–61. PubMed PMID: 23275372. Pubmed Central PMCID: 3661802. Epub 2013/01/01.eng.
48. Thorburn AW, Crapo PA, Griver K, Wallace P, Henry RR. Long-term effects of dietary fructose on carbohydrate metabolism in non-insulin-dependent diabetes mellitus. *Metabolism*. 1990;39(1):58–63.
49. Fabbrini E, Magkos F, Mohammed BS, Pietka T, Abumrad NA, Patterson BW et al. Intrahepatic fat, not visceral fat, is linked with metabolic complications of obesity. *Proc Natl Acad Sci USA*. 2009;106(36):15430–5.
50. Fabbrini E, Mohammed BS, Magkos F, Korenblat KM, Patterson BW, Klein S. Alterations in adipose tissue and hepatic lipid kinetics in obese men and women with nonalcoholic fatty liver disease. *Gastroenterology*. 2008;134(2):424–31.
51. Ouyang X, Cirillo P, Sautin Y, McCall S, Bruchette JL, Diehl AM et al. Fructose consumption as a risk factor for non-alcoholic fatty liver disease. *J Hepatol*. 2008;48(6):993–9.

52. Kim JS, Le KA, Mahurkar S, Davis JN, Goran MI. Influence of elevated liver fat on circulating adipocytokines and insulin resistance in obese Hispanic adolescents. *Pediatric Obesity*. 2012;7(2):158–64.
53. Kumashiro N, Yoshimura T, Cantley JL, Majumdar SK, Guebre-Egziabher F, Kursawe R et al. The role of patatin-like phospholipase domain-containing 3 on lipid-induced hepatic steatosis and insulin resistance in rats. *Hepatology*. 2013;57(5):1763–72. Epub 2012/11/24.Eng.
54. Romeo S, Kozlitina J, Xing C, Pertsemlidis A, Cox D, Pennacchio LA et al. Genetic variation in PNPLA3 confers susceptibility to nonalcoholic fatty liver disease. *Nature Genet*. 2008;40(12):1461–5.
55. Li JZ, Huang Y, Karaman R, Ivanova PT, Brown HA, Roddy T et al. Chronic overexpression of PNPLA3I148M in mouse liver causes hepatic steatosis. *J Clin Invest*. 2012;122:4130–44.
56. Goran MI, Walker R, Le KA, Mahurkar S, Vikman S, Davis JN et al. Effects of PNPLA3 on liver fat and metabolic profile in Hispanic children and adolescents. *Diabetes*. 2010;59(12):3127–30.
57. Hyysalo J, Gopalacharyulu P, Bian H, Hyotylainen T, Leivonen M, Jaser N et al. Circulating triacylglycerol signatures in nonalcoholic fatty liver disease associated with the I148M variant in PNPLA3 and with obesity. *Diabetes*. 2014;63(1):312–22.
58. Le KA, Ith M, Kreis R, Faeh D, Bortolotti M, Tran C et al. Fructose overconsumption causes dyslipidemia and ectopic lipid deposition in healthy subjects with and without a family history of type 2 diabetes. *Am J Clin Nutr*. 2009;89(6):1760–5.
59. Tappy L, Le KA. Does fructose consumption contribute to non-alcoholic fatty liver disease? *Clin Res Hepatol Gastroenterol*. 2012;36:554–60.
60. Johnson RJ, Segal MS, Sautin Y, Nakagawa T, Feig DI, Kang DH et al. Potential role of sugar (fructose) in the epidemic of hypertension, obesity and the metabolic syndrome, diabetes, kidney disease, and cardiovascular disease. *Am J Clin Nutr*. 2007;86(4):899–906.
61. Reaven GM, Ho H, Hoffman BB. Effects of a fructose-enriched diet on plasma insulin and triglyceride concentration in SHR and WKY rats. *Horm Metab Res*. 1990;22:363–5.
62. Perez-Pozo SE, Schold J, Nakagawa T, Sanchez-Lozada LG, Johnson RJ, Lillo JL. Excessive fructose intake induces the features of metabolic syndrome in healthy adult men: Role of uric acid in the hypertensive response. *Int J Obesity*. 2010;34(3):454–61.
63. Galipeau D, Verma S, McNeill JH. Female rats are protected against fructose-induced changes in metabolism and blood pressure. *Am J Physiol Heart Circulatory Physiol*. 2002;283(6):H2478–84.
64. Couchepin C, Le KA, Bortolotti M, da Encarnacao JA, Oboni JB, Tran C et al. Markedly blunted metabolic effects of fructose in healthy young female subjects compared with male subjects. *Diabetes Care*. 2008;31(6):1254–6.
65. Stanhope KL, Schwarz JM, Keim NL, Griffen SC, Bremer AA, Graham JL et al. Consuming fructose-sweetened, not glucose-sweetened, beverages increases visceral adiposity and lipids and decreases insulin sensitivity in overweight/obese humans. *J Clin Invest*. 2009;119(5):1322–34.
66. Mayes PA. Intermediary metabolism of fructose. *Am J Clin Nutr*. 1993;58(5 Suppl):754S–65S.
67. Shmueli O, Horn-Saban S, Chalifa-Caspi V, Shmoish M, Ophir R, Benjamin-Rodrig H et al. GeneNote: Whole genome expression profiles in normal human tissues. *Comptes Rendus Biologies*. 2003;326(10–11):1067–72.
68. Tappy L, Le KA. Metabolic effects of fructose and the worldwide increase in obesity. *Physiol Rev*. 2010;90(1):23–46.
69. Bjorkman O, Felig P. Role of the kidney in the metabolism of fructose in 60-hour fasted humans. *Diabetes*. 1982;31(6 Pt 1):516–20.
70. Acheson KJ, Schutz Y, Bessard T, Ravussin E, Jequier E, Flatt JP. Nutritional influences on lipogenesis and thermogenesis after a carbohydrate meal. *Am J Physiol*. 1984;246(1 Pt 1):E62–70.
71. Suarez RK, Herrera ML, Welch KC, Jr. The sugar oxidation cascade: Aerial refueling in hummingbirds and nectar bats. *J Exp Biol*. 2011;214:172–8.
72. Egli L, Lecoultre V, Theytaz F, Campos V, Hodson L, Schneiter P et al. Exercise prevents fructose-induced hypertriglyceridemia in healthy young subjects. *Diabetes*. 2013; 62:2259–65.
73. Hermier D. Lipoprotein metabolism and fattening in poultry. *J Nutr*. 1997;127(5 Suppl):805S–8S.

14 Satiating Effects of Fructose and Glucose

Yada Treesukosol and Timothy H. Moran

CONTENTS

KEY POINTS

- Fructose and glucose share taste signaling pathways, yet differ in a number of other significant ways.
- On a molar basis, compared to glucose, fructose appears sweeter and less effective at altering feeding-related gut peptides. Fructose and glucose have opposite effects on AMP-activated protein kinase, a central energy sensor, and differential effects on activation of feeding-related cortical areas.
- In long-term tests, intake of fructose is less than that of glucose.
- Overall, preload experiments comparing the relative effects of glucose and fructose on subsequent food intake find no differences or greater suppression on intake in response to a fructose preload.

INTRODUCTION

Fructose, like glucose, is a monosaccharide, and together they make up the disaccharide sucrose. However, glucose and fructose do differ in a number of important ways. These saccharides appear to share taste-signaling pathways but on a molar basis elicit different intensities. Does this in turn lead to differences in relative intake? What are the consequences of long-term exposure to these compounds? How do these saccharides contribute to potentially differential effects on satiety and metabolism? How do glucose and fructose affect appetite-associated neural signals? In this chapter, we will review the literature in the context of these questions.

TASTE TRANSDUCTION OF GLUCOSE AND FRUCTOSE

Recent discoveries in rodents have contributed to evidence supporting the necessity of the T1R2 and T1R3 proteins (encoded by the genes *Tas1r2* and *Tas1r3*, respectively) in the mediation of "sweet" taste. Based on intracellular calcium imaging responses in HEK-293-derived cells transfected with rat, mouse, or human T1R2 and T1R3, it has been shown that the subunits combine to form a heterodimer broadly tuned to bind with a range of compounds that humans describe as sweet and for which rodents show a preference [1–3]. These stimuli include glucose and fructose [2] although there is evidence that fructose elicits a more robust effect than glucose [1]. Consistent with this view, there is a high degree of co-expression of T1R3 with T1R2 (or T1R1) in taste receptor cells [1,4–6]. Electrophysiological recordings from the chorda tympani (CT) nerve, which innervates the anterior tongue, and the glossopharyngeal (GL) nerve, which innervates the posterior tongue, show that T1R2 KO and T1R3 KO mice have markedly reduced responses to natural sugars including glucose and fructose compared with WT mice, but display weak residual responses, particularly at higher concentrations [7–10].

Electrophysiological measures in rats have shown that both 0.5 M fructose and 0.5 M glucose evoke responses in the greater superficial petrosal (GSP; a branch of the facial nerve that innervates taste receptor fields of the soft palate) and the CT nerve. Consistent with findings from calcium imaging in transfected cells, controlling for relative concentration, fructose elicits a larger response than glucose [11] for both the tonic and phasic components of response [12]. Both stimuli elicit larger responses in the GSP compared to the CT.

Similarly, central electrophysiological recordings reveal that sweeteners including fructose and glucose elicit similar neural responses across S-neurons in hamster parabrachial neurons (second-order relay in the rodent gustatory pathway) [13]. Although both fructose and glucose elicit responses in the rat nucleus of the solitary tract (NST; the first central relay for ascending gustatory information), fructose has relatively higher effectiveness than glucose [14]. In regards to neural profiles, sucrose appears to elicit a response closer to that of fructose than to glucose in the NST [15] and in ventroposteromedial nucleus of the thalamus [16] in rats. Thus, while the transduction of signaling elicited by glucose and fructose is similar, fructose is a relatively more effective stimulus.

BEHAVIORAL: QUALITATIVE IDENTIFICATION OF FRUCTOSE AND GLUCOSE

Intake measures in rats also suggest that the relative "sweetness" of fructose is higher than that of glucose [17] although in studies that render intensity a less salient cue, this difference is not apparent. Based on data generated from rats and hamsters conditioned to avoid particular compounds, it appears that both glucose and fructose generalize to sucrose [18]. Similarly, measures arranged in a three-dimensional space by two multidimensional scaling procedures in humans show that glucose and fructose tend to fall near each other [19]. Glucose and fructose appear to elicit unitary percepts in both humans [20] and mice [21], with evidence in both studies of discrimination based on intensity.

Relative overall ingestion of glucose and fructose depends on the testing paradigms employed. Examining lick rates in brief-access tests in which satiety influences are minimized has revealed that rats show a small but consistent increased rate of ingestion of fructose relative to glucose across concentrations suggestive of increased fructose palatability or preference [22]. Such a finding is consistent with results from measures of perceived sweetness of the sugars dating back to 1925 [23]. Thus, although fructose and glucose activate the same receptor and signaling pathways and appear to elicit similar sensations, both electrophysiological and behavioral data demonstrate that fructose is sweeter on a molar basis.

CONSEQUENCES OF LONG-TERM SACCHARIDE EXPOSURE

However, longer ingestion tests that compared the overall ingestion of saccharide solutions suggest that while fructose is sweeter, this does not necessarily lead to greater ingestion. In tests in which saccharide solutions were always available, rats consumed more glucose, maltose, and sucrose relative to fructose, suggesting that factors other than relative sweetness or palatability were ultimately controlling intake [24]. Chronic access to saccharide solutions, in general, has been associated with increased food intake and body weight gain in rodent studies and there is the suggestion that access to fructose leads to greater weight gain. For example, a study that compared the effects of chronic access to high concentrations of glucose, sucrose, or fructose demonstrated that while all three saccharides resulted in excess caloric intake, weight gain, and increased fat deposition, rats with fructose access gained the most weight [25]. Jurgens et al. [26] have demonstrated that mice with access to a 15% fructose solution gained significantly more weight and had significantly higher percentages of body fat. Interpretations from this study are complicated by the different concentrations of sucrose and fructose and the absence of a glucose-only condition. Similarly, the interpretation by Bocarsly et al. [27] that 55% high-fructose corn syrup leads to greater weight gain than sucrose in rats with 12-h daily access are complicated by differential results in short- and long-term studies and different concentrations of the saccharides.

GASTROINTESTINAL EFFECTS OF GLUCOSE AND FRUCTOSE

Glucose and fructose are differently absorbed in the gastrointestinal tract, and their ingestion results in very different endocrine and metabolic states. Glucose is mainly absorbed from the duodenum via the sodium-dependent glucose transporter (SGLT-1), whereas fructose is absorbed by a facilitated diffusion via GLUT-5 [28] that is primarily expressed in the duodenum and jejunum. GLUT-2, a low-affinity transporter, plays some role with both fructose and glucose via facilitative diffusion [28]. These differential transport mechanisms and the endocrine and neural responses they trigger may contribute to the different rates of gastric emptying for glucose and fructose [29]. The gastric emptying of glucose solutions is characterized by two phases, an initial rapid rate of emptying affected primarily by the gastric volume and rate of stomach filling [30]. This is followed by a slower linear phase of emptying that is sensitive to the glucose concentration such that emptying is slower with more concentrated solutions, allowing an equivalent rate of glucose delivery from the stomach to the intestine over a wide range of glucose concentrations [31]. The gastric emptying of fructose is more rapid and less linear. Emptying does slow with increasing fructose concentration but the overall rate of delivery of fructose from the stomach to the intestine is more exponential in character and almost twice the rate of glucose [29].

The gastrointestinal presence of glucose and fructose results in differing profiles of hormones that affect food intake. Teff et al. [32] monitored 24-h plasma profiles of a variety of endocrine parameters in response to subjects consuming three meals in which 30% of the total energy intake was in the form of free glucose or free fructose. Consistent with the known effects of glucose and fructose on insulin secretion, the high-glucose meals elevated plasma glucose and insulin significantly more than did the high-fructose diet. The high-glucose meals also resulted in higher levels of the adiposity hormone leptin that signals the availability of nutrient stores. These higher levels were maintained throughout most of the day. The high-glucose meals were also more effective in producing greater postprandial decreases in plasma levels of the gastric orexigenic hormone ghrelin. This overall profile of decreased elevations in the adiposity signals such as insulin and leptin, and smaller postprandial decreases in the orexigenic peptide ghrelin has been suggested to have the potential to result in decreased satiety and increased food intake during long-term fructose consumption. In a longer study in rats, Lindqvist et al. [33] monitored the effects of access to sugar solutions of glucose, fructose, or sucrose. Access to all three saccharides decreased chow intake although less fructose was consumed than glucose or sucrose. Fructose was less effective at elevating serum leptin and resulted in higher levels of serum ghrelin than either glucose or sucrose. Thus, even though the lower fructose consumption may have contributed to the diminished effects on leptin and ghrelin levels, the findings are similar to those from the study of Teff et al. [32]—lower levels of adiposity signals and relatively higher levels of the feeding stimulatory hormone ghrelin.

The ability of glucose and fructose to differentially affect the secretion of the lower gut hormones glucagon like peptide 1 (GLP-1) and peptide YY (PYY) has also been investigated. These peptides are secreted from intestinal L-cells that are found mainly in the distal intestine. Both peptides, when exogenously administered, decrease food intake and slow gastric emptying. In the Lindqvist et al. [33] study reported above, both sucrose and glucose consumption resulted in increased levels of serum PYY following consumption for 24 h, whereas fructose did not. In a study examining the ability of gastric loads of a range of sweeteners to affect fullness and gut hormone levels, Steinert et al. [34] demonstrated that although both glucose and fructose loads resulted in increased ratings of satiety and fullness, glucose resulted in significantly greater plasma levels of the satiety hormones GLP-1 and PYY. Gastric glucose also resulted in a greater decrease in plasma ghrelin than did gastric fructose. Some interpretational caution is necessary here as the glucose and fructose loads were not equivalent but were equated based on ratings of sweetness resulting in twice as much glucose in the gastric load as there was for fructose.

In a study that compared the effects of equal amounts of glucose and fructose consumed as a beverage on appetite hormones, Bowen et al. [35] found no differences in the ability of the glucose and fructose drinks to elevate the plasma levels of GLP-1 or of the duodenal satiety hormone cholecystokinin in obese subjects. In this study, the total loads of glucose and fructose were relatively small (50 g) and it may be the case that higher levels of ingestion are necessary to identify differences in gut hormone levels. Using a larger load (75 g) of fructose and glucose given orally to normal weight subjects, Kong et al. [36] found that fructose was less effective at elevating plasma GLP-1.

One study has examined the effects of intraduodenal fructose and glucose on plasma GLP-1 levels [37]. The intraduodenal route of administration gets around differential nutrient delivery that would occur as the solutions emptied from the stomach. In this case, no differences were found in the ability of slow infusions (2 mL) of 25% glucose and fructose to elevate plasma GLP-1, suggesting that differences in studies using oral or gastric administration may depend upon differences in gastric emptying rate.

A few studies have looked at potential differences between the effects of sucrose and high-fructose corn syrup on satiety hormones. Yet, no significant differences have been detected [38,39].

EFFECTS OF GLUCOSE AND FRUCTOSE ON NEURAL SIGNALS AFFECTING APPETITE

Lindqvist et al. [33] have also investigated whether glucose and fructose access results in differential effects on hypothalamic peptides and receptors involved in feeding control. Similar effects on the expression of the orexigenic peptide NPY and the anorexigenic prepropeptide POMC were found. Fructose did have a differential effect of increasing the hypothalamic expression of the type 1 cannabinoid receptor, a finding that could be interpreted as reflecting increased reward signaling. Fructose has also been shown to affect hypothalamic signing differently than does glucose. Central glucose suppresses food intake mediated by the hypothalamic AMP-kinase/malonyl-CoA signaling system. Unlike glucose, centrally administered fructose activates AMP-activated protein kinase (AMPK) and fails to increase malonyl-CoA resulting in increases in food intake [40]. Similarly, central GLP-1 signaling depends upon the suppression of AMPK activation and the presence of fructose impairs this suppression [41]. Although these latter effects have only been demonstrated in response to central fructose administration, such actions have been proposed as ways that dietary fructose may negatively impact overall energy balance. Preliminary evidence for differential central effects of glucose and fructose have been provided in a neuroimaging study by Purnell et al. [42], demonstrating that intravenous fructose reduces activity in cortical areas involved in feeding control, while similar glucose infusions do not.

RESPONSES TO FRUCTOSE AND GLUCOSE PRELOADS

Short-term effects of glucose and fructose on subsequent ingestion have been evaluated in a variety of testing situations. The results have been mixed with some data suggesting differences, while others have found similar satiating potential for the two saccharides. The differences may relate to differences in the testing protocol or experimental subjects.

The different rates of gastric emptying between glucose and fructose and the resulting differences in gastric distention were used as a test for the relevance of potential pre-absorptive and absorptive events in the production of satiety [29]. Nonhuman primates received gastric preloads of glucose or fructose immediately before daily 4-h access to food, and the effects on cumulative food intake were monitored. In this case, the overall effects of glucose and fructose on total food intake did not differ. However, the dynamics of feeding through the 4-h period differed markedly. Despite a more rapid delivery from the stomach to the intestine, fructose was less effective at suppressing food intake at early time points, suggesting the possibility that fructose was less satiating than glucose. However, this period of more rapid ingestion was followed by a period in which ingestion rate was significantly reduced relative to that following the glucose preloads, resulting in almost identical feeding suppression across the days in total intake and suggesting that monitoring intake at different intervals could lead to different conclusions.

Differential time courses of the effects of fructose and glucose preloads on subsequent intake have also been found in rodent studies. Warwick and Weingarten [43] examined the effects of glucose and fructose preloads administered at various intervals prior to a scheduled meal. In their hands, glucose and fructose preloads resulted in equivalent suppression on intake when the interval between the preload and the meal was relatively short but fructose had a greater suppressive effect than glucose, as the intervals between the preload and meal were extended. The authors interpreted these data as suggesting that responses to glucose and fructose preloads were differentially affected by test condition and the state of the animal but that there was no overall tendency for one saccharide to be more or less satiating than the other.

Comparisons of the ability of fructose and glucose preloads to reduce test meal intake have also been studied in human subjects. Rodin and her colleagues [44–46] carried out a series of experiments comparing the satiating effects of fructose and glucose preloads. Small (50 g) preloads of fructose and glucose had a differential effect on buffet test meal intake when administered either 35 min or 2 h prior to lunch. In these experiments, fructose reduced intake by 500 kcal more than glucose did, suggesting an overall greater appetite suppressive effect for fructose and an effect that was significantly beyond the energy content of the preload.

Follow-up studies demonstrated a similar greater suppressive effect of fructose preloads on lean and obese subjects and the authors suggested a role for plasma insulin in the differential effects—glucose loads elevated plasma glucose and insulin levels, while the fructose preload did not [46]. Importantly, the differences in test meal intake were lost when the fructose and glucose preloads were given as a part of a mixed breakfast meal rather than as single nutrient preloads [44].

Guss et al. [47] examined the effects of glucose and fructose solutions on gastric emptying and subsequent food intake in nonobese women. This study involved using two different saccharide amounts (5 and 50 g) and two different intervals between the preloads and the test meals (30 and 135 min). As in the nonhuman primate studies, fructose emptied from the stomach more rapidly than glucose as determined by the disappearance of a radioactive tracer from the stomach. At the 30-min delay, the higher concentrations of both sugars significantly reduced intake relative to the more dilute solutions. At the 135-min interval, only the fructose preload resulted in a significant suppression of food intake. These data again suggest differential timing of satiating influences of the two sugars.

These results are not consistent with those of Rodin in which the timing of the preload relative to the test meal did not seem to matter. Guss et al. [47] have suggested that a remaining difference between the paradigms was the physiological state of the subjects at the time of the preload. In the

Rodin experiments, subjects were food-deprived from the evening before, while in the Guss experiments, subjects consumed a standard breakfast. Such state effects would be consistent with the rodent findings of Warwick and Weingarten.

The addition of glucose or fructose to a cereal preload produced a trend for differential timing of effects [48]. Equicaloric cereal preloads containing either fructose or glucose resulted in equivalent effects on intake in a test meal scheduled 30 min following the preload but there was a trend for a greater effect of the fructose on test meal intake 2 h later. Overall, these experiments examining the relative effectiveness of individual loads of fructose and glucose on subsequent food intake either found no differences or greater feeding suppression in response to the fructose preloads.

SATIETY EFFECTS OF SACCHARIDE COMBINATIONS

Work from Anderson and colleagues has produced a different conclusion about the relative satiety effects of glucose and fructose [39,49]. They examined the relative effects of oral preloads of differing glucose:fructose combinations on subsequent food intake. In these experiments, 1 kcal/mL liquid preloads containing varying mixtures of glucose and fructose were consumed 80 min prior to a test meal. Glucose:fructose concentrations ranged from 80% glucose:20% fructose to 20% glucose:80% fructose. Overall, the higher the relative glucose concentration, the greater the feeding suppression.

CONCLUSIONS

Examination of the physiological consequences of fructose and glucose ingestion and the degree to which they affect neural mechanisms involved in energy balance would lead to the prediction that fructose would be much less satiating than glucose. By multiple measures, fructose is sweeter than glucose and is less effective at altering the release of gut peptides that contribute to feeding control. Fructose ingestion does increase hypothalamic CB1 receptor expression, a result that would be expected to increase food intake since CG1 antagonists reduce food intake. Furthermore, the central effects of local increases in fructose and glucose concentrations have differential effects on AMPK, a central energy sensor. Glucose reduces AMPK activation resulting in decreased food intake, whereas fructose has the opposite effect. Finally, increasing the circulating levels of fructose results in reduced activation of cortical areas involved in feeding control.

However, in tests of long-term access, less fructose is consumed relative to glucose and the majority of the data from preload experiments directly assessing the relative effects of glucose and fructose on subsequent food intake either find no differences or greater suppression in response to fructose. The greater effects with fructose could be secondary to metabolic factors, or, as raised by some investigators, a negative influence on intake due to gastrointestinal malaise from the tendency for concentrated fructose solutions to draw water into the GI tract [39,50,51]. Fructose absorption from the GI tract is improved in the presence of glucose [51] providing a potential explanation for why fructose effects appear to disappear when the glucose:fructose mixtures are used or when fructose is given as part of a mixed meal.

REFERENCES

1. Nelson G, Hoon MA, Chandrashekar J, Zhang Y, Ryba NJP, Zuker CS. Mammalian sweet taste receptors. *Cell*. 2001;106:381–90.
2. Li X, Staszewski L, Xu H, Durick K, Zoller M, Adler E. Human receptors for sweet and umami taste. *Proc Natl Acad Sci USA*. 2002;99(7):4692–6.
3. Xu H, Straszewski L, Tang H, Adler E, Zoller M, Li X. Different functional roles of T1r subunits in the heteromeric taste receptors. *Proc Natl Acad Sci USA*. 2004;101(39):14258–63.
4. Kitagawa M, Kusakabe Y, Miura H, Ninomiya Y, Hino A. Molecular genetic identification of a candidate receptor gene for sweet taste. *Biochem Biophys Res Commun*. 2001;283:236–42.

5. Max M, Shanker YG, Huang L, Rong M, Liu Z, Campagne F et al. Tas1r3, encoding a new candidate taste receptor, is allelic to the sweet responsiveness locus sac. *Nat Genet.* 2001;28(1):58–63.
6. Montmayeur J-P, Liberles SD, Matsunami H, Buck LB. A candidate taste receptor gene near a sweet taste locus. *Nat Neurosci.* 2001;4(5):492–7.
7. Zukerman S, Glendinning JI, Margolskee RF, Sclafani A. T1r3 taste receptor is critical for sucrose but not polycose taste. *Am J Physiol Regul Integr Comp Physiol.* 2009;296(4):R866–76.
8. Damak S, Rong M, Yasumatsu K, Kokrashvili Z, Varadarajan V, Zou S et al. Detection of sweet and umami taste in the absence of taste receptor T1r3. *Science.* 2003;301:850–3.
9. Zhao GQ, Zhang Y, Hoon MA, Chandrashekar J, Erlenbach I, Ryba NJP et al. The receptors for mammalian sweet and umami taste. *Cell.* 2003;115:255–66.
10. Ohkuri T, Yasumatsu K, Horio N, Jyotaki M, Margolskee RF, Ninomiya Y. Multiple sweet receptors and transduction pathways reveal in knockout mice by temperature dependence and gurmarin sensitivity. *Am J Physiol Regul Integr Comp Physiol.* 2009;296(4):R960–71.
11. Nejad MS. The neural activities of the greater superficial petrosal nerve of the rat in response to chemical stimulation of the palate. *Chem Senses.* 1986;11:283–93.
12. Harada S, Yamamoto T, Yamaguchi K, Kasahara Y. Different characteristics of gustatory responses between the greater superficial petrosal and chorda tympani nerves in the rat. *Chem Senses.* 1997;22 (2):133–40.
13. Smith DV, Van Buskirk RL, Travers JB, Bieber SL. Coding of taste stimuli by hamster brain stem neurons. *J Neurophysiol.* 1983;50(2):541–58. Epub 1983/08/01.
14. Travers SP, Norgren R. Coding the sweet taste in the nucleus of the solitary tract: Differential roles for anterior tongue and nasoincisor duct gustatory receptors in the rat. *J Neurophysiol.* 1991;65(6):1372–80.
15. Giza BK, Scott TR, Sclafani A, Antonucci RF. Polysaccharides as taste stimuli: Their effect in the nucleus tractus solitarius of the rat. *Brain Res.* 1991;555(1):1–9.
16. Verhagen JV, Giza BK, Scott TR. Responses to taste stimulation in the ventroposteromedial nucleus of the thalamus in rats. *J Neurophysiol.* 2003;89(1):265–75. Epub 2003/01/11.
17. Cagan RH, Maller O. Taste of sugars: Brief exposure single-stimulus behavioral method. *J Coomp Physiol Psychol.* 1974;87(1):47–55.
18. Nowlis GH, Frank ME, Pfaffman C. Specificity of acquired aversions to taste qualities in hamsters and rats. *J Comp Physiol Psychol.* 1980;94(5):932–42.
19. Schiffman SS, Reilly DA, Clark TBI. Qualitative differences among sweeteners. *Physiol Behav.* 1979;23(1):1–9.
20. Breslin PA, Beauchamp GK, Pugh EN. Monogeusia for fructose, glucose, sucrose, and maltose. *Percept Psychophys.* 1996;58(3):327–41.
21. Dotson CD, Spector AC. Behavioral discrimination between sucrose and other natural sweeteners in mice: Implications for the neural coding of T1r ligands. *J Neurosci.* 2007;27(42):11242–53.
22. Davis JD. The effectiveness of some sugars in stimulating licking behavior in the rat. *Physiol Behav.* 1973;11(1):39–45.
23. Biester A, Wood MW, Wahlin CS. Carbohydrate studies. I. The relative sweetness of pure sugars. *Am J Physiol.* 1925;73:387–95.
24. Richter CP. Six common sugars and tools for the study of appetite for sugar. In: Weiffenbach JM, editor. *Taste and Development: The Genesis of Sweet Preference.* Bethesda, MD: US Department of Health, Education and Welfare; 1977.
25. Kanarek RB, Orthen-Gambill N. Differential effects of sucrose, fructose and glucose on carbohydrate-induced obesity in rats. *J Nutr.* 1982;112(8):1546–54. Epub 1982/08/01.
26. Jurgens H, Haas W, Castaneda TR, Schurmann A, Koebnick C, Dombrowski F et al. Consuming fructose-sweetened beverages increases body adiposity in mice. *Obes Res.* 2005;13(7):1146–56.
27. Bocarsly ME, Powell ES, Avena NM, Hoebel BG. High-fructose corn syrup causes characteristics of obesity in rats: Increased body weight, body fat and triglyceride levels. *Pharmacol Biochem Behav.* 2010;97(1):101–6. Epub 2010/03/12.
28. Drozdowski LA, Thomson AB. Intestinal sugar transport. *World J Gastroenterol.* 2006;12(11):1657–70. Epub 2006/04/06.
29. Moran TH, McHugh PR. Distinctions among three sugars in their effects on gastric emptying and satiety. *Am J Physiol.* 1981;241(1):R25–30. Epub 1981/07/01.
30. Moran TH, Knipp S, Schwartz GJ. Gastric and duodenal features of meals mediate controls of liquid gastric emptying during fill in rhesus monkeys. *Am J Physiol.* 1999;277(5 Pt 2):R1282–90. Epub 1999/11/24.

31. McHugh PR, Moran TH. Calories and gastric emptying: A regulatory capacity with implications for feeding. *Am J Physiol*. 1979;236(5):R254–60. Epub 1979/05/01.
32. Teff KL, Elliot SS, Tschop M, Kieffer TJ, Rader D, Heiman M et al. Dietary fructose reduces circulating insulin and leptin, attenuates postprandial suppresion of ghrelin, and increases triglycerides in women. *J Clin Endocrinol Metab*. 2004;89(6):2963–73.
33. Lindqvist A, Baelemans A, Erlanson-Albertsson C. Effects of sucrose, glucose and fructose on peripheral and central appetite signals. *Regul Pept*. 2008;150(1–3):26–32. Epub 2008/07/17.
34. Steinert RE, Frey F, Topfer A, Drewe J, Beglinger C. Effects of carbohydrate sugars and artificial sweeteners on appetite and the secretion of gastrointestinal satiety peptides. *Br J Nutr*. 2011;105(9):1320–8.
35. Bowen J, Noakes M, Clifton PM. Appetite hormones and energy intake in obese men after consumption of fructose, glucose and whey protein beverages. *Int J Obes (Lond)*. 2007;31(11):1696–703. Epub 2007/06/28.
36. Kong MF, Chapman I, Goble E, Wishart J, Wittert G, Morris H et al. Effects of oral fructose and glucose on plasma Glp-1 and appetite in normal subjects. *Peptides*. 1999;20(5):545–51. Epub 1999/08/28.
37. Rayner CK, Park HS, Wishart JM, Kong M, Doran SM, Horowitz M. Effects of intraduodenal glucose and fructose on antropyloric motility and appetite in healthy humans. *Am J Physiol Regul Integr Comp Physiol*. 2000;278(2):R360–6. Epub 2000/02/09.
38. Melanson KJ, Zukley L, Lowndes J, Nguyen V, Angelopoulos TJ, Rippe JM. Effects of high-fructose corn syrup and sucrose consumption on circulating glucose, insulin, leptin, and ghrelin and on appetite in normal-weight women. *Nutrition*. 2007;23(2):103–12. Epub 2007/01/20.
39. Akhavan T, Anderson GH. Effects of glucose-to-fructose ratios in solutions on subjective satiety, food intake, and satiety hormones in young men. *Am J Clin Nutr*. 2007;86(5):1354–63.
40. Cha SH, Wolfgang M, Tokutake Y, Chohnan S, Lane MD. Differential effects of central fructose and glucose on hypothalamic Malonyl-Coa and food intake. *Proc Natl Acad Sci USA*. 2008;105(44):16871–5. Epub 2008/10/31.
41. Burmeister MA, Ayala J, Drucker DJ, Ayala JE. Central glucagon-like peptide 1 receptor-induced anorexia requires glucose metabolism-mediated suppression of AMPK and is impaired by central fructose. *Am J Physiol Endocrinol Metab*. 2013;304(7):E677–85. Epub 2013/01/24.
42. Purnell JQ, Klopfenstein BA, Stevens AA, Havel PJ, Adams SH, Dunn TN et al. Brain functional magnetic resonance imaging response to glucose and fructose infusions in humans. *Diabetes Obes Metab*. 2011;13(3):229–34. Epub 2011/01/06.
43. Warwick ZS, Weingarten HP. Dynamics of intake suppression after a preload: Role of calories, volume, and macronutrients. *Am J Physiol*. 1994;266(4 Pt 2):R1314–8.
44. Rodin J. Comparative effects of fructose, aspartame, glucose, and water preloads on calorie and macronutrient intake. *Am J Clin Nutr*. 1990;51(3):428–35.
45. Spitzer L, Rodin J. Effects of fructose and glucose preloads on subsequent food intake. *Appetite*. 1987;8(2):135–45. Epub 1987/04/01.
46. Rodin J, Reed DR, Jamner L. Metabolic effects of fructose and glucose: Implications for food intake. *Am J Clin Nutr*. 1988;47(4):683–9.
47. Guss JL, Kissileff HR, Pi-Sunyer FX. Effects of glucose and fructose solutions on food intake and gastric emptying in nonobese women. *Am J Physiol*. 1994;267(6 Pt 2):R1537–44.
48. Stewart SL, Black RM, Wolever TMS, Anderson GH. The relationship between the glycaemic response to breakfast cereals and subjective appetite and food intake. *Nutr Res*. 1997;17(8):1249–60.
49. Anderson GH, Catherine NLA, Woodend DM, Wolever TMS. Inverse association between the effect of carbohydrates on blood glucose and subsequent short-term food intake in young men. *Am J Clin Nutr*. 2002;76(5):1023–30.
50. Henry RR, Crapo PA, Thorburn AW. Current issues in fructose metabolism. *Annu Rev Nutr*. 1991;11:21–39.
51. Rumessen JJ, Gudmand-Hoyer E. Absorption capacity of fructose in healthy adults: Comparison with sucrose and its constituent monosaccharides. *Gut*. 1986;27(10):1161–8.

15 Sugars in the Brain

Jonathan Q. Purnell

CONTENTS

KEY POINTS

- Glucose is the major fuel source for the brain and energetic interactions between the neurons, and glia sustain synaptic function. These metabolic pathways serve as the basis for advanced imaging methodologies.
- Changes in blood glucose levels can be sensed by specialized neurons in the hypothalamus and brainstem, resulting in counter-regulatory responses during hypoglycemia and appetitive behaviors that govern body weight.
- Transducing changes of blood glucose levels into behavioral and metabolic outcomes occur through action of neuronal glucokinase, K_{ATP} channel closure, and AMP-kinase activity, as well as systems that do not directly rely on glucose metabolism.
- Fructose delivered directly to key brain centers has been shown to be alternatively metabolized and to elicit contrasting effects on food intake (increased) than glucose (decreased), thus providing a biological basis for epidemiological and ad libitum interventional studies linking high intakes of dietary fructose and weight gain in the population.

INTRODUCTION

Glucose plays one of its most important roles in the body as the primary source of fuel for the brain. However, glucose serves several other important roles in the brain as well. Metabolites of glucose become substrates for neurotransmitter production and alternative energy sources. Also, glucose can be "sensed" by the brain, triggering or inhibiting specialized neurons responding to changes in blood glucose levels and, in turn, affecting peripheral regulation of glucose levels, feeding behavior, and energy expenditure. Sugars other than glucose can also be metabolized and sensed by the brain.

As will be discussed later in this chapter, the common dietary additive, fructose, undergoes both alternative metabolism and is sensed differently from glucose by neural tissue, resulting in divergent behavioral consequences.

SUGARS AND BRAIN ENERGETICS

Brain neurons generate signals that are transmitted across both complex regional networks and over long distances, such as from the brain to the spinal cord and beyond. Glial cells act as supportive tissue for the neurons, provide insulation for axons, and play a key role in maintaining functional neuronal coupling. Unlike other organs such as the liver and muscle, which are metabolically flexible in their ability to switch between carbohydrates and fat for energy, the brain relies almost exclusively on a constant supply of glucose to meet its cellular energy needs, increasing blood flow when enhanced neuronal firing demands more oxygen and glucose. In now classic and often quoted studies of brain blood flow and glucose uptake by Kety and Schmidt [1] and Sokoloff [2,3], it has been estimated that although the human brain represents only 2% of body mass, it accounts for 20% of total body oxygen consumption and 25% of total body glucose utilization (for excellent reviews, see References 4 and 5). How much glucose is utilized is directly proportional to early development [6], brain size and activity [7,8], and is inversely proportional to age [9].

Blood Levels and Transport of Simple Sugars into the Brain

In the absence of disease, when not absorbing glucose from dietary carbohydrates, blood glucose levels are maintained at nearly constant levels through the day between roughly 4.0 and 6.7 mmol/L by regulatory hormones (insulin, glucagon, catecholamine, cortisol, and growth hormone) that adjust endogenous glucose production by the liver and kidney. In order to enter the brain, circulating glucose must pass through a specialized endothelium, known as the blood–brain barrier, designed to limit diffusion of large molecules and allow passage of small (such as O_2, CO_2) and hydrophobic molecules. This is accomplished by specialized transporters known collectively as glucose transporters (GLUTs) [10]. GLUT-1 resides on the lumenal and ablumenal surfaces of the brain capillaries and through a passively facilitated process, transports glucose into the brain extracellular fluid space. GLUT-1 are saturable and, although there is some evidence that basal insulin has some stimulatory role in whole-brain glucose uptake [11], above basal levels glucose uptake via GLUT-1 is thought to be largely insulin-independent [12,13]. Using magnetic resonance spectroscopy and continuous glucose infusion, it has been demonstrated in humans that there is a linear relationship between blood glucose levels ranging from 4 to 30 mmol/L and corresponding brain glucose levels and that the maximum transport capacity through the blood–brain barrier is nearly twofold higher than maximal brain glucose utilization [14] (Figure 15.1). This and other studies [15,16] demonstrate that brain extracellular glucose levels are in the range of 20–30% of blood glucose levels across the physiological range.

Other monosaccharides found in the diet include mannose, a C-2 epimer of glucose, galactose, and fructose. Mannose occurs naturally in small amounts in fruits, but most of the mannose in humans is thought to be derived endogenously from glucose and is ultimately used in formation of glycoproteins [17]. Mannose that does make it into circulation is transported readily into the brain in a similar manner to glucose [18] and can be used alternatively to glucose as a brain energy substrate by being metabolized to fructose-6-phosphate with subsequent entry into the tricarboxylic acid cycle [19,20]. Galactose is commonly found in fruits and dairy products combined with glucose to form the disaccharide lactose. Following absorption, galactose is readily converted into glucose by the liver [21], but in contrast to glucose and mannose, galactose is poorly transported across the blood–brain barrier [18] and is not thought to contribute to neural energetics. Fructose is inherently sweeter than other sugars and is found commonly in fruits, some vegetables (e.g., sugar beets), and plants (e.g., sugarcane). Because the sweet taste of this monosaccharide enhances food

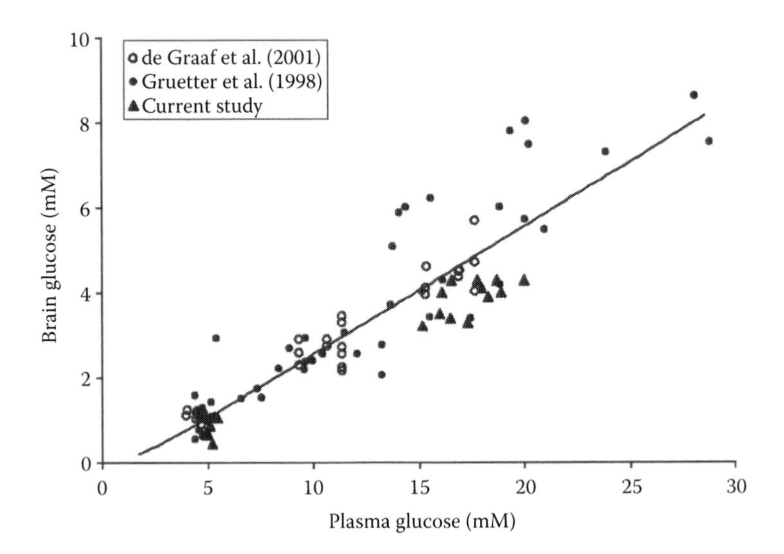

FIGURE 15.1 Steady-state brain versus plasma glucose concentrations in humans. (Adapted from Shestov AA et al. *Am J Physiol Endocrinol Metab.* 2011;301(5):E1040–9. Epub 2011/07/28.)

desirability, fructose is commonly added to processed foods and sweetened beverages, both alone and combined with glucose to form the disaccharide sucrose. After ingestion, fructose is readily and nearly completely taken up by the liver and metabolized to lactate [22]. However, some fructose does pass into the circulation. Within an hour of ingestion of a sugar-sweetened beverage, baseline fructose levels of near zero increase to reach up to 300 μmol/L [23]. From the bloodstream, fructose can be transported into the brain [24,25] by GLUT-5 receptors, which have been detected in endothelial cells of human brain microvasculature [26] and in glial cells of humans [27] and rodents [10,25,28]. Ultimately, fructose in the brain can also be metabolized to glyceraldehyde-3-phosphate or lactate and enter into the tricarboxylic acid cycle to serve as an energy substrate alternative to glucose [20].

Despite the possibility of utilizing both mannose and fructose as alternative fuels, during prolonged glucoprivation, ketone bodies produced by the liver are the primary fuel source the body uses to maintain normal brain function [29].

Fate of Sugars in the Brain: The Neurovascular Unit and the BOLD Response in Neuroimaging

Neuronal bodies communicate with one another via dendritic and axonal extensions. Astrocytes, one of the most abundant of are glial cells, are positioned anatomically between the capillaries traversing the brain and neurons, connecting the vascular endothelium by way of their specialized "endfeet" [30], on the one hand, and with neuronal dendritic and axonal projections, including synaptic junctions, by filamentous projections [31], on the other hand (Figure 15.2). The endothelium, astrocytes, and neurons comprise what can be energetically referred to as a neurovascular unit.

Maintaining normal brain function requires a constant supply of energy, which rises and falls with states of mental alertness and activity. Neuronal activation triggers cerebral arteriolar vasodilation through direct production and release of nitrous oxide and indirectly by stimulating astrocyte production of prostaglandins and epoxyeicosatienoic acids [32] (Figure 15.3). Increased blood flow enhances delivery of both glucose and oxygen to the activated brain region. Glucose leaves the circulation and enters the brain's extracellular space by GLUT-1 transportation across the blood–brain barrier and subsequently is taken up into neuronal cells by facilitated transport via

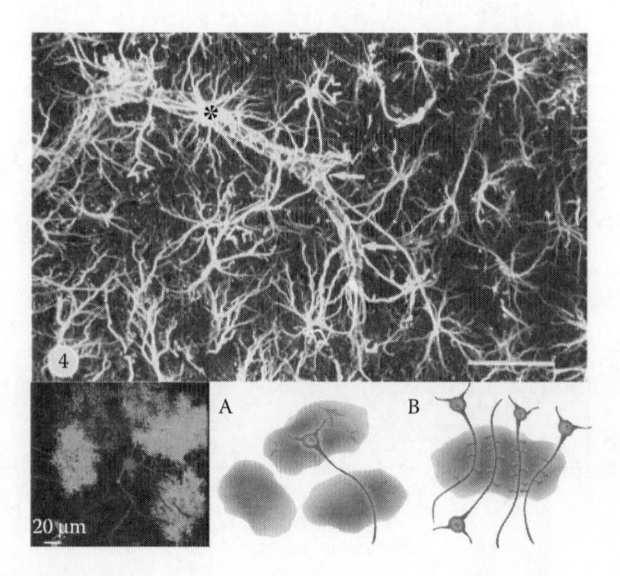

FIGURE 15.2 (See color insert.) Top: Coronal sections of a brain showing the features of the astrocyte–cerebral capillary relationships. The asterisk indicates an astrocyte close to the capillary, outlined arrows indicate one astrocyte contacting several vascular sites via multiple feet, and solid arrow indicates a single site receiving feet from several astrocytes. Scale bar: 50 µm. (Taken from Kacem K et al. *Glia*. 1998;23(1):1–10. Epub 1998/04/30). Bottom: Leftmost figure shows regions of EGFP expression corresponding to one (green) astrocyte. Part A shows schematic figure of three astrocytes. The holes are filled with neurons, one of which is shown to have its processes extending out to other astrocytes pointing to the potential of different neuronal compartments being modulated by different astrocytes. Part B shows schematic of functional synaptic islands: a group of dendrites from several neurons are enwrapped by a single astrocyte. Synapses localized within the territory of this astrocyte have the potential to be modulated in a coordinated manner by gliotransmitter(s) released from this glial cell. (Taken from Halassa MM et al. *J Neurosci*. 2007;27(24):6473–7. Epub 2007/06/15.)

GLUT-3 [10]. In some neurons containing insulin receptors, glucose can be actively taken up by insulin-sensitive GLUT-4 transporters [10]. Glucose that is taken up by the neuron undergoes glycolysis, entry into the tricarboxylic acid cycle, and in the presence of oxygen, oxidative phosphorylation for adenosine triphosphate (ATP) production. This energy production allows for restoration of the sodium and potassium gradients and membrane resting potential following depolarization [4]. Glucose is simultaneously taken up by astrocytes via GLUT-1 and -2 transporters [10] where it has two fates (Figure 15.3). When neurons are at rest, small amounts of glucose can be stored as glycogen (brain glycogen is reported to be located exclusively in astrocytes) [33]. On the other hand, when neuronal energy demand increases, glucose broken down from stored glycogen or directly taken up by the astrocyte from the circulating pool undergoes glycolysis to form lactate [4]. Energy generated during this glycolytic process is used to maintain the NA^+/K^+-ATPase pump of fibrillar astrocytic processes responsible for taking up glutamate released transynaptically from adjacent excitatory neurons, as well as converting this glutamate to glutamine, which is then shuttled back to neurons to be converted back into glutamate for use during the next activation episode (glutamine–glutamate shuttle) (Figure 15.3) [4]. Lactate generated in the astrocyte during glycolysis is shuttled to the neighboring neuron to be converted back into pyruvate and enter into oxidative phosphorylation for ATP production (astrocyte–neuron lactate shuttle) (Figure 15.3). In this model of neuronal energetics, astrocytic glycolysis is an important immediate source of ATP that maintains synaptic readiness following neuronal activation, much of which comes immediately from cellular glycogen stores [4].

Establishing the underlying pathways of this neural-astrocyte coupling helped to explain an observation noted from early studies of brain energy metabolism that not all neuronal energy

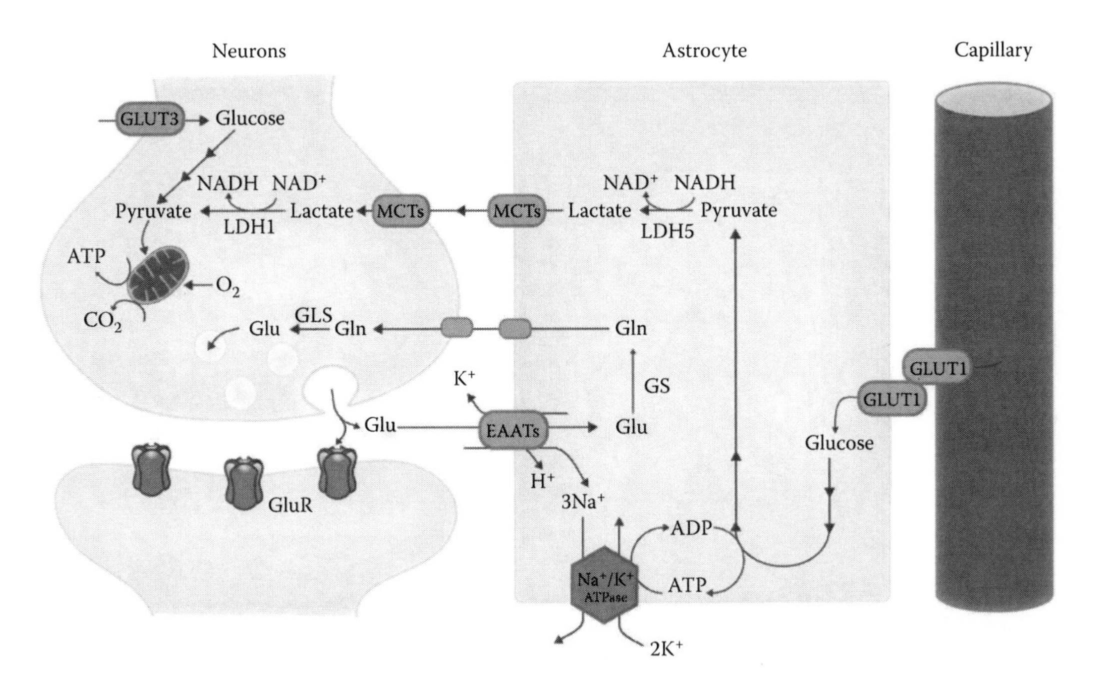

FIGURE 15.3 Schematic representation of the astrocyte–neuron lactate shuttle (ANLS). Glutamate (Glu) released at the synapse activates glutamatergic receptors (GluR) and is associated with important energy expenditures in neuronal compartments. A large proportion of the glutamate released at the synapse is taken up by astrocytes via excitatory amino acid transporters (EAATs, more specifically GLT-1 and GLAST) together with three Na^+ ions. This Na^+ is extruded by the action of the Na^+/K^+ ATPase, consuming ATP. This triggers nonoxidative glucose utilization in astrocytes and glucose uptake from the circulation through the glucose transporter GLUT-1 expressed by both capillary endothelial cells and astrocytes. Glycolytically derived pyruvate is converted into lactate by lactate dehydrogenase 5 (LDH5; mainly expressed in astrocytes) and shuttled to neurons through monocarboxylate transporters (mainly MCT1 and MCT4 in astrocytes and MCT2 in neurons). In neurons, this lactate can be used as an energy substrate following its conversion to pyruvate (Pyr) by LDH1 (mainly expressed in neurons). Neurons can also take up glucose via the neuronal glucose transporter 3 (GLUT-3). Concomitantly, astrocytes participate in the recycling of synaptic glutamate via the glutamate–glutamine cycle. Following its uptake by astrocytes, glutamate is converted into glutamine (gln) by the action of glutamine synthetase (GS) and shuttled to neurons, where it is converted back into glutamate by glutaminases (GLS). (Taken from Belanger M, Allaman I, Magistretti PJ. *Cell Metab.* 2011;14(6):724–38. Epub 2011/12/14.)

needs were met through oxidative phosphorylation and that the brain relied on excess glycolysis [34]. In addition, this neuronal unit, including regulation of cerebral blood flow, is also the basis for current understanding of the blood oxygen level-dependent signal (BOLD) generated during functional magnetic resonance imaging (fMRI) [35,36]. In short, when performing a mental task, enhanced blood flow delivers both increased glucose and oxygen to the active neurons. Oxygenated and deoxygenated hemoglobin have differing magnetic polarization characteristics when placed in a magnetic field that is detected by the magnetic resonance (MR) machine. When changes in concentrations of oxygenated and deoxygenated hemoglobin occur in the capillaries of activated brain, this "contrast" in magnetic field behavior can be picked up as a change in MR signal. Thus, during neuronal activation, the combination of increased glycolysis and blood flow leading to availability without utilization of oxygen is what accounts for increases in BOLD fMRI signal changes [36] (Figure 15.4). Conversely, when neuronal activity is inhibited, oxidative phosphorylation is reduced but there is proportionally greater reductions in blood flow and glycolysis, leading to a reduction in BOLD signal [36] (Figure 15.4).

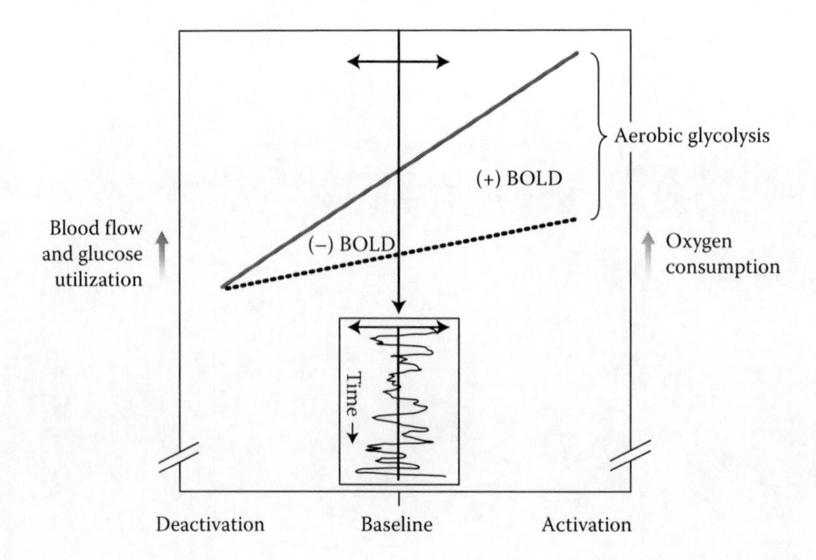

FIGURE 15.4 A schematic representation of the relationship of blood flow and glucose utilization to oxygen consumption and cellular activity (*x*-axis) at baseline and during increases (activation) and decreases (deactivation) in neuronal activity. The presence of aerobic glycolysis causes activity-dependent variations in oxygen availability in the brain that are detectable by fMRI. Activations as seen by fMRI result from a disproportionate increase in blood flow and glucose utilization, whereas deactivations result from the opposite. At baseline, time-varying fluctuations in neuronal activity are seen as spontaneous fluctuations in the fMRI BOLD signal (inset). (Taken from Raichle ME, Mintun MA. *Annu Rev Neurosci.* 2006;29:449–76. Epub 2006/06/17)

SUGARS AND BRAIN SENSING

In addition to (and presumably because of) its importance as an energy substrate, the possibility that blood glucose levels can be detected, or "sensed," by specialized cells in the body has been supported by two lines of evidence. The first is the detection of hypoglycemia (low to very low glucose levels) and activation of a cascade of hormonal and neurological responses that restore blood glucose levels to normal. The second evolved from the theory that food intake and body weight is regulated and involves cellular detection and responses to changes in blood glucose levels within normal, or physiological, ranges.

Of these two lines of evidence supporting glucose sensing, the first involving detection and response to critically low blood glucose levels has been extensively studied in animals and humans. As blood glucose levels fall, characteristic "counter-regulatory" responses occur that initially reduces glucose disposal and then progressively activates systems to enhance glucose appearance so as to restore levels to normal. In healthy subjects, this includes a reduction in insulin secretion as glucose levels in the blood approach 4.4 mmol/L, followed by increases in secretion of epinephrine and glucagon, as well as growth hormone and cortisol as levels approach 3.6 mmol/L. Finally, neurological impairment occurs characteristically at glucose levels below 2.8 mmol/L [37–40]. Specialized glucose-sensing cells that mediate these responses have been described in peripheral organs such as the pancreas [41–43], carotid body [44], portal vein [45–47], and in the brain [48,49].

The second line of evidence linking the brain with glucose sensing arose from observations of hyperphagia and spontaneous obesity in humans with hypothalamic destruction at the turn of the twentieth century (for review, see References 50 and 51). Lesioning studies in animals then demonstrated that destruction of the ventromedial nucleus in the hypothalamus [52–54] led to uncontrolled hunger and food intake. This region was referred to a "satiety" center because the observed unregulated food

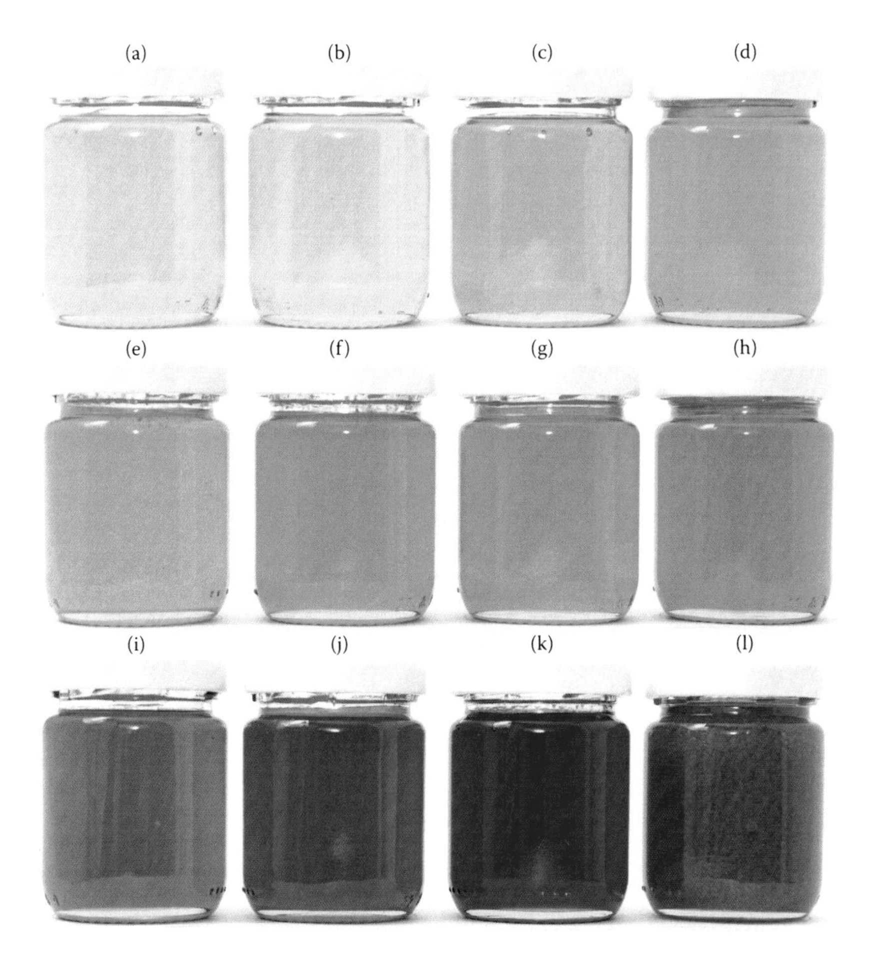

FIGURE 5.1 Colors of unifloral honeys. Examples of unifloral honeys: (a) robinia, (b) citrus, (c) clover, (d) rape, (e) tilia, (f) leatherwood, (g) dandelion, (h) sunflower, (i) chestnut, (j) eucalyptus, (k) honeydew, (l) manuka. The honeys were liquefied (except manuka honey). The color of any type of unifloral honey may vary to a certain extent, especially when a honey crystallizes, for example, a crystallized rape honey is whitish-yellow.

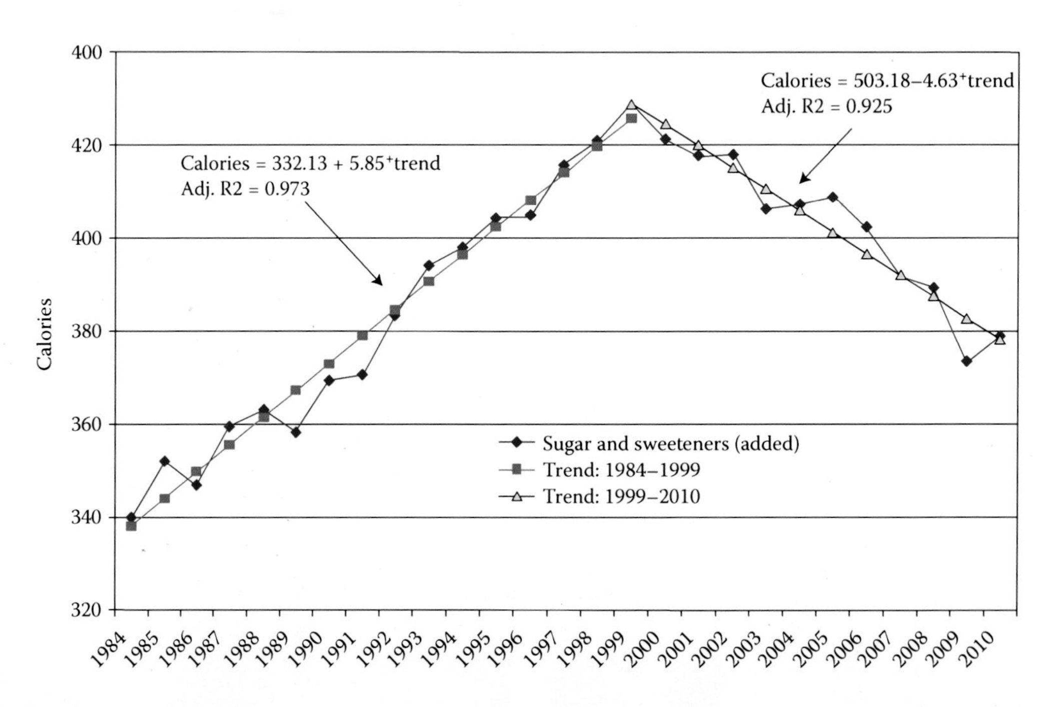

FIGURE 10.1 Average daily per capita calories from added sugar and sweeteners availability, adjusted for spoilage and other waste.

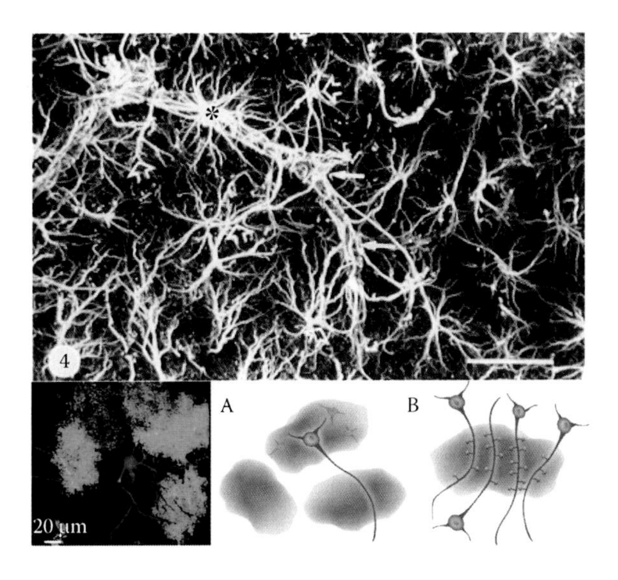

FIGURE 15.2 Top: Coronal sections of a brain showing the features of the astrocyte–cerebral capillary relationships. The asterisk indicates an astrocyte close to the capillary, outlined arrows indicate one astrocyte contacting several vascular sites via multiple feet, and solid arrow indicates a single site receiving feet from several astrocytes. Scale bar: 50 μm. (Taken from Kacem K et al. *Glia*. 1998;23(1):1–10. Epub 1998/04/30.) Bottom: Leftmost figure shows regions of EGFP expression corresponding to one (green) astrocyte. Part A shows schematic figure of three astrocytes. The holes are filled with neurons, one of which is shown to have its processes extending out to other astrocytes pointing to the potential of different neuronal compartments being modulated by different astrocytes. Part B shows schematic of functional synaptic islands: a group of dendrites from several neurons are enwrapped by a single astrocyte. Synapses localized within the territory of this astrocyte have the potential to be modulated in a coordinated manner by gliotransmitter(s) released from this glial cell. (Taken from Halassa MM et al. *J Neurosci*. 2007;27(24):6473–7. Epub 2007/06/15.)

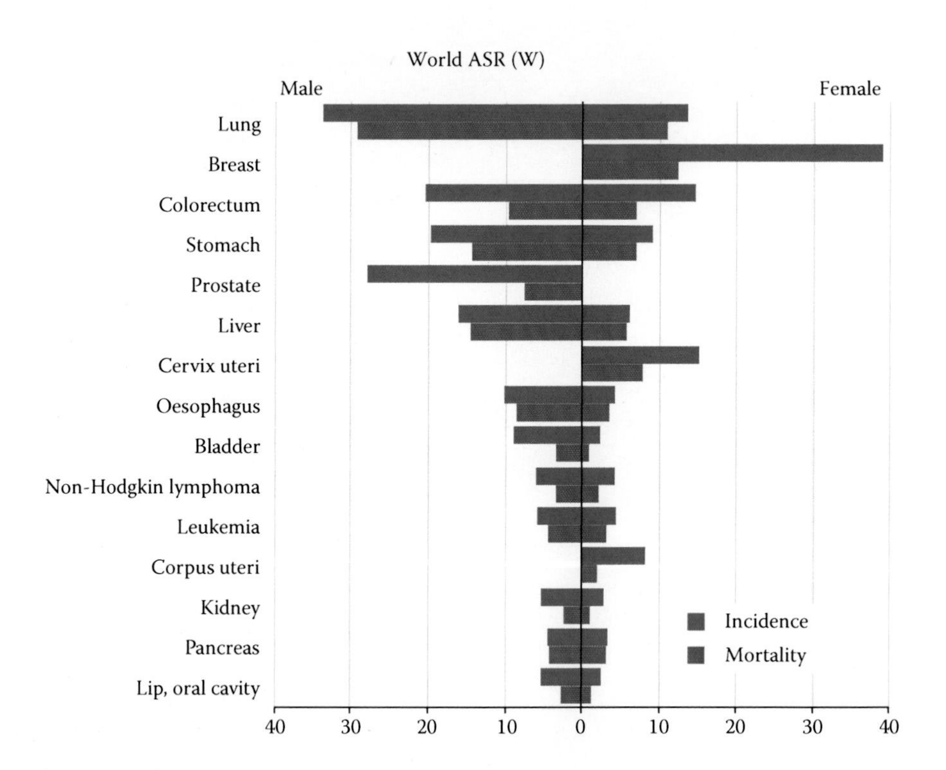

FIGURE 24.1 Risks of cancer worldwide.

intake that ensued was postulated to be due to a failure to experience meal-related satiation. This was confirmed when electrical stimulation from chronically implanted electrodes in this nucleus resulted in suppressed food intake [55]. Conversely, lesioning studies of the lateral hypothalamus resulted in failure to eat and weight loss. This region became referred to as a "feeding" center of the brain, since its destruction resulted in failure to initiate meal intake and death from starvation [53,54]. Again, electrical stimulation from implanted electrodes confirmed the importance of this nucleus by eliciting feeding behaviors [56]. Additional control centers that govern long-term feeding behaviors and body weight have also been localized to the amygdala [57] and the ventral noradrenergic bundle in the brainstem [58], and detailed neuroanatomical studies have shown that there are extensive connections between these regions and the hypothalamus, effectively creating an integrated network governing weight regulation.

Accompanying these discoveries were theories regarding the existence of circulating factors constituting afferent signals in a feedback loop that regulate the activity of these brain centers and govern both meal-to-meal food intake and long-term body weight [59]. One such theory, called the "glucostatic" hypothesis, held that the brain could detect fluctuations of glucose within the physiological range between fasting and postprandial levels, regulating appetite on a meal-to-meal basis [60]. In this model, a postprandial rise in glucose would elicit a satiety response, whereas the drop in glucose utilization or postprandial levels (several hours after a meal) would trigger hunger and food intake [61–63]. The observation that gold thioglucose injected peripherally could result in selective destruction of the ventromedial hypothalamus and expression of obesity in rodents [64] and that this effect was specific for gold attached to a glucose molecule [65] strengthened this hypothesized link between glucose-sensing cells in the brain and appetite control.

Glucose Sensing: Pancreatic β-Cell Model

Before discussing glucose sensing in the brain, however, it is worthwhile reviewing the cellular mechanisms that allow detection of glucose fluctuations by the pancreatic β-cell [43]. With rising glucose levels, such as that occurs following a meal, pancreatic β-cells increase release of insulin. As insulin acts to reduce glucose appearance from the liver and kidney as well as promote uptake and utilization into the liver and adipose tissue, the subsequent fall in glucose levels is paralleled by a reduction in pancreatic β-cell insulin secretion. In order to respond within this narrow range of glucose levels (4.4–7.8 mmol/L), pancreatic β-cells possess high-capacity, low-affinity glucose transporters (GLUT-2) that allow free exchange of glucose inward from the extracellular space. This ensures that intracellular levels continuously reflect changes in blood levels. However, in order to translate fluctuations in glucose levels into a cellular signal (insulin secretion in this case), a "transducing" mechanism is needed. The pancreatic β-cell transducer is made up of a specialized hexokinase, glucokinase (GK), and an inwardly rectifying potassium (K^+) channel that is sensitive to ATP (K_{ATP} channel). Pancreatic GK activity is optimal during fluctuations in glucose that mirror the physiological range in the blood and is not inhibited by its product, glucose-6-phosphate (G-6-P) [43]. With little or no capacity to form glycogen, conversion of glucose to G-6-P commits this molecule to undergo glycolysis and enter the tricarboxylic acid cycle (TCA) and oxidative phosphorylation pathways, generating ATP. The increase in [ATP]/[ADP][Pi] ratio then results in closure of the K_{ATP} channels and depolarization of the cell membrane that promotes an inward flux of calcium and subsequent exocytosis of insulin-laden micelles for release into the circulation. Metabolism of free fatty acids and amino acids that raise β-cell ATP concentrations also couple insulin secretion to increases in blood levels of these nutrients [43]. Since increases and decreases in glucose metabolism and cellular energy level (ATP, ADP, Pi) presumably parallel change in blood glucose levels outside the optimal activity range for GK, it has been postulated that subcellular microdomain sequestration of this transducing apparatus is key to normal β-cell glucose sensing [66]. Such a compartmentalization would be important for neurons, which are nearly exclusively dependent on glucose as an energy source.

Glucose-Sensing Neurons in the Brain

By focusing on the brain regions found to regulate food intake from the lesioning studies and postulated to be sites of "glucostatic" regulation as described above, the existence of specialized neurons that respond to increases and decreases in glucose levels by parallel changes in firing rates was first reported in the ventromedial and lateral nuclei of the hypothalamus in 1964 [67,68]. Further investigations have shown that with a few exceptions [69,70], glucose-sensing neurons are mostly concentrated in these two sites: the brainstem [48,71] and the hypothalamus [72–74]. These sites are anatomically situated in proximity to brain regions that connect directly to sympathetic nervous system outflow tracts, the pituitary (to control secretion of hormone products by gonadotrophic, corticotrophic, and somatrophic neurons), and to feeding centers, making them ideal regions to regulate counter-regulatory hormones during hypoglycemia and to be involved in body weight regulation.

Subsequent studies estimated that ~40% of ventromedial nuclear and ~30% of lateral hypothalamic neurons increase firing rates during increases in glucose levels between 3.6 and 17 mmol/L [75,76] (glucose excitatory, or GE, neurons), whereas ~20–30% of lateral hypothalamic neurons became inhibited when glucose levels rose above 5.6 mmol/L (glucose inhibitory, or GI, neurons) and showed maximal firing rates below this level [75,76]. Increases and decreases in units of 0.2–0.3 mmol/L could affect neuronal firing rates [76], consistent with a "sensing" function. As previously mentioned, however, brain glucose levels in humans range between 20 and 30% of blood glucose levels (Figure 15.1), so that when blood glucose levels are in the normal range between 4.4 and 7.8 mmol/L, brain glucose levels range as low as 0.88–2.5 mmol/L. Using extracellular glucose levels between 0.10 and 10 mmol/L to better reflect physiological levels, approximately 14% of ventromedial nucleus cells were GE (increasing their firing rates when extracellular glucose levels rise from 0.10 to 2.5 mmol/L) [77] and 30–40% were found to be GI (decreasing their firing rates when glucose levels increase from 0.10 to 2.5 mmol/L) [78]. Within the more medial arcuate nucleus of the hypothalamus, these GE and GI neurons cluster near to each other [79].

Mechanisms of Glucose Sensing by Brain Neurons: Energetics

Because neurons rely on a continuous supply of glucose for energy needs and have little or no capacity to store glucose as glycogen, a cellular transducing mechanism that would translate fluctuations in physiological glucose levels, similar to the pancreatic β-cell, was sought [80]. Indeed, the inwardly rectifying K_{ATP} channels (made up of multimeric Kir6.1-6.2 and sulfonylurea receptor, SUR, subunits) responsive to increases in cellular [ATP]/[ADP][Pi] levels [81] and to sulfonylureas [82] were found in GE neurons of the hypothalamic ventromedial nucleus, but the gene expression of these channels was reported to be ubiquitously distributed throughout the brain [83–85] (Figure 15.5). Instead, what was subsequently reported to be uniquely distributed in the hypothalamus and hindbrain where glucose-sensing neurons are primarily located is the pancreatic form of GK [80,86]. Cellular studies confirmed that GK gene expression is found in GE (64%) neurons of the ventromedial nucleus, that these cells respond to changes reflecting physiological levels of brain extracellular glucose levels [77,79,87,88], and that disrupted GK function in ventromedial nuclear cells leads to impaired GE function [86,88] and reduced counter-regulatory responses to hypoglycemia [89].

In terms of the initial "sensing" of extracellular glucose levels, many GI neurons (43%) in the ventromedial hypothalamus, like the GE neurons, express glucokinase [90]. The importance for GK function in GI cells was demonstrated when induced impairment of this enzyme led to near-silencing of these cells [86,88]. However, the analogy of the pancreatic β-cell model where rising glucose levels and subsequent cellular energy content increases membrane depolarization (activation) via K_{ATP} channels does not explain the mechanisms underlying increased neuronal firing by GI neurons during reductions in glucose levels. Under such conditions, a transducer would need to be sensitive to lower cellular energy content. AMP-activated kinase (AMP-K) is a cellular heterotrimeric protein that is allosterically activated by rising [AMP]/[ATP] levels and had been suggested as a nutrient

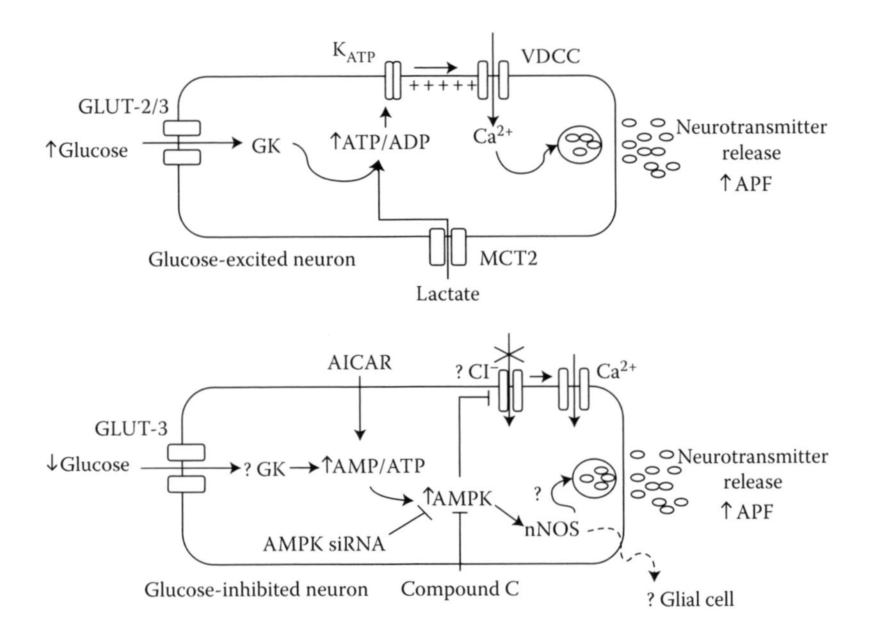

FIGURE 15.5 Top: Hypothetical sensing mechanism of GE neurons. Glucose enters the GE neuron through GLUT-2 or -3 and is phosphorylated by glucokinase (GK), acting as the gatekeeper, and regulating the production of cytosolic ATP in a subcellular compartment. The ATP closes K_{ATP} channels in the plasma membrane, causing depolarization. In turn, this leads to Ca^{2+} influx through VDCCs, stimulating neurotransmitter release and/or increased APF. Lactate, produced locally by astrocytes or arriving systemically, enters the neuron via MCT2 and can then be metabolized to form ATP. Bottom: Hypothetical sensing mechanism of GI neurons. In GI neurons, GK may once again act as the gatekeeper. A falling glucose results in an increase in the AMP: ATP ratio, an effect that can be mimicked pharmacologically by AICAR. AMP-K, once activated, stimulates the formation of NOS, which may diffuse out to adjacent neurons or glial cells. In addition, AMP-K may act on chloride channels leading to neuronal depolarization and neurotransmitter release and/or increased APF. This action of AMP-K can be blocked pharmacologically by compound C. (Taken from McCrimmon R. *Diabet Med.* 2008;25(5):513–22.)

sensor sensitive to periods of low energy states, such as starvation and hypoxia [91]. Cellular studies confirmed that AMP-K is present in the brain and hypothalamus [92,93] and that glucose effects on GI neurons in the ventromedial hypothalamus are mediated by AMP-K activity [78,94,95] (Figure 15.5). During hypoglycemia, therefore, it is thought that when ATP levels fall and AMP levels rise in GI neurons, AMP-K becomes activated [78,96]. Increased AMP-K, in turn, generates nitrous oxide [78,97], closes the cystic fibrosis transmembrane regulator (CFTR), and depolarizes the cell [98]. This proposed mechanism is consistent with studies that show hypothalamic AMP-K to be an important regulator nutrient-induced hepatic glucose production [99,100] and, through central activation, plays a key role in hepatic glucose counter-regulation during hypoglycemia [101].

Other Glucose-Sensing Mechanisms

A sizable number of GE and GI cells do not express glucokinase, a key first step in the transduction of blood glucose levels into a change in neuronal activation [102]. Several studies have also demonstrated glucose-induced changes in hypothalamic neuronal activity that are independent of glucose metabolism of intracellular [ATP] [103,104]. Alternative cellular mechanisms for sensing and responding with changes in neuronal firing that do not rely on changing cellular energetics have been proposed [103]. In cellular studies in which neuronal [ATP] content is kept constant [103] or in which lactate is used as an alternative to glucose [87], evidence is found for neuronal activation by an ATP-independent closure of the K_{ATP} channels. Although the mechanism(s) for this effect have not been determined, one study has identified that a nonmetabolizable substrate (α-methylgluopyranoside) for the sodium-glucose transporter (SGLT) can mimic the effect of high glucose levels on GE cells in the hypothalamus. SGLT has previously been shown to be a candidate glucose sensor in a cell line that secretes glucagon-like peptide 1 (GLP-1) [105] and, when inhibited, impairs activation of GE neurons [80].

Glucose Excitatory and Inhibited Neurons: Roles in Body Weight Regulation

Since the 1950s, the "glucostatic" hypothesis that meal-to-meal appetite is regulated by fluctuations in blood glucose levels has given way to a more complicated model that integrates both satiety signals (meal-to-meal, including nutrient signals and gut hormones) and circulating factors reflecting body fat stores [106]. This latter concept was embodied in the "lipostatic" hypothesis of Kennedy [107], which postulated the existence of a signal factor secreted by fat tissue into the blood that directly bound to receptors in these key brain centers to govern weight long-term, anticipating the discovery of leptin [108] and its receptor [109] in the early 1990s.

Following those reports, leptin was found to regulate distinct neuronal populations within the hypothalamus and brainstem in the control of food intake and body weight [59,110]. In the arcuate nucleus of the hypothalamus, leptin-regulating neurons containing neuropeptide-Y (NPY) and agouti-related peptide (AgRP) were found to stimulate food intake and reduce energy expenditure, while neurons containing pro-opiomelanocortin (POMC) inhibited these processes [59,110]. In keeping with its role as a "feeding" center, distinct populations of neurons within the lateral hypothalamus expressing the peptides orexin [111] and melanin-concentrating hormone (MCH) [112] were found that increase food intake and affect wakefulness. Each of these sites contain leptin receptors [113] as well as extensive projections to and from other hypothalamic nuclei (paraventricular nucleus), dopaminergic "reward" pathways [114], and executive function sites [59,115]. Functionally, as leptin levels fall (such as during periods of starvation and weight loss), POMC neuron activity is reduced and activities of NPY and orexin cells increase, leading to increased food intake [59]. With restoration of body weight, leptin levels rise, reducing activity in NPY and orexin neurons and stimulating POMC neurons to return food intake and body weight to baseline.

There is also extensive overlap between leptin-responsive cells governing food intake and body weight and glucose-sensing cell populations in the hypothalamus. For example, subpopulations of GI neurons in the hypothalamus have been shown to express neuropeptide-Y [95,96,116,117]. On the other hand, subpopulations of hypothalamic GE and GI neurons express POMC [94,117–119]. Glucose sensing has also been described in neurons containing MCH [120,121] and orexin [121–123]. Given that NPY [124] and orexin [111] stimulate food intake and the responsiveness of these cells to changes in glucose levels [96,116,122], it has been suggested that this pathway may mediate, in part, glucoprivic feeding.

From these studies, it is evident that neurons in these key hypothalamic centers that regulate body weight in response to leptin also sense and respond to glucose. In addition, both glucose-sensing and POMC/NPY/orexin cells reside independent of one another in these same sites. Although from the studies cited above, evidence can be found in animal models supporting roles for glucose-sensing neurons in counter-regulatory hormonal and feeding responses to low glucose levels [125], given the interconnectedness and shared signaling systems between glucose-sensing cells and those responding to leptin and insulin, it has been difficult to determine the relative roles that glucose and leptin sensing in these neurons play in regulating short- and long-term body weight [126]. In support of glucose sensing playing a key role in body weight regulation are studies that show impaired glucose sensing in animal models of obesity [77,119,127–129].

A confounding factor in determining the role of glucose on appetitive behaviors in animals and humans is the fact that when glucose is consumed under normal conditions, insulin secretion is also triggered. This is important because many of the same neuronal populations that respond to leptin also contain insulin receptors and insulin has been shown to have similar effects on food intake and body weight (including a shared signaling system) as leptin [130–132]. Human studies have shown that insulin delivered intranasally so as to allow rapid penetration into CSF near the hypothalamus [133] without alterations in peripheral insulin or glucose levels results in reduced appetite and weight loss in men [134]. This is consistent with reports of an inverse association between postprandial insulin secretion in response to one meal and a reduction in subsequent food intake with the next [135]. It is notable that insulin-stimulated [ATP] levels in the brains of the study subjects correlated with reductions in food intake [136]. This is consistent with reports of expression of the insulin-dependent GLUT-4 transporter in glucose-sensing neurons of the ventromedial nucleus [90,137] and of insulin's ability to activate K_{ATP} channels in hypothalamic neurons in rodents [138]. Another confounding factor to consider is that glucose is seldom consumed by itself during a meal and that "sensing" mechanisms in hypothalamic neurons have been described for both lipids and amino acids that have been postulated to mediate changes in food intake and body weight by affecting the ratios of [ATP] to [ADP] and [AMP] in a similar manner to glucose [139–142], and, in fact, are likely exerting effects in the same cells [143,144].

One approach to selectively study the effects of glucose on hypothalamic centers without these confounders is to administer glucose directly to these hypothalamic centers by an intracerebroventricular (ICV) injection. When this was performed in rodents, ICV glucose increased hypothalamic [ATP], reduced AMP-K phosphorylation, reduced NPY/AgRP gene expression, and reduced food intake [145]. This is in contrast to the effects of a similar ICV injection of fructose. Fructose given ICV to rodents increases food intake [145,146] and has the opposite effects of ICV glucose on hypothalamic neurons: it reduces [ATP], increases AMP-K phosphorylation, and reduces POMC expression [145]. Subsequent studies have confirmed that compared to centrally administered glucose, ICV fructose increases AMP-K phosphorylation in the ventromedial hypothalamus [147,148] as well as food intake and hepatic gluconeogenesis [147], and impairs the ability of a glucagon-like peptide (GLP-1) to suppress both AMP-K phosphorylation and food intake (presumably by increasing AMP-K phosphorylation) [147]. Although both glucose and fructose can be metabolized for ATP production in the brain and should therefore equally inhibit AMP-K activity, it has been suggested that because fructose bypasses the glycolysis step that glucose undergoes (with subsequent net ATP generation) and requires an initial energy-consuming phosphorylation by 2-ketohexokinase before metabolism to glyceraldehyde 3-phosphate, [ATP] is rapidly depleted and [AMP] increases, thereby activating AMP-K [149] (Figure 15.6).

Several studies have also attempted to address a role for glucose in brain signaling associated with food intake using fMRI by describing the temporal response to glucose ingestion or infusion. Consistently, these studies have found suppression of hypothalamic BOLD signaling after administration of glucose to rats [150] and humans [25,151–154]. Obese subjects have been reported to have diminished attenuation of the BOLD signal suppression to glucose ingestion compared with lean subjects [155] and patients with type 2 diabetes have been shown to show no hypothalamic signal change compared to nondiabetic people [153]. However, consuming a meal results in potential brain responses to taste [156] and changes in levels of gut hormones that have been shown to have receptors in hypothalamic neurons (ghrelin, GLP-1, PYY) [157]. In one study in which glucose was injected, thus bypassing neuronal inputs from the GI system, hypothalamic BOLD signal was suppressed, but not to the extent that it was after ingestion [154]. In another study, no significant changes in hypothalamic BOLD response were seen to injected glucose, but cortical BOLD signal increased [158]. This finding contrasted with the cortical brain BOLD response to a similar injection of fructose, which resulted in significant suppression of BOLD signal [158]. In this latter condition (fructose injection), insulin levels were blunted and lactate levels increased quite a bit, whereas insulin levels increased in parallel with the glucose infusion. While technical limitations of imaging the hypothalamus (susceptibility artifact, head movement, and resolution) may explain the differences in hypothalamic results between these studies [154,158], the contrasting BOLD responses in the cortex were interpreted to be consistent with opposing effects on [ATP], [AMP], and AMP-K activities by glucose (and insulin) and fructose (Figure 15.6) [149].

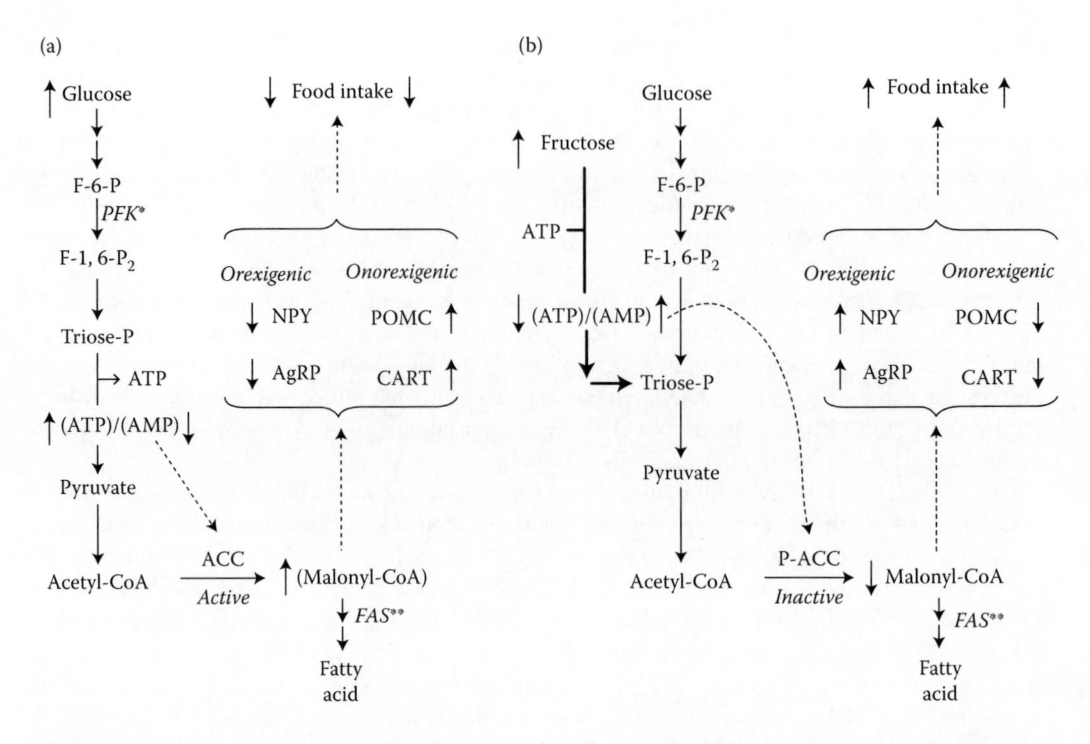

FIGURE 15.6 Hypothalamic signaling pathways triggered by metabolism of (A) glucose and (B) fructose leading to inverse effects on food intake. PFK* refers to phosphofructokinase and FAS** to fatty acid synthase. (Taken from Lane MD, Cha SH. *Biochem Biophys Res Commun*. 2009;382(1):1–5. Epub 2009/03/07.)

CONCLUSIONS

Glucose plays a dual role in the brain. The first is as an energy source that maintains normal neuronal activity through direct neuronal uptake as well as by the glial cells, which form a functional unit involving the dendrites, a lactate shuttle to provide additional energy to the neuron, and a glutamine–glutamate shuttle that clears the synaptic cleft and readies the neuron for the next activation. This neuronal–glial unit forms the anatomic basis for the BOLD response during fMRI brain imaging. The second involves "sensing" changes in blood glucose levels by specialized circumventricular brain regions and subsequent neuronal and behavioral responses. The best understood of these responses is the counter-regulatory response elicited by progressively worsening hypoglycemia in both animal and human studies. Animal models also suggest a role for sensing changes in blood glucose levels within the physiological range that govern feeding and metabolic responses. Transduction of this glucose signal into feeding behaviors and metabolic responses involves alterations in neuronal energetics and activation of ATP and AMP responsive enzymes, cellular systems that do not require glucose metabolism, and modulation of neuronal responses to weight regulatory hormones such as insulin and leptin. Alterations in cellular energetics is also thought to play a major role in "nutrient sensing" that governs food intake and body weight in response to changes in dietary intake of fats, protein, and alternative dietary sugars, such as fructose.

The potentially greatest public health impact from sensing sugars in the brain is in the role that added sugars, and specifically the role of increased fructose consumption, in the American diet have played in the increase in body weight over the past 40 years [159,160]. From the 1970s to 2004, added sugars in the form of high-fructose corn syrup (HFCS) increased from <1% to 42% of all sweeteners available for consumption in the USA [161,162], and while the rates of added sugar consumption (including sucrose, a disaccharide made up of one molecule of glucose and one molecule of fructose) has recently declined slightly to 14% of total daily energy consumption [163], intake still remains higher than recommended (10% or less of total calories) [164]. As reviewed in other chapters, epidemiological [160,165], genetic [166], and interventional studies [167] in humans support a contributing role for added sugars in the weight gain experienced by the American public over the last several decades, especially amongst susceptible subpopulations [166,168]. Data from animal studies suggest that it is the greater exposure to the sugar fructose, specifically, that diminishes the normal brain-sensing responses and leads to increased food intake and body weight [145–148,169,170], which is supported by a limited number of human intervention studies under ad libitum feeding conditions [171] and brain responses by fMRI [25,158]. If so, then major considerations in policy will be needed to address America's current emphasis on processed foods, especially those with added sugars, because the weight of the evidence supports the conclusion that the taste engineering that enhances food "likability" also alters our appetitive responses in such a way that satiety is not fully felt until higher total caloric intakes are achieved.

OPEN QUESTIONS/RECOMMENDATIONS OF FUTURE RESEARCH AND/OR NEEDS IN THE FIELD

FUTURE RESEARCH NEEDS

- Establishment of relevant levels of glucose and fructose in the diet, blood, and brain when studying metabolic effects of sugars in both animals and humans.
- Better understanding of the molecular mechanisms associated with nutrient sensing in animals and humans, especially the relative contribution of sugar sensing to long-term body weight by weight regulatory peptides.
- More studies examining the effects of sugar sensing during in utero exposure and effect on programming and epigenetic predisposition to chronic diseases of adulthood.
- Development of imaging techniques that allow better spatial resolution and include molecular imaging of intermediate sugar metabolism in animals and humans.
- Attention in dietary studies to control diets that reflect "real-world" conditions in which people would be free to consume alternatives such as water, milk, and foods free of added sugars in addition to the requisite glucose control.
- Inclusion in human studies of subpopulations at increased risk for obesity, followed long term.

Current and future research needs fall into three categories: establishing relevant blood and brain levels of sugars that influence brain sensing, utilizing novel imaging techniques to study animal and human brain metabolism in real time as it relates to sugar sensing and behavioral responses, and design of human studies to reflect realistic food intakes (not just of sugar but also other macro- and micronutrients) and powered adequately to detect long-term outcomes.

While much work has addressed relevant levels of blood glucose in the brain for glucose sensing, far less is known regarding relevant levels of fructose in extracellular fluid (especially in humans) and what levels occur following consumption of a sugar-sweetened beverage or added-sugar meal. In addition, free living populations do not consume only one or another sugar, but rather consume sugars together and in combination with other dietary macronutrients that may have independent effects (either directly or indirectly) on study outcomes (such as central brain metabolism, control of food intake, and regulation of peripheral metabolism). Accounting for these sometimes subtle differences will be important to understand the relevance of study findings to populations.

The majority of our current understanding of brain sugar metabolism and sensing comes from animal models that allow direct testing using brain tissue. However, human studies of similar scientific voracity will require better use of current technologies (fMRI, MRS, PET, etc.) and development of novel brain imaging techniques—specifically development of the ability to quantify and track individual metabolic and molecular intermediates in vivo, in real time. Outstanding questions include, for example: Are circumferential nuclei (VMH, brainstem) truly outside of the blood–brain barrier in humans? On a cellular level, which organelles are involved in glucose sensing and does glucose sensing require subcellular compartmentalization of glucose (or fructose) metabolism? Can the rate of change in glucose levels elicit physiological responses, or are changes in the absolute levels sufficient and necessary? What sensing mechanisms allow for detection of changes in extracellular glucose levels that do not involve active glucose metabolism? What are the effects of weight gain and obesity, weight loss (such as after bariatric surgery or with pharmacological treatment), and comorbid diseases and their treatments on brain sugar sensing?

Finally, to be informative for public health decision-making, studies are needed that include sufficient numbers of obese and "at-risk" for obesity groups the study population will need to be large enough and followed long enough (>1 year) to detect potentially small changes in food intake and body weight, especially in susceptible subgroups. Also, attention needs to be paid to ensure that people are free to consume alternatives such as water, milk, and foods free of added sugars.

REFERENCES

1. Kety SS, Schmidt CF. The nitrous oxide method for the quantitative determination of cerebral blood flow in man: Theory, procedure and normal values. *J Clin Invest*. 1948;27(4):476–83. Epub 1948/07/01.
2. Sokoloff L, Reivich M, Kennedy C, Des Rosiers MH, Patlak CS, Pettigrew KD et al. The [^{14}C]deoxyglucose method for the measurement of local cerebral glucose utilization: Theory, procedure, and normal values in the conscious and anesthetized albino rat. *J Neurochem*. 1977;28(5):897–916. Epub 1977/05/01.
3. Reivich M, Kuhl D, Wolf A, Greenberg J, Phelps M, Ido T et al. The [^{18}F]fluorodeoxyglucose method for the measurement of local cerebral glucose utilization in man. *Circ Res*. 1979;44(1):127–37. Epub 1979/01/01.
4. Belanger M, Allaman I, Magistretti PJ. Brain energy metabolism: Focus on astrocyte-neuron metabolic cooperation. *Cell Metab*. 2011;14(6):724–38. Epub 2011/12/14.
5. Rolfe DF, Brown GC. Cellular energy utilization and molecular origin of standard metabolic rate in mammals. *Physiol Rev*. 1997;77(3):731–58. Epub 1997/07/01.
6. Erecinska M, Cherian S, Silver IA. Energy metabolism in mammalian brain during development. *Prog Neurobiol*. 2004;73(6):397–445. Epub 2004/08/18.
7. Attwell D, Laughlin SB. An energy budget for signaling in the grey matter of the brain. *J Cereb Blood Flow Metab*. 2001;21(10):1133–45. Epub 2001/10/13.
8. Howarth C, Gleeson P, Attwell D. Updated energy budgets for neural computation in the neocortex and cerebellum. *J Cereb Blood Flow Metab*. 2012;32(7):1222–32. Epub 2012/03/22.
9. De Santi S, de Leon MJ, Convit A, Tarshish C, Rusinek H, Tsui WH et al. Age-related changes in brain: II. Positron emission tomography of frontal and temporal lobe glucose metabolism in normal subjects. *Psychiatr Q*. 1995;66(4):357–70. Epub 1995/01/01.
10. McEwen BS, Reagan LP. Glucose transporter expression in the central nervous system: Relationship to synaptic function. *Eur J Pharmacol*. 2004;490(1–3):13–24. Epub 2004/04/20.
11. Bingham EM, Hopkins D, Smith D, Pernet A, Hallett W, Reed L et al. The role of insulin in human brain glucose metabolism: An ^{18}fluoro-deoxyglucose positron emission tomography study. *Diabetes*. 2002;51(12):3384–90. Epub 2002/11/28.
12. Seaquist ER, Damberg GS, Tkac I, Gruetter R. The effect of insulin on in vivo cerebral glucose concentrations and rates of glucose transport/metabolism in humans. *Diabetes*. 2001;50(10):2203–9. Epub 2001/09/28.
13. Hasselbalch SG, Knudsen GM, Videbaek C, Pinborg LH, Schmidt JF, Holm S et al. No effect of insulin on glucose blood–brain barrier transport and cerebral metabolism in humans. *Diabetes*. 1999;48(10):1915–21. Epub 1999/10/08.

14. Shestov AA, Emir UE, Kumar A, Henry PG, Seaquist ER, Oz G. Simultaneous measurement of glucose transport and utilization in the human brain. *Am J Physiol Endocrinol Metab.* 2011;301(5):E1040–9. Epub 2011/07/28.
15. Silver IA, Erecinska M. Extracellular glucose concentration in mammalian brain: Continuous monitoring of changes during increased neuronal activity and upon limitation in oxygen supply in normo-, hypo-, and hyperglycemic animals. *J Neurosci.* 1994;14(8):5068–76. Epub 1994/08/01.
16. Abi-Saab WM, Maggs DG, Jones T, Jacob R, Srihari V, Thompson J et al. Striking differences in glucose and lactate levels between brain extracellular fluid and plasma in conscious human subjects: Effects of hyperglycemia and hypoglycemia. *J Cereb Blood Flow Metab.* 2002;22(3):271–9. Epub 2002/03/14.
17. Herman RH. Mannose metabolism I. *Am J Clin Nutr.* 1971;24(4):488–98. Epub 1971/04/01.
18. Pardridge WM, Oldendorf WH. Kinetics of blood–brain transport of hexoses. *Biochim Biophys Acta.* 1975;382(3):377–92. Epub 1975/03/25.
19. Sloviter HA, Kamimoto T. The isolated, persed rat brain preparation metabolizes mannose but not maltose. *J Neurochem.* 1970;17(7):1109–11. Epub 1970/07/01.
20. Wada H, Okada Y, Uzuo T, Nakamura H. The effects of glucose, mannose, fructose and lactate on the preservation of neural activity in the hippocampal slices from the guinea pig. *Brain Res.* 1998;788(1–2):144–50. Epub 1998/05/21.
21. Coss-Bu JA, Sunehag AL, Haymond MW. Contribution of galactose and fructose to glucose homeostasis. *Metab Clin Exp.* 2009;58(8):1050–8. Epub 2009/06/02.
22. Elliott SS, Keim NL, Stern JS, Teff K, Havel PJ. Fructose, weight gain, and the insulin resistance syndrome. *Am J Clin Nutr.* 2002;76(5):911–22. Epub 2002/10/26.
23. Le MT, Frye RF, Rivard CJ, Cheng J, McFann KK, Segal MS et al. Effects of high-fructose corn syrup and sucrose on the pharmacokinetics of fructose and acute metabolic and hemodynamic responses in healthy subjects. *Metabolism.* 2012;61(5):641–51. Epub 2011/12/14.
24. Thurston JH, Levy CA, Warren SK, Jones EM. Permeability of the blood–brain barrier to fructose and the anaerobic use of fructose in the brains of young mice. *J Neurochem.* 1972;19(7):1685–96.
25. Page KA, Chan O, Arora J, Belfort-Deaguiar R, Dzuira J, Roehmholdt B et al. Effects of fructose vs glucose on regional cerebral blood flow in brain regions involved with appetite and reward pathways. *JAMA.* 2013;309(1):63–70. Epub 2013/01/03.
26. Mantych GJ, James DE, Devaskar SU. Jejunal/kidney glucose transporter isoform (Glut-5) is expressed in the human blood–brain barrier. *Endocrinology.* 1993;132(1):35–40. Epub 1993/01/01.
27. Horikoshi Y, Sasaki A, Taguchi N, Maeda M, Tsukagoshi H, Sato K et al. Human Glut5 immunolabeling is useful for evaluating microglial status in neuropathological study using paraffin sections. *Acta Neuropathol.* 2003;105(2):157–62.
28. Payne J, Maher F, Simpson I, Mattice L, Davies P. Glucose transporter Glut 5 expression in microglial cells. *Glia.* 1997;21(3):327–31. Epub 1997/12/31 23:38.
29. Sokoloff L. Metabolism of ketone bodies by the brain. *Annu Rev Med.* 1973;24:271–80. Epub 1973/01/01.
30. Kacem K, Lacombe P, Seylaz J, Bonvento G. Structural organization of the perivascular astrocyte endfeet and their relationship with the endothelial glucose transporter: A confocal microscopy study. *Glia.* 1998;23(1):1–10. Epub 1998/04/30.
31. Halassa MM, Fellin T, Takano H, Dong JH, Haydon PG. Synaptic islands defined by the territory of a single astrocyte. *J Neurosci.* 2007;27(24):6473–7. Epub 2007/06/15.
32. Attwell D, Buchan AM, Charpak S, Lauritzen M, Macvicar BA, Newman EA. Glial and neuronal control of brain blood flow. *Nature.* 2010;468(7321):232–43. Epub 2010/11/12.
33. Cataldo AM, Broadwell RD. Cytochemical identification of cerebral glycogen and glucose-6-phosphatase activity under normal and experimental conditions. II. Choroid plexus and ependymal epithelia, endothelia and pericytes. *J Neurocytol.* 1986;15(4):511–24. Epub 1986/08/01.
34. Norberg K, Siesjo BK. Metabolism of oxygen, glucose, lactate and pyruvate in the rat brain in situ. *J Neurochem.* 1974;22(6):1127–9. Epub 1974/06/01.
35. Magistretti PJ, Pellerin L, Rothman DL, Shulman RG. Energy on demand. *Science.* 1999;283(5401):496–7. Epub 1999/02/13.
36. Raichle ME, Mintun MA. Brain work and brain imaging. *Annu Rev Neurosci.* 2006;29:449–76. Epub 2006/06/17.
37. Mitrakou A, Ryan C, Veneman T, Mokan M, Jenssen T, Kiss I et al. Hierarchy of glycemic thresholds for counterregulatory hormone secretion, symptoms, and cerebral dysfunction. *Am J Physiol.* 1991;260(1 Pt 1):E67–74.

38. Schwartz NS, Clutter WE, Shah SD, Cryer PE. Glycemic thresholds for activation of glucose counterregulatory systems are higher than the threshold for symptoms. *J Clin Invest*. 1987;79(3):777–81.
39. Fanelli C, Pampanelli S, Epifano L, Rambotti AM, Ciofetta M, Modarelli F et al. Relative roles of insulin and hypoglycaemia on induction of neuroendocrine responses to, symptoms of, and deterioration of cognitive function in hypoglycaemia in male and female humans. *Diabetologia*. 1994;37(8):797–807.
40. Rizza RA, Cryer PE, Gerich JE. Role of glucagon, catecholamines, and growth hormone in human glucose counterregulation: Effects of somatostatin and combined alpha- and beta-adrenergic blockade on plasma glucose recovery and glucose flux rates after insulin-induced hypoglycemia. *J Clin Invest*. 1979;64(1):62–71.
41. Barg S, Galvanovskis J, Gopel SO, Rorsman P, Eliasson L. Tight coupling between electrical activity and exocytosis in mouse glucagon-secreting alpha-cells. *Diabetes*. 2000;49(9):1500–10.
42. Quoix N, Cheng-Xue R, Mattart L, Zeinoun Z, Guiot Y, Beauvois MC et al. Glucose and pharmacological modulators of ATP-sensitive K+ channels control $[Ca^{2+}]C$ by different mechanisms in isolated mouse alpha-cells. *Diabetes*. 2009;58(2):412–21.
43. Matschinsky FM. Banting lecture 1995. A lesson in metabolic regulation inspired by the glucokinase glucose sensor paradigm. *Diabetes*. 1996;45(2):223–41.
44. Pardal R, Lopez-Barneo J. Low glucose-sensing cells in the carotid body. *Nat Neurosci*. 2002;5(3):197–8.
45. Niijima A. Glucose-sensitive afferent nerve fibres in the hepatic branch of the vagus nerve in the guinea-pig. *J Physiol*. 1982;332:315–23.
46. Hevener AL, Bergman RN, Donovan CM. Hypoglycemic detection does not occur in the hepatic artery or liver: Findings consistent with a portal vein glucosensor locus. *Diabetes*. 2001;50(2):399–403.
47. Hevener AL, Bergman RN, Donovan CM. Novel glucosensor for hypoglycemic detection localized to the portal vein. *Diabetes*. 1997;46(9):1521–5.
48. Ritter RC, Slusser PG, Stone S. Glucoreceptors controlling feeding and blood glucose: Location in the hindbrain. *Science*. 1981;213(4506):451–2.
49. Frizzell RT, Jones EM, Davis SN, Biggers DW, Myers SR, Connolly CC et al. Counterregulation during hypoglycemia is directed by widespread brain regions. *Diabetes*. 1993;42(9):1253–61.
50. Brobeck JR, Tepperman J, Long CN. Experimental hypothalamic hyperphagia in the albino rat. *Yale J Biol Med*. 1943;15(6):831–53.
51. Bray GA, Gallagher Jr. TF. Manifestations of hypothalamic obesity in man: A comprehensive investigation of eight patients and a review of the literature. *Medicine (Baltimore)*. 1975;54(4):301–30. Epub 1975/07/11.
52. Kennedy GC. The hypothalamic control of food intake in rats. *Proc R Soc Lond B Biol Sci*. 1950;137(889):535–49. Epub 1950/11/01.
53. Anand BK, Dua S, Shoenberg K. Hypothalamic control of food intake in cats and monkeys. *J Physiol*. 1955;127(1):143–52.
54. Anand BK, Brobeck JR. Hypothalamic control of food intake in rats and cats. *Yale J Biol Med*. 1951;24(2):123–40.
55. Anand BK, Dua S. Feeding responses induced by electrical stimulation of the hypothalamus in cat. *Indian J Med Res*. 1955;43(1):113–22.
56. Delgado JM, Anand BK. Increase of food intake induced by electrical stimulation of the lateral hypothalamus. *Am J Physiol*. 1953;172(1):162–8.
57. King BM. Amygdaloid lesion-induced obesity: Relation to sexual behavior, olfaction, and the ventromedial hypothalamus. *Am J Physiol Regul Integr Comp Physiol*. 2006;291(5):R1201–14. Epub 2006/06/17.
58. Ahlskog JE, Hoebel BG. Overeating and obesity from damage to a noradrenergic system in the brain. *Science*. 1973;182(108):166–9. Epub 1973/10/12.
59. Morton GJ, Cummings DE, Baskin DG, Barsh GS, Schwartz MW. Central nervous system control of food intake and body weight. *Nature*. 2006;443(7109):289–95. Epub 2006/09/22.
60. Mayer J. Glucostatic mechanism of regulation of food intake. *N Engl J Med*. 1953;249(1):13–6. Epub 1953/07/02.
61. Smith GP, Epstein AN. Increased feeding in response to decreased glucose utilization in the rat and monkey. *Am J Physiol*. 1969;217(4):1083–7.
62. Louis-Sylvestre J, Le Magnen J. Fall in blood glucose level precedes meal onset in free-feeding rats. *Neurosci Biobehav Rev*. 1980;4(Suppl. 1):13–5.
63. Campfield LA, Smith FJ. Functional coupling between transient declines in blood glucose and feeding behavior: Temporal relationships. *Brain Res Bull*. 1986;17(3):427–33.
64. Waxler SH, Brecher G. Obesity and food requirements in albino mice following administration of gold thioglucose. *Am J Physiol*. 1950;162(2):428–33.

65. Marshall NB, Mayer J. Specificity of gold thioglucose for ventromedial hypothalamic lesions and hyperphagia. *Nature*. 1956;178(4547):1399–400.
66. Kennedy HJ, Pouli AE, Ainscow EK, Jouaville LS, Rizzuto R, Rutter GA. Glucose generates sub-plasma membrane ATP microdomains in single islet beta-cells. Potential role for strategically located mitochondria. *J Biol Chem*. 1999;274(19):13281–91.
67. Oomura Y, Kimura K, Ooyama H, Maeno T, Iki M, Kuniyoshi M. Reciprocal activities of the ventromedial and lateral hypothalamic areas of cats. *Science*. 1964;143(3605):484–5.
68. Anand BK, Chhina GS, Sharma KN, Dua S, Singh B. Activity of single neurons in the hypothalamic feeding centers: Effect of glucose. *Am J Physiol*. 1964;207:1146–54.
69. Shoji S. Glucose regulation of synaptic transmission in the dorsolateral septal nucleus of the rat. *Synapse*. 1992;12(4):322–32.
70. Nakano Y, Oomura Y, Lenard L, Nishino H, Aou S, Yamamoto T et al. Feeding-related activity of glucose- and morphine-sensitive neurons in the monkey amygdala. *Brain Res*. 1986;399(1):167–72.
71. Ritter S, Dinh TT, Zhang Y. Localization of hindbrain glucoreceptive sites controlling food intake and blood glucose. *Brain Res*. 2000;856(1–2):37–47. Epub 2000/03/10.
72. Borg WP, During MJ, Sherwin RS, Borg MA, Brines ML, Shulman GI. Ventromedial hypothalamic lesions in rats suppress counterregulatory responses to hypoglycemia. *J Clin Invest*. 1994;93(4):1677–82.
73. Borg WP, Sherwin RS, During MJ, Borg MA, Shulman GI. Local ventromedial hypothalamus glucopenia triggers counterregulatory hormone release. *Diabetes*. 1995;44(2):180–4.
74. Borg MA, Sherwin RS, Borg WP, Tamborlane WV, Shulman GI. Local ventromedial hypothalamus glucose perfusion blocks counterregulation during systemic hypoglycemia in awake rats. *J Clin Invest*. 1997;99(2):361–5.
75. Oomura Y, Ono T, Ooyama H, Wayner MJ. Glucose and osmosensitive neurones of the rat hypothalamus. *Nature*. 1969;222(5190):282–4.
76. Silver IA, Erecinska M. Glucose-induced intracellular ion changes in sugar-sensitive hypothalamic neurons. *J Neurophysiol*. 1998;79(4):1733–45.
77. Song Z, Levin BE, McArdle JJ, Bakhos N, Routh VH. Convergence of pre- and postsynaptic influences on glucosensing neurons in the ventromedial hypothalamic nucleus. *Diabetes*. 2001;50(12):2673–81.
78. Canabal DD, Song Z, Potian JG, Beuve A, McArdle JJ, Routh VH. Glucose, insulin, and leptin signaling pathways modulate nitric oxide synthesis in glucose-inhibited neurons in the ventromedial hypothalamus. *Am J Physiol Regul Integr Comp Physiol*. 2007;292(4):R1418–28.
79. Wang R, Liu X, Hentges ST, Dunn-Meynell AA, Levin BE, Wang W et al. The regulation of glucose-excited neurons in the hypothalamic arcuate nucleus by glucose and feeding-relevant peptides. *Diabetes*. 2004;53(8):1959–65.
80. Yang XJ, Kow LM, Funabashi T, Mobbs CV. Hypothalamic glucose sensor: Similarities to and differences from pancreatic beta-cell mechanisms. *Diabetes*. 1999;48(9):1763–72.
81. Ashford ML, Boden PR, Treherne JM. Glucose-induced excitation of hypothalamic neurones is mediated by ATP-sensitive K+ channels. *Pflugers Arch*. 1990;415(4):479–83.
82. Ashford ML, Boden PR, Treherne JM. Tolbutamide excites rat glucoreceptive ventromedial hypothalamic neurones by indirect inhibition of ATP-K+ channels. *Br J Pharmacol*. 1990;101(3):531–40.
83. Karschin C, Ecke C, Ashcroft FM, Karschin A. Overlapping distribution of K(ATP) channel-forming Kir6.2 subunit and the sulfonylurea receptor Sur1 in rodent brain. *FEBS Lett*. 1997;401(1):59–64.
84. Karschin C, Schreibmayer W, Dascal N, Lester H, Davidson N, Karschin A. Distribution and localization of a G protein-coupled inwardly rectifying K+ channel in the rat. *FEBS Lett*. 1994;348(2):139–44.
85. Dunn-Meynell AA, Rawson NE, Levin BE. Distribution and phenotype of neurons containing the ATP-sensitive K+ channel in rat brain. *Brain Res*. 1998;814(1–2):41–54.
86. Dunn-Meynell AA, Routh VH, Kang L, Gaspers L, Levin BE. Glucokinase is the likely mediator of glucosensing in both glucose-excited and glucose-inhibited central neurons. *Diabetes*. 2002; 51(7):2056–65.
87. Song Z, Routh VH. Differential effects of glucose and lactate on glucosensing neurons in the ventromedial hypothalamic nucleus. *Diabetes*. 2005;54(1):15–22.
88. Kang L, Dunn-Meynell AA, Routh VH, Gaspers LD, Nagata Y, Nishimura T et al. Glucokinase is a critical regulator of ventromedial hypothalamic neuronal glucosensing. *Diabetes*. 2006;55(2):412–20.
89. Levin BE, Becker TC, Eiki J, Zhang BB, Dunn-Meynell AA. Ventromedial hypothalamic glucokinase is an important mediator of the counterregulatory response to insulin-induced hypoglycemia. *Diabetes*. 2008;57(5):1371–9.
90. Kang L, Routh VH, Kuzhikandathil EV, Gaspers LD, Levin BE. Physiological and molecular characteristics of rat hypothalamic ventromedial nucleus glucosensing neurons. *Diabetes*. 2004;53(3):549–59.

91. Kahn BB, Alquier T, Carling D, Hardie DG. AMP-activated protein kinase: Ancient energy gauge provides clues to modern understanding of metabolism. *Cell Metab*. 2005;1(1):15–25.
92. Culmsee C, Monnig J, Kemp BE, Mattson MP. AMP-activated protein kinase is highly expressed in neurons in the developing rat brain and promotes neuronal survival following glucose deprivation. *J Mol Neurosci*. 2001;17(1):45–58.
93. Turnley AM, Stapleton D, Mann RJ, Witters LA, Kemp BE, Bartlett PF. Cellular distribution and developmental expression of AMP-activated protein kinase isoforms in mouse central nervous system. *J Neurochem*. 1999;72(4):1707–16.
94. Claret M, Smith MA, Batterham RL, Selman C, Choudhury AI, Fryer LG et al. AMPK is essential for energy homeostasis regulation and glucose sensing by POMC and AGRP neurons. *J Clin Invest*. 2007;117(8):2325–36.
95. Mountjoy PD, Bailey SJ, Rutter GA. Inhibition by glucose or leptin of hypothalamic neurons expressing neuropeptide Y requires changes in AMP-activated protein kinase activity. *Diabetologia*. 2007;50(1):168–77.
96. Murphy BA, Fioramonti X, Jochnowitz N, Fakira K, Gagen K, Contie S et al. Fasting enhances the response of arcuate neuropeptide Y-glucose-inhibited neurons to decreased extracellular glucose. *Am J Physiol Cell Physiol*. 2009;296(4):C746–56.
97. Fioramonti X, Marsollier N, Song Z, Fakira KA, Patel RM, Brown S et al. Ventromedial hypothalamic nitric oxide production is necessary for hypoglycemia detection and counterregulation. *Diabetes*. 2010;59(2):519–28.
98. Murphy BA, Fakira KA, Song Z, Beuve A, Routh VH. AMP-activated protein kinase and nitric oxide regulate the glucose sensitivity of ventromedial hypothalamic glucose-inhibited neurons. *Am J Physiol Cell Physiol*. 2009;297(3):C750–8.
99. Yang CS, Lam CK, Chari M, Cheung GW, Kokorovic A, Gao S et al. Hypothalamic AMP-activated protein kinase regulates glucose production. *Diabetes*. 2010;59(10):2435–43.
100. Lam CK, Chari M, Rutter GA, Lam TK. Hypothalamic nutrient sensing activates a forebrain-hindbrain neuronal circuit to regulate glucose production in vivo. *Diabetes*. 2011;60(1):107–13.
101. McCrimmon RJ, Fan X, Ding Y, Zhu W, Jacob RJ, Sherwin RS. Potential role for AMP-activated protein kinase in hypoglycemia sensing in the ventromedial hypothalamus. *Diabetes*. 2004;53(8):1953–8.
102. Gonzalez JA, Reimann F, Burdakov D. Dissociation between sensing and metabolism of glucose in sugar sensing neurones. *J Physiol*. 2009;587(Pt 1):41–8.
103. Ainscow EK, Mirshamsi S, Tang T, Ashford ML, Rutter GA. Dynamic imaging of free cytosolic ATP concentration during fuel sensing by rat hypothalamic neurones: Evidence for ATP-independent control of ATP-sensitive K(+) channels. *J Physiol*. 2002;544(Pt 2):429–45.
104. Gonzalez JA, Jensen LT, Fugger L, Burdakov D. Metabolism-independent sugar sensing in central orexin neurons. *Diabetes*. 2008;57(10):2569–76.
105. Gribble FM, Williams L, Simpson AK, Reimann F. A novel glucose-sensing mechanism contributing to glucagon-like peptide-1 secretion from the glutag cell line. *Diabetes*. 2003;52(5):1147–54.
106. Woods SC. Metabolic signals and food intake. Forty years of progress. *Appetite*. 2013;71:440–4.
107. Kennedy GC. The role of depot fat in the hypothalamic control of food intake in the rat. *Proc R Soc Lond B Biol Sci*. 1953;140(901):578–96.
108. Zhang Y, Proenca R, Maffei M, Barone M, Leopold L, Friedman JM. Positional cloning of the mouse obese gene and its human homologue. *Nature*. 1994;372(6505):425–32.
109. Tartaglia LA, Dembski M, Weng X, Deng N, Culpepper J, Devos R et al. Identification and expression cloning of a leptin receptor, Ob-R. *Cell*. 1995;83(7):1263–71.
110. Sohn JW, Elmquist JK, Williams KW. Neuronal circuits that regulate feeding behavior and metabolism. *Trends Neurosci*. 2013;36(9):504–12.
111. Sakurai T, Amemiya A, Ishii M, Matsuzaki I, Chemelli RM, Tanaka H et al. Orexins and orexin receptors: A family of hypothalamic neuropeptides and G protein-coupled receptors that regulate feeding behavior. *Cell*. 1998;92(4):573–85.
112. Qu D, Ludwig DS, Gammeltoft S, Piper M, Pelleymounter MA, Cullen MJ et al. A role for melanin-concentrating hormone in the central regulation of feeding behaviour. *Nature*. 1996;380(6571):243–7.
113. Myers Jr. MG, Munzberg H, Leinninger GM, Leshan RL. The geometry of leptin action in the brain: More complicated than a simple arc. *Cell Metab*. 2009;9(2):117–23.
114. Figlewicz DP, Evans SB, Murphy J, Hoen M, Baskin DG. Expression of receptors for insulin and leptin in the ventral tegmental area/substantia nigra (Vta/Sn) of the rat. *Brain Res*. 2003;964(1):107–15. Epub 2003/02/08.
115. Volkow ND, Wang GJ, Tomasi D, Baler RD. Obesity and addiction: Neurobiological overlaps. *Obes Rev*. 2013;14(1):2–18. Epub 2012/09/29.

116. Muroya S, Yada T, Shioda S, Takigawa M. Glucose-sensitive neurons in the rat arcuate nucleus contain neuropeptide Y. *Neurosci Lett*. 1999;264(1–3):113–6.
117. Fioramonti X, Contie S, Song Z, Routh VH, Lorsignol A, Penicaud L. Characterization of glucosensing neuron subpopulations in the arcuate nucleus: Integration in neuropeptide Y and Pro-Opio melanocortin networks? *Diabetes*. 2007;56(5):1219–27.
118. Ibrahim N, Bosch MA, Smart JL, Qiu J, Rubinstein M, Ronnekleiv OK et al. Hypothalamic proopiomelanocortin neurons are glucose responsive and express K(ATP) channels. *Endocrinology*. 2003;144(4):1331–40.
119. Parton LE, Ye CP, Coppari R, Enriori PJ, Choi B, Zhang CY et al. Glucose sensing by Pomc neurons regulates glucose homeostasis and is impaired in obesity. *Nature*. 2007;449(7159):228–32.
120. Kong D, Vong L, Parton LE, Ye C, Tong Q, Hu X et al. Glucose stimulation of hypothalamic Mch neurons involves K(ATP) channels, is modulated by Ucp2, and regulates peripheral glucose homeostasis. *Cell Metab*. 2010;12(5):545–52.
121. Burdakov D, Gerasimenko O, Verkhratsky A. Physiological changes in glucose differentially modulate the excitability of hypothalamic melanin-concentrating hormone and orexin neurons in situ. *J Neurosci*. 2005;25(9):2429–33.
122. Yamanaka A, Beuckmann CT, Willie JT, Hara J, Tsujino N, Mieda M et al. Hypothalamic orexin neurons regulate arousal according to energy balance in mice. *Neuron*. 2003;38(5):701–13.
123. Muroya S, Uramura K, Sakurai T, Takigawa M, Yada T. Lowering glucose concentrations increases cytosolic Ca^{2+} in orexin neurons of the rat lateral hypothalamus. *Neurosci Lett*. 2001;309(3):165–8.
124. Billington CJ, Levine AS. Hypothalamic neuropeptide Y regulation of feeding and energy metabolism. *Curr Opin Neurobiol*. 1992;2(6):847–51.
125. Routh VH. Glucose-sensing neurons: Are they physiologically relevant? *Physiol Behav*. 2002;76(3):403–13.
126. Levin BE. Neuronal glucose sensing: Still a physiological orphan? *Cell Metab*. 2007;6(4):252–4.
127. Levin BE, Govek EK, Dunn-Meynell AA. Reduced glucose-induced neuronal activation in the hypothalamus of diet-induced obese rats. *Brain Res*. 1998;808(2):317–9.
128. Yang XJ, Mastaitis J, Mizuno T, Mobbs CV. Glucokinase regulates reproductive function, glucocorticoid secretion, food intake, and hypothalamic gene expression. *Endocrinology*. 2007;148(4):1928–32.
129. Levin BE, Routh VH, Kang L, Sanders NM, Dunn-Meynell AA. Neuronal glucosensing: What do we know after 50 years? *Diabetes*. 2004;53(10):2521–8.
130. Niswender KD, Morrison CD, Clegg DJ, Olson R, Baskin DG, Myers Jr. MG et al. Insulin activation of phosphatidylinositol 3-kinase in the hypothalamic arcuate nucleus: A key mediator of insulin-induced anorexia. *Diabetes*. 2003;52(2):227–31.
131. Morton GJ, Gelling RW, Niswender KD, Morrison CD, Rhodes CJ, Schwartz MW. Leptin regulates insulin sensitivity via phosphatidylinositol-3-Oh kinase signaling in mediobasal hypothalamic neurons. *Cell Metab*. 2005;2(6):411–20.
132. Banks WA, Owen JB, Erickson MA. Insulin in the brain: There and back again. *Pharmacol Ther*. 2012;136(1):82–93.
133. Born J, Lange T, Kern W, McGregor GP, Bickel U, Fehm HL. Sniffing neuropeptides: A transnasal approach to the human brain. *Nat Neurosci*. 2002;5(6):514–6. Epub 2002/05/07.
134. Hallschmid M, Benedict C, Schultes B, Fehm HL, Born J, Kern W. Intranasal insulin reduces body fat in men but not in women. *Diabetes*. 2004;53(11):3024–9. Epub 2004/10/27.
135. Verdich C, Toubro S, Buemann B, Lysgard Madsen J, Juul Holst J, Astrup A. The role of postprandial releases of insulin and incretin hormones in meal-induced satiety—Effect of obesity and weight reduction. *Int J Obesity Rel Metab Disorders: J Int Assoc Study Obesity*. 2001;25(8):1206–14. Epub 2001/07/31.
136. Jauch-Chara K, Friedrich A, Rezmer M, Melchert UH, H GS-E, Hallschmid M et al. Intranasal insulin suppresses food intake via enhancement of brain energy levels in humans. *Diabetes*. 2012;61(9):2261–8. Epub 2012/05/16.
137. Diggs-Andrews KA, Zhang X, Song Z, Daphna-Iken D, Routh VH, Fisher SJ. Brain insulin action regulates hypothalamic glucose sensing and the counterregulatory response to hypoglycemia. *Diabetes*. 2010;59(9):2271–80.
138. Spanswick D, Smith MA, Mirshamsi S, Routh VH, Ashford ML. Insulin activates ATP-sensitive K+ channels in hypothalamic neurons of lean, but not obese rats. *Nat Neurosci*. 2000;3(8):757–8.
139. Blouet C, Schwartz GJ. Hypothalamic nutrient sensing in the control of energy homeostasis. *Behav Brain Res*. 2010;209(1):1–12.
140. Grill HJ, Hayes MR. Hindbrain neurons as an essential hub in the neuroanatomically distributed control of energy balance. *Cell Metab*. 2012;16(3):296–309.

141. Lam TK. Neuronal regulation of homeostasis by nutrient sensing. *Nat Med*. 2010;16(4):392–5.
142. Obici S, Rossetti L. Minireview: Nutrient sensing and the regulation of insulin action and energy balance. *Endocrinology*. 2003;144(12):5172–8.
143. Wang R, Cruciani-Guglielmacci C, Migrenne S, Magnan C, Cotero VE, Routh VH. Effects of oleic acid on distinct populations of neurons in the hypothalamic arcuate nucleus are dependent on extracellular glucose levels. *J Neurophysiol*. 2006;95(3):1491–8.
144. Le Foll C, Irani BG, Magnan C, Dunn-Meynell AA, Levin BE. Characteristics and mechanisms of hypothalamic neuronal fatty acid sensing. *Am J Physiol Regul Integr Comp Physiol*. 2009;297(3):R655–64.
145. Cha SH, Wolfgang M, Tokutake Y, Chohnan S, Lane MD. Differential effects of central fructose and glucose on hypothalamic Malonyl-Coa and food intake. *Proc Natl Acad Sci USA*. 2008;105(44):16871–5. Epub 2008/10/31.
146. Miller CC, Martin RJ, Whitney ML, Edwards GL. Intracerebroventricular injection of fructose stimulates feeding in rats. *Nutr Neurosci*. 2002;5(5):359–62. Epub 2002/10/19.
147. Kinote A, Faria JA, Roman EA, Solon C, Razolli DS, Ignacio-Souza LM et al. Fructose-induced hypothalamic AMPK activation stimulates hepatic Pepck and gluconeogenesis due to increased corticosterone levels. *Endocrinology*. 2012;153(8):3633–45.
148. Burmeister MA, Ayala J, Drucker DJ, Ayala JE. Central glucagon-like peptide 1 receptor-induced anorexia requires glucose metabolism-mediated suppression of AMPK and is impaired by central fructose. *Am J Physiol Endocrinol Metab*. 2013;304(7):E677–85.
149. Lane MD, Cha SH. Effect of glucose and fructose on food intake via Malonyl-Coa signaling in the brain. *Biochem Biophys Res Commun*. 2009;382(1):1–5. Epub 2009/03/07.
150. Mahankali S, Liu Y, Pu Y, Wang J, Chen CW, Fox PT et al. In vivo FMRI demonstration of hypothalamic function following intraperitoneal glucose administration in a rat model. *Magn Reson Med: Off J Soc Magn Reson Med/Soc Magn Reson Med*. 2000;43(1):155–9.
151. Liu Y, Gao JH, Liu HL, Fox PT. The temporal response of the brain after eating revealed by functional MRI. *Nature*. 2000;405(6790):1058–62. Epub 2000/07/13.
152. Smeets PA, de Graaf C, Stafleu A, van Osch MJ, van der Grond J. Functional MRI of human hypothalamic responses following glucose ingestion. *Neuroimage*. 2005;24(2):363–8. Epub 2005/01/04.
153. Vidarsdottir S, Smeets PA, Eichelsheim DL, van Osch MJ, Viergever MA, Romijn JA et al. Glucose ingestion fails to inhibit hypothalamic neuronal activity in patients with type 2 diabetes. *Diabetes*. 2007;56(10):2547–50. Epub 2007/08/03.
154. Smeets PA, Vidarsdottir S, de Graaf C, Stafleu A, van Osch MJ, Viergever MA et al. Oral glucose intake inhibits hypothalamic neuronal activity more effectively than glucose infusion. *Am J Physiol Endocrinol Metab*. 2007;293(3):E754–8. Epub 2007/06/15.
155. Matsuda M, Liu Y, Mahankali S, Pu Y, Mahankali A, Wang J et al. Altered hypothalamic function in response to glucose ingestion in obese humans. *Diabetes*. 1999;48(9):1801–6. Epub 1999/09/10.
156. Haase L, Cerf-Ducastel B, Murphy C. Cortical activation in response to pure taste stimuli during the physiological states of hunger and satiety. *Neuroimage*. 2009;44(3):1008–21. Epub 2008/11/15.
157. Wren AM, Bloom SR. Gut hormones and appetite control. *Gastroenterology*. 2007;132(6):2116–30. Epub 2007/05/15.
158. Purnell JQ, Klopfenstein BA, Stevens AA, Havel PJ, Adams SH, Dunn TN et al. Brain functional magnetic resonance imaging response to glucose and fructose infusions in humans. *Diabetes, Obesity Metab*. 2011;13(3):229–34. Epub 2011/01/06.
159. Bray GA, Nielsen SJ, Popkin BM. Consumption of high-fructose corn syrup in beverages may play a role in the epidemic of obesity. *Am J Clin Nutr*. 2004;79(4):537–43. Epub 2004/03/31.
160. Malik VS, Pan A, Willett WC, Hu FB. Sugar-sweetened beverages and weight gain in children and adults: A systematic review and meta-analysis. *Am J Clin Nutr*. 2013;98(4):1084–102.
161. Duffey KJ, Popkin BM. High-fructose corn syrup: Is this what's for dinner? *Am J Clin Nutr*. 2008;88(6):1722S–32S.
162. Marriott BP, Cole N, Lee E. National estimates of dietary fructose intake increased from 1977 to 2004 in the United States. *J Nutr*. 2009;139(6):1228S–35S. Epub 2009/05/01.
163. Welsh JA, Sharma AJ, Grellinger L, Vos MB. Consumption of added sugars is decreasing in the United States. *Am J Clin Nutr*. 2011;94(3):726–34. Epub 2011/07/15.
164. Nishida C, Uauy R, Kumanyika S, Shetty P. The joint who/FAO expert consultation on diet, nutrition and the prevention of chronic diseases: Process, product and policy implications. *Public Health Nutr*. 2004;7(1A):245–50.
165. Mozaffarian D, Hao T, Rimm EB, Willett WC, Hu FB. Changes in diet and lifestyle and long-term weight gain in women and men. *N Engl J Med*. 2011;364(25):2392–404. Epub 2011/06/24.

166. Qi Q, Chu AY, Kang JH, Jensen MK, Curhan GC, Pasquale LR et al. Sugar-sweetened beverages and genetic risk of obesity. *N Engl J Med*. 2012;367(15):1387–96. Epub 2012/09/25.
167. de Ruyter JC, Olthof MR, Seidell JC, Katan MB. A trial of sugar-free or sugar-sweetened beverages and body weight in children. *N Engl J Med*. 2012;367(15):1397–406. Epub 2012/09/25.
168. Ebbeling CB, Feldman HA, Chomitz VR, Antonelli TA, Gortmaker SL, Osganian SK et al. A randomized trial of sugar-sweetened beverages and adolescent body weight. *N Engl J Med*. 2012;367(15):1407–16. Epub 2012/09/25.
169. Cha SH, Lane MD. Central lactate metabolism suppresses food intake via the hypothalamic AMP kinase/Malonyl-Coa signaling pathway. *Biochem Biophys Res Commun*. 2009;386(1):212–6. Epub 2009/06/16.
170. Shu HJ, Isenberg K, Cormier RJ, Benz A, Zorumski CF. Expression of fructose sensitive glucose transporter in the brains of fructose-fed rats. *Neuroscience*. 2006;140(3):889–95.
171. Sievenpiper JL, de Souza RJ, Mirrahimi A, Yu ME, Carleton AJ, Beyene J et al. Effect of fructose on body weight in controlled feeding trials: A systematic review and meta-analysis. *Ann Intern Med*. 2012;156(4):291–304. Epub 2012/02/22.
172. McCrimmon R. The mechanisms that underlie glucose sensing during hypoglycaemia in diabetes. *Diabet Med*. 2008;25(5):513–22.

16 Sugars, Obesity, and Chronic Diseases in Adults

Vasanti S. Malik and Frank B. Hu

CONTENTS

KEY POINTS

- Intake of added sugars has increased markedly in the past few decades in parallel with rising rates of obesity and related chronic diseases.
- Sugar-sweetened beverages (SSBs) are the single largest source of calories and added sugars in the US diet, with consumption levels exceeding recommendations for all added sugars.
- Prospective cohort studies and trials have provided strong evidence for a causal link between intake of SSBs and weight gain or risk obesity and related chronic diseases, especially diabetes.
- SSBs promote weight gain because liquid calories are not filling and people do not reduce their food intake at subsequent meals following ingestion of liquid calories. These beverages can lead to diabetes and cardiovascular disease through excess adiposity, but also independently through glycemic effects and metabolic consequences of fructose.
- Based on the totality of the available evidence, intake of SSBs should be limited for obesity and chronic disease prevention and replaced by healthy alternatives such as water, coffee, tea, and low-fat milk.

- Public policy and regulatory strategies to reduce intake of SSBs are already in place or are being considered. These strategies should combine education and public health campaigns with regulations and laws to change social norms and improve consumption patterns.
- Scientific evidence should continue to evolve regarding the health effects of SSBs and be used to guide and update recommendations and policy strategies.

INTRODUCTION

The adverse health effects of dietary sugars have long been a matter of much public and scientific interest. For decades, it has been thought that high intake of dietary sugars is associated with the development of obesity, type 2 diabetes, cardiovascular disease, fatty liver disease, and some cancers. However, inconsistent findings have precluded the ability to draw definitive conclusions regarding many of these associations. A major challenge has been a lack of consensus on how sugars are defined. Naturally occurring sugars such as fructose, sucrose, and lactose are found intrinsically in fruits, vegetables, and dairy. In contrast, added or extrinsic sugars refer to sugars and syrups that are added to foods and beverages during processing and preparation, for example, high-fructose corn syrup (HFCS), the most common sweetener used in soda. To enable a more standardized approach to examining potential adverse health effects, the World Health Organization and the Food and Agriculture Organization of the United Nations have adopted a classification of carbohydrates based on polymer chain length and clarified definitions of various groups of sugars including free sugars, which includes all monosaccharaides and disaccharides added to foods plus those naturally present in honey, syrups, and fruit juices.

Time-trend data over the last three to four decades have shown a close parallel between the rise in intake of added sugars and the obesity and diabetes epidemics in the USA [1,2]. National survey data have estimated that the per capita intake of added sugars increased from 235 kcal/day in the late 1970s to 318 kcal/day in 1995 [2]. Largely driving this trend has been the dramatic increase in the consumption of sugar-sweetened beverages (SSBs), which are the single largest source of calories and added sugars in the US diet [3,4], as shown in Table 16.1. SSBs include the full spectrum of soft drinks, fruit drinks, and energy and vitamin water drinks, which are sweetened by caloric sweeteners such as HFCS, sucrose, or fruit juice concentrates that are added to the beverages by manufacturers, establishments, or individuals. HFCS is the sweetener most commonly used in SSBs in the USA, and usually contains 55% fructose, 40% glucose, and 5% other sugars, while sucrose or table sugar, the predominant sweetener in Europe, consists of 50% fructose and 50% glucose. Consumption of SSBs in the USA appears to have decreased modestly in the past decade [5] but data from the National Health and Nutrition Examination Survey (2005–2008) show that half of the US population consumes SSBs on a given day with one in four obtaining at least 200 calories from these beverages and 5% obtaining at least 567 calories, equivalent to four cans of soda [6]. These values exceed American Heart Association recommendations for no more than 100–150 kcal/day from all added sugars for most men and women [7]. In other parts of the world, particularly developing countries, intake of SSBs is on the rise, due to widespread urbanization and heavy marketing [8].

Over the past decade, a large body of evidence has accumulated, which shows a strong association between SSBs and obesity and related chronic diseases [9–11]. For this reason and because they provide "empty" calories and almost no nutritional value, SSBs have been identified as a suitable target for public health interventions. However, controversy remains whether the associations are causal (see Chapter 21), and whether public action should be taken on the basis of the existing evidence. In this chapter, we examine the epidemiological evidence evaluating the relationship between sugars and obesity, diabetes, and cardiovascular risk in adults, focusing on SSBs since they are the most abundant and well-characterized source of added sugars in the diet. We also examine whether the available evidence linking SSB intake to obesity and diabetes meets the criteria for causality commonly used in noncommunicable disease epidemiology. Although not a main focus

TABLE 16.1
Mean Intake of Added Sugars and Mean Contribution (Teaspoons) of Various Foods among US Population, by Age, National Health and Nutrition Examination Survey 2005–2006

		All Persons	2–18 Years	19+ Years
Sample size		**8272**	**3553**	**4719**
Mean intake of added sugars (tsp.)		**21**	**23**	**20**
Rank[a]	**Food Group**			
1	Soda/energy/sports drinks	**7.5**	**7.3**	**7.6**
2	Grain-based desserts	**2.7**	**2.5**	**2.8**
3	Fruit drinks	**2.2**	**3.4**	**1.8**
4	Dairy desserts	**1.4**	**1.8**	**1.2**
5	Candy	**1.3**	**1.6**	**1.2**
6	Ready-to-eat cereals	0.8	1.5	0.6
7	Sugars/honey	0.7	0.3	0.9
8	Tea	0.7	0.5	0.8
9	Yeast breads	0.4	0.4	0.4
10	Syrups/toppings	0.4	0.7	0.3

Source: From http://riskfactor.cancer.gov/diet/foodsources/added_sugars.

[a] Rank for all persons only. Columns for other age groups are ordered by this ranking. The top five food groups for each age group are in bold.

of this chapter, we briefly discuss potential biological mechanisms underlying these associations. Since the majority of evidence we review is from prospective cohort studies, we also consider some methodological issues inherent in observational data. Finally, we discuss healthier alternatives to SSBs, implications for public health policies, and areas for future research.

SSBs AND OBESITY

Observational Evidence

Numerous epidemiological studies have evaluated the relationship between consumption of SSBs and the development of obesity in adults. Among the various study designs, ecological studies, which make cross-population comparisons, are most susceptible to confounding and other biases. Cross-sectional studies, which evaluate the exposure and outcome at the same point in time, are also highly prone to confounding and reverse causation bias. Because these designs are not able to establish a temporal sequence and infer causality, they have limited utility in nutritional epidemiology outside of hypothesis generation. Thus, evidence from these types of studies is not discussed in this chapter. Instead, we consider carefully conducted and analyzed prospective cohort studies, which study a group of people over time, and are considered the strongest nonrandomized study design, able to capture long-term diet and disease relationships.

The majority [3,9,10,12,13] but not all [14] of systematic reviews have reported positive associations between SSBs and weight gain or risk of overweight or obesity. We recently conducted a comprehensive systematic review and meta-analysis of cohort studies and randomized controlled trials of SSBs and weight gain in children and adults [10]. For this analysis, we included estimates that were not adjusted for total energy intake. Because SSBs add extra calories to the diet, total energy intake is likely to mediate the association between SSB intake and weight gain. Thus, adjusting for total energy intake would be equivalent to assessing the effects of SSB intake on body weight that do not occur through a change in total energy intake. This type of analysis would artificially underestimate the association between SSBs and body weight. Based on seven cohort studies in adults, with 174,252 participants, a one-serving per day increase in SSBs was associated with an additional weight gain of 0.22 kg (95% CI: 0.09–0.34 kg) and 0.12 kg (95% CI: 0.10–0.14 kg) over 1 year, in random- and fixed-effects models, respectively (Figure 16.1). The estimate from the fixed-effects model was not as strong as that from the random-effects model most likely because the random-effects model gives greater weight to smaller studies compared to the fixed-effects model and there were a couple of small studies that were outliers included in the analysis, which could have impacted the overall summary estimate. Although these estimates seem modest, adult weight gain in the general population is a gradual process, occurring over decades and averaging about 1 pound per year [15]. Thus, eliminating SSBs from the diet could be an effective way to prevent age-related weight gain. All of the studies included in the meta-analysis had repeated measurements of diet and weight and utilized a "change-on-change" analysis strategy. This type of analysis has some of the features of a quasi-experimental design, although it lacks the element of randomization in a clinical trial. An advantage of this design is the generalizability to a real-world setting, relative to a controlled laboratory setting, because participants are able to change their diet and lifestyle without investigator-driven intervention. Looking at individual studies in the meta-analysis, the largest and most influential was conducted among 120,877 initially non-obese men and women in the three Harvard longitudinal cohorts [the Nurses' Health study (NHS), Nurses' Health Study 11 (NHS II), and Health Professionals Follow-up study (HPFS)] [15]. This study examined the relationships between changes in diet and lifestyle factors with weight change using repeated measurements every 4 years and found that SSB was most strongly associated with 4-year weight change after potato chips and potatoes. Each daily increase in one 12-oz. serving of SSBs was associated with approximately 0.5 kg greater weight gain every 4 years (or 0.13 kg per

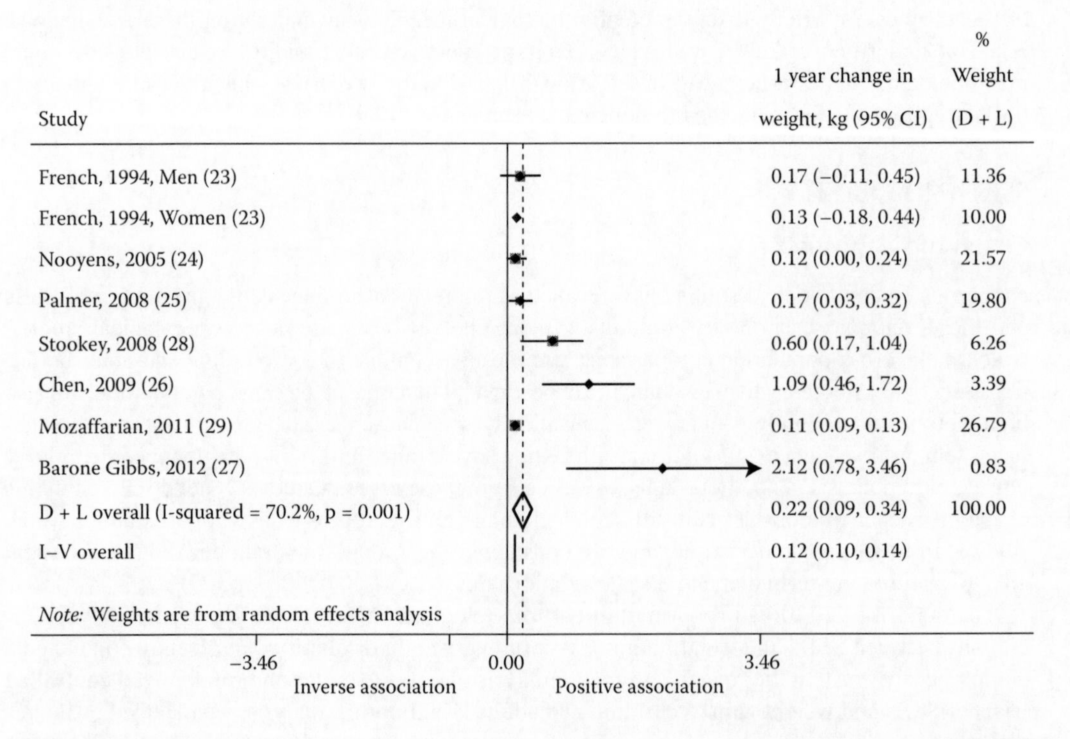

FIGURE 16.1 Forest plot of 1-year changes (95% CI) in weight (kg) per 1 serving/day increase in SSBs from prospective cohort studies in adults using a change versus change analysis strategy. (From Malik VS et al. *The American Journal of Clinical Nutrition*. 2013;98(4):1084–102. Epub 2013/08/24.).

year), in the multivariable adjusted model, which is similar to our results from the meta-analysis. Other obesogenic foods identified in this study included red and processed meat, refined grains, and desserts. In contrast, greater consumption of fruits, vegetables, whole grains, nuts, and yogurt was associated with less weight gain. These results suggest that obesity prevention should focus on improving overall diet quality by consuming more healthy foods and beverages and limiting unhealthy ones. Since a large number of individuals consume multiple servings of SSBs daily, reducing consumption of SSBs is an important step in improving diet quality and reducing long-term weight gain. In an earlier study conducted in over 50,000 participants in the NHS II, women who increased their SSB consumption and maintained a high level of intake gained on average 8.0 kg over 8 years, while women who decreased their SSB intake and maintained a low level of intake gained on average 2.8 kg [16]. Similar results have been observed in other populations including over 40,000 women in the Black Women's Health Study [17] and in a cohort of over 43,000 Chinese men and women in Singapore [18]. Among studies that were excluded from the meta-analysis and reviewed qualitatively, the majority [18–21] found positive associations between SSBs and weight gain in either primary analysis or subgroup findings, while two studies [22,23] did not find significant associations.

The association between SSBs and obesity is strengthened by our recent analysis of gene–SSB interactions, which examined whether consumption of SSBs can modify the genetic risk of obesity, using a genetic predisposition score based on 32 obesity genes identified from genome-wide association studies [24]. Based on data from three large cohorts (NHS, HPFS, and the Women's Genome Health Study), we found that greater consumption of SSBs was associated with a more pronounced genetic effect on elevated body mass index (BMI) and an increased risk of obesity. Individuals who consumed one or more servings of SSBs per day had genetic effects on BMI and obesity risk that were approximately twice as large as those who consumed less than one serving per month. These data suggest that regular consumers of SSBs may be more susceptible to genetic effects on obesity, implying that a genetic predisposition to obesity can be partly offset by healthier beverage choices. Alternatively, persons with a greater genetic predisposition to obesity may be more susceptible to the deleterious effects of SSBs on BMI. These findings may partly explain individual differences in the metabolic response to intake of SSBs.

Randomized Clinical Trials

Compared to observational studies, evidence from randomized clinical trials (RCTs) is limited, and the majority of trials are designed to evaluate short-term effects of specific interventions on weight change rather than long-term patterns. In our recent meta-analysis of five trials including 292 adults, we found that adding SSBs to the diet significantly increased body weight (Figure 16.2) [10]. The weighted mean difference (WMD) in the change in body weight (kg) from baseline to the end of follow-up between intervention and control groups was 0.85 (95% CI: 0.50–1.20). All of the studies in the analysis observed significantly greater weight gain or trends towards greater weight gain in intervention compared with control regimens, and there was no evidence of between-study heterogeneity. Similarly, another meta-analysis of seven RCTs found a significant dose-dependent increase in body weight when SSBs were added to participants' diets [14]. However, in their meta-analysis of another eight trials aiming to reduce SSB consumption (for prevention of weight gain), there was no overall effect on BMI, but a significant benefit was observed among individuals who were initially overweight [14]. This meta-analysis included two recent large and rigorously conducted RCTs in children and adolescents [25,26], which have overcome many of the limitations of previous trials and provide strong evidence that decreasing consumption of SSBs significantly reduces weight gain and obesity in this age group. In the trial by Ebbeling et al. [25], there were significant between-group differences for changes in BMI (−0.57, $P = 0.045$) and weight (−1.9 kg, $P = 0.04$) comparing intervention and control groups after 1 year and in the trial by de Ruyter et al. [26], weight increased by 6.35 kg in the sugar-free beverage group as compared with 7.37 kg in

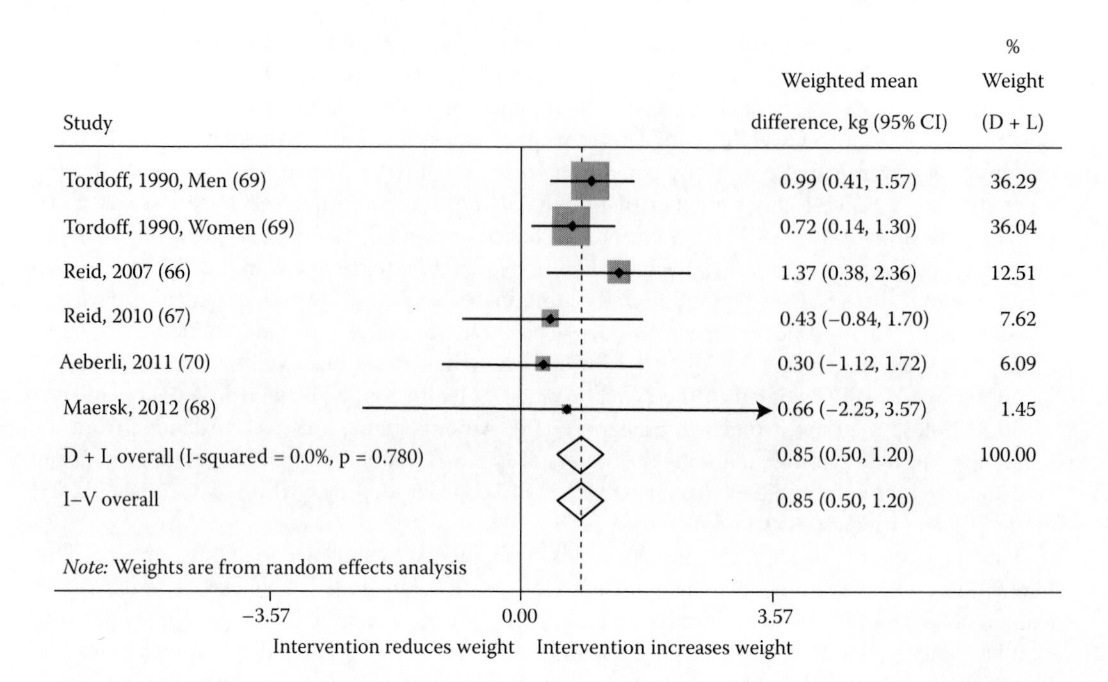

FIGURE 16.2 Forest plot of WMD (95% CI) in weight change (kg) between the intervention and control regimens from randomized controlled trials in adults. Interventions evaluated the effect of adding SSBs. (From Malik VS et al. *The American Journal of Clinical Nutrition*. 2013;98(4):1084–102. Epub 2013/08/24.).

the SSB group (95% CI for the difference, −1.54 to −0.48) after 18 months. It should be noted that these meta-analyses combined studies in adults and children and as pointed out by the authors, many of the trials had methodological limitations including small sample sizes, short duration, poor compliance, lack of randomization at the individual level, lack of blinding and the overstating of subgroup findings, the two recent RCTs in children and adolescents notwithstanding. It should also be noted that some of these trials are "effectiveness" trials of behavioral modification, which evaluate intervention modalities more so than causal relations because their findings are greatly affected by intervention intensity and adherence. Thus, a lack of benefit does not mean that the relation between SSBs and weight gain is not causal but rather that the given modality might not be effective at changing behaviors.

Among trials of SSBs and body weight, it is important to distinguish between those that evaluate weight gain and weight loss. From a public health point of view, identifying dietary determinants of weight gain is more important than short-term weight loss in reducing obesity prevalence in the population [27]. This is because once an individual becomes obese, it is difficult to achieve and maintain weight loss. For this reason, fewer studies have evaluated the impact of SSB restriction on weight loss. Tate et al. [28] recently evaluated replacement of caloric beverages with water or diet beverages as a strategy for weight loss, in a 6-month RCT among overweight and obese adults. At the end of follow-up, all intervention groups showed statistically significant weight loss but there were no differences between groups. However, participants who were assigned to caloric beverage replacement, compared with attention controls (who made dietary changes of their choosing), were twice as likely to have achieved a 5% weight loss over the course of the study. Interestingly, the control group also reduced their caloric beverage consumption despite not being informed about the true study purpose. Thus, a smaller caloric difference between the two beverage substitution groups and the control group was observed, which can explain the lack of significant effects on the amount of weight loss between groups.

Meta-Analysis of Added Sugar

Recently, the World Health Organization commissioned a systematic review and meta-analysis to address the effects of added sugars on body weight and to determine whether the existing evidence supports its current recommendation to limit added sugar intake to less than 10% of total energy [29]. They included 30 RCTs and 38 prospective cohort studies in children and adults that reported the intake of total sugars, a component of total sugars or sugar-containing foods and beverages and at least one measure of body fatness. Of the 16 cohort studies in adults, 11 reported one or more significantly positive associations between a sugar exposure and measure of adiposity and one study reported both significantly positive and negative associations. Possible reasons for the variable findings in this study include too short a duration of follow-up (2 years) and the small increment of sweets or SSBs (100 g/day) used for estimating risk in the estimates. The meta-analysis found that in trials of adults with ad libitum diets, decreased intake of added sugars by comparison with no reduction or an increase in sugar intakes (differences in sugar intakes between intervention and control groups ranged from less than 1% to 14% of total energy intake) significantly reduced body weight (0.80 kg, 95% CI: 0.39–1.21; $P < 0.001$) in studies ranging from 10 weeks to 8 months, whereas increased consumption led to a comparable weight increase (0.75 kg, 95% CI: 0.30–1.19; $P = 0.001$). The authors concluded that "Among free living people involving ad libitum diets, intake of free sugars or SSBs is a determinant of body weight." Furthermore, the authors noted, "When considering the rapid weight gain that occurs after an increased intake of sugars, it seems reasonable to conclude that advice relating to sugar intake is a relevant component of a strategy to reduce the high risk of overweight and obesity in most countries."

SSBs AND DIABETES

A growing body of evidence indicates that SSB consumption is associated with increased risk of diabetes through effects on adiposity and independently through other metabolic effects. Although experimental evidence from RCTs is lacking due to high cost and other feasibility considerations, findings from prospective cohort studies have shown a relatively strong and consistent association in well-powered studies. We conducted a meta-analysis of eight prospective cohort studies evaluating SSB intake and risk of diabetes [11] (Figure 16.3). Based on 310,819 participants and 15,043 cases, individuals in the highest category of SSB intake (usually 1–2 servings per day) had a 26% (RR:

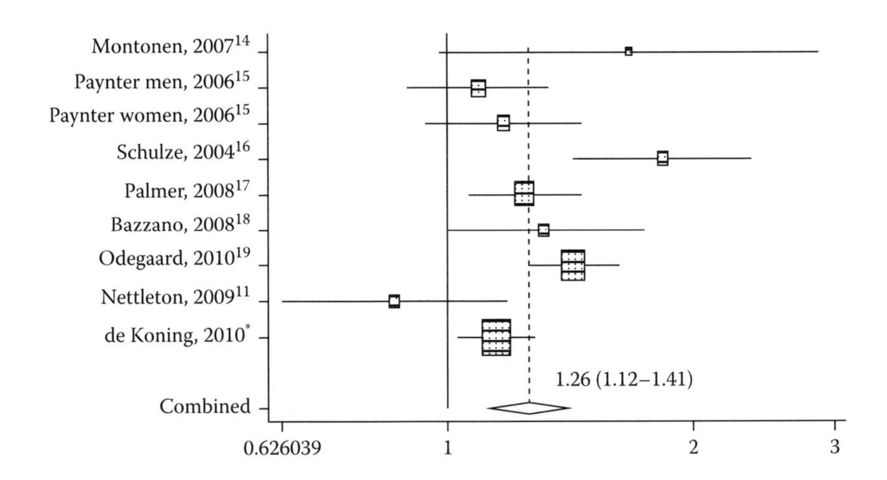

FIGURE 16.3 Forest plot of studies evaluating SSB consumption and risk of type 2 diabetes, comparing extreme categories of intake. Random-effects estimate (DerSimonian and Laird method). *Personal communication. (From Malik VS et al. *Diabetes Care*. 2010;33(11):2477–83.)

1.26; 95% CI: 1.12–1.41) greater risk of developing diabetes compared to those in the lowest category (none or less than one per month). A one serving per day increase in SSB was associated with about 15% increased risk for diabetes (RR: 1.15; 95% CI: 1.11–1.20). This association is consistent across ethnic groups (Caucasians, African-Americans, and Asians), gender, and age groups. As with our meta-analysis on weight gain, we selected estimates that did not adjust for potential intermediates in the causal chain such as total energy intake and BMI. A similar association was recently found in a subcohort of 15,374 participants and 11,684 incident cases from eight cohorts participating in the European Prospective Investigation into Cancer and Nutrition (EPIC) study [30]. In adjusted models, a one serving per day increase in SSB was associated with a 22% increased risk of diabetes (RR: 1.22; 95% CI: 1.09–1.38). As expected, the association was attenuated after further adjustment for total energy intake and BMI (RR: 1.18; 95% CI: 1.06–1.32). In a separate study, the French component of EPIC, which included 66,118 women and 1369 incident cases, found that women in the highest quartile of SSB intake had a 34% increase of diabetes compared to nonconsumers (RR: 1.34; 95% CI: 1.05–1.71) [31]. In sensitivity analyses, associations were partly mediated by BMI, although there was still a strong significant independent effect.

A recent systematic review of cohort studies and RCTs evaluated the effect of sugar intake including SSBs, sucrose, and fructose on risk of diabetes, cardiovascular disease, and related metabolic risk factors [32]. This review was part of the fifth version of the Nordic Nutrition Recommendations (NNR) project, with the aim of reviewing and updating the scientific basis of the fourth edition of the NNR issued in 2004, which like the WHO recommends a maximal intake of 10% of total energy from added sugars. Nine cohort studies were identified for incidence of diabetes. Of these, four of six studies found significant positive associations for SSBs. In general, larger studies with longer durations of follow-up reported stronger associations, and BMI seemed to mediate part of the increased risk, which supports findings from our meta-analysis [11] and previous reviews [3,9,12,33]. Intake of total sugars, glucose, or fructose was not consistently associated with diabetes. The authors suggested that one reason for this might be that a significant proportion of the sugars consumed were not added sugar but naturally occurring sugars in fruits, for example. Some studies have shown beneficial effects of fruit consumption on risk of diabetes [34].

As previously mentioned, trial data on SSBs and diabetes as an endpoint is limited, however short-term mechanistic studies have established a biologic rationale with biomarkers of diabetes risk such as insulin resistance and chronic inflammation. These studies in combination with findings from cohort studies make a strong case for causality [27].

SSBS, OBESITY, AND DIABETES: ARE THE ASSOCIATIONS CAUSAL?

RCTs are generally considered the gold standard in epidemiology for establishing a causal relationship between an exposure and an outcome. However, most trials of SSBs and obesity have been short-term and it is not feasible to examine the relationship between SSB consumption and risk of chronic diseases such as diabetes through RCTs because of cost and compliance issues. Realistically, an ideal RCT may never be conducted in free-living populations for dietary behavioral changes since almost all trials, no matter how well designed, will suffer from one or more major limitations, such as reduced compliance over time and infeasibility of blinding the interventions. On the other hand, large cohort studies, particularly those with repeated measures that carefully adjust for potential confounders, are powerful tools to investigate long-term associations between dietary exposures and chronic disease risk. Therefore, to make inferences about causality between SSBs and obesity and diabetes, it is essential to consider evidence from both RCTs and prospective cohort studies.

To answer the question whether the associations between SSB consumption and obesity and diabetes are causal, we applied the Bradford Hill criteria for causality to the available evidence [27,33]. This set of conditions commonly used in noncommunicable disease epidemiology evaluates an evidence-base according to nine criteria [35].

1. *Strength of the association*: Our meta-analysis of cohort studies found that a one serving per day increase in SSBs was associated with an additional weight gain of 0.12–0.22 kg over 1 year [10]. Although the effect size seems modest, the unit of exposure is relatively small (i.e., one serving per day). RCTs have shown greater short-term weight gain with the addition of SSBs to the diet and clinically significant benefits of reducing SSBs or added sugar consumption on body weight. From our meta-analysis of cohort studies on diabetes, we found that daily consumers of SSBs had a 26% greater risk of developing diabetes compared to infrequent or nonconsumers (RR: 1.26; 95% CI: 1.12–1.41) [11]. Experimental studies of SSBs and biomarkers of diabetes risk support this association [33].
2. *Consistency of the association*: The evidence from prospective cohort studies and RCTs for obesity and risk of diabetes is highly consistent.
3. *Specificity of the association*: Consumption of SSBs increases the risk of related metabolic conditions and unrelated conditions such as dental caries. This criterion has limited utility since causes of a given effect cannot be expected to lack other effects on any logical grounds.
4. *Temporality of the association*: The temporal relationships between SSBs and obesity and diabetes risk are well established, given that the evidence reviewed here is derived from prospective cohort studies and RCTs.
5. *Biological gradient or dose–response*: As SSB intake increases, the amount of weight gain increases in a dose–response manner. Similarly as SSB increases, risk of diabetes too increases.
6. *Biological plausibility*: SSBs contain large amounts of energy from rapidly absorbable sugars. Consumption of these calories in liquid form is associated with less satiety and an incomplete compensatory reduction in energy intake at subsequent meals, leading to the overconsumption of total daily calories [9]. SSBs lead to diabetes through obesity and independently through glycemic effects from postprandial spikes in blood glucose and insulin and also from the metabolic consequences of fructose [9].
7. *Biological coherence*: The interpretation of the associations between SSBs and obesity and diabetes risk does not conflict with what is currently known about the natural history of these conditions.
8. *Experimental evidence*: RCTs have shown that reducing consumption of SSBs or added sugars significantly decreases weight gain and that adding SSBs to the diet significantly increases weight gain. Short-term mechanistic studies have shown that SSB consumption increases visceral adiposity, dyslipidemia, insulin resistance, and plasma concentrations of uric acid and inflammatory cytokines.
9. *Analogous evidence or alternate explanations*: The positive associations between SSBs and obesity and diabetes risk found in observational studies may be due to confounding by other correlated dietary and lifestyle factors. However, these factors were carefully adjusted for in multivariable analyses in most studies. Results from RCTs are not susceptible to such confounding and support conclusions from observational studies.

Taken together, the current evidence on SSBs and obesity and diabetes meets all of the key criteria commonly used to evaluate causal relationships in epidemiology. Thus, there is compelling evidence that SSB intake is causally related to increased risk of obesity and diabetes. This does not mean that work in this area is complete. The scientific evidence should continue to evolve regarding the health effects of SSBs and be used to guide and update nutritional policy. As Sir Austin Bradford Hill wrote several decades ago [35]:

> All scientific work is incomplete—whether it be observational or experimental. All scientific work is liable to be upset or modified by advancing knowledge. That does not confer upon us a freedom to ignore the knowledge we already have, or to postpone the action it appears to demand at a given time.

SSBs AND CARDIOVASCULAR RISK

There is increasing evidence that higher SSB consumption increases cardiovascular risk by contributing to the development of hypertension, dyslipidemia, inflammation, coronary heart disease, and stroke. We pooled findings from three prospective cohort studies evaluating SSBs and risk of metabolic syndrome, which is a clustering of metabolic risk factors including central obesity, elevated triglycerides, reduced HDL cholesterol, elevated fasting plasma glucose, and elevated blood pressure [11]. Based on 19,431 participants and 5803 cases, we observed a 20% increased risk of metabolic syndrome comparing highest to lowest categories of intake. In the Coronary Artery Risk Development in Young Adults (CARDIA) study, higher SSB consumption was associated with a number of cardiometabolic outcomes: high waist circumference (RR: 1.09; 95% CI: 1.04–1.14), high LDL cholesterol (RR: 1.18; 95% CI: 1.02–1.35), high triglycerides (RR: 1.06; 95% CI: 1.01–1.13), and hypertension (RR: 1.06; 95% CI: 1.01–1.12) [36].

Findings for hypertension are supported by stronger associations in the NHS and NHS II cohorts. Women who consumed ≥4 servings per day of SSBs had a 44% (RR: 1.44; 95% CI: 0.98–2.11) and 28% (RR: 1.28; 95% CI: 1.01–1.62) greater risk of developing hypertension, respectively, compared with infrequent consumers [37]. In a post hoc analysis of an 18-month behavioral intervention trial, a reduction in consumption of SSBs was significantly associated with reduced blood pressure, even after adjustment for weight change [38]. Regarding lipid parameters, Dhingra et al. [19] found that daily soft drink consumers had a 22% greater risk of developing hypertriglyceridemia (≥1.7 mmol L^{-1} or on treatment; RR = 1.22, 95% CI: 1.07–1.41) and low–high-density lipoprotein (HDL) cholesterol (<1.03 mmol L^{-1} for men and <1.3 mmol L^{-1} for women or on treatment; RR = 1.22, 95% CI: 1.04–1.44) compared with non-consumers. Similarly, among participants in the Multi-Ethnic Study of Atherosclerosis, daily SSB consumers had a 28% greater risk of developing hypertriglyceridemia (RR = 1.28, 95% CI: 1.02–1.60) and low-HDL cholesterol (RR = 1.28, 95% CI: 0.99–1.64) than non-consumers [39].

Data from short-term trials also provide important evidence linking SSBs with cardiovascular risk. Raben et al. [40] found that a sucrose-rich diet consumed for 10 weeks resulted in significant elevations of postprandial glycemia, insulinemia, and lipidemia compared to a diet rich in artificial sweeteners in overweight healthy subjects. A randomized crossover trial among normal weight healthy men found that after 3 weeks, SSBs consumed in small-to-moderate quantities (600 mL SSB/day containing 40–80 g of sugar) significantly impaired glucose and lipid metabolism and promoted inflammation [41]. Specifically, LDL particle size was reduced for high-fructose and high-sucrose SSBs and a more atherogenic LDL subclass distribution was seen when fructose and high-sucrose-containing SSBs were consumed [41]. Fasting glucose and high-sensitivity C-reactive protein (CRP) increased significantly after fructose, glucose, and sucrose interventions and leptin increased during interventions with SSBs containing glucose [41]. A 10-week intervention comparing effects of sucrose and artificially sweetened food/beverages on markers of inflammation found that serum levels of haptoglobin, transferrin, and CRP were elevated in the sucrose group compared to the sweetener group [42].

SSBs may affect risk of coronary heart disease (CHD) in just a few years through effects on inflammation, which influences atherosclerosis, plaque stability, and thrombosis. In the NHS, we found that regular SSB intake was significantly associated with increased incidence of CHD (nonfatal myocardial infarction or fatal CHD) [43]. In over 88,000 women followed for 24 years, those who consumed ≥2 servings per day of SSBs had a 35% greater risk of CHD compared with infrequent consumers, after adjusting for other unhealthy lifestyle factors (RR: 1.35; 95% CI: 1.10, 1.20) [43]. Additional adjustment for potential mediating factors (including BMI, total energy intake, and incident diabetes) attenuated the associations, but they remained statistically significant, suggesting that the effect of SSBs may not be entirely mediated by these factors. Similar results were found in the HPFS among 42,883 men [44]. In this study, intake of SSBs was also significantly associated with increased plasma concentrations of inflammatory cytokines, including CRP, interleukin-6, and tumor necrosis factor receptors [44].

Recent evidence has also emerged linking intake of SSBs to increased risk of stroke. Among 84,085 women and 43,371 men in the Harvard cohorts followed for 28 and 22 years, respectively, ≥1 serving of SSB per day was associated with 16% increased risk of total stroke (RR: 1.16; 95% CI: 1.00–1.34) compared with none in multivariable adjusted models [45]. An association of a similar magnitude was also observed for diet soda. However, as mentioned by the authors, the association between diet drinks and stroke should be interpreted with caution since they did not find associations between diet drinks and weight gain, diabetes, or CHD in their study population, which are risk factors for stroke, and a clear biologic mechanism between diet drink consumption and stroke is not known [45]. In the multiethnic cohort of 2564 residents in Northern Manhattan followed for a mean of 10 years, daily soft drink consumption was associated with an increased risk of vascular events (stroke, MI, and vascular death) only in participants free of obesity, diabetes, and metabolic syndrome [46]. This study also found a significant association with diet drinks that warrants further investigation. A Japanese cohort of 39,786 men and women followed for 18 years found significant positive associations between SSB intake and total and ischemic stroke in women but not in men [47]. Adjustment for BMI and total energy intake had little effect, suggesting that these factors are not major mediators. SSB intake was not associated with risk of ischemic heart disease or hemorrhagic stroke for either sex [47].

Lastly, intake of both added sugars and SSBs was associated with an increased risk for CVD mortality in a recent analysis of National Health and Nutrition Examination Survey III Linked Morality cohort data [48]. After a median of 14.6 years of follow-up, added sugar intake was associated with a two-fold (RR: 2.03; 95% CI: 1.26–3.27) greater risk of CVD death comparing extreme quintiles of intake in the fully adjusted model including BMI, systolic blood pressure, total serum cholesterol, and total energy intake. Participants who consumed seven or more servings per week of SSB had a 29% greater risk of CVD mortality compared to those who consumed 1 serving per week or less. In contrast, a recent analysis from the NIH-AARP Diet and Health Study, a prospective cohort of older US adults aged 50–71 years at baseline, found that intake of total fructose but not of added sugar was associated with a modest increase in risk of all-cause mortality in men and women [49]. However, all investigated sugars from beverages, including added sugars, were positively associated with risk of all-cause, CVD, and other cause mortality in women, while only fructose from beverages was positively associated with risk of all-cause and CVD mortality in men. Additional confirmatory studies evaluating the impact of added sugars and SSBs on mortality are warranted.

SSBs AND OTHER METABOLIC DISEASES

SSBs contain large amounts of fructose from added sugars, which is known to increase serum uric acid levels. Regular consumption of SSBs has been associated with hyperuricemia as well as with gout, which is a common form of inflammatory arthritis arising from deposition of uric acid in articular cartilage, in our cohorts [50,51]. Men and women who consumed ≥2 SSBs per day had an 85% (RR: 1.85; 95% CI: 1.08–3.16) [50] and over two-fold (RR: 2.39; 95% CI: 1.34–4.26) [51] increased risk of developing gout compared to infrequent consumers, respectively. Consumption of SSBs, particularly cola-type soft drinks which usually contain caramel color, has also been associated with development of albuminuria, a marker of early kidney damage, formation of kidney stones, and increased risk of chronic kidney disease [52,53]. In the NHS II, sucrose consumption was associated with an increased risk of incident kidney stones [54]. Women in the highest quintile of sucrose intake had a 31% increased risk of developing kidney stones compared to infrequent consumers [54]. Observational studies have also found that a higher intake of sucrose and fructose and a higher dietary glycemic load, of which SSB is a large contributor, is associated with a higher frequency of gallstones [55,56]. It has been estimated that the equivalent of 40 g of sugar per day doubles the risk of symptomatic gallstones [57].

BIOLOGICAL MECHANISMS

The prevailing mechanisms linking SSB intake to weight gain are decreased satiety and an incomplete compensatory reduction in energy intake at subsequent meals following ingestion of liquid calories [9]. A typical 12 oz. serving of soda contains on average 140–150 cal and 35–37.5 g of dietary sugars, which is equivalent to about 10 teaspoons of table sugar. If these calories are added to the typical diet without compensation for the additional calories, one can of soda per day, could in theory lead to a weight gain of 5 pounds in 1 year [33]. Short-term feeding studies comparing SSBs to artificially sweetened beverages in relation to energy intake [58] and weight change [40,58–61] illustrate this point. Additional evidence supporting incomplete compensation for liquid calories has been provided by studies showing greater energy intake and weight gain after isocaloric consumption of beverages compared to solid food [62,63]. These studies argue that sugar or HFCS in liquid beverages may not suppress intake of solid foods to the level needed to maintain energy balance; however, the mechanisms responsible for the weaker compensatory response to fluids is largely unknown.

SSBs may contribute to the development of diabetes and cardiovascular risk, in part, through the caloric effects and ability to induce weight gain, but there are also likely noncalorically related effects arising from the high amounts of rapidly absorbable sugars or HFCS in these beverages. [9] (Figure 16.4). Consumption of SSBs has been shown to induce rapid spikes in blood glucose and insulin levels [40,64], which in combination with the large volumes consumed contribute to a high dietary glycemic load. High-GL diets are thought to stimulate appetite and promote weight gain due to the higher postprandial insulin response following ingestion of a high-GL meal [65]. High-GL diets have also been shown to stimulate insulin secretion due to postprandial hyperglycemia leading to hyperinsulinemia and insulin resistance [65]. An increase in GL has also been shown to exacerbate levels of inflammatory biomarkers such as CRP [66]. Inflammation is known to influence atherosclerosis, plaque stability, and thrombosis; therefore, SSB consumption may affect CHD risk within just a few years. High-dietary GL has also been associated with greater risk of CHD [43,44]. In addition, the caramel coloring used in cola-type soft drinks is high in advanced glycation end products, which may further increase insulin resistance and inflammation [67,68]. Habitual consumption of diets with a high GL may also influence cancer risk via hyperinsulinemia and the insulin-like growth factor axis [69].

Some evidence also suggests that consuming fructose, a constituent of sucrose, and in slightly higher amounts from HFCS and fruit juices may exert additional adverse cardiometabolic effects, as reviewed in Chapter 19. Fructose is preferentially metabolized to lipid in the liver, leading to increased hepatic de novo lipogenesis, atherogenic dyslipidemia, and insulin resistance [70]. Fructose has also

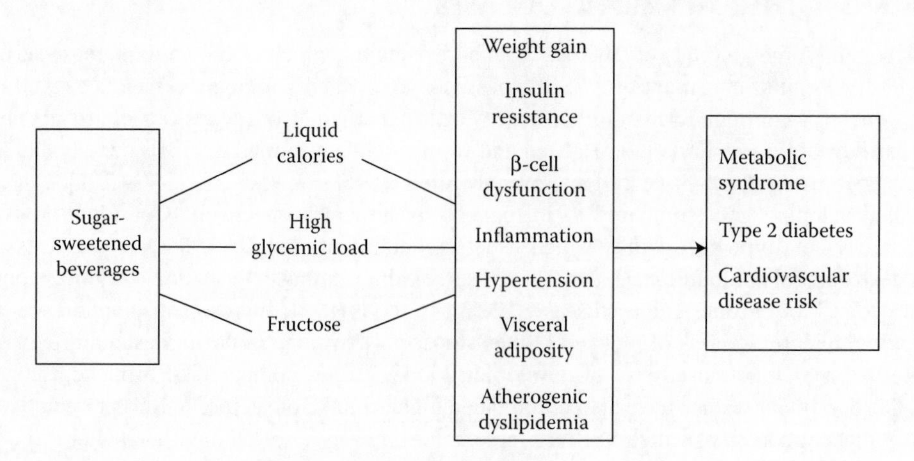

FIGURE 16.4 Biological mechanisms linking SSBs to weight gain and related chronic diseases. (From Malik VS et al. *Circulation*. 2010;121(11):1356–64.).

been shown to promote the accumulation of visceral adiposity and the deposition of ectopic fat [71–74]. Fructose is the only sugar known to increase serum uric acid levels by increasing adenosine triphosphate degradation to adenosine monophosphate, a precursor of uric acid [75]. The production of uric acid in the liver may reduce endothelial nitric oxide, which may partly explain the association between SSBs and CHD [76]. Fructose may also increase cancer risk through oxidative stress [77].

METHODOLOGICAL CONSIDERATIONS IN OBSERVATIONAL STUDIES

As previously mentioned, prospective cohort studies are powerful tools in capturing long-term patterns of diet and disease since, in contrast to most trials, they are of sufficient duration for causal action and disease initiation to occur. However, certain limitations inherent in these studies are important to consider when interpreting the evidence. Most of the prospective cohort studies discussed in this chapter adjusted their analyses for potential confounding by various diet and lifestyle factors, and for the majority, a positive association persisted, suggesting an independent effect of SSBs. However, residual confounding by unmeasured or imperfectly measured factors may still exist. Higher SSBs or sugar intake could be a marker of a globally unhealthy diet. Therefore, incomplete adjustment for various lifestyle factors could lead to an overestimation of the association. Because results are consistent across different cohorts, this reduces the likelihood that residual confounding is responsible for the findings.

Another issue that can seriously impact results is whether a study has adjusted for intermediate factors in the causal chain such as adjusting for total energy intake when evaluating SSBs and body weight. In these scenarios, associations will be attenuated since adjusting for an intermediate is equivalent to removing its effects from the disease process. Still, some studies have shown positive associations between SSBs and obesity and diabetes after adjusting for mediating factors like total energy intake and BMI, which supports an effect of SSBs that is not entirely mediated through these factors [16,78]. Measurement error in dietary assessment is inevitable, but in the setting of prospective cohort studies, the misclassification of SSB intake does not likely differ by case status. Such nondifferential misclassification of exposure may actually attenuate the associations. Awareness of weight status could, however, result in systematic underreporting of SSB intake, which could weaken associations between SSBs and weight gain.

Longitudinal studies evaluating diet and body weight or chronic diseases may also be prone to reverse causation (i.e., people change their diet in response to their weight or health, which could result in spurious associations). Ascertainment of repeated measures of exposure and outcome or stable exposure patterns during long periods of follow-up may reduce the likelihood of this bias. For this reason, in our recent meta-analysis of SSBs and weight gain, we included only studies with repeated measures [10].

HEALTHY ALTERNATIVES TO SSBs

Several beverages have been suggested as alternatives to SSBs including water, 100% fruit juice, coffee, tea, and artificially sweetened drinks. Unlike SSBs, water does not contain liquid calories, and small short-term studies have shown that water consumption before a meal is associated with an increase in satiety and a subsequent lower energy intake [79–81]. In a recent analysis in the Harvard cohorts, we found that replacement of 1 serving per day of SSBs with one serving of water was associated with 0.49 kg (95% CI: 0.32–0.65) less weight gain over each 4-year period [82]. Substitution of SSBs with other beverages (coffee, tea, diet beverages, low-fat milk) was also associated with significantly less weight gain [82]. In the NHS II, substituting water for SSBs was also associated with a significantly lower risk of diabetes [83]. For most people with access to safe drinking water, water is the optimal calorie-free beverage because it is cheap and readily accessible.

One hundred percent fruit juices could be perceived to be a healthy alternative to SSBs, since juices contain some vitamins and other nutrients. However, fruit juices also contain a relatively high number of calories from natural sugars, with likely greater amounts of fructose, and should therefore be consumed in moderation. Previous cohort studies have found positive associations between consumption of fruit juice and greater weight gain [16] and diabetes [84]. Thus, it has been recommended that daily intake of fruit juices be limited to 4–6 oz.

Numerous prospective cohort studies have shown that regular consumption of coffee (decaffeinated or regular) and tea can have favorable effects on diabetes and cardiovascular disease risk (85–88) possibly because of their high polyphenol content. Thus, coffee and tea are healthy alternatives to SSBs for individuals without contraindications provided that caloric sweeteners and creamers are used sparingly. In NHS II, substituting one serving of SSBs with one cup of coffee daily was associated with a 17% lower risk of diabetes [78].

Artificially sweetened beverages such as diet soda may be a reasonable alternative to SSBs since they provide few to no calories, however little is known about the long-term consequences of consuming any artificial sweeteners such as aspartame, sucralose, saccharine, acesulfame potassium, and neotame [89]. As reviewed in more detail in Chapter 7, some studies have reported positive associations between diet soda consumption and weight gain and risk of metabolic syndrome and diabetes [19,39,90]. However, these findings may be due to reverse causation or residual confounding since individuals who consume diet soda are more likely to have higher BMI and a greater prevalence of comorbidities and dieting behaviors. In our cohorts, we found nonsignificant associations between diet soda and diabetes [16,78] and CHD [43] after adjustment for baseline weight and comorbidities. In contrast, some evidence suggests that the intense sweetness of artificial sweeteners [91] may condition towards a greater preference for sweets and enhance appetite [23]. Consumers of diet soda may also use this choice as rationale for consuming other unhealthy high-calorie foods, ultimately leading to weight gain [89]. Although consumption of artificially sweetened beverages is preferable to the use of SSBs, further studies are needed to evaluate the long-term metabolic consequences of artificial sweeteners.

IMPLICATIONS FOR PUBLIC HEALTH POLICY

In light of the mounting evidence linking regular consumption of SSBs to obesity and related chronic diseases, national and international organizations have already called for reductions in intake of these beverages to help prevent obesity and improve overall health [92]. Both the WHO, and American Heart Association recommend limiting intake of all added sugars and numerous associations including the American Diabetes Association, American Academy of Pediatrics, Institute of Medicine of the National Academies, American Medical Association, Centers for Disease Control and Prevention and United States Department of Agriculture specifically recommend limiting intake of SSBs. In addition to strong and widespread public health recommendations, public policy interventions are often required to change consumption patterns and individual behaviors because they can bring about rapid and effective changes in the food environment [8]. A combination of strategies across multiple levels are thus needed to reduce intake of SSBs, as illustrated in Box 16.1. Implementing and evaluating these types of strategies should be a priority for the scientific community and policymakers.

Combining incentives and disincentives can be an effective strategy to encourage consumption of healthy alternatives in the place of SSBs. Taxation of SSBs is one approach that is being considered by some governments as a means of reducing intake of SSBs in the place of healthier alternatives and offset some of the high healthcare costs attributed to obesity. For cigarette smoking, imposing steep taxes has been successful in reducing their use, particularly among young people who are more sensitive to the price of cigarettes than adults. Current taxes on SSBs in most states are probably too low to have an appreciable impact on purchasing behaviors [93]. For this reason, additional tax increases around 20% have been suggested, based on econometric and modeling studies [94–96]. Restrictions on access to SSBs with a large-portion size have also been considered by some governments and some experts have proposed limiting the use of Supplemental Nutrition Assistance Program (SNAP) benefits for SSBs or subsidizing SNAP purchases of healthier foods.

BOX 16.1 POLICY STRATEGIES FOR REDUCING SSBs

- Social marketing and public health campaigns are needed to raise awareness about the health effects of SSBs and added sugars and about healthy alternatives.
- Governments should impose financial incentives such as taxation of SSBs, and implement limits for use of Supplemental Nutrition Assistance Program (SNAP) benefits for SSBs or subsidizing SNAP purchases of healthier foods, to encourage healthier beverages choices.
- Regulations are needed to reduce exposure to marketing of SSBs in the media and at sports events or other activities.
- Policies should be put in place to reduce the availability of SSBs in the workplace, health-care facilities, government institutions, and other public places and ensure access to safe water and healthy alternatives. Restrictions should also be put in place on large portion sizes.
- Educational campaigns about the health risks associated with overconsumption of SSBs should be aimed at health-care professionals and clinical populations.
- National and international campaigns targeting obesity and chronic disease prevention should include the health risks associated with overconsumption of SSBs.
- National and international dietary recommendations should include specific guidelines for healthy beverage consumption.

These types of regulations and laws, together with education and social marketing or public health campaigns, are an important approach to changing social norms and improving food and beverage consumption patterns on the population level.

CONCLUSIONS AND FUTURE DIRECTIONS

Intake of added sugars, predominantly from SSBs, has increased markedly in recent decades, in parallel with the upsurge in obesity and related chronic diseases. The totality of the available evidence from observational studies and experimental trials is sufficient to conclude that consumption of SSBs causes excess weight gain and diabetes in adults and that these beverages are unique dietary contributors to obesity and related chronic diseases. Several public policy and regulatory strategies to reduce intake of SSBs are already in place or are being considered. Implementing and evaluating such policies are important areas for scientists and policymakers. However, the scientific evidence should continue to evolve regarding the health effects of SSBs and be used to guide and update nutritional recommendations and policy.

Key areas that warrant future research include establishing a consensus on the definition of added sugars and SSBs, examining the effects of different sugars (glucose vs. fructose vs. sucrose) on health outcomes, investigating the health effects of sugar consumed in solid form in comparison to liquid sugar and further elucidating the biological mechanism by which intake of liquid calories induces an incomplete compensatory intake of energy at subsequent meals. There is also a need for additional studies to examine the impact of reducing SSB intake on weight loss and to explore the biological and behavioral mechanisms underlying this relationship. More studies evaluating SSBs and cancer risk are warranted as well as those evaluating the long-term health effects of consuming artificial sweeteners as a substitute for sugar. Lastly, more and higher-quality RCTs are needed to identify effective strategies to reduce SSB consumption at the individual and population level. Although reducing consumption of SSBs or added sugars alone is unlikely to solve the obesity epidemic entirely, limiting intake is one simple change that could have a measurable impact on weight control and prevention of chronic diseases.

REFERENCES

1. Gross LS, Li L, Ford ES, Liu S. Increased consumption of refined carbohydrates and the epidemic of type 2 diabetes in the United States: An ecologic assessment. *The American Journal of Clinical Nutrition*. 2004;79(5):774–9. Epub 2004/04/29.
2. Bray GA, Nielsen SJ, Popkin BM. Consumption of high-fructose corn syrup in beverages may play a role in the epidemic of obesity. *The American Journal of Clinical Nutrition*. 2004;79(4):537–43. Epub 2004/03/31.
3. Hu FB, Malik VS. Sugar-sweetened beverages and risk of obesity and type 2 diabetes: Epidemiologic evidence. *Physiology & Behavior*. 2010;100(1):47–54.
4. National Cancer Institute. Sources of Calories from Added Sugars among the US population, 2005–2006. Risk Factor Monitoring and Methods Branch Web site. Applied Research Program. Mean intake of added sugars & percentage contribution of various foods among us population. http://riskfactor.cancer.gov/diet/foodsources/added_sugars/ (accessed 10 February 2013).
5. Welsh JA, Sharma AJ, Grellinger L, Vos MB. Consumption of added sugars is decreasing in the United States. *The American Journal of Clinical Nutrition*. 2011;94(3):726–34.
6. Ogden CL, Kit BK, Carroll MD, Park S. Consumption of sugar drinks in the United States, 2005–2008. *NCHS Data Brief*. 2011(71):1–8. Epub 2012/05/24.
7. Johnson RK, Appel LJ, Brands M, Howard BV, Lefevre M, Lustig RH et al. Dietary sugars intake and cardiovascular health: A scientific statement from the American Heart Association. *Circulation*. 2009;120(11):1011–20.
8. Malik VS, Willett WC, Hu FB. Global obesity: Trends, risk factors and policy implications. *Nature Reviews Endocrinology*. 2013;9(1):13–27. Epub 2012/11/21.
9. Malik VS, Popkin BM, Bray GA, Despres JP, Hu FB. Sugar-sweetened beverages, obesity, type 2 diabetes mellitus, and cardiovascular disease risk. *Circulation*. 2010;121(11):1356–64.
10. Malik VS, Pan A, Willett WC, Hu FB. Sugar-sweetened beverages and weight gain in children and adults: A systematic review and meta-analysis. *The American Journal of Clinical Nutrition*. 2013;98(4):1084–102. Epub 2013/08/24.
11. Malik VS, Popkin BM, Bray GA, Despres JP, Willett WC, Hu FB. Sugar-sweetened beverages and risk of metabolic syndrome and type 2 diabetes: A meta-analysis. *Diabetes Care*. 2010;33(11):2477–83.
12. Malik VS, Schulze MB, Hu FB. Intake of sugar-sweetened beverages and weight gain: A systematic review. *The American Journal of Clinical Nutrition*. 2006;84(2):274–88.
13. Vartanian LR, Schwartz MB, Brownell KD. Effects of soft drink consumption on nutrition and health: A systematic review and meta-analysis. *American Journal of Public Health*. 2007;97(4):667–75.
14. Kaiser KA, Shikany JM, Keating KD, Allison DB. Will reducing sugar-sweetened beverage consumption reduce obesity? Evidence supporting conjecture is strong, but evidence when testing effect is weak. *Obesity Reviews: An Official Journal of the International Association for the Study of Obesity*. 2013;14(8):620–33. Epub 2013/06/08.
15. Mozaffarian D, Hao T, Rimm EB, Willett WC, Hu FB. Changes in diet and lifestyle and long-term weight gain in women and men. *The New England Journal of Medicine*. 2011;364(25):2392–404.
16. Schulze MB, Manson JE, Ludwig DS, Colditz GA, Stampfer MJ, Willett WC et al. Sugar-sweetened beverages, weight gain, and incidence of type 2 diabetes in young and middle-aged women. *JAMA: The Journal of the American Medical Association*. 2004;292(8):927–34.
17. Palmer JR, Boggs DA, Krishnan S, Hu FB, Singer M, Rosenberg L. Sugar-sweetened beverages and incidence of type 2 diabetes mellitus in African American women. *Archives of Internal Medicine*. 2008;168(14):1487–92.
18. Odegaard AO, Koh WP, Arakawa K, Yu MC, Pereira MA. Soft drink and juice consumption and risk of physician-diagnosed incident type 2 diabetes: The Singapore Chinese Health Study. *American Journal of Epidemiology*. 2010;171(6):701–8.
19. Dhingra R, Sullivan L, Jacques PF, Wang TJ, Fox CS, Meigs JB et al. Soft drink consumption and risk of developing cardiometabolic risk factors and the metabolic syndrome in middle-aged adults in the community. *Circulation*. 2007;116(5):480–8.
20. Bes-Rastrollo M, Sanchez-Villegas A, Gomez-Gracia E, Martinez JA, Pajares RM, Martinez-Gonzalez MA. Predictors of weight gain in a Mediterranean cohort: The Seguimiento Universidad de Navarra Study 1. *The American Journal of Clinical Nutrition*. 2006;83(2):362–70; quiz 94–5.
21. Inoue M, Toyokawa S, Inoue K, Suyama Y, Miyano Y, Suzuki T et al. Lifestyle, weight perception and change in body mass index of Japanese workers: MY Health Up Study. *Public Health*. 2010;124(9):530–7.

22. Kvaavik E, Meyer HE, Tverdal A. Food habits, physical activity and body mass index in relation to smoking status in 40–42-year-old Norwegian women and men. *Preventive Medicine*. 2004;38(1):1–5.
23. Fowler SP, Williams K, Resendez RG, Hunt KJ, Hazuda HP, Stern MP. Fueling the obesity epidemic? Artificially sweetened beverage use and long-term weight gain. *Obesity (Silver Spring)*. 2008;16(8):1894–900.
24. Qi Q, Chu AY, Kang JH, Jensen MK, Curhan GC, Pasquale LR et al. Sugar-sweetened beverages and genetic risk of obesity. *The New England Journal of Medicine*. 2012;367(15):1387–96.
25. Ebbeling CB, Feldman HA, Chomitz VR, Antonelli TA, Gortmaker SL, Osganian SK et al. A randomized trial of sugar-sweetened beverages and adolescent body weight. *The New England Journal of Medicine*. 2012;367(15):1407–16.
26. de Ruyter JC, Olthof MR, Seidell JC, Katan MB. A trial of sugar-free or sugar-sweetened beverages and body weight in children. *The New England Journal of Medicine*. 2012;367(15):1397–406.
27. Hu FB. Resolved: There is sufficient scientific evidence that decreasing sugar-sweetened beverage consumption will reduce the prevalence of obesity and obesity-related diseases. *Obesity Reviews: An Official Journal of the International Association for the Study of Obesity*. 2013;14(8):606–19. Epub 2013/06/15.
28. Tate DF, Turner-McGrievy G, Lyons E, Stevens J, Erickson K, Polzien K et al. Replacing caloric beverages with water or diet beverages for weight loss in adults: Main results of the Choose Healthy Options Consciously Everyday (CHOICE) Randomized Clinical Trial. *The American Journal of Clinical Nutrition*. 2012;95(3):555–63. Epub 2012/02/04.
29. Te Morenga L, Mallard S, Mann J. Dietary sugars and body weight: Systematic review and meta-analyses of randomised controlled trials and cohort studies. *British Medical Journal*. 2013;346:e7492. Epub 2013/01/17.
30. InterAct Consortium. Consumption of sweet beverages and type 2 diabetes incidence in European adults: Results from EPIC-InterAct. *Diabetologia*. 2013;56(7):1520–30. Epub 2013/04/27.
31. Fagherazzi G, Vilier A, Saes Sartorelli D, Lajous M, Balkau B, Clavel-Chapelon F. Consumption of artificially and sugar-sweetened beverages and incident type 2 diabetes in the Etude Epidemiologique aupres des femmes de la Mutuelle Generale de l'Education Nationale-European Prospective Investigation into Cancer and Nutrition cohort. *The American Journal of Clinical Nutrition*. 2013;97(3):517–23. Epub 2013/02/01.
32. Sonestedt E, Overby NC, Laaksonen DE, Birgisdottir BE. Does high sugar consumption exacerbate cardiometabolic risk factors and increase the risk of type 2 diabetes and cardiovascular disease? *Food & Nutrition Research*. 2012;56. Epub 2012/08/03.
33. Malik VS, Hu FB. Sweeteners and Risk of Obesity and Type 2 Diabetes: The Role of Sugar-Sweetened Beverages. *Current Diabetes Reports*. 2012;12:195–203. Epub 2012/02/01.
34. Muraki I, Imamura F, Manson JE, Hu FB, Willett WC, van Dam RM et al. Fruit consumption and risk of type 2 diabetes: Results from three prospective longitudinal cohort studies. *British Medical Journal*. 2013;347:f5001. Epub 2013/08/31.
35. Hill AB. The environment and disease: Association or causation? *Proceedings of the Royal Society of Medicine*. 1965;58:295–300. Epub 1965/05/01.
36. Duffey KJ, Gordon-Larsen P, Steffen LM, Jacobs Jr. DR, Popkin BM. Drinking caloric beverages increases the risk of adverse cardiometabolic outcomes in the Coronary Artery Risk Development in Young Adults (CARDIA) Study. *The American Journal of Clinical Nutrition*. 2010;92(4):954–9. Epub 2010/08/13.
37. Winkelmayer WC, Stampfer MJ, Willett WC, Curhan GC. Habitual caffeine intake and the risk of hypertension in women. *JAMA: The Journal of the American Medical Association*. 2005;294(18):2330–5. Epub 2005/11/10.
38. Chen L, Caballero B, Mitchell DC, Loria C, Lin PH, Champagne CM et al. Reducing consumption of sugar-sweetened beverages is associated with reduced blood pressure: A prospective study among United States adults. *Circulation*. 2010;121(22):2398–406. Epub 2010/05/26.
39. Nettleton JA, Lutsey PL, Wang Y, Lima JA, Michos ED, Jacobs Jr. DR. Diet soda intake and risk of incident metabolic syndrome and type 2 diabetes in the Multi-Ethnic Study of Atherosclerosis (MESA). *Diabetes Care*. 2009;32(4):688–94.
40. Raben A, Moller BK, Flint A, Vasilaris TH, Christina Moller A, Juul Holst J et al. Increased postprandial glycaemia, insulinemia, and lipidemia after 10 weeks' sucrose-rich diet compared to an artificially sweetened diet: A randomised controlled trial. *Food & Nutrition Research*. 2011;55. Epub 2011/07/30.
41. Aeberli I, Gerber PA, Hochuli M, Kohler S, Haile SR, Gouni-Berthold I et al. Low to moderate sugar-sweetened beverage consumption impairs glucose and lipid metabolism and promotes inflammation

in healthy young men: A randomized controlled trial. *The American Journal of Clinical Nutrition*. 2011;94(2):479–85.

42. Sorensen LB, Raben A, Stender S, Astrup A. Effect of sucrose on inflammatory markers in overweight humans. *The American Journal of Clinical Nutrition*. 2005;82(2):421–7.
43. Fung TT, Malik V, Rexrode KM, Manson JE, Willett WC, Hu FB. Sweetened beverage consumption and risk of coronary heart disease in women. *The American Journal of Clinical Nutrition*. 2009;89(4):1037–42.
44. de Koning L, Malik VS, Kellogg MD, Rimm EB, Willett WC, Hu FB. Sweetened beverage consumption, incident coronary heart disease, and biomarkers of risk in men. *Circulation*. 2012;125(14):1735–41, S1.
45. Bernstein AM, de Koning L, Flint AJ, Rexrode KM, Willett WC. Soda consumption and the risk of stroke in men and women. *The American Journal of Clinical Nutrition*. 2012;95(5):1190–9. Epub 2012/04/12.
46. Gardener H, Rundek T, Markert M, Wright CB, Elkind MS, Sacco RL. Diet soft drink consumption is associated with an increased risk of vascular events in the Northern Manhattan Study. *Journal of General Internal Medicine*. 2012;27(9):1120–6. Epub 2012/01/28.
47. Eshak ES, Iso H, Kokubo Y, Saito I, Yamagishi K, Inoue M et al. Soft drink intake in relation to incident ischemic heart disease, stroke, and stroke subtypes in Japanese men and women: The Japan Public Health Centre-based study cohort I. *The American Journal of Clinical Nutrition*. 2012;96(6):1390–7. Epub 2012/10/19.
48. Yang Q, Zhang Z, Gregg EW, Flanders WD, Merritt R, Hu FB. Added sugar intake and cardiovascular diseases mortality among US adults. *JAMA Internal Medicine*. 2014;174(4):516–24. Epub 2014/02/05.
49. Tasevska N, Park Y, Jiao L, Hollenbeck A, Subar AF, Potischman N. Sugars and risk of mortality in the NIH-AARP Diet and Health Study. *The American Journal of Clinical Nutrition*. 2014;99(5);1077–88. Epub 2014/02/21.
50. Choi HK, Curhan G. Soft drinks, fructose consumption, and the risk of gout in men: Prospective cohort study. *British Medical Journal*. 2008;336(7639):309–12.
51. Choi HK, Willett W, Curhan G. Fructose-rich beverages and risk of gout in women. *JAMA: The Journal of the American Medical Association*. 2010;304(20):2270–8.
52. Saldana TM, Basso O, Darden R, Sandler DP. Carbonated beverages and chronic kidney disease. *Epidemiology*. 2007;18(4):501–6.
53. Shoham DA, Durazo-Arvizu R, Kramer H, Luke A, Vupputuri S, Kshirsagar A et al. Sugary soda consumption and albuminuria: Results from the National Health and Nutrition Examination Survey, 1999–2004. *PloS One*. 2008;3(10):e3431.
54. Curhan GC, Willett WC, Knight EL, Stampfer MJ. Dietary factors and the risk of incident kidney stones in younger women: Nurses' Health Study II. *Archives of Internal Medicine*. 2004;164(8):885–91.
55. Cuevas A, Miquel JF, Reyes MS, Zanlungo S, Nervi F. Diet as a risk factor for cholesterol gallstone disease. *The Journal of the American College of Nutrition*. 2004;23(3):187–96.
56. Tsai CJ, Leitzmann MF, Willett WC, Giovannucci EL. Dietary carbohydrates and glycaemic load and the incidence of symptomatic gall stone disease in men. *Gut*. 2005;54(6):823–8.
57. Scragg RK, McMichael AJ, Baghurst PA. Diet, alcohol, and relative weight in gall stone disease: A case–control study. *British Medical Journal (Clinical Research Ed.)*. 1984;288(6424):1113–9.
58. DellaValle DM, Roe LS, Rolls BJ. Does the consumption of caloric and non-caloric beverages with a meal affect energy intake? *Appetite*. 2005;44(2):187–93.
59. Raben A, Vasilaras TH, Moller AC, Astrup A. Sucrose compared with artificial sweeteners: Different effects on ad libitum food intake and body weight after 10 wk of supplementation in overweight subjects. *The American Journal of Clinical Nutrition*. 2002;76(4):721–9.
60. Tordoff MG, Alleva AM. Effect of drinking soda sweetened with aspartame or high-fructose corn syrup on food intake and body weight. *The American Journal of Clinical Nutrition*. 1990;51(6):963–9.
61. Reid M, Hammersley R, Hill AJ, Skidmore P. Long-term dietary compensation for added sugar: Effects of supplementary sucrose drinks over a 4-week period. *British Journal of Nutrition*. 2007;97(1):193–203.
62. DiMeglio DP, Mattes RD. Liquid versus solid carbohydrate: Effects on food intake and body weight. *International Journal of Obesity and Related Metabolic Disorders*. 2000;24(6):794–800.
63. Pan A, Hu FB. Effects of carbohydrates on satiety: Differences between liquid and solid food. *Current Opinion in Clinical Nutrition and Metabolic Care*. 2011;14(4):385–90. Epub 2011/04/27.
64. Janssens JP, Shapira N, Debeuf P, Michiels L, Putman R, Bruckers L et al. Effects of soft drink and table beer consumption on insulin response in normal teenagers and carbohydrate drink in youngsters. *European Journal of Cancer Prevention*. 1999;8(4):289–95.
65. Ludwig DS. The glycemic index: Physiological mechanisms relating to obesity, diabetes, and cardiovascular disease. *JAMA: The Journal of the American Medical Association*. 2002;287(18):2414–23.

66. Liu S, Manson JE, Buring JE, Stampfer MJ, Willett WC, Ridker PM. Relation between a diet with a high glycemic load and plasma concentrations of high-sensitivity C-reactive protein in middle-aged women. *The American Journal of Clinical Nutrition*. 2002;75(3):492–8.
67. Vlassara H, Cai W, Crandall J, Goldberg T, Oberstein R, Dardaine V et al. Inflammatory mediators are induced by dietary glycotoxins, a major risk factor for diabetic angiopathy. *Proceedings of the National Academy of Sciences of the United States of America*. 2002;99(24):15596–601.
68. Hofmann SM, Dong HJ, Li Z, Cai W, Altomonte J, Thung SN et al. Improved insulin sensitivity is associated with restricted intake of dietary glycoxidation products in the db/db mouse. *Diabetes*. 2002;51(7):2082–9.
69. Gnagnarella P, Gandini S, La Vecchia C, Maisonneuve P. Glycemic index, glycemic load, and cancer risk: A meta-analysis. *The American Journal of Clinical Nutrition*. 2008;87(6):1793–801. Epub 2008/06/11.
70. Bray GA. How bad is fructose? *The American Journal of Clinical Nutrition*. 2007;86(4):895–6.
71. Teff KL, Grudziak J, Townsend RR, Dunn TN, Grant RW, Adams SH et al. Endocrine and metabolic effects of consuming fructose- and glucose-sweetened beverages with meals in obese men and women: Influence of insulin resistance on plasma triglyceride responses. *The Journal of Clinical Endocrinology and Metabolism*. 2009;94(5):1562–9.
72. Stanhope KL, Schwarz JM, Keim NL, Griffen SC, Bremer AA, Graham JL et al. Consuming fructose-sweetened, not glucose-sweetened, beverages increases visceral adiposity and lipids and decreases insulin sensitivity in overweight/obese humans. *The Journal of Clinical Investigation*. 2009;119(5):1322–34.
73. Stanhope KL, Griffen SC, Bair BR, Swarbrick MM, Keim NL, Havel PJ. Twenty-four-hour endocrine and metabolic profiles following consumption of high-fructose corn syrup-, sucrose-, fructose-, and glucose-sweetened beverages with meals. *The American Journal of Clinical Nutrition*. 2008;87(5):1194–203.
74. Stanhope KL, Havel PJ. Endocrine and metabolic effects of consuming beverages sweetened with fructose, glucose, sucrose, or high-fructose corn syrup. *The American Journal of Clinical Nutrition*. 2008;88(6):1733S–7S.
75. Johnson RJ, Segal MS, Sautin Y, Nakagawa T, Feig DI, Kang DH et al. Potential role of sugar (fructose) in the epidemic of hypertension, obesity and the metabolic syndrome, diabetes, kidney disease, and cardiovascular disease. *The American Journal of Clinical Nutrition*. 2007;86(4):899–906.
76. Nakagawa T, Tuttle KR, Short RA, Johnson RJ. Hypothesis: Fructose-induced hyperuricemia as a causal mechanism for the epidemic of the metabolic syndrome. *Nature Clinical Practice Nephrology*. 2005;1(2):80–6.
77. Port AM, Ruth MR, Istfan NW. Fructose consumption and cancer: Is there a connection? *Current Opinion in Endocrinology, Diabetes, and Obesity*. 2012;19(5):367–74. Epub 2012/08/28.
78. de Koning L, Malik VS, Rimm EB, Willett WC, Hu FB. Sugar-sweetened and artificially sweetened beverage consumption and risk of type 2 diabetes in men. *The American Journal of Clinical Nutrition*. 2011;93(6):1321–7. Epub 2011/03/25.
79. Stookey JD, Constant F, Popkin BM, Gardner CD. Drinking water is associated with weight loss in overweight dieting women independent of diet and activity. *Obesity (Silver Spring)*. 2008;16(11):2481–8.
80. Dennis EA, Dengo AL, Comber DL, Flack KD, Savla J, Davy KP et al. Water consumption increases weight loss during a hypocaloric diet intervention in middle-aged and older adults. *Obesity (Silver Spring)*. 2010;18(2):300–7.
81. Popkin BM, Barclay DV, Nielsen SJ. Water and food consumption patterns of U.S. adults from 1999 to 2001. *Obesity Research*. 2005;13(12):2146–52.
82. Pan A, Malik VS, Hao T, Willett WC, Mozaffarian D, Hu FB. Changes in water and beverage intake and long-term weight changes: Results from three prospective cohort studies. *International Journal of Obesity (London)*. 2013;37(10):1378–85. Epub 2013/01/16.
83. Pan A, Malik VS, Schulze MB, Manson JE, Willett WC, Hu FB. Plain-water intake and risk of type 2 diabetes in young and middle-aged women. *The American Journal of Clinical Nutrition*. 2012;95(6):1454–60. Epub 2012/05/04.
84. Bazzano LA, Li TY, Joshipura KJ, Hu FB. Intake of fruit, vegetables, and fruit juices and risk of diabetes in women. *Diabetes Care*. 2008;31(7):1311–7.
85. Huxley R, Lee CM, Barzi F, Timmermeister L, Czernichow S, Perkovic V et al. Coffee, decaffeinated coffee, and tea consumption in relation to incident type 2 diabetes mellitus: A systematic review with meta-analysis. *Archives of Internal Medicine*. 2009;169(22):2053–63. Epub 2009/12/17.
86. van Dam RM. Coffee consumption and risk of type 2 diabetes, cardiovascular diseases, and cancer. *Applied Physiology, Nutrition, and Metabolism*. 2008;33(6):1269–83.

87. van Dieren S, Uiterwaal CS, van der Schouw YT, van der AD, Boer JM, Spijkerman A et al. Coffee and tea consumption and risk of type 2 diabetes. *Diabetologia*. 2009;52(12):2561–9.
88. Bhupathiraju SN, Pan A, Malik VS, Manson JE, Willett WC, van Dam RM et al. Caffeinated and caffeine-free beverages and risk of type 2 diabetes. *The American Journal of Clinical Nutrition*. 2013;97(1):155–66. Epub 2012/11/16.
89. Mattes RD, Popkin BM. Nonnutritive sweetener consumption in humans: Effects on appetite and food intake and their putative mechanisms. *The American Journal of Clinical Nutrition*. 2009;89(1):1–14.
90. Lutsey PL, Steffen LM, Stevens J. Dietary intake and the development of the metabolic syndrome: The Atherosclerosis Risk in Communities study. *Circulation*. 2008;117(6):754–61.
91. Brown RJ, de Banate MA, Rother KI. Artificial sweeteners: A systematic review of metabolic effects in youth. *International Journal of Pediatric Obesity: IJPO: An Official Journal of the International Association for the Study of Obesity*. 2010;5(4):305–12. Epub 2010/01/19.
92. Yale Rudd Center for Food Policy and Obesity. SUgar-Sweetened Beverage Taxes and Sugar Intake: Policy Statements, Endorsements, and Recommendations. http://www.yaleruddcenter.org/resources/upload/docs/what/policy/SSBtaxes/SSBTaxStatements.pdf (accessed 10 January 2013).
93. Fletcher JM, Frisvold D, Tefft N. Taxing soft drinks and restricting access to vending machines to curb child obesity. *Health Affairs (Millwood)*. 2010;29(5):1059–66. Epub 2010/04/03.
94. Andreyeva T, Chaloupka FJ, Brownell KD. Estimating the potential of taxes on sugar-sweetened beverages to reduce consumption and generate revenue. *Preventive Medicine*. 2011;52(6):413–6. Epub 2011/03/30.
95. Finkelstein EA, Zhen C, Nonnemaker J, Todd JE. Impact of targeted beverage taxes on higher- and lower-income households. *Archives of Internal Medicine*. 2010;170(22):2028–34. Epub 2010/12/15.
96. Wang YC, Coxson P, Shen YM, Goldman L, Bibbins-Domingo K. A penny-per-ounce tax on sugar-sweetened beverages would cut health and cost burdens of diabetes. *Health Affairs (Millwood)*. 2012;31(1):199–207. Epub 2012/01/11.

17 Dietary Sugars, Obesity, and Chronic Diseases in Children

Jaimie N. Davis and Stacey Lee

CONTENTS

KEY POINTS

- Although intake of dietary sugars, including added sugars and sugar-sweetened beverage (SSB) intake, has recently started to decline in US children in the last decade, dietary sugar intake still far exceeds current recommendations and is still much higher now than in prior generations.
- High levels of dietary sugars, specifically SSB intake, are linked to increased energy intake, obesity, and metabolic disturbances in children, with these effects beginning early in life.
- Current interventions targeting dietary sugar reduction, specifically SSBs, show promising results on reducing obesity and metabolic disease risk; however, much more intervention research is needed.

INTRODUCTION

Although the prevalence of childhood obesity in the USA has appeared to plateau somewhat in the past decade [1], it has dramatically increased over the past three decades and is on the rise in almost every country [2]. Recent NHANES data show that among children and adolescents, 2–19 years of age, 17% were obese and 32% were overweight in 2009–2010 [1]. Of note, 12.3% were at or above the 97th percentile for BMI, indicating a shift to a greater degree of obesity within our pediatric population. Minority groups are disproportionately affected by overweight and obesity, with 39% of Hispanics and non-Hispanic Black (NHB) children (2–19 years) being overweight compared to 28% of non-Hispanic White (NHW) children [1]. The spread of obesity is also occurring much younger in life, with almost 10% of US children from birth to 2 years of age having high weight-for-recumbent length. Overweight or obese children have a twofold higher risk for becoming overweight as adults [3]. Obesity is a major cause of death and is a contributor to many other types of diseases, including cardiovascular disease, metabolic syndrome, type 2 diabetes, fatty liver, and various types of cancers. These obesity-related metabolic diseases also disproportionally affect minority pediatric groups [4–7]. This ethnic disparity is partly mediated by lower socioeconomic status (SES), genetics, obesogenic environments, and behaviors. Given that changing SES, genetics, and an established environment is challenging, ample amounts of research have focused on what behaviors, specifically dietary behaviors, are most linked to pediatric obesity and related metabolic disorders.

In this chapter, we will review the evidence linking consumption of dietary sugars during infancy and childhood, particularly sugar-sweetened beverages (SSBs; including sodas, fruit drinks, juices, and sports drink), to pediatric obesity. There is a growing amount of evidence from interventions that target reductions in added sugar intake and SSBs, showing efficacy for decreasing childhood obesity rates. Some evidence exists to examine the effects of different dietary sugars on metabolic health in children, but few intervention studies have been conducted in this area. This chapter will include the following: (a) Discussion on national and international consumption trends in dietary sugar intake consumption in pediatric populations; (b) examination of how dietary sugar intake and its different forms are linked to obesity and related metabolic disorders in youth; and (c) effects of interventions focusing on reductions in dietary sugar intake on obesity and related metabolic outcomes in children and adolescents.

TRENDS IN CONSUMPTION OF DIETARY SUGARS IN CHILDREN

As outlined in previous chapters, consumption of added sugars, which are defined as sugars or syrups added to foods/beverages during processing or preparation, in the US diet has steadily increased from the 1950s through the mid-1990s. While cane and beet sugar has decreased in the USA in the last 50 years, corn sweeteners, notably high-fructose corn syrup, have increased eightfold, going from 11 to 85 pounds per capita, dry weight, which accounts for about 52 teaspoons of added sugar per day per person in 2000 [8]. Reedy and Kreb-Smith [9] using National Health and Nutrition Examination Survey (NHANES) data from children (2–18 years) from 2003 to 2006 show that SSBs contribute 45–50% of added sugar intake in all racial/ethnic and income groups. Top sources of added sugar intake were soda, fruit drinks, grain desserts, and candy for all children (2–18 years). NHANES data from 1988 to 2004 showed that 79% of all US youth consumed SSBs on a typical day [10]. SSB intake increased from 204 kcal/day in 1988 to 224 kcal/day in 2004, and 100% juice intake increased from 38 to 48 kcal/day, with the largest increases among children aged 6 to 11 years (~20% increase) [10]. Increases in SSBs were largest among the Black and Mexican American youth and among the low-income populations. When examining the younger children (2–3 years), the top sources of added sugar were identical [9]. The Feeding Infant and Toddler Study showed that 46% of children (2–3 years) consumed some type of sweetened beverage intake on the survey day, with the fruit-flavored drinks being the most common. These data suggest that patterns of added sugar intake consumption are consistent across childhood and start at very early ages.

Similar trends in dietary sugar intake are seen in other countries as well. Nearly 60% of Greek kindergarten children consumed SSBs on a daily basis [11]. Another study with Bahraini school children (6–18 years), consisting of 11 different populated regions around Saudi Arabia, found that almost 50% of children consumed at least one soda drink per day [12]. Two national representative dietary intake surveys from Mexico showed the caloric beverages accounted for 28% of energy intake for preschoolers and 21% for school children [13]. These data suggest that SSB intake is high among children of all different ages and ethnicities.

However, several recent national studies have shown a decline in added sugar intake in both adults and children over the past decade. Data from five national studies found that energy intake from added sugar intake actually decreased in US children (2–19 years) going from 18% in 1994 to 14% in 2010 [14]. Similarly, Welsh et al. [15] examined the NHANES data and found that added sugar intake, and more specifically soda consumption, decreased significantly from 1999 to 2008 in US residents ≥2 years of age. Decreases in SSB consumption, both in the home and away from home and in both meals and snacks, also decreased in the past decade. In 1999–2000, 10.9% of energy intake per day came from SSB intake, whereas in 2009–2010 this decreased to 8.0% of energy intake per day from SSB [16]. Despite these small national decreases, added sugar intake, particularly SSB consumption, of youth around the world still far exceeds current recommendations and is still much higher now than in prior generations. In addition, the reduction in SSB intake is offset by an increase in 100% juice intake and flavored milk consumption, particularly in the younger children [17]. According to recent NHANES data, 100% juice intake has increased by 20% and flavored milk has increased by 14% in the last decade in children from birth to 5 years of age [17].

INTAKE OF ADDED SUGARS AND OBESITY

Data linking total or added dietary sugar intake to increased childhood obesity levels is somewhat mixed, with some studies showing a positive relationship while others show no association (and no study has found any beneficial effects). A cross-sectional study with 1294 British youth (7–18 years) found that percentage of energy of non-milk extrinsic sugars in the diet were inversely correlated with BMI z-scores [18]. Longitudinal data on 216 children found that an increase in total added sugar intake in the second year of life was associated with higher BMI at age 7 [19]. Several studies have shown a link with total dietary sugar intake and increased adiposity measures, beyond BMI parameters. In a cross-sectional analysis with 169 Swedish female adolescents (16–17 years), sugar intake was positively associated with percent body fat, as measured by BodPod [20]. In another cross-sectional analysis with 120 overweight Hispanic children (10–17 years), sugar intake was associated with increased BMI parameters and total body fat, as measured by DXA [21]. Pollock et al. found that total fructose intake, which included both free fructose plus one-half of free sucrose, was associated with increased visceral adiposity, as measured by MRI in 559 White and Black adolescents [22].

In contrast, several studies using national data sets have not found any association with total or added sugar intake and obesity in children. Nicklas et al. [23] using data from NHANES 2003–2006 with 3136 children (6–18 years) found no association with added sugar intake and weight or adiposity measures. Data from NHANES with nearly 20,000 children and adolescents (1–18 years) found no association of total or added sugar intake with BMI [24]. Similarly, Storey et al. [25] using data from the Continuing Survey of Food Intake 1994–1998 (CSFII) and NHANES with over 16,000 children and adolescents did not find an association of total or added sugar intake with BMI parameters. However, this study did find that carbohydrates (less added sugars) were inversely related to BMI among adolescents [25]. This lack of an association with sugars and childhood obesity may be due in part to underreporting of food intake, which is more prevalent in obese adolescents compared to lean counterparts [26]. In addition, foods higher in added sugar intake have been shown to be selectively underreported [27]. Although there appears to be somewhat mixed findings, no study has shown that high levels of dietary sugars are beneficial to pediatric health.

SSB INTAKE AND OBESITY

Numerous studies exists identifying SSB intake as a leading culprit contributing to the pediatric obesity epidemic. A prospective cohort with 11,654 boys and girls (9–14 years) from the US Growing Up Today Study showed that SSB intake was associated with weight gain during corresponding years [28]. Adjustments for energy intake attenuated the results, but this is likely due to the contributions of SSB to total energy intake. Findings from the NHANES data showed that consumption of soft drinks contributed a higher proportion of energy in overweight than in normal-weight subjects in each age and sex group [29]. A notable study by Ludwig et al. with 548 ethnically diverse schoolchildren reported that with each additional serving of SSBs, the odds of obesity increased by 60% [30]. Similar findings, although not as dramatic, were seen in a study of 319 Mexican American children (8–10 years), which found that each additional serving of soda was linked to a 29% increase in the odds of obesity, but consumption of diet soda, other SSBs, or 100% juice was not associated [31].

Several studies have found a link between SSBs and adiposity measures, beyond BMI measures. A longitudinal study by Fiorito et al. [32] with 170 NHW found that SSB at age 5, but not milk or fruit juice intake, was positively associated with increased body fat percentage and waist circumference, as well as weight status from 5 to 15 years. A large cross-sectional study conducted with 9433 Saudi school children (10–19 years) showed that sugar-sweetened carbonated beverage intake was linked to increased obesity and waist circumference in boys only [33]. A long-term study with 269 Danish children found a weak association between sweet drink intake, which included soft drink, fruit juice, chocolate milk, and drinkable yogurts, at age 9 years with changes in skin-fold thickness from the age of 9–13 years [34].

This link between SSB intake and obesity is evident early in life. A longitudinal study conducted by Weijs et al. [35] showed that higher consumption of SSBs in the first year of life was associated with a 13% increase in overweight at age 8. Another longitudinal study in 365 low-income African-American preschool children (3–5 years) found that soda and all SSB intake was linked to baseline and changes in overweight prevalence over 2 years [36]. In a longitudinal study of 1944 Canadian children, those that consumed at least one serving of SSBs daily between the ages of 2.5 and 4.5 were three times more likely to be overweight at age 4.5 years compared to children who did not consume any SSB [37]. In a study with 1483 Hispanic children (2–4 years) from a Los Angeles Women, Infants and Children (WIC) cohort, children who consumed at least two SSBs per day had a 31% increase in the odds of obesity prevalence compared to children who did not consume SSB [38]. In a retrospective study of 10,904 WIC children (2–3 years) from Missouri, children who were overweight at baseline and consumed at least one SSB per day were twice more likely to remain overweight one year later [39].

Although the majority of the literature has shown a positive association of SSBs with obesity, a few studies have shown no association at all [40,41]. A longitudinal study by Blum et al. [40] with 166 children (8–10 years) showed no association with consumption of SSBs and BMI *z*-scores; however, the overweight subjects and subjects who gained weight had significantly higher diet soda consumption than normal weight subjects. Another prospective study conducted by Newby et al. [41] with 1345 WIC children from North Dakota with at least two visits between 6 and 12 months apart, found that SSB intake was not linked to obesity or changes in weight over time. Nevertheless, no study has ever shown any kind of protective effect of SSB intake on health.

JUICE INTAKE AND OBESITY

Some of the above studies have included juices within the definition of SSB, therefore making it difficult look at the separate or unique effects of 100% juice consumption on obesity parameters. As previously discussed, fruit juice consumption, particularly in young children, has dramatically increased over the past three decades. Young children have the highest consumption of fruit juices of all age groups in the USA [42]. Data supporting a link between 100% juice intake and obesity is conflicting. Dennison et al. [43] showed that young children (2–5 years) consuming 12 fl. oz. or more of 100% fruit juices had a higher overweight prevalence than those consuming less than 12 fl. oz. a day (32% vs. 9%). This study also showed that children who were high consumers of 100% juice consumed compared to low consumers consumed higher amounts of daily energy, fructose, and glucose intake. In a case–control study with 53 Puerto Rican children (7–10 years), 100% fruit juice consumption was positively associated with BMI and tricep skinfolds [44].

In contrast, in the NHANES data from 1999 to 2002 with 3618 children (2–11 years), there was no association between100% juice intake and weight status, but 100% juice intake was linked with better nutrient intake [45]. Similarly, O'Connor et al. [46] using the NHANES 1999–2002 data set, showed that 100% juice intake in young children (2–5 years) was associated with increased energy intake but not BMI parameters. A more recent analyses of NHANES data from 2003 to 2006 showed that consumption of 100% orange juice was linked to higher energy intake in children, but no association with overweight or obese risk was found [47].

Despite the inconclusive evidence directly linking fruit juice to obesity, the evidence does support that increased juice intake is linked to increased daily energy intake, which is subsequently linked to increased obesity levels. Also, none of the above studies found a protective effect of juice consumption against obesity. Based on this evidence, the Institute of Medicine (IOM) has recently recommended limiting children's consumption of fruit juice, with no fruit juice for infants under 1 year, and a maximum amount of fruit juice of 4 fl. oz./day for children ≥1 year [48]. WIC also recently changed its food package to eliminate 100% juice provisions for infants <12 months and no more than 4 fl. oz./day for children over 1 year [49].

A possible disadvantage for children drinking SSBs and/or juices at an early age is that they may develop a preference for sweet beverages or foods. Literature has shown that early exposure to sugar-sweetened foods and beverages (which includes 100% juice) leads to increased preferences for sweetened items, and this preference is developed early in life [50,51]. One study showed that children that were exposed to more added sugars during the first year of life were more likely to prefer juices with added sugars and chose cereals higher in sugar at age 4–7 [50]. Another study with 59 children (8–10 years) showed that 8-day exposure of sweet orangeades increased children's preference for this orangeade [52]. Also, research shows that children who have a preference for SSBs also have a preference for sweet and savory snacks and a lower preference for fruits and vegetables [51].

CONSUMPTION OF DIETARY SUGARS AND METABOLIC DISEASE RISK IN CHILDREN

Data from numerous studies show that consumption of added sugars, mainly in the form of SSB, is related to increased risk for numerous metabolic diseases in children. A recent cross-sectional study by Welsh et al. [15] using 2157 US adolescents from the NHANES 1999–2004 data found that added sugar was inversely linked to high-density lipoprotein (HDL) cholesterol levels and positively linked to low-density lipoprotein (LDL) cholesterol and triglycerides (TGs). Among the overweight/obese adolescents, added sugar intake was linked to increased insulin resistance, as measured by homeostasis model (HOMA-IR). Another study using the NHANES data with 4880 children (3–11 years) showed that SSB intake was linked to increased C-reactive protein concentrations and waist circumference and decreased HDL-cholesterol levels [53]. In a large European study with 546 adolescents [54], those who consumed SSB >5 times/week compared with those consuming less frequently had higher HOMA-IR values. In a study of 63 overweight Hispanic youth (9–13 years), total sugar intake and SSBs were linked to decreased acute insulin response and beta-cell function, as measured by a frequently sampled intravenous glucose tolerance test (FSIVGTT), and these results remained after controlling for pubertal stage and body composition [55]. Davis et al. [21] with 120 overweight Hispanic youth (10–17 years) showed that total sugar intake was inversely correlated with insulin sensitivity and beta-cell function, as measured by FSIVGTT, however, no association was found with SSB intake. Another study with 185 Mexican children (9–13 years) showed that soft drinks and SSBs were linked to increased fasting glucose levels and diastolic blood pressure [56]. All of the above studies suggest that sugar intake, specifically SSBs, exacerbates the risk of type 2 diabetes and cardiovascular diseases in children. These findings also suggest that added sugar intake, specifically SSBs, may be more problematic for metabolic risk in children who are already overweight or obese.

As discussed in some of the other chapters, fructose, in particular, has been shown to have more metabolically damaging effects than glucose, and the impact of fructose on metabolic outcomes may be more pronounced in growing infants and children, as discussed in Chapter 18. A relatively small study with 38 children (5–19 years) showed that fructose intake was linked to increased HOMA-IR and decreased adiponectin [57]. A much larger study by Pollock et al. [22] with 559 adolescents found that total fructose consumption (free fructose plus one-half the intake of free sucrose) was linked to increased visceral adipose tissue (VAT), as measured by MRI, but not associated with subcutaneous adipose tissue. Fructose intake was also linked to higher systolic blood pressure, fasting glucose, HOMA-IR and C-reactive protein, and lower HDL-cholesterol and adiponectin. However, these associations were attenuated when VAT was added to the models, suggesting that the effect of dietary sugars on promoting increased VAT stores plays an important role in the mechanism behind other metabolic risk factors.

High fructose consumption has been associated with NAFLD in adult studies [58,59], but studies on the effect of added sugars and fructose intake on liver fat in children are lacking. In a 2-day, cross-over feeding study with nine children with NAFLD and 10 matched controls without NAFLD [60], the intake of a fructose-sweetened beverage, compared to a glucose beverage, induced postprandial and overnight increases in plasma TG and decreases in HDL-cholesterol levels in children with and without NAFLD. Nonesterified fatty acids were not impacted by either beverage group but were significantly higher in children with NAFLD. These data suggest that dietary fructose induced a dyslipidemic effect in both healthy children and those with NAFLD; however, children with NAFLD demonstrated an increased sensitivity to the impact of dietary fructose. In a study with 149 children (2–17 years) with known or suspected NAFLD, uric acid, which may reflect total fructose consumption, was significantly associated with nonalcoholic steatohepatitis (NASH) [61]. Goran et al. [7] have examined the relationship with genetic factors, liver fat, and dietary sugar in Hispanic youth. Hispanic children with the GG genotype in the PNPLA3 gene have a two-fold higher liver fat fraction compared to other genotypes. Hispanic youth with this GG variant were also more susceptible to increased hepatic fat when dietary carbohydrate, specifically total and added sugar, was high [62]. These data suggest that interventions focusing on reductions in added sugar, fructose, and SSB intake may have profound effects on reducing liver fat in children. However, clinical interventions in this area are warranted.

SSB AND OBESOGENIC ENVIRONMENTS

Evidence is fairly convincing that SSB intake is linked to obesity and related metabolic diseases, but children who consume SSBs also tend to live in more obesogenic environments. Children and adolescents who live and go to school in areas with more convenient fast food restaurants rather than healthier outlets, such as grocery stores, are more likely to consume SSBs [63]. Several studies have shown that children who consume SSBs also have higher fast food consumption [64]. In a multicountry study, children (2–9 years) who consume high sugar foods were more likely to have high-risk television behaviors, including eating in front of the TV, watching more than 1 h of TV per day, and having a TV in their room [65]. A study with over 16,000 high school students (grades 9–12) found that consuming one or more SSB per day was linked to the following: (a) watching more than 2 h of TV per day; (b) playing video games at least 2 h per day; (c) being physically active less than five times per week; and (d) being a current tobacco user [66]. It is possible and likely that children who drink excessive amounts of SSBs are also the ones that live in obesogenic environments. These children exhibit other unhealthy dietary behaviors and tend to be more sedentary. However, many of these other factors are considered and controlled for in the above studies, and added sugar intake, specifically SSBs, still has an independent and strong effect on increased obesity and metabolic disease risk in youth.

PEDIATRIC INTERVENTIONS FOCUSED ON SUGAR REDUCTION

Over the past decade, a few obesity interventions targeting sugar reductions have been conducted in children. Ebbeling et al. [67] conducted a randomized controlled 25-week pilot study with 103 adolescents (13–18 years), which relied largely on home deliveries of noncaloric beverages to displace SSBs. Although there was no overall intervention effect, among overweight or obese subjects, the intervention was successful at reducing BMI compared to the control group (–0.63 ± 0.23 kg/m^2 vs. +0.12 ± 0.34 kg/m^2; $P = 0.03$). More recently, Ebbeling et al. [68] conducted a randomized trial where 224 overweight and obese adolescents, who were regular SSB consumers, were either randomized to a 1-year intervention designed to decrease SSBs, with a 1-year follow-up, or a control group. The 1-year intervention consisted of home delivery of noncaloric beverages every 2 weeks, monthly motivational telephone calls with parents, and three check-in visits with participants. The experimental group, compared to controls, had significant reductions in energy, sugar, and SSB intake at years 1 and 2. The experimental group compared to controls had smaller increases in BMI (0.06 ± 0.20 vs. 0.63 ± 0.20 kg/m^2; $P = 0.045$) and weight gain (1.6 ± 0.6 vs. 3.5 ± 0.6 kg; $P = 0.04$) at year 1, but significant differences were not maintained at year 2. There was also a significant ethnic effect, with Hispanics in the experimental group compared to Hispanics controls, having smaller increases in BMI and slower weight gains at both years 1 and 2. Another recent 18-month trial in Holland where 641 normal weight children (4–11 years) were randomized to either receive 250 mL (8 fl. oz) per day of sugar-free, artificially sweetened beverage (sugar-free group) or a similar sugar-containing beverage (sugar group) [69]. The sugar group compared to the sugar-free group had greater increases in BMI *z*-score (mean difference in change of –0.13 SD; $P = 0.001$) in weight (mean difference in change of 1.01 kg; $P < 0.001$), skinfold thickness measurements (mean difference in change of —2.2 mm; $P = 0.02$), waist-to-height ratio, and more fat mass (mean difference in change of –1.07% body fat; $P = 0.02$). A smaller pilot study with 15 overweight/obese German children (5–8 years) showed that a 3-month dietary intervention focused on fructose reduction resulted in significant reductions in energy intake, fructose, sucrose, and glucose intake as well as reductions in BMI parameters; however, this study did not have a control group [70].

To date, only a few interventions have examined the effects of reducing sugar and SSB intake on metabolic outcomes. In a 16-week randomized nutrition and strength training intervention with 100 African American and Hispanic adolescents, the nutrition-only group (which focused on reductions in sugar and SSB intake) had significant improvements in insulin sensitivity and beta- cell function [71]. Secondary analyses from this 16-week intervention with the Hispanic adolescents found that those participants who decreased added sugar intake (mean decrease of 47 g/day, equivalent to one soda per day) compared to those who increased sugar intake had significant improvements in glucose control and insulin secretion [72]. More interventions targeting reductions in added sugar intake and SSBs that examine the effects on metabolic disease outcomes are warranted in pediatric populations.

CONCLUSION

Consumption of added sugars and SSB's in infants, children, and adolescents is much higher than current dietary recommendations and higher than that compared to previous generations. Current evidence also suggests that higher levels of dietary sugars, specifically SSB intake, are linked to increased energy intake, obesity, and metabolic disturbances in children, with these effects beginning early in life. Convincing evidence exists to show that sugar exposure early in life, in utero, and infancy plays a critical role in promoting obesity, adiposity, and disease development. As discussed in this and other chapters, not all sugars have the same effect on health. Fructose intake, in particular, either from sucrose, HFCS (which is the most common sweetener used in our food/beverage supply), or free fructose, is linked to metabolic diseases, such as dyslipidemia and NAFLD in pediatric populations. However, more clinical and experimental research is warranted to fully understand the effects of fructose on metabolic health in children.

Current interventions targeting SSB reduction show promising results on reducing obesity and metabolic disease risk; however, much more intervention research is needed. Of note, targeting one key dietary behavior, such as SSBs, is a very concise and easy-to-follow behavior change compared to many of the obesity interventions that target multiple behavior changes. This focused approach might be easier for children and parents to grasp and achieve. There is also a need for interventions targeting sugar reduction to be conducted with infants and young children and their parents.

There is a need for public health messages targeting dietary sugar reduction to be implemented in the schools, communities, hospitals/health clinics, etc. These public health messages should be geared toward both children and parents. Nutrition education programs in federal services, such as Supplemental Nutrition Assistance Program (SNAP) and WIC programs, should teach parents and children to choose no or low-sugar foods/beverages and discourage consumption of high-sugar foods/beverages, including 100% fruit juices. Food vouchers for these programs should incentivize low-sugar foods, such as fresh fruits and vegetables, and limit the vouchers available for high-sugar foods/beverages.

Decreasing dietary sugars in childhood is going to be very challenging without the support of the food and beverage industries. Food and beverage industries should have to comply with recommendations to decrease sugar intake in foods and beverages, particularly those marketed to children. There should also be stricter guidelines put on what foods and beverages can be advertised to children and when and where these advertisements can occur. The most common and easiest reaction to this excessive sugar problem is to place the blame on the food and beverage industries. It very evident that the food and beverage industries are extremely powerful, rather permanent, and very influential in policy development; therefore, in order to decrease dietary sugar in our food supply, enlisting the help and support of industry will be more effective than simply challenging them. Given that many of the food and beverage companies have healthier low-sugar options, including bottled and sparkling waters, the development, availability, and marketing of these low-sugar products to children and their families should be incentivized and encouraged by industries and supported by the government.

Decreasing availability and consumption of added sugars, particularly SSBs, has the potential to have profound effects on reducing obesity and related metabolic diseases in pediatric populations.

REFERENCES

1. Ogden CL, Carroll MD, Kit BK, Flegal KM. Prevalence of obesity and trends in body mass index among US children and adolescents, 1999–2010. *JAMA*. 2012;307(5):483–90. Epub 2012/01/19.
2. Wang Y, Lobstein T. Worldwide trends in childhood overweight and obesity. *Int J Pediatr Obes*. 2006;1(1):11–25.
3. Serdula MK, Ivery D, Coates RJ, Freedman DS, Williamson DF, Byers T. Do obese children become obese adults? A review of the literature. *Prev Med*. 1993;22(2):167–77. Epub 1993/03/01.
4. Goran MI, Lane C, Toledo-Corral C, Weigensberg MJ. Persistence of pre-diabetes in overweight and obese hispanic children: Association with progressive insulin resistance, poor beta-cell function, and increasing visceral fat. *Diabetes*. 2008;57(11):3007–12. Epub 2008/08/06.
5. Goran MI, Gower BA. Longitudinal study on pubertal insulin resistance. *Diabetes*. 2001;50(11):2444–50.
6. Cruz ML, Bergman RN, Goran MI. Unique effect of visceral fat on insulin sensitivity in obese hispanic children with a family history of type 2 diabetes. *Diabetes Care*. 2002;25(9):1631–6.
7. Goran MI, Walker R, Le KA, Mahurkar S, Vikman S, Davis JN et al. Effects of Pnpla3 on liver fat and metabolic profile in hispanic children and adolescents. *Diabetes*. 2010;59(12):3127–30.
8. United States Department of Agriculture. Economic Research Service. Food Availability (Per Capita) Dat System, 2013. http://www.ers.usda.gov/data-products/food-availability (accessed 2 January).
9. Reedy J, Krebs-Smith SM. Dietary sources of energy, solid fats, and added sugars among children and adolescents in the United States. *J Am Diet Assoc*. 2010;110(10):1477–84.
10. Wang YC, Bleich SN, Gortmaker SL. Increasing caloric contribution from sugar-sweetened beverages and 100% fruit juices among US children and adolescents, 1988–2004. *Pediatrics*. 2008;121(6):e1604–14.
11. Linardakis M, Sarri K, Pateraki MS, Sbokos M, Kafatos A. Sugar-added beverages consumption among kindergarten children of crete: Effects on nutritional status and risk of obesity. *BMC Public Health*. 2008;8:279.
12. Gharib N, Rasheed P. Energy and macronutrient intake and dietary pattern among school children in Bahrain: A cross-sectional study. *Nutr J*. 2011;10:62.

13. Barquera S, Campirano F, Bonvecchio A, Hernandez-Barrera L, Rivera JA, Popkin BM. Caloric beverage consumption patterns in Mexican children. *Nutr J.* 2010;9:47.
14. Slining MM, Popkin BM. Trends in intakes and sources of solid fats and added sugars among U.S. children and adolescents: 1994–2010. *Pediatr Obes.* 2013;8(4):307–24. Epub 2013/04/05.
15. Welsh JA, Sharma AJ, Grellinger L, Vos MB. Consumption of added sugars is decreasing in the United States. *Am J Clin Nutr.* 2011;94(3):726–34. Epub 2011/07/15.
16. Kit BK, Fakhouri TH, Park S, Nielsen SJ, Ogden CL. Trends in sugar-sweetened beverage consumption among youth and adults in the United States: 1999–2010. *Am J Clin Nutr.* 2013;98(1):180–8.
17. Fulgoni III VL, Quann EE. National trends in beverage consumption in children from birth to 5 years: Analysis of Nhanes across three decades. *Nutr J.* 2012;11:92.
18. Gibson S, Neate D. Sugar intake, soft drink consumption and body weight among British children: Further analysis of national diet and nutrition survey data with adjustment for under-reporting and physical activity. *Int J Food Sci Nutr.* 2007;58(6):445–60.
19. Herbst A, Diethelm K, Cheng G, Alexy U, Icks A, Buyken AE. Direction of associations between added sugar intake in early childhood and body mass index at age 7 years may depend on intake levels. *J Nutr.* 2011;141(7):1348–54.
20. Vagstrand K, Barkeling B, Forslund HB, Elfhag K, Linne Y, Rossner S et al. Eating habits in relation to body fatness and gender in adolescents—Results from the 'Swedes' study. *Eur J Clin Nutr.* 2007;61(4):517–25.
21. Davis JN, Alexander KE, Ventura EE, Kelly LA, Lane CJ, Byrd-Williams CE et al. Associations of dietary sugar and glycemic index with adiposity and insulin dynamics in overweight Latino youth. *Am J Clin Nutr.* 2007;86(5):1331–8. Epub 2007/11/10.
22. Pollock NK, Bundy V, Kanto W, Davis CL, Bernard PJ, Zhu H et al. Greater fructose consumption is associated with cardiometabolic risk markers and visceral adiposity in adolescents. *J Nutr.* 2012;142(2):251–7. Epub 2011/12/23.
23. Nicklas TA, O'Neil CE, Liu Y. Intake of added sugars is not associated with weight measures in children 6 to 18 years: National health and nutrition examination surveys 2003–2006. *Nutr Res.* 2011;31(5):338–46.
24. Song WO, Wang Y, Chung CE, Song B, Lee W, Chun OK. Is obesity development associated with dietary sugar intake in the U.S.? *Nutrition.* 2012;28(11–12):1137–41.
25. Storey ML, Forshee RA, Weaver AR, Sansalone WR. Demographic and lifestyle factors associated with body mass index among children and adolescents. *Int J Food Sci Nutr.* 2003;54(6):491–503.
26. Johnson RK. Changing eating and physical activity patterns of US children. *Proc Nutr Soc.* 2000;59(2):295–301.
27. Krebs-Smith SM, Graubard BI, Kahle LL, Subar AF, Cleveland LE, Ballard-Barbash R. Low energy reporters vs others: A comparison of reported food intakes. *Eur J Clin Nutr.* 2000;54(4):281–7.
28. Berkey CS, Rockett HR, Field AE, Gillman MW, Colditz GA. Sugar-added beverages and adolescent weight change. *Obes Res.* 2004;12(5):778–88.
29. Troiano RP, Briefel RR, Carroll MD, Bialostosky K. Energy and fat intakes of children and adolescents in the United States: Data from the national health and nutrition examination surveys. *Am J Clin Nutr.* 2000;72(5 Suppl):1343S–53S.
30. Ludwig DS, Peterson KE, Gortmaker SL. Relation between consumption of sugar-sweetened drinks and childhood obesity: A prospective, observational analysis. *Lancet.* 2001;357(9255):505–8.
31. Beck AL, Tschann J, Butte NF, Penilla C, Greenspan LC. Association of beverage consumption with obesity in Mexican American children. *Public Health Nutr.* 2013:1–7.
32. Fiorito LM, Marini M, Francis LA, Smiciklas-Wright H, Birch LL. Beverage intake of girls at age 5 y predicts adiposity and weight status in childhood and adolescence. *Am J Clin Nutr.* 2009;90(4):935–42.
33. Collison KS, Zaidi MZ, Subhani SN, Al-Rubeaan K, Shoukri M, Al-Mohanna FA. Sugar-sweetened carbonated beverage consumption correlates with BMI, waist circumference, and poor dietary choices in school children. *BMC Public Health.* 2010;10:234.
34. Jensen BW, Nielsen BM, Husby I, Bugge A, El-Naaman B, Andersen LB et al. Association between sweet drink intake and adiposity in Danish children participating in a long-term intervention study. *Pediatr Obes.* 2013;8(4):259–70. Epub 2013/05/01.
35. Weijs PJ, Kool LM, van Baar NM, van der Zee SC. High beverage sugar as well as high animal protein intake at infancy may increase overweight risk at 8 years: A prospective longitudinal pilot study. *Nutr J.* 2011;10:95.
36. Lim S, Zoellner JM, Lee JM, Burt BA, Sandretto AM, Sohn W et al. Obesity and sugar-sweetened beverages in African-American preschool children: A longitudinal study. *Obesity (Silver Spring).* 2009;17(6):1262–8.

37. Dubois L, Farmer A, Girard M, Peterson K. Regular sugar-sweetened beverage consumption between meals increases risk of overweight among preschool-aged children. *J Am Diet Assoc*. 2007;107(6):924–34; discussion 34–5.
38. Davis JN, Whaley SE, Goran MI. Effects of breastfeeding and low sugar-sweetened beverage intake on obesity prevalence in Hispanic toddlers. *Am J Clin Nutr*. 2012;95(1):3–8. Epub 2011/12/16.
39. Welsh JA, Cogswell ME, Rogers S, Rockett H, Mei Z, Grummer-Strawn LM. Overweight among low-income preschool children associated with the consumption of sweet drinks: Missouri, 1999–2002. *Pediatrics*. 2005;115(2):e223–9. Epub 2005/02/03.
40. Blum JW, Jacobsen DJ, Donnelly JE. Beverage consumption patterns in elementary school aged children across a two-year period. *J Am Coll Nutr*. 2005;24(2):93–8.
41. Newby PK, Peterson KE, Berkey CS, Leppert J, Willett WC, Colditz GA. Beverage consumption is not associated with changes in weight and body mass index among low-income preschool children in North Dakota. *J Am Diet Assoc*. 2004;104(7):1086–94.
42. Commision on Nutrition. American Academy of Pediatrics: The use and misuse of fruit juice in pediatrics. *Pediatrics*. 2001;107(5):1210–3.
43. Dennison BA, Rockwell HL, Baker SL. Excess fruit juice consumption by preschool-aged children is associated with short stature and obesity. *Pediatrics*. 1997;99(1):15–22.
44. Tanasescu M, Ferris AM, Himmelgreen DA, Rodriguez N, Perez-Escamilla R. Biobehavioral factors are associated with obesity in Puerto Rican children. *J Nutr*. 2000;130(7):1734–42.
45. Nicklas TA, O'Neil CE, Kleinman R. Association between 100% juice consumption and nutrient intake and weight of children aged 2 to 11 years. *Arch Pediatr Adolesc Med*. 2008;162(6):557–65.
46. O'Connor TM, Yang SJ, Nicklas TA. Beverage intake among preschool children and its effect on weight status. *Pediatrics*. 2006;118(4):e1010–8.
47. O'Neil CE, Nicklas TA, Rampersaud GC, Fulgoni III VL. One hundred percent orange juice consumption is associated with better diet quality, improved nutrient adequacy, and no increased risk for overweight/obesity in children. *Nutr Res*. 2011;31(9):673–82.
48. Smith U. Carbohydrates, Fat, and Insulin Action. *Am J Clin Nutr*. 1994;59(Suppl. 3):686S–9S.
49. Toubro S, Astrup A. Day-to-day variability of 24-H energy expenditure, respiratory quotient, macronutrient oxidation, and physical activity measured in a respiratory chamber. *Am J Clin Nutr*. 1994;59(Suppl.):775S.
50. Liem DG, Mennella JA. Sweet and sour preferences during childhood: Role of early experiences. *Dev Psychobiol*. 2002;41(4):388–95.
51. Rodenburg G, Oenema A, Kremers SP, van de Mheen D. Clustering of diet- and activity-related parenting practices: Cross-sectional findings of the INPACT study. *Int J Behav Nutr Phys Act*. 2013;10:36.
52. Liem DG, de Graaf C. Sweet and sour preferences in young children and adults: Role of repeated exposure. *Physiol Behav*. 2004;83(3):421–9.
53. Kosova EC, Auinger P, Bremer AA. The relationships between sugar-sweetened beverage intake and cardiometabolic markers in young children. *J Acad Nutr Diet*. 2013;113(2):219–27.
54. Kondaki K, Grammatikaki E, Jimenez-Pavon D, De Henauw S, Gonzalez-Gross M, Sjostrom M et al. Daily sugar-sweetened beverage consumption and insulin resistance in European adolescents: The Helena (Healthy Lifestyle in Europe by Nutrition in Adolescence) Study. *Public Health Nutr*. 2013;16(3):479–86.
55. Davis J, Ventura E, Weigensberg M, Ball G, ML C, Shaibi G et al. The relation of sugar intake to beta-cell function in overweight Latino children. *Am J Clin Nutr*. 2005;82:1004–10.
56. Perichart-Perera O, Balas-Nakash M, Rodriguez-Cano A, Munoz-Manrique C, Monge-Urrea A, Vadillo-Ortega F. Correlates of dietary energy sources with cardiovascular disease risk markers in Mexican school-age children. *J Am Diet Assoc*. 2010;110(2):253–60.
57. Mager DR, Patterson C, So S, Rogenstein CD, Wykes LJ, Roberts EA. Dietary and physical activity patterns in children with fatty liver. *Eur J Clin Nutr*. 2010;64(6):628–35.
58. Thuy S, Ladurner R, Volynets V, Wagner S, Strahl S, Konigsrainer A et al. Nonalcoholic fatty liver disease in humans is associated with increased plasma endotoxin and plasminogen activator inhibitor 1 concentrations and with fructose intake. *J Nutr*. 2008;138(8):1452–5.
59. Ouyang X, Cirillo P, Sautin Y, McCall S, Bruchette JL, Diehl AM et al. Fructose consumption as a risk factor for non-alcoholic fatty liver disease. *J Hepatol*. 2008;48(6):993–9.
60. Jin R, Le NA, Liu S, Farkas Epperson M, Ziegler TR, Welsh JA et al. Children with Nafld are more sensitive to the adverse metabolic effects of fructose beverages than children without Nafld. *J Clin Endocrinol Metab*. 2012;97(7):E1088–98.

61. Vos MB, Colvin R, Belt P, Molleston JP, Murray KF, Rosenthal P et al. Correlation of vitamin E, uric acid, and diet composition with histologic features of pediatric Nafld. *J Pediatr Gastroenterol Nutr.* 2012;54(1):90–6.
62. Davis JN, Le KA, Walker RW, Vikman S, Spruijt-Metz D, Weigensberg MJ et al. Increased hepatic fat in overweight hispanic youth influenced by interaction between genetic variation in Pnpla3 and high dietary carbohydrate and sugar consumption. *Am J Clin Nutr.* 2010;92(6):1522–7.
63. Babey SH, Wolstein J, Diamant AL. Food environments near home and school related to consumption of soda and fast food. *Policy Brief UCLA Cent Health Policy Res.* 2011(PB2011-6):1–8.
64. Powell LM, Nguyen BT. Fast-food and full-service restaurant consumption among children and adolescents: Effect on energy, beverage, and nutrient intake. *JAMA Pediatr.* 2013;167(1):14–20.
65. Lissner L, Habicht JP, Strupp BJ, Levitsky DA, Haas JD, Roe DA. Body composition and energy intake: Do overweight women overeat and underreport? *Am J Clin Nutr.* 1989;49:320–5.
66. Park S, Blanck HM, Sherry B, Brener N, O'Toole T. Factors associated with sugar-sweetened beverage intake among United States high school students. *J Nutr.* 2012;142(2):306–12.
67. Ebbeling CB, Feldman HA, Osganian SK, Chomitz VR, Ellenbogen SJ, Ludwig DS. Effects of decreasing sugar-sweetened beverage consumption on body weight in adolescents: A randomized, controlled pilot study. *Pediatrics.* 2006;117(3):673–80. Epub 2006/03/03.
68. Ebbeling CB, Feldman HA, Chomitz VR, Antonelli TA, Gortmaker SL, Osganian SK et al. A randomized trial of sugar-sweetened beverages and adolescent body weight. *N Engl J Med.* 2012;367(15):1407–16.
69. de Ruyter JC, Olthof MR, Seidell JC, Katan MB. A trial of sugar-free or sugar-sweetened beverages and body weight in children. *N Engl J Med.* 2012;367(15):1397–406. Epub 2012/09/25.
70. Maier IB, Stricker L, Ozel Y, Wagnerberger S, Bischoff SC, Bergheim I. A low fructose diet in the treatment of pediatric obesity: A pilot study. *Pediatr Int.* 2011;53(3):303–8.
71. Hasson RE, Adam TC, Davis JN, Kelly LA, Ventura EE, Byrd-Williams CE et al. Randomized controlled trial to improve adiposity, inflammation, and insulin resistance in obese African-American and Latino youth. *Obesity (Silver Spring).* 2012;20(4):811–8. Epub 2011/02/05.
72. Ventura E, Davis J, Byrd-Williams C, Alexander K, McClain A, Lane CJ et al. Reduction in risk factors for type 2 diabetes mellitus in response to a low-sugar, high-fiber dietary intervention in overweight Latino adolescents. *Arch Pediatr Adolesc Med.* 2009;163(4):320–7. Epub 2009/04/08.

18 Impact of Dietary Sugars on Obesity and Metabolic Risk during Critical Periods of Growth and Development

Michael I. Goran

CONTENTS

KEY POINTS

- Changes in the food supply over the last 50 years have disrupted the balance of fructose to glucose in the environment and this may have effects on obesity during developmental periods.
- Dietary fructose has different metabolic effects than glucose but the impact of these differences during development has not been broadly considered.
- Exposure to dietary fructose during critical periods of development may act as an obesogen favoring long-term development of obesity and associated metabolic risks.
- Critical periods of development include fetal development and breastfeeding where exposure may occur through maternal transmission or via direct consumption during infancy.
- The limited studies, mostly animal models, indicate that the negative programming impact of sugars on obesity and metabolic pathways during developmental periods are similar to those observed in children and adults and likely driven by the impact of fructose.
- Mechanisms of effect include disruption of neuroendocrine function, appetite control, and feeding behavior, promotion of adipogenesis, and accumulation of ectopic fat.

INTRODUCTION

Growing evidence supports the link between maternal nutrition during critical periods of development and obesity in the offspring, with a major focus surrounding the potential obesogenic effect of fructose, as reviewed elsewhere [1,2]. Studies in several animal models and limited human data suggest that fructose-induced metabolic disruptions during critical periods of development, including pregnancy and lactation, may be possible mechanisms that predispose offspring to long-term metabolic, neuroendocrine, and behavioral dysfunction [3–6]. For example, limited human data suggest that poor diet during pregnancy is associated with development of similar poor dietary habits in offspring [7]. As outlined in previous chapters, there is a strong impact of elevated sugar consumption during early childhood on obesity and metabolic risk [8]. However, consumption of high levels of dietary sugars and sweetened beverages is not uncommon during pregnancy and lactation [9], and in some studies this is associated with poor pregnancy outcomes [9–11]. This chapter provides an overview of the evidence linking excess dietary sugars, especially fructose, during critical periods of development to increased obesity and metabolic disease and summarizes the limited evidence and potential mechanisms of these effects.

Obesogenic Effects of Dietary Sugars During Critical Periods of Early Growth

The developing fetus and rapidly growing infant are not immune to the potential hazardous effects of high levels of maternal consumption of dietary sugars. McCurdy et al. [12] studied the concept of critical periods in pregnant female primates fed a chronic high-fat diet and looked at the impact on the development of fetal metabolic systems. They found fetal offspring from both lean and obese mothers fed a high-fat diet had a three-fold increase in liver triglycerides, increased hepatic oxidative stress, increased serum triglycerides, and a two-fold increase in body fat, consistent with the development of nonalcoholic fatty liver disease [12]. The adverse effects of excess fuel consumption during pregnany on fetal development may be due to a lack of white adipose tissue in most species until late in pregnancy (typically third trimester). White adiopose tissue is critical for the storage of excess lipids and thus failure to develop strucutrally or functionally sufficient adipose tissue depots to handle excess lipid leads to ectopic lipid storage that can induce whole body insulin resistance and suceptibility to fatty liver disease in adulthood [5,6].

After birth, rapid weight gain during the first 4–6 months of life has been associated with greater odds of child overweight at age 4 or 7 years [13–15] and as a teenager [13,16–19]. Child-feeding practices and early nutritional experiences play a causal role in children's energy regulation and weight outcomes [20,21]. Mothers who are overweight or obese may inadvertently expose their children to an obesogenic food environment. For example, in a study of 718 parents of children ages 3–5 years, parents with an indulgent feeding style (e.g., offering sugary beverages to placate) had children with a higher child body mass index [22]. Another emerging finding is that children with a "difficult" temperament may be more prone to obesity [23], and this may be due to parental use of sugary treats and sugary beverages to placate their child [24].

Although the deleterious effects of excess sugars and fructose throughout life are well researched, there are only limited data regarding the impact of excess sugars/fructose consumption during critical periods of development that largely set the stage for lifelong health. Emerging research suggests that fructose consumption both by mothers and offspring during gestation, lactation, and early-life can lead to persistent neuroendocrine and metabolic dysfunction. Appetite, energy balance, and metabolism are regulated by the central nervous system. The important components of this neural network include neurons located in the arcuate nucleus (ARC) of the hypothalamus, particularly those that produce proopiomelanocortin (POMC), neuropeptide Y (NPY), and agouti-related peptide (AgRP). The hypothalamus primarily regulates the homeostatic drive to eat, while other regions such as the ventral striatum, insula, amygdala, and hippocampus form the behavioral pathway that controls the hedonic drive to eat [25]. The homeostatic and hedonic feeding regions are tightly interconnected and form an integrated network that dictates feeding behavior. This network that is recruited (activated) in the hunger state and its activity normally decreases in response to food intake [25]. The hypothalamus undergoes a tremendous growth beginning early in gestation, which continues during the postnatal period. These developmental windows represent periods of vulnerability, during which alterations in the environment may perturb hypothalamic development and subsequent function.

Evidence from animal and human studies support the notion that compared to glucose, fructose has very different effects on the brain that favor an increase in food intake and obesity (see Chapter 15).

In animal studies, direct administration of fructose versus glucose into the brain has been shown to have opposing effects on obesity and food intake regulation [26]. Essentially, these studies show that fructose metabolism in the brain is less controlled and more rapidly depletes hypothalamic adenosine triphosphate (ATP), whereas glucose metabolism is more regulated and increases ATP levels in the hypothalamus. Consequently, fructose leads to a reduction in malonyl-CoA in the brain and this has been shown to be a contributor to increased food intake [26]. In another study, rats fed a very high-fructose diet demonstrated leptin resistance and reduced hypothalamic pSTAT3 activation by 6 months. These leptin-resistant animals gained more weight and had greater fat pad weights than control animals when switched to a high-fat diet for 2 weeks [27]. Such leptin resistance would be particularly relevant during early-life, as other work has shown that leptin is a critical neurotrophic factor for the developing hypothalamus [28], and leptin resistance during this critical period could impair energy balance throughout life [29,30].

In other work relative to newborn animals before weaning, Alzamendi et al. [31] examined fructose exposure by feeding lactating rats either a 10% fructose-rich diet or tap water starting postnatal day 1. Offspring of fructose-fed rats showed increased body weight, decreased hypothalamic sensitivity to exogenous leptin, increased food intake, insulin resistance, and increased retroperitoneal adipose tissue, with an increase in mass and cell size [31]. Data from animal studies show that exposure to 10% fructose during pregnancy increases risk of gestational diabetes [32,33] and liver fat infiltration during pregnancy [34]. Additional studies have teased apart the impact of the fructose moiety during critical periods, by comparative analysis with different sugar concentrations. Jen et al. fed female rats either 40% fructose or 50% sucrose diet with a control ad libitum diet during gestation and lactation. During gestation, fructose induces elevated levels of circulating glucose and triglycerides, which led offspring of fructose-fed dams to be hyperglycemic at birth. Follow-up studies using a similar model showed that only the fructose-fed mothers and their offspring had hyperglycemia during pregnancy and after birth, suggesting that a possible mechanism may be the increased concentration of the fructose moiety [35]. Another study randomly assigned female rats to a deionized distilled water diet or a deionized distilled water diet sweetened with 13% glucose, sucrose, fructose, or HFCS for 8 weeks. Thirteen percent was used to mimic common sweetener concentrations found in the human diet. No difference was found in energy intake; however, the type of caloric sweetener added to beverages influenced body fat mass. Only HFCS 55 promoted adiposity in rats, suggesting that the type of added sweetener is critical, consistent with Sullivan et al.'s conclusions with types of fats, discussed above [36].

Additional studies have used maternal rat diets of 10% fructose versus 10% glucose and showed that fructose-fed dams ate more food and drank less water compared to dams fed glucose. The offspring of fructose-fed dams had almost double the fasting insulin at weaning compared to the offspring of glucose fed dams [37]. In some cases, offspring of fructose-fed dams just showed increased plasma leptin and plasma glucose with no change in insulin [38]. Other studies show that increased fructose consumption, but not glucose during pregnancy, was associated with increased circulating triglycerides in offspring [39]. Furthermore, when examining impact of successive generations, female rats were weaned onto diets containing either starch (no fructose) or sucrose (50% fructose and 50% glucose) and maintained the diet through breeding. Offspring from the first generation born to sucrose-fed dams were heavier with increased body fat, higher circulation glucose, and triglycerides compared to those born to starch-fed dams who would have had no fructose exposure [40].

Other studies have focused on understanding the role of maternal nutrition on the development of taste preferences in offspring as a potential mechanism. Sweet flavor preferences were hypothesized to develop before weaning, suggesting that nutrient conditioning (i.e., the development of flavor preferences) from the maternal diet is transmitted through breast milk [41]. Human studies showed that maternal intake of protein, fat, and carbohydrates during preganancy was associated with child intake at 10 years of age [42]. During the period of lacation, there is some evidence to show that fructose negatively impacts milk quality with greater milk fat [43]. Furthermore, 10-week-old rat pups born to mothers fed a junk food diet (high fat, sugar, salt) during gestation and lactation showed a greater preference for fatty, sugary, and salty foods, compared to pups whose mothers were fed a balanced chow diet [44]. Follow-up studies revealed that offspring whose mothers were fed the junk food diet during gestation and lactation developed more obesity, elevated glucose, and insulin, increased risk for fatty liver disease, and signs of steatosis and liver damage compared to rats given free access to the same diet, but whose mothers had a normal chow diet [45].

MECHANISMS OF EXCESS FRUCTOSE EXPOSURE DURING CRITICAL PERIODS OF DEVELOPMENT

There are several potential mechanisms that might explain the negative impact of high-fructose exposure during critical perinatal developmental periods that merit further investigation. From an evolutionary perspective, infants would not be typically exposed to high levels of fructose since sugar from human milk is lactose (glucose bonded to galactose), and although 30 or more oligosaccharides are also present [46], fructose is not a natural component. Under normal conditions in animal models, it has been shown that the abundance of mRNAs encoding the sodium-dependent and facilitative transporter proteins for sugars are developmentally modulated, with the highest levels in adult intestines [47]. This suggests that the mechanism for fructose absorption may not be fully or even partially functioning during gestation and early life [47]. In some ways, this may be protective since an infant might not have the ability to absorb fructose. However, in animal models, excess fructose [48] as well as induced hyperglycemia and type 2 diabetes have been shown to upregulate Glut-5 expression in the intestine [49,50]. It is unknown whether this upregulation can occur during fetal development or infancy, but this is plausible since fructose does cross the placenta into the developing fetus and infants would be exposed to fructose through maternal transmission in breast milk or via direct consumption by the infant. Studies in sheep have shown that fetal blood contains appreciable amounts of fructose throughout gestation. Subsequent studies revealed a difference in fructose concentration of maternal and fetal blood, showing that the sheep placenta actively transfers fructose to the fetal circulation [51,52]. Thus, fetal and infant exposure to fructose either through maternal transmission or direct consumption is possible and would have detrimental metabolic effects on fetal and infant metabolism. However, there is very limited human data related to the important topic of transport of different sugars across the placenta with initial evidence for a role of variations in the GLUT-9 transporter in the placenta in diabetic pregnancies [53].

Another hypothesis is that fructose directly promotes adipogenesis during critical periods when adipose tissue is rapidly expanding. This is supported by a recent study showing that fructose induced adipocyte differentiation in 3T3-L1 preadipocytes [54] and that blocking fructose uptake in vivo using Glut5−/− mice led to a dramatic reduction in epididymal fat mass compared to Glut+/+ controls [54]. Another possible mechanism through which excess fructose could promote obesity during development is by disrupting cross-talk between adipose tissue and the hypothalamus. The arcuate nucleus (ARC) of the hypothalamus contains neurons that respond to various circulating factors, including glucose, insulin, and leptin [55]. By acting on the ARC, leptin conveys the level of adiposity to the brain, thereby promoting energy expenditure and reducing food intake [56]. A previous study in mice showed that leptin acts as a critical growth factor for connecting the ARC to other hypothalamic nuclei during brain development [28]. However, since fructose does not stimulate leptin release, an imbalance in fetal fructose:glucose exposure could potentially limit the effects of leptin on these important brain development pathways. This seems plausible given that other studies have shown that prenatal or early-life overnutrition leads to hypothalamic leptin insensitivity, impaired pSTAT3 signaling, and obesity in adulthood [57,58]. Collectively, this evidence supports the concept that excess fructose during development could promote obesity by direct action of fructose on the adipose tissue, direct or indirect action on the developing hypothalamus, or by disrupting the “adipocyte-hypothalamic axis” during critical periods.

SUMMARY AND CONCLUSION

Evidence from humans and animals suggest differential metabolic effects of fructose that favor the development of obesity likely drive the link between dietary sugars and obesity. These effects are operational and relevant during critical periods of development such as gestation and early infancy, when rapid growth and development occurs in both brain and adipose tissue. It is hypothesized that exposure to excess fructose in utero (placental transfer arising from maternal consumption) and/or during infancy (transfer through breast milk arising from maternal consumption, or by direct consumption by the infant) promotes obesity during periods of adipose tissue development and expansion. In addition, since fructose has differential and more adverse effects on the brain that favor obesity, exposure to excess fructose during development could result in obesity by direct action of fructose on the developing hypothalamus, or by disrupting the "adipocyte-hypothalamic axis" during critical developmental periods. Given that fructose has a unique metabolic fate that favors the development of obesity, there is no reason to believe that the developing fetus, neonate, and infant would be protected from these well-known adverse effects. Thus, exposure to fructose, which is not a natural component of an infant's diet, in conjunction with the ability for fructose to cross the placental barrier, likely increases the risk for fructose to cause metabolic and developmental dysfunction and requires further investigation of the impact of excessive fructose consumption during critical periods of gestation and lactation.

CONFLICTS OF INTEREST

Michael Goran's research has been or is currently supported by the National Institutes of Health, the American Diabetes Association, the Thrasher Research Fund, and the Dr Robert C and Veronica Atkins Foundation. The author has no other conflicts of interest.

REFERENCES

1. Regnault TR, Gentili S, Sarr O, Toop CR, Sloboda DM. Fructose, pregnancy and later life impacts. *Clin Exp Pharmacol Physiol*. 2013;40(11):824–37. Epub 2013/09/17.
2. Goran MI, Dumke K, Bouret SG, Kayser B, Walker RW, Blumberg B. The obesogenic effect of high fructose exposure during early development. *Nat Rev Endocrinol*. 2013;9(8):494–500. Epub 2013/06/05.
3. Kral JG, Biron S, Simard S, Hould FS, Lebel S, Marceau S et al. Large maternal weight loss from obesity surgery prevents transmission of obesity to children who were followed for 2 to 18 years. *Pediatrics*. 2006;118(6):e1644–9. Epub 2006/12/05.
4. Taylor GM, Alexander FE, D'Souza SW. Interactions between fetal Hla-Dq alleles and maternal smoking influence birthweight. *Paediatr Perinat Epidemiol*. 2006;20(5):438–48. Epub 2006/08/17.
5. Lawlor DA, Smith GD, O'Callaghan M, Alati R, Mamun AA, Williams GM et al. Epidemiologic evidence for the fetal overnutrition hypothesis: Findings from the mater-university study of pregnancy and its outcomes. *Am J Epidemiol*. 2007;165(4):418–24. Epub 2006/12/13.
6. Knight B, Shields BM, Hill A, Powell RJ, Wright D, Hattersley AT. The impact of maternal glycemia and obesity on early postnatal growth in a nondiabetic caucasian population. *Diabetes Care*. 2007;30(4):777–83. Epub 2007/01/26.
7. Brion M-JA, Ness AR, Rogers I, Emmett P, Cribb V, Smith GD et al. Maternal macronutrient and energy intakes in pregnancy and offspring intake at 10 y: Exploring parental comparisons and prenatal effects. *Am J Clin Nutr*. 2010;91(3).
8. Davis JN, Whaley SE, Goran MI. Effects of breastfeeding and low sugar-sweetened beverage intake on obesity prevalence in hispanic toddlers. *Am J Clin Nutr*. 2012;95(1):3–8. Epub 2011/12/16.
9. Englund-Ogge L, Brantsaeter AL, Haugen M, Sengpiel V, Khatibi A, Myhre R et al. Association between intake of artificially sweetened and sugar-sweetened beverages and preterm delivery: A large prospective cohort study. *Am J Clin Nutr*. 2012;96(3):552–9. Epub 2012/08/03.
10. Wong AC, Ko CW. Carbohydrate intake as a risk factor for biliary sludge and stones during pregnancy. *J Clin Gastroenterol*. 2013;47(8):700–5. Epub 2013/02/28.
11. Borgen I, Aamodt G, Harsem N, Haugen M, Meltzer HM, Brantsaeter AL. Maternal sugar consumption and risk of preeclampsia in nulliparous Norwegian women. *Eur J Clin Nutr*. 2012;66(8):920–5. Epub 2012/06/21.

12. McCurdy CE, Bishop JM, Williams SM, Grayson BE, Smith MS, Friedman JE et al. Maternal high-fat diet triggers lipotoxicity in the fetal livers of nonhuman primates. *J Clin Invest*. 2009;119(2):323–35. Epub 2009/01/17.
13. Stettler N, Zemel BS, Kumanyika S, Stallings VA. Infant weight gain and childhood overweight status in a multicenter, cohort study. *Pediatrics*. 2002;109(2):194–9.
14. Ong KK. Size at birth, postnatal growth and risk of obesity. *Horm Res*. 2006;65(Suppl. 3):65–9. Epub 2006/04/14.
15. Ong KK, Loos RJ. Rapid infancy weight gain and subsequent obesity: Systematic reviews and hopeful suggestions. *Acta Paediatr*. 2006;95(8):904–8. Epub 2006/08/03.
16. Taveras EM, Rifas-Shiman SL, Belfort MB, Kleinman KP, Oken E, Gillman MW. Weight status in the first 6 months of life and obesity at 3 years of age. *Pediatrics*. 2009;123(4):1177–83. Epub 2009/04/02.
17. Ekelund U, Ong K, Linne Y, Neovius M, Brage S, Dunger DB et al. Upward weight percentile crossing in infancy and early childhood independently predicts fat mass in young adults: The Stockholm Weight Development Study (SWEDES). *Am J Clin Nutr*. 2006;83(2):324–30. Epub 2006/02/14.
18. Dennison BA, Edmunds LS, Stratton HH, Pruzek RM. Rapid infant weight gain predicts childhood overweight. *Obesity (Silver Spring)*. 2006;14(3):491–9. Epub 2006/05/02.
19. Stettler N, Stallings VA, Troxel AB, Zhao J, Schinnar R, Nelson SE et al. Weight gain in the first week of life and overweight in adulthood: A cohort study of European American subjects fed infant formula. *Circulation*. 2005;111(15):1897–903. Epub 2005/04/20.
20. Birch LL, Davison KK. Family environmental factors influencing the developing behavioral controls of food intake and childhood overweight. *Pediatr Clin North Am*. 2001;48(4):893–907.
21. Birch LL. Development of food preferences. *Annu Rev Nutr*. 1999;19:41–62.
22. Hughes SO, Shewchuk RM, Baskin ML, Nicklas TA, Qu H. Indulgent feeding style and children's weight status in preschool. *J Dev Behav Pediatr*. 2008;29(5):403–10. Epub 2008/08/21.
23. Carey WB, Hegvik RL, McDevitt SC. Temperamental factors associated with rapid weight gain and obesity in middle childhood. *J Dev Behav Pediatr*. 1988;9(4):194–8. Epub 1988/08/01.
24. Vollrath ME, Tonstad S, Rothbart MK, Hampson SE. Infant temperament is associated with potentially obesogenic diet at 18 months. *Int J Pediatr Obes*. 2011;6(2–2):e408–14. Epub 2010/09/22.
25. Malik S, McGlone F, Bedrossian D, Dagher A. Ghrelin modulates brain activity in areas that control appetitive behavior. *Cell Metab*. 2008;7(5):400–9. Epub 2008/05/08.
26. Cha SH, Wolfgang M, Tokutake Y, Chohnan S, Lane MD. Differential effects of central fructose and glucose on hypothalamic malonyl-CoA and food intake. *Proc Natl Acad Sci USA*. 2008;105(44):16871–5. Epub 2008/10/31.
27. Shapiro A, Mu W, Roncal C, Cheng KY, Johnson RJ, Scarpace PJ. Fructose-induced leptin resistance exacerbates weight gain in response to subsequent high-fat feeding. *Am J Physiol Regul Integr Comp Physiol*. 2008;295(5):R1370–5. Epub 2008/08/16.
28. Bouret SG, Draper SJ, Simerly RB. Trophic action of leptin on hypothalamic neurons that regulate feeding. *Science*. 2004;304(5667):108–10. Epub 2004/04/06.
29. Bouret SG. Role of early hormonal and nutritional experiences in shaping feeding behavior and hypothalamic development. *J Nutr*. 2010;140(3):653–7. Epub 2010/01/29.
30. Bouret SG, Simerly RB. Minireview: Leptin and development of hypothalamic feeding circuits. *Endocrinology*. 2004;145(6):2621–6. Epub 2004/03/27.
31. Alzamendi A, Castrogiovanni D, Gaillard RC, Spinedi E, Giovambattista A. Increased male offspring's risk of metabolic-neuroendocrine dysfunction and overweight after fructose-rich diet intake by the lactating mother. *Endocrinology*. 2010;151(9).
32. Alzamendi A, Del Zotto H, Castrogiovanni D, Romero J, Giovambattista A, Spinedi E. Oral metformin treatment prevents enhanced insulin demand and placental dysfunction in the pregnant rat fed a fructose-rich diet. *ISRN Endocrinol*. 2012;2012. Article ID: 757913. Epub 2012/09/08.
33. Alzamendi A, Giovambattista A, Garcia ME, Rebolledo OR, Gagliardino JJ, Spinedi E. Effect of pioglitazone on the fructose-induced abdominal adipose tissue dysfunction. *PPAR Res*. 2012;2012. Article ID: 259093. Epub 2012/10/24.
34. Zou M, Arentson EJ, Teegarden D, Koser SL, Onyskow L, Donkin SS. Fructose consumption during pregnancy and lactation induces fatty liver and glucose intolerance in rats. *Nutr Res*. 2012;32(8):588–98. Epub 2012/09/01.
35. Jen KLC, Rochon C, Zhong S, Whitcomb L. Fructose and sucrose feeding during pregnancy and lactation in rats changes maternal and pup fuel metabolism. *J Nutr*. 1991;121(12):1999–2005.

36. Light HR, Tsanzi E, Gigliotti J, Morgan K, Tou JC. The type of caloric sweetener added to water influences weight gain, fat mass, and reproduction in growing Sprague-Dawley female rats. *Exp Biol Med.* 2009;234(6):651–61. Epub 2009/04/11.
37. Rawana S, Clark K, Zhong SB, Buison A, Chackunkal S, Jen KLC. Low-dose fructose ingestion during gestation and lactation affects carbohydrate-metabolism in rat dams and their offspring. *J Nutr.* 1993;123(12):2158–65.
38. Vickers MH, Clayton ZE, Yap C, Sloboda DM. Maternal fructose intake during pregnancy and lactation alters placental growth and leads to sex-specific changes in fetal and neonatal endocrine function. *Endocrinology.* 2011;152(4).
39. Rodriguez L, Panadero MI, Roglans N, Otero P, Alvarez-Millan JJ, Laguna JC et al. Fructose during pregnancy affects maternal and fetal leptin signaling. *J Nutr Biochem.* 2013;24(10):1709–16. Epub 2013/05/07.
40. GhusainChoueiri AA, Rath EA. Effect of carbohydrate source on lipid metabolism in lactating mice and on pup development. *British Journal of Nutrition.* 1995;74(6):821–31.
41. Myers KP, Sclafani A. Development of learned flavor preferences. *Dev Psychobiol.* 2006;48(5):380–8. Epub 2006/06/14.
42. Brion MJ, Ness AR, Rogers I, Emmett P, Cribb V, Davey Smith G et al. Maternal macronutrient and energy intakes in pregnancy and offspring intake at 10 y: Exploring parental comparisons and prenatal effects. *Am J Clin Nutr.* 2010;91(3):748–56. Epub 2010/01/08.
43. Campbell WJ, Brendemuhl JH, Bazer FW. Effect of fructose consumption during lactation on sow and litter performance and sow plasma constituents. *J Anim Sci.* 1990;68(5):1378–88. Epub 1990/05/01.
44. Bayol SA, Farrington SJ, Stickland NC. A maternal 'junk food' diet in pregnancy and lactation promotes an exacerbated taste for 'junk food' and a greater propensity for obesity in rat offspring. *Br J Nutr.* 2007;98(4):843–51. Epub 2007/08/19.
45. Bayol SA, Simbi BH, Bertrand JA, Stickland NC. Offspring from mothers fed a 'junk food' diet in pregnancy and lactation exhibit exacerbated adiposity that is more pronounced in females. *J Physiol.* 2008;586(13):3219–30. Epub 2008/05/10.
46. Jenness R. The composition of human milk. *Semin Perinatol.* 1979;3(3):225–39. Epub 1979/07/01.
47. Davidson NO, Hausman AM, Ifkovits CA, Buse JB, Gould GW, Burant CF et al. Human intestinal glucose transporter expression and localization of Glut5. *Am J Physiol.* 1992;262(3 Pt 1):C795–800. Epub 1992/03/01.
48. Burant CF, Saxena M. Rapid reversible substrate regulation of fructose transporter expression in rat small intestine and kidney. *Am J Physiol.* 1994;267(1 Pt 1):G71–9. Epub 1994/07/01.
49. Douard V, Choi HI, Elshenawy S, Lagunoff D, Ferraris RP. Developmental reprogramming of rat Glut5 requires glucocorticoid receptor translocation to the nucleus. *J Physiol.* 2008;586(Pt 15):3657–73. Epub 2008/06/17.
50. Douard V, Ferraris RP. Regulation of the fructose transporter Glut5 in health and disease. *Am J Physiol Endocrinol Metab.* 2008;295(2):E227–37. Epub 2008/04/10.
51. Holmberg NG, Kaplan B, Karvonen MJ, Lind J, Malm M. Permeability of human placenta to glucose, fructose, and xylose. *Acta Physiol Scand.* 1956;36(4):291–9. Epub 1956/05/31.
52. Hagerman DD, Villee CA. The transport of fructose by human placenta. *J Clin Invest.* 1952;31(10):911–3. Epub 1952/10/01.
53. Bibee KP, Illsley NP, Moley KH. Asymmetric syncytial expression of Glut9 splice variants in human term placenta and alterations in diabetic pregnancies. *Reprod Sci.* 2011;18(1):20–7. Epub 2010/10/12.
54. Du L, Heaney AP. Regulation of adipose differentiation by fructose and Glut5. *Mol Endocrinol.* 2012;26(10):1773–82. Epub 2012/07/26.
55. Sandoval D, Cota D, Seeley RJ. The integrative role of CNS fuel-sensing mechanisms in energy balance and glucose regulation. *Annu Rev Physiol.* 2008;70:513–35.
56. Elmquist JK, Coppari R, Balthasar N, Ichinose M, Lowell BB. Identifying hypothalamic pathways controlling food intake, body weight, and glucose homeostasis. *J Comp Neurol.* 2005;493(1):63–71.
57. Kirk SL, Samuelsson AM, Argenton M, Dhonye H, Kalamatianos T, Poston L et al. Maternal obesity induced by diet in rats permanently influences central processes regulating food intake in offspring. *PLoS One.* 2009;4(6):e5870.
58. Glavas MM, Kirigiti MA, Xiao XQ, Enriori PJ, Fisher SK, Evans AE et al. Early overnutrition results in early-onset arcuate leptin resistance and increased sensitivity to high-fat diet. *Endocrinology.* 2010;151(4):1598–610.

19 Mechanisms by Which Dietary Sugars Influence Lipid Metabolism, Circulating Lipids and Lipoproteins, and Cardiovascular Risk

Kimber L. Stanhope and Peter J. Havel

CONTENTS

KEY POINTS

- The uptake of dietary glucose by the liver is regulated by hepatic energy status, whereas the uptake of dietary fructose is unregulated.
- The unregulated hepatic uptake of fructose results in increased production of lipogenic precursors, thereby leading to increased de novo lipogenesis (DNL), inhibited fatty acid oxidation, and increased hepatic lipid supply.

- Increased hepatic lipid supply is associated with increased production of large very-low-density lipoprotein 1 (VLDL1) particles and dyslipidemia.
- Increased hepatic lipid accumulation is associated with hepatic insulin resistance.
- Fructose-induced hepatic insulin resistance has the potential to set up a vicious cycle by causing increased activation of DNL → increased hepatic lipid content → increased insulin resistance → further activation of DNL.
- Fructose-induced hepatic insulin resistance may increase VLDL1 production directly via impaired insulin suppression of apolipoprotein B (apoB) degradation, microsomal triglyceride-transfer protein expression and apolipoprotein CIII expression, and also indirectly via increased hepatic lipid supply.
- Fructose-induced increases in uric acid production and inflammatory factors may also exacerbate VLDL production.
- Sustained hypertriglyceridemia may lead to intramyocellular lipid accumulation, which is associated with reduced whole-body insulin sensitivity.
- Intervention studies in human subjects consuming high-fructose or -sugar diets have documented adverse effects including increased DNL and inhibited fatty acid oxidation; increased hepatic lipid content; increased circulating levels of triglyceride, cholesterol, low-density lipoprotein (LDL) cholesterol, very low LDL, apoB, and remnant lipoprotein-triglyceride and -cholesterol; hepatic insulin resistance; intramyocellular lipid accumulation; and reduced whole-body insulin sensitivity.
- There are plausible mechanisms and both epidemiological and direct experimental evidence to support a causal relationship between the consumption of excessive amounts of dietary sugars and the development of metabolic disease.

INTRODUCTION

There is considerable epidemiological evidence suggesting intake of added sugars and/or sugar-sweetened beverages is associated with the presence of unfavorable lipid/lipoprotein levels [1–3], insulin resistance [4,5], fatty liver [6,7], type 2 diabetes [8–12], cardiovascular disease [13,14], metabolic syndrome [15–18], and increased visceral adiposity [19,20]. However, these studies do not provide definitive evidence that consumption of excessive sugars leads to the development of these adverse metabolic states. For that, direct experimental evidence demonstrating that consumption of diets high in sugars alters risk factors for metabolic disease compared with isocaloric diets that are low in sugar is needed. It is also necessary to demonstrate that there are plausible mechanisms to mediate a causal relationship between sugar and metabolic disease.

FRUCTOSE—POTENTIAL LINK BETWEEN SUGAR CONSUMPTION AND METABOLIC DISEASE

Our group has reported that overweight to obese adult men and women (40–72 years of age) consuming fructose-sweetened beverages at 25% of energy requirements for 10 weeks exhibited increased visceral adipose deposition and de novo lipogenesis (DNL), decreased fatty acid oxidation, dyslipidemia, and decreased glucose tolerance/insulin sensitivity. However, subjects consuming glucose-sweetened beverages did not demonstrate any of these changes, even though both groups of subjects gained comparable amounts of body weight (~1.4 kg) [21,22]. Since foods are not sweetened with pure fructose or pure glucose, these results have limited direct relevance to the effects of sugars as they are normally consumed in the diet. However, they are important in that they suggest that fructose consumption has effects on the development of metabolic disease that are independent of body weight gain and markedly different from the effects of glucose consumption. They are also important in that they suggest that fructose may be the link explaining the associations between consumption of sugars and the development of metabolic risk factors and disease. The potential

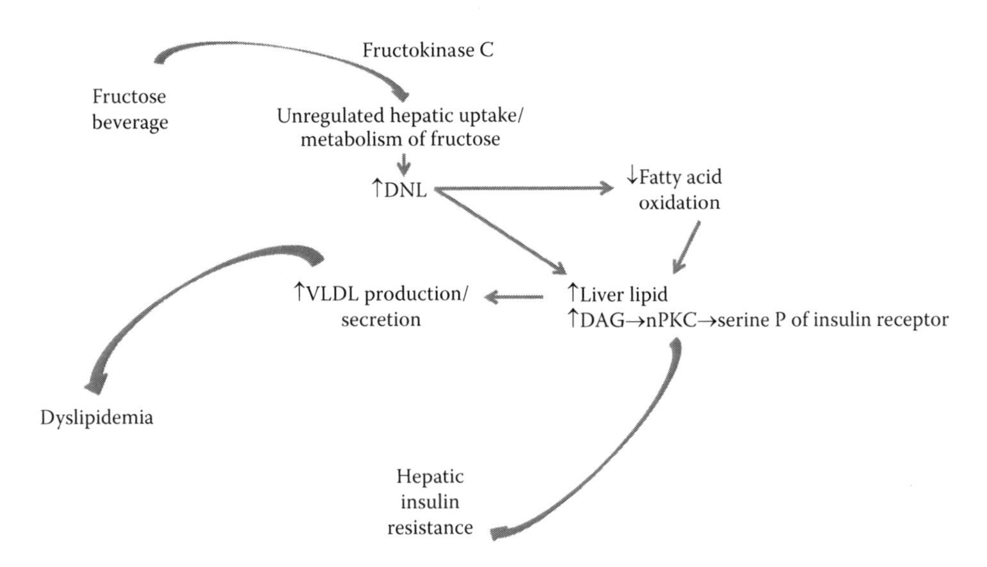

FIGURE 19.1 Potential mechanism by which consumption of fructose affects lipid metabolism and hepatic insulin sensitivity: Unregulated fructose uptake by the liver, mediated primarily by phosphorylation via fructokinase C, leads to increased DNL. DNL increases the intrahepatic lipid supply directly, via synthesis of fatty acids, and indirectly, by inhibiting fatty acid oxidation. Increased levels of intrahepatic lipid content promote VLDL production and secretion, which leads to dyslipidemia. Increased levels of hepatic lipids may also promote hepatic insulin resistance by increasing levels of DAG, which activates nPKC and leads to serine phosphorylation of the insulin receptor and IRS-1 and impaired insulin action. DNL: de novo lipogenesis; VLDL: very-low-density lipoprotein; DAG: diacylglycerol; nPKC: novel protein kinase C; serine P: serine phosphorylation; IRS-1, insulin receptor substrate 1.

mechanisms [23–27] by which the consumption of fructose leads to lipid dysregulation, liver lipid accumulation, and insulin resistance are described below and summarized in Figures 19.1 and 19.2. The direct experimental evidence that supports the plausibility of these mechanisms and the causal relationship between sugar consumption and risk factors for metabolic disease is also described.

REGULATION OF HEPATIC GLUCOSE METABOLISM

Hepatic glucose uptake is dependent on glucose transport into hepatic cells by a facilitative glucose transporter (GLUT2), followed by glucose phosphorylation to glucose-6-phosphate by glucokinase; this enzyme has a high K_m for glucose, and its activity is essentially regulated by portal glycemia; furthermore, its expression is increased by insulin. Glucose-6-phosphate is further metabolized in glycolysis, and this pathway is mainly regulated by phosphofructokinase (PFK). PFK is inhibited by adenosine triphosphate (ATP) and citrate when hepatic energy status is elevated, thereby limiting hepatic uptake of dietary glucose. Altogether, this regulation of hepatic glucose metabolism by insulin and hepatic energy allows much of ingested glucose arriving via the portal vein to bypass the liver and reach the systemic circulation. Thus, consumption of glucose-sweetened beverages with meals leads to increased plasma glucose and insulin excursions compared with consumption of the baseline complex carbohydrate diet [28,29].

REGULATION OF HEPATIC FRUCTOSE UPTAKE

The initial phosphorylation of dietary fructose is largely catalyzed by fructokinase, which is not regulated by hepatic energy status. The result is unregulated fructose uptake by the liver with little

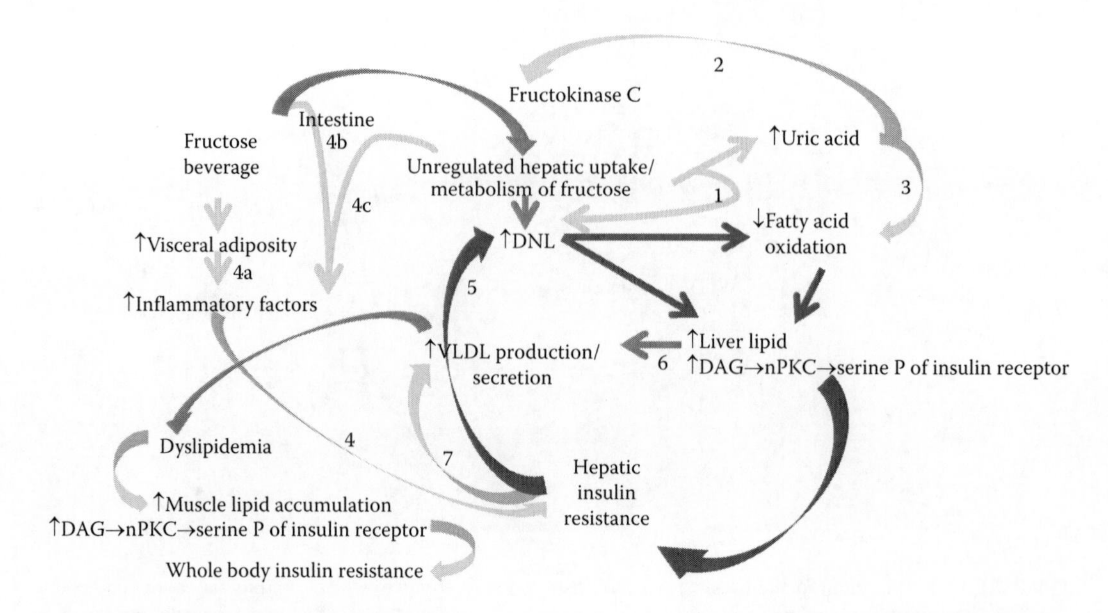

FIGURE 19.2 Potential exacerbation of the effects of fructose: the pathway depicted in Figure 19.1 may be exacerbated at the seven sites labeled 1–7. The unregulated fructose uptake by the liver, mediated by fructokinase C, also leads to increased production of uric acid via the purine degradation pathway. (1) This pathway may indirectly contribute to the liver lipid supply by concurrently generating mitochondrial oxidants that upregulate DNL. (2) Uric acid may also promote fructose uptake into the liver by upregulating expression of fructokinase C. (3) Uric acid may contribute to the accumulation of lipid in the liver by inhibiting AMP-activated kinase, an activator of fatty acid oxidation. (4) Fructose-induced increases of visceral adipose (4a), or fructose exposure to intestine (4b) or hepatocytes (4c), may promote inflammatory responses that impair hepatic insulin signaling or increase hepatic lipid levels. (5) Due to selective insulin resistance, DNL is even more strongly activated in the insulin-resistant liver DNL, which has the potential to generate a vicious cycle (darkest arrows). (6) This cycle would be expected to further exacerbate VLDL production and secretion by increasing the intrahepatic lipid supply. (7) Hepatic insulin resistance also exacerbates VLDL production/secretion by increasing apoB availability. The potential exacerbation of the adverse effects of fructose at sites 1–7 may contribute to increased exposure to circulating triglyceride, leading to the accumulation of intramyocellular lipid in skeletal muscle, impaired insulin signaling, and whole-body insulin resistance. DNL: de novo lipogenesis; VLDL: very-low-density lipoprotein; apoB: apolipoprotein B.

of the ingested fructose reaching the systemic circulation. This is illustrated in the 24-h fructose and glucose profiles in subjects who consumed fructose- or glucose-sweetened beverages with three meals in a 24-h crossover trial [30]. When the subjects consumed the glucose-sweetened beverages, postmeal glucose peaks increased over fasting levels by 4–5 mmol; when they consumed the fructose-sweetened beverages, postmeal fructose peaks increased by less than 0.4 mmol [30]. Accordingly, postprandial increases of plasma glucose and insulin concentrations were substantially lower when subjects consumed fructose along with mixed meals compared with a baseline complex carbohydrate diet [28,29].

FRUCTOKINASE C

Ishimoto et al. [31] have recently provided compelling evidence highlighting the importance of fructokinase in mediating the adverse effects of fructose. They report that fructokinase exists as two isoforms: fructokinase A which is widely distributed and has low affinity for fructose; and fructokinase C, which is expressed primarily in the liver, intestine, and kidney and has high affinity for fructose. They demonstrated that the adverse metabolic changes induced by fructose consumption are prevented in knockout mice lacking both isoforms, but are exacerbated in fructokinase A knockout mice compared with wild-type mice [31]. These results indicate that fructokinase C is the key isoform driving the adverse effects of dietary fructose, whereas fructokinase A may offer some protection against the adverse effects by allowing increased fructose metabolism in extrahepatic tissues.

DE NOVO LIPOGENESIS

The unlimited hepatic uptake of fructose results in increased production of lipogenic precursors, thereby leading to increased DNL. The rate of fractional DNL was increased in subjects consuming meals containing 25% of energy as fructose-sweetened beverages under steady-state conditions compared with when they consumed meals high in complex carbohydrate, and also compared with subjects consuming 25% of energy as glucose-sweetened beverages [22]. The actual percentage of fructose converted into very-low-density lipoprotein (VLDL) triglyceride under physiologically relevant meal-fed conditions is yet to be determined. Accurate estimations will require assessments of DNL and VLDL production, secretion, and clearance using nonsteady-state tracer kinetic models. The seminal study from Donnelly et al. [32] demonstrates that in patients with nonalcoholic fatty liver disease (NAFLD), 26% of both intrahepatic fat and VLDL-triglyceride are made de novo.

FATTY ACID OXIDATION

Additionally, upregulation of hepatic DNL limits fatty acid oxidation in the liver via production of malonyl-CoA, which reduces the entry of fatty acids into the mitochondria [33]. Thus, the same subjects who exhibited fructose-induced increases of fractional DNL also exhibited markedly inhibited postmeal fatty acid oxidation compared with the subjects consuming glucose [21].

Hepatic lipid: The data suggest that fructose promotes hepatic lipid accumulation directly by increased production of fatty acids via DNL [22] and indirectly by DNL-induced inhibition of oxidation of endogenous and exogenous fatty acids [21]. Thus, in subjects who consumed 3-week diets that were supplemented with 1000 kcal/day, provided as candy and sugar-sweetened beverage, the increase in liver fat was proportional to the increase in DNL (as indexed by the palmitate to linoleate (18:2n−6) ratio) [34]. The best evidence to date that consumption of fructose increases levels of liver lipid comes from a study in which subjects consumed 1 L/day of sucrose-sweetened soda at ~20% energy requirements, isocaloric amounts of low-fat milk, 1 L/day aspartame-sweetened beverages, or 1 L/day water for 6 months. Body weight at the end of the intervention period was not significantly different from baseline in any group, but subjects consuming sucrose exhibited increased liver lipid content compared with baseline levels and with the three control groups [35].

HEPATIC LIPID AND VLDL PRODUCTION

Hepatic lipid content is involved in the regulation of VLDL production and secretion, which is not surprising given it is the role of VLDL to transport excess triglyceride out of the liver [36]. Specifically, increased levels of hepatic triglyceride not only provides the lipid substrate that is packaged into VLDL, but also leads to reduced posttranslational degradation of apolipoprotein B100 (apoB) [37]. ApoB is essential for the intracellular assembly of triglyceride into VLDL. Unlike other apolipoproteins, it is nonexchangeable and, therefore, remains with the lipoprotein particle from the time it is formed in the liver (usually as a VLDL) until it is taken up (often as an LDL) and catabolized by cells [37]. ApoB is the ligand for the LDL receptor [38] and elevated plasma levels of LDL-apoB100 are strongly associated with increased risk of coronary artery disease [37]. This risk involves the retention of LDL within the arterial wall due to an ionic interaction between basic amino acids in apoB and negatively charged sulfate groups on the artery wall proteoglycans [39]. Increased availability of hepatic lipid has also been described as a driver of the overproduction of large VLDL particle (VLDL1) [40]. VLDL1 is a triglyceride-rich lipoprotein, as opposed to

VLDL2, which is a smaller lipoprotein containing significantly less triglyceride. It has been suggested that triglyceride derived from DNL increases the size of VLDL, whereas triglyceride derived from exogenous fatty acids promotes the production of VLDL2 [36]. Overproduction of VLDL1 has been described as the underlying defect that leads to the dyslipidemia that is characteristic of patients with type-2 diabetes and metabolic syndrome [41].

DYSLIPIDEMIA

Increased secretion of VLDL1 into the circulation, reduced lipoprotein lipase (LPL) activation by insulin, and competition for LPL-mediated triglyceride hydrolysis by chylomicrons can all contribute to a longer VLDL residence time, resulting in increased postprandial triglyceride concentrations following consumption of fructose. Six separate studies, with dietary interventions ranging from 24 h to 10 weeks, conducted by our research group demonstrate that consumption of fructose markedly increases postprandial triglyceride concentrations compared with isocaloric consumption of glucose in human subjects [22,28,30,42–44]. Interestingly, and in contrast to the consistent effect of fructose to increase postprandial triglyceride levels, the subjects in the short-term studies all exhibited fructose-induced increases of fasting triglyceride concentrations [30,42,44], but the subjects in the longer studies (2–10 weeks) did not [22,28,43]. This indicates that the change in fasting triglyceride level is not a reliable indicator of fructose-induced dyslipidemia [25]. Several studies have shown that consumption of sucrose [45–47] or high-fructose corn syrup (HFCS) [28,42] also increases postprandial triglyceride concentrations compared with consumption of starch, glucose, or nonnutritive sweeteners. Our studies in both older [22] and younger [28] subjects indicate that the differential effects of fructose and fructose-containing sugars compared with complex carbohydrate on 24-h triglyceride profiles are apparent shortly after lunch and are most marked in the late evening, approximately 4 and 6 h after dinner.

POSTPRANDIAL TRIGLYCERIDE AND PROATHEROGENIC CONDITIONS

There is evidence linking increases of postprandial triglyceride concentrations with a proatherogenic state [48–53]; however, the possible mechanism(s) remain controversial [54]. Potential mechanisms include [1] increased levels of VLDL1 induce lipoprotein remodeling that is mediated by cholesteryl ester transfer protein and hepatic lipase and generates increased levels of small dense LDL (sdLDL) [55,56]; [2] increased lipolysis of triglyceride-rich lipoprotein generates remnant particles which are more able to enter the vessel wall than nascent triglyceride-rich lipoprotein, have a high rate of retention, and contain 5–20 times more cholesterol per particle than LDL [57,58]; [3] increases of apolipoprotein CIII (apoCIII), a component of VLDL which inhibits clearance of triglyceride-rich lipoprotein, promotes channeling of VLDL1 to sdLDL [59] and also activates the proinflammatory signal transduction in vascular cells [60].

Whatever the mechanism, a number of studies have documented increases of established and potential risk factors for cardiovascular disease in subjects consuming fructose or fructose-containing sugars compared with glucose or complex carbohydrate [22,28,61–64]. These risk factors include fasting and postprandial concentrations of apoB, LDL, sdLDL, oxidized LDL, and postprandial concentrations of remnant lipoprotein-triglyceride and -cholesterol.

HEPATIC LIPID AND INSULIN SENSITIVITY

The increase in hepatic lipid may also lead to hepatic insulin resistance [65], possibly through increased intrahepatic levels of diacylglycerol (DAG), which activates novel-PKC [66]. Novel-PKC decreases tyrosine phosphorylation and/or increases serine phosphorylation of the insulin receptor and insulin receptor substrate-1 (IRS-1) and other downstream proteins, resulting in impaired insulin action in the liver (Figure 19.1) [66]. Aeberli et al. [62] have reported that hepatic insulin sensitivity, indexed by endogenous glucose production during euglycemic-hyperinsulinemic clamps, was decreased in healthy young men who consumed 80 g of fructose/day for 3 weeks, compared with when they consumed 80 g of glucose/day. These results are important, because an average man will consume approximately 80 g of fructose/day when consuming added sugar at 25% of energy, the maximal intake level of added sugar suggested in the Report of the Dietary Guidelines Advisory Committee (DGAC) on the Dietary Guidelines for Americans 2010 [67]. Importantly, Aeberli et al. [62] also reported that these young men did not exhibit decreases of whole-body insulin sensitivity, as indexed by peripheral glucose disposal. This suggests that the development of hepatic insulin resistance on high-sugar diets occurs prior to the development of whole-body insulin resistance.

WHOLE-BODY INSULIN SENSITIVITY

Figure 19.1 summarizes the potential mechanisms by which fructose may mediate liver lipid accumulation, dyslipidemia, and hepatic insulin resistance. It is possible that these events in themselves are sufficient to eventually lead to impairments in whole-body insulin sensitivity when the fructose exposure exceeds 3 weeks and/or 80 g/day. In older overweight and obese men and women who consumed an average of 167 g of fructose/day for 9 weeks, whole-body insulin sensitivity decreased by 17% [22] (hepatic insulin sensitivity was not assessed in this study). However, it is more likely that other factors, including other direct effects of fructose, exacerbate the sequence of events depicted in Figure 19.1 and are therefore important contributors to the eventual development of whole-body insulin resistance (Figure 19.2). These other direct effects of fructose include increased production of uric acid and possibly inflammation.

URIC ACID

One of the most marked and significant effects of fructose consumption are increases of both fasting uric acid and 24-h uric acid exposure (the mean plasma concentration of samples collected every 30–60 min over a 24-h period). After 10 weeks of fructose consumption, both fasting uric acid concentrations and 24-h uric acid exposure were significantly increased in older, overweight subjects [68]. In younger, normal, and overweight subjects, who consumed 25% of energy requirements as fructose, HFCS, or sucrose for 2 weeks, fasting levels and 24-h exposure of uric acid were also significantly increased (unpublished results).

As with the pathways presented in Figure 19.1, the mechanism by which fructose consumption leads to increased uric acid concentrations involves the unregulated uptake and metabolism of fructose (Figure 19.2). The first step in the metabolic pathway, the fructokinase-catalyzed phosphorylation of fructose to fructose-1-P, results in conversion of ATP to adenosine monophosphate (AMP) and a depletion of inorganic phosphate. The degradation of AMP leads to increased uric acid production [69]. While uric acid is a potent and physiologically relevant antioxidant, recent evidence suggests that elevated levels may be associated with increased oxidative stress, and there is still considerable debate as to which of these roles is more important in the context of metabolic disease [70]. However, it is well known that increased circulating levels of uric acid can lead to gout, and extensive recent work by Richard Johnson and co-workers suggests that the fructose-induced increases of uric acid may amplify the lipogenic effects of fructose by several mechanisms. The sites of these mechanisms are shown in Figure 19.2 as 1, 2, and 3, and are explained below.

1. The purine degradation pathway, which generates uric acid, also upregulates DNL via the generation of mitochondrial oxidants. Mitochondrial oxidative stress results in the inhibition of aconitase in the Krebs cycle, resulting in the accumulation of citrate and the activation of ATP citrate lyase and fatty-acid synthase leading to an enhancement of DNL [71].
2. Uric acid promotes fructose overload in the liver by upregulating fructokinase expression. In cultured human hepatocytes exposed to fructose, uric acid activates the transcription

factor ChREBP, which in turn results in the transcriptional activation of fructokinase by binding to a specific sequence within its promoter [72].
3. Uric acid contributes to the accumulation of lipid in the liver by inhibiting AMP-activated kinase, an activator of fatty acid oxidation [73].

In vivo evidence supports the suggestion that fructose-induced increases of uric acid contribute to the adverse effects of fructose. Rats treated with uricase inhibitor to increase uric acid levels and/or fed sucrose-sweetened beverage exhibited the following [74]:

- Uricase inhibitor induced glomerular hypertension
- Sucrose-sweetened beverage induced insulin resistance
- Uricase inhibitor plus sucrose-sweetened beverage produced both effects, plus synergistic effects on systemic blood pressure, intraglomerular pressure, plasma glucose concentrations, hepatic triglyceride content, and oxidative stress [74]

INFLAMMATORY FACTORS

As illustrated in Figure 19.2 at site 4, inflammation may be an important contributor or exacerbator of the adverse effects of fructose and the eventual development of whole-body insulin resistance. There is considerable data from studies in rodents suggesting that fructose increases levels or expression of inflammatory factors in the liver [75–78]. These in turn may adversely affect hepatic insulin signaling or increase hepatic lipid levels [79]. In humans, direct experimental data that dietary fructose induces inflammation and oxidative stress are limited due to constraints regarding clinical liver sampling. However, and despite the fact that plasma levels of inflammatory markers may not adequately reflect tissue-specific inflammation, we have reported that fasting concentrations of markers of inflammation, monocyte chemoattractant protein-1 (MCP-1), plasminogen activator inhibitor-1 (PAI-1), and E-selectin, as well as retinol binding protein-4 and the liver enzyme, gamma glutamyl transferase, were increased in older, overweight/obese subjects consuming fructose for 10 weeks [68,80]. We also observed significant increases of intra-abdominal fat deposition in these same subjects [22]. In humans, visceral adipose mass has been shown to be a primary determinant of PAI-1 levels [81], and PAI-1 has been shown to be preferentially secreted by visceral adipose tissue compared with subcutaneous adipose tissue [82]. In addition, Bruun et al. [83] investigated the relationship between adipose tissue resident macrophages, adiposity, and MCP-1 in human adipose tissue and demonstrated that MCP-1 is preferentially secreted from visceral adipose tissue compared with subcutaneous adipose tissue. Thus, the increased deposition of visceral adipose tissue in subjects consuming fructose may help to explain the observed increases in PAI-1 and MCP-1 in these subjects (Figure 19.2, site 4a).

It is also possible that inflammatory responses to fructose are mediated through its direct exposure to the intestine (Figure 19.2, site 4b) or hepatocytes (Figure 19.2, site 4c). Fructose consumption has been shown to lead to increased intestinal translocation of bacterial endotoxin, induction of hepatic tumor necrosis factor-α, and liver lipid accumulation in mice, while treatment with antibiotics has been shown to almost completely block these effects [84]. Portal blood concentrations of endotoxin were increased by 31% in nonhuman primates consuming an energy-balanced diet containing 24% of energy as fructose compared with those consuming a low-fructose control diet [85]. Increased circulating concentrations of endotoxin were noted in patients with NAFLD, who consumed more fructose and also had higher circulating concentrations and hepatic expression of PAI-1 than control patients [86]. In isolated hepatocytes, fructose exposure, compared with glucose exposure, leads to activation of c-jun NH_2-terminal kinase, increased serine phosphorylation of IRS-1, and reduced insulin-stimulated tyrosine phosphorylation of IRS-1 and IRS-2 [87]. These acute in vitro effects of fructose could potentially be mediated by increased cellular concentrations of methylglyoxal [88].

HEPATIC INSULIN RESISTANCE AND DNL

The factor with the greatest potential to exacerbate the effects of fructose presented in Figure 19.1 may be hepatic insulin resistance. While the effects of insulin resistance on hepatic metabolism are numerous, Figure 19.2 focuses on just two, starting with upregulation of DNL (see Figure 19.2, site 5). DNL is an insulin-activated process in the normal liver that is even more strongly activated in the insulin resistant liver [89]. A number of mechanisms have been proposed to explain this paradoxical effect of hepatic insulin resistance [90]. The mechanism appears to involve the insulin receptor, because, while mice lacking hepatic insulin receptors exhibit hyperglycemia, circulating triglyceride concentrations are quite low in these animals [91]. Thus, the selective insulin resistance that allows for continued activation of DNL by insulin results in more severely compromised metabolism, consisting of both hyperglycemia/hyperinsulinemia and hypertriglyridemia, than that seen when all insulin-regulated processes are impaired due to insulin receptor knockout [92]. Increased activation of DNL due to fructose-induced hepatic insulin resistance has the potential to set up a vicious cycle (Figure 19.2; see darkest arrows) in which the resulting increase in hepatic lipid content exacerbates the insulin resistance which further activates DNL and further increases hepatic lipid accumulation.

HEPATIC INSULIN RESISTANCE AND VLDL PRODUCTION

This vicious cycle may also exacerbate VLDL production/secretion due to the increasing liver lipid accumulation (Figure 19.2, site 6). However, VLDL production/secretion is also increased in the insulin-resistant liver due to mechanisms independent of hepatic lipid supply (Figure 19.2, site 7). There is evidence to suggest that insulin decreases apoB availability by inhibiting its synthesis [93], and, even more importantly, by targeting apoB for posttranslational degradation [94,95]. Insulin also inhibits microsomal triglyceride-transfer protein (MTP) expression via an insulin response element on the MTP gene [96]. MTP is essential for assembly of triglyceride and apoB into VLDL and secretion of VLDL [97]. Thus, increased availability of apoB and chronic upregulation of MTP expression and protein levels may further promote increased production of VLDL in the insulin-resistant liver [89,98]. A third mechanism by which hepatic insulin resistance may lead to increased VLDL production/secretion, specifically increased VLDL1 production/secretion, involves apoCIII [98]. It is known that apoCIII promotes hypertriglyceridemia by inhibiting LPL activity and clearance of triglyceride-rich lipoproteins by hepatic receptors [59]. More recent evidence suggests that apoCIII plays a role in the second-step incorporation of lipid into VLDL, which converts VLDL2 into VLDL1 [99,100]. Since expression of apoCIII is suppressed by insulin [101], upregulation of apoCIII may be involved in the increased production/secretion of VLDL1 associated with insulin resistance [98].

A mechanism that is often implicated in the increased production of VLDL by insulin resistance is increased fatty acid flux into the liver due to unsuppressed lipolysis in adipose tissue [98]. A recent review, however, concludes that kinetic studies show a lack of relationship between free fatty acid flux and availability and VLDL production [102]. We have previously questioned the importance of this mechanism in the insulin resistance induced by fructose [26] based on the observation that 24-h free fatty acid exposure is not increased in subjects consuming fructose for 10 weeks [22].

MUSCLE LIPID ACCUMULATION

Increased VLDL secretion increases 24-h exposure to triglyceride and intramyocellular lipid accumulation. In the study already described, in which subjects consumed 1 L/day of sucrose-sweetened cola, low-fat milk, aspartame-sweetened cola, or water for 6 months, muscle lipid content increased compared with baseline only in subjects consuming sucrose [35]. Intramyocellular lipid concentrations are correlated with reduced whole-body insulin sensitivity in humans [103]. It is possible,

TABLE 19.1
Questions for Future Research

Question	Objective	Model	Duration	Primary Outcomes
Does a high-sugar diet increase risk factors compared to a high-complex carbohydrate diet under a strict dietary protocol, that is, experimental diets are formulated to achieve an identical macronutrient intake and eliminate outpatient dietary variations and are provided to the subjects throughout the entire investigation?	To obtain definitive evidence that is not limited by potential diet variations between experimental groups	Healthy adults	Two weeks to demonstrate increase in CVD risk factors 8+ weeks to demonstrate changes in whole-body insulin sensitivity	Circulating lipids, live lipid content, hepatic insulin sensitivity, whole-body insulin sensitivity
Does a high-sugar diet increase risk factors compared to a high-complex carbohydrate diet under a strict dietary protocol that does not allow for weight gain?	To determine if sugar consumption has effects on risk factors for metabolic disease that are independent of body weight gain	Healthy adults	Two weeks to demonstrate increase in CVD risk factors 8+ weeks to demonstrate changes in whole body insulin sensitivity	Circulating lipids, live lipid content, hepatic insulin sensitivity, whole-body insulin sensitivity
Does a high-sugar diet that is provided in quantities that allow for weight gain increase risk factors compared with an identical diet that is provided in quantities that do not allow for weight gain?	To determine if weight gain exacerbates the independent effects of sugar consumption	Healthy adults	Two weeks to demonstrate increase in CVD risk factors 8+ weeks to demonstrate changes in whole-body insulin sensitivity	Circulating lipids, live lipid content, hepatic insulin sensitivity, whole-body insulin sensitivity
Does a high-sugar diet increase DNL and VLDL production compared to a high-complex carbohydrate diet when assessed during meal-fed conditions? What percentage of the ingested fructose is converted into VLDL-TG?	To use nonsteady-state modeling to accurately determine DNL and VLDL production under a relevant feeding protocol	Healthy adults	1+ week	DNL, VLDL production
Does a high-sugar diet increase hepatic and muscle levels of inflammation, oxidative stress, and lipid intermediates that impair insulin signaling compared with a high-complex carbohydrate diet in obese rhesus macaques, a relevant model of metabolic syndrome?	To test the proposed mechanisms in a model that allows for multiple sampling of liver and muscle	Obese rhesus macaques	6+ months	Liver and muscle metabolomic/ lipidom profiles

but not definite [104], that this relationship is mediated by the same mechanism described for the development of hepatic insulin resistance; DAG-mediated activation of nPKC resulting in serine phosphorylation of the insulin receptor or IRS-1 [105]. It is also possible that other factors such as inflammation and oxidative stress [106] are contributors to, or possibly mediators of, muscle insulin resistance [107].

SUMMARY

The unregulated uptake/metabolism of fructose by the liver increases triglyceride synthesis via DNL resulting in accumulation of triglycerides in the liver, increased VLDL production/secretion, dyslipidemia, and hepatic insulin resistance. Increases in the production of uric acid resulting from fructose consumption, and possibly inflammatory and oxidative stress factors, may exacerbate these effects. Sustained exposure to fructose may lead to a vicious cycle in which hepatic insulin resistance exacerbates DNL, leading to increased hepatic lipid content, which in turn worsens hepatic insulin resistance. The increased lipid content in the liver and the insulin resistance exacerbates VLDL production/secretion, resulting in sustained exposure to circulating triglyceride that leads to muscle lipid accumulation and whole-body insulin resistance.

CONCLUSION

The intervention studies with dietary sugars cited above provide support for the plausibility of these proposed mechanism by which consumption of fructose and fructose-containing sugars may increase risk factors for metabolic disease. While each of these studies has limitations which precludes its being definitive [108], together they constitute a strong body of direct experimental evidence that support a causal relationship between the consumption of excessive amounts of sugar and the development of metabolic disease. Table 19.1 lists the future research that is needed to provide the definitive proof of this relationship and also the research that is needed to support the proposed mechanisms. The necessary clinical studies will be costly and will take more than 5 years to complete. This projection leads to the question as to whether it is in the best interest of public health to wait until this definitive evidence is available to begin educating the public about the potential adverse effects of consuming high-sugar diets and initiating public health policies to reduce sugar consumption. Coming up with the best answer to this question is not difficult when considering that there are no health risks associated with decreasing the added sugar content of the diet, while the risks in waiting for all of the definitive evidence to be generated could include further increases in the prevalence of metabolic syndrome, cardiovascular disease, diabetes, and NAFLD, and an increased burden to the health-care system.

REFERENCES

1. Duffey KJ, Gordon-Larsen P, Steffen LM, Jacobs Jr. DR, Popkin BM. Drinking caloric beverages increases the risk of adverse cardiometabolic outcomes in the Coronary Artery Risk Development in Young Adults (CARDIA) study. *Am J Clin Nutr*. 2010;92(4):954–9. Epub 2010/08/13.
2. Welsh JA, Sharma A, Abramson JL, Vaccarino V, Gillespie C, Vos MB. Caloric sweetener consumption and dyslipidemia among US adults. *JAMA*. 2010;303(15):1490–7. Epub 2010/04/22.
3. Welsh JA, Sharma A, Cunningham SA, Vos MB. Consumption of added sugars and indicators of cardiovascular disease risk among US adolescents. *Circulation*. 2011;123(3):249–57. Epub 2011/01/12.
4. Bremer AA, Auinger P, Byrd RS. Sugar-sweetened beverage intake trends in US adolescents and their association with insulin resistance-related parameters. *J Nutr Metab*. 2010; Epub 2009 Sep 6. Epub 2010/08/12.
5. Yoshida M, McKeown NM, Rogers G, Meigs JB, Saltzman E, D'Agostino R et al. Surrogate markers of insulin resistance are associated with consumption of sugar-sweetened drinks and fruit juice in middle and older-aged adults. *J Nutr*. 2007;137(9):2121–7. Epub 2007/08/22.
6. Assy N, Nasser G, Kamayse I, Nseir W, Beniashvili Z, Djibre A et al. Soft drink consumption linked with fatty liver in the absence of traditional risk factors. *Can J Gastroenterol*. 2008;22(10):811–6. Epub 2008/10/18.
7. Ouyang X, Cirillo P, Sautin Y, McCall S, Bruchette JL, Diehl AM et al. Fructose consumption as a risk factor for non-alcoholic fatty liver disease. *J Hepatol*. 2008;48(6):993–9. Epub 2008/04/09.
8. Bhupathiraju SN, Pan A, Malik VS, Manson JE, Willett WC, van Dam RM et al. Caffeinated and caffeine-free beverages and risk of type 2 diabetes. *Am J Clin Nutr*. 2013;97(1):155–66. Epub 2012/11/16.

9. de Koning L, Malik VS, Rimm EB, Willett WC, Hu FB. Sugar-sweetened and artificially sweetened beverage consumption and risk of type 2 diabetes in men. *Am J Clin Nutr*. 2011;93(6):1321–7. Epub 2011/03/25.
10. Montonen J, Jarvinen R, Knekt P, Heliovaara M, Reunanen A. Consumption of sweetened beverages and intakes of fructose and glucose predict type 2 diabetes occurrence. *J Nutr*. 2007;137(6):1447–54. Epub 2007/05/22.
11. Palmer JR, Boggs DA, Krishnan S, Hu FB, Singer M, Rosenberg L. Sugar-sweetened beverages and incidence of type 2 diabetes mellitus in African American women. *Arch Intern Med*. 2008;168(14):1487–92. Epub 2008/07/30.
12. Schulze MB, Manson JE, Ludwig DS, Colditz GA, Stampfer MJ, Willett WC et al. Sugar-sweetened beverages, weight gain, and incidence of type 2 diabetes in young and middle-aged women. *JAMA*. 2004;292(8):927–34. Epub 2004/08/26.
13. de Koning L, Malik VS, Kellogg MD, Rimm EB, Willett WC, Hu FB. Sweetened beverage consumption, incident coronary heart disease, and biomarkers of risk in men. *Circulation*. 2012;125(14):1735–41, S1. Epub 2012/03/14.
14. Fung TT, Malik V, Rexrode KM, Manson JE, Willett WC, Hu FB. Sweetened beverage consumption and risk of coronary heart disease in women. *Am J Clin Nutr*. 2009;89(4):1037–42. Epub 2009/02/13.
15. Denova-Gutierrez E, Talavera JO, Huitron-Bravo G, Mendez-Hernandez P, Salmeron J. Sweetened beverage consumption and increased risk of metabolic syndrome in Mexican adults. *Public Health Nutr*. 2010;13(6):835–42. Epub 2010/02/11.
16. Dhingra R, Sullivan L, Jacques PF, Wang TJ, Fox CS, Meigs JB et al. Soft drink consumption and risk of developing cardiometabolic risk factors and the metabolic syndrome in middle-aged adults in the community. *Circulation*. 2007;116(5):480–8.
17. Hosseini-Esfahani F, Bahadoran Z, Mirmiran P, Hosseinpour-Niazi S, Hosseinpanah F, Azizi F. Dietary fructose and risk of metabolic syndrome in adults: Tehran lipid and glucose study. *Nutr Metab (Lond)*. 2011;8(1):50. Epub 2011/07/14.
18. Hostmark AT. The Oslo health study: Soft drink intake is associated with the metabolic syndrome. *Appl Physiol Nutr Metab*. 2010;35(5):635–42. Epub 2010/10/22.
19. Odegaard AO, Choh AC, Czerwinski SA, Towne B, Demerath EW. Sugar-sweetened and diet beverages in relation to visceral adipose tissue. *Obesity (Silver Spring)*. 2012;20(3):689–91. Epub 2011/09/09.
20. Pollock NK, Bundy V, Kanto W, Davis CL, Bernard PJ, Zhu H et al. Greater fructose consumption is associated with cardiometabolic risk markers and visceral adiposity in adolescents. *J Nutr*. 2012;142(2):251–7. Epub 2011/12/23.
21. Cox CL, Stanhope KL, Schwarz JM, Graham JL, Hatcher B, Griffen SC et al. Consumption of fructose-sweetened beverages for 10 weeks reduces net fat oxidation and energy expenditure in overweight/obese men and women. *Eur J Clin Nutr*. 2012;66(2):201–8. Epub 2011/09/29.
22. Stanhope KL, Schwarz JM, Keim NL, Griffen SC, Bremer AA, Graham JL et al. Consuming fructose-sweetened, not glucose-sweetened, beverages increases visceral adiposity and lipids and decreases insulin sensitivity in overweight/obese humans. *J Clin Invest*. 2009;119(5):1322–34. Epub 2009/04/22.
23. Stanhope KL. Role of fructose-containing sugars in the epidemics of obesity and metabolic syndrome. *Annu Rev Med*. 2012;63:329–43. Epub 2011/11/01.
24. Stanhope KL, Havel PJ. Endocrine and metabolic effects of consuming beverages sweetened with fructose, glucose, sucrose, or high-fructose corn syrup. *Am J Clin Nutr*. 2008;88(6):1733S–7S. Epub 2008/12/10.
25. Stanhope KL, Havel PJ. Fructose consumption: Considerations for future research on its effects on adipose distribution, lipid metabolism, and insulin sensitivity in humans. *J Nutr*. 2009;139:1236S–41S. Epub 2009/05/01.
26. Stanhope KL, Havel PJ. Fructose consumption: Potential mechanisms for its effects to increase visceral adiposity and induce dyslipidemia and insulin resistance. *Curr Opin Lipidol*. 2008;19(1):16–24.
27. Stanhope KL, Havel PJ. Fructose consumption: Recent results and their potential implications. *Ann NY Acad Sci*. 2010;1190(2010):15–24.
28. Stanhope KL, Bremer AA, Medici V, Nakajima K, Ito Y, Nakano T et al. Consumption of fructose and high fructose corn syrup increase postprandial triglycerides, LDL-cholesterol, and apolipoprotein-B in young men and women. *J Clin Endocrinol Metab*. 2011;96(10):E1596–605. Epub 2011/08/19.
29. Stanhope KL, Griffen SC, Bremer AA, Vink RG, Schaefer EJ, Nakajima K et al. Metabolic responses to prolonged consumption of glucose- and fructose-sweetened beverages are not associated with postprandial or 24-H glucose and insulin excursions. *Am J Clin Nutr*. 2011;94(1):112–9. Epub 2011/05/27.

30. Teff KL, Grudziak J, Townsend RR, Dunn TN, Grant RW, Adams SH et al. Endocrine and metabolic effects of consuming fructose- and glucose-sweetened beverages with meals in obese men and women: Influence of insulin resistance on plasma triglyceride responses. *J Clin Endocrinol Metab.* 2009;94(5):1562–9. Epub 2009/02/12.
31. Ishimoto T, Lanaspa MA, Le MT, Garcia GE, Diggle CP, Maclean PS et al. Opposing effects of fructokinase c and a isoforms on fructose-induced metabolic syndrome in mice. *Proc Natl Acad Sci USA.* 2012;109(11):4320–5. Epub 2012/03/01.
32. Donnelly KL, Smith CI, Schwarzenberg SJ, Jessurun J, Boldt MD, Parks EJ. Sources of fatty acids stored in liver and secreted via lipoproteins in patients with nonalcoholic fatty liver disease. *J Clin Invest.* 2005;115(5):1343–51.
33. McGarry JD. Malonyl-Coa and carnitine palmitoyltransferase I: An expanding partnership. *Biochem Soc Trans.* 1995;23(3):481–5. Epub 1995/08/01.
34. Sevastianova K, Santos A, Kotronen A, Hakkarainen A, Makkonen J, Silander K et al. Effect of short-term carbohydrate overfeeding and long-term weight loss on liver fat in overweight humans. *Am J Clin Nutr.* 2012;96(4):727–34. Epub 2012/09/07.
35. Maersk M, Belza A, Stodkilde-Jorgensen H, Ringgaard S, Chabanova E, Thomsen H et al. Sucrose-sweetened beverages increase fat storage in the liver, muscle, and visceral fat depot: A 6-Mo randomized intervention study. *Am J Clin Nutr.* 2012;95(2):283–9. Epub 2011/12/30.
36. Choi SH, Ginsberg HN. Increased very low density lipoprotein (VLDL) secretion, hepatic steatosis, and insulin resistance. *Trends Endocrinol Metab.* 2011;22(9):353–63. Epub 2011/05/28.
37. Olofsson SO, Boren J. Apolipoprotein B secretory regulation by degradation. *Arterioscler Thromb Vasc Biol.* 2012;32(6):1334–8. Epub 2012/05/18.
38. Boren J, Lee I, Zhu W, Arnold K, Taylor S, Innerarity TL. Identification of the low density lipoprotein receptor-binding site in apolipoprotein B100 and the modulation of its binding activity by the carboxyl terminus in familial defective Apo-B100. *J Clin Invest.* 1998;101(5):1084–93. Epub 1998/04/16.
39. Boren J, Olin K, Lee I, Chait A, Wight TN, Innerarity TL. Identification of the principal proteoglycan-binding site in LDL: A single-point mutation in apo-b100 severely affects proteoglycan interaction without affecting ldl receptor binding. *J Clin Invest.* 1998;101(12):2658–64. Epub 1998/06/24.
40. Adiels M, Taskinen MR, Packard C, Caslake MJ, Soro-Paavonen A, Westerbacka J et al. Overproduction of large VLDL particles is driven by increased liver fat content in man. *Diabetologia.* 2006;49(4):755–65. Epub 2006/02/08.
41. Adiels M, Olofsson SO, Taskinen MR, Boren J. Overproduction of very low-density lipoproteins is the hallmark of the dyslipidemia in the metabolic syndrome. *Arterioscler Thromb Vasc Biol.* 2008;28(7):1225–36. Epub 2008/06/21.
42. Stanhope KL, Griffen SC, Bair BR, Swarbrick MM, Keim NL, Havel PJ. Twenty-four-hour endocrine and metabolic profiles following consumption of high-fructose corn syrup-, sucrose-, fructose-, and glucose-sweetened beverages with meals. *Am J Clin Nutr.* 2008;87(5):1194–203.
43. Swarbrick MM, Stanhope KL, Elliott SS, Graham JL, Krauss RM, Christiansen MP et al. Consumption of fructose-sweetened beverages for 10 weeks increases postprandial triacylglycerol and apolipoprotein-B concentrations in overweight and obese women. *Br J Nutr.* 2008;100(5):947–52.
44. Teff KL, Elliott SS, Tschop M, Kieffer TJ, Rader D, Heiman M et al. Dietary fructose reduces circulating insulin and leptin, attenuates postprandial suppression of ghrelin, and increases triglycerides in women. *J Clin Endocrinol Metab.* 2004;89(6):2963–72. Epub 2004/06/08.
45. Mann JI, Truswell AS. Effects of isocaloric exchange of dietary sucrose and starch on fasting serum lipids, postprandial insulin secretion and alimentary lipaemia in human subjects. *Br J Nutr.* 1972;27(2):395–405. Epub 1972/03/01.
46. Raben A, Moller BK, Flint A, Vasilaris TH, Christina Moller A, Juul Holst J et al. Increased postprandial glycaemia, insulinemia, and lipidemia after 10 weeks' sucrose-rich diet compared to an artificially sweetened diet: A randomised controlled trial. *Food Nutr Res.* 2011;55. Epub 2011/07/30.
47. Raben A, Vasilaras TH, Moller AC, Astrup A. Sucrose compared with artificial sweeteners: Different effects on ad libitum food intake and body weight after 10 wk of supplementation in overweight subjects. *Am J Clin Nutr.* 2002;76(4):721–9. Epub 2002/09/27.
48. Bansal S, Buring JE, Rifai N, Mora S, Sacks FM, Ridker PM. Fasting compared with nonfasting triglycerides and risk of cardiovascular events in women. *JAMA.* 2007;298(3):309–16.
49. Hyson D, Rutledge JC, Berglund L. Postprandial lipemia and cardiovascular disease. *Curr Atheroscler Rep.* 2003;5(6):437–44.
50. Karpe F. Postprandial lipoprotein metabolism and atherosclerosis. *J Intern Med.* 1999;246(4):341–55.

51. Lopez-Miranda J, Perez-Martinez P, Marin C, Moreno JA, Gomez P, Perez-Jimenez F. Postprandial lipoprotein metabolism, genes and risk of cardiovascular disease. *Curr Opin Lipidol.* 2006;17(2):132–8.
52. Nordestgaard BG, Benn M, Schnohr P, Tybjaerg-Hansen A. Nonfasting triglycerides and risk of myocardial infarction, ischemic heart disease, and death in men and women. *JAMA.* 2007;298(3):299–308.
53. Stalenhoef AF, de Graaf J. Association of fasting and nonfasting serum triglycerides with cardiovascular disease and the role of remnant-like lipoproteins and small dense LDL. *Curr Opin Lipidol.* 2008;19(4):355–61. Epub 2008/07/09.
54. Goldberg IJ, Eckel RH, McPherson R. Triglycerides and heart disease: Still a hypothesis? *Arterioscler Thromb Vasc Biol.* 2011;31(8):1716–25. Epub 2011/04/30.
55. Chapman MJ, Le Goff W, Guerin M, Kontush A. Cholesteryl ester transfer protein: At the heart of the action of lipid-modulating therapy with statins, fibrates, niacin, and cholesteryl ester transfer protein inhibitors. *Eur Heart J.* 2010;31(2):149–64. Epub 2009/10/15.
56. Packard CJ. Triacylglycerol-rich lipoproteins and the generation of small, dense low-density lipoprotein. *Biochem Soc Trans.* 2003;31(Pt 5):1066–9.
57. Nakajima K, Nakano T, Tanaka A. The oxidative modification hypothesis of atherosclerosis: The comparison of atherogenic effects on oxidized LDL and remnant lipoproteins in plasma. *Clin Chim Acta.* 2006;367(1–2):36–47.
58. Schwartz EA, Reaven PD. Lipolysis of triglyceride-rich lipoproteins, vascular inflammation, and atherosclerosis. *Biochim Biophys Acta.* 2012;1821(5):858–66. Epub 2011/10/18.
59. Zheng C, Khoo C, Furtado J, Sacks FM. Apolipoprotein C-Iii and the metabolic basis for hypertriglyceridemia and the dense low-density lipoprotein phenotype. *Circulation.* 2010;121(15):1722–34. Epub 2010/04/07.
60. Kawakami A, Yoshida M. Apolipoprotein Ciii links dyslipidemia with atherosclerosis. *J Atheroscler Thromb.* 2009;16(1):6–11. Epub 2009/03/06.
61. Aeberli I, Gerber PA, Hochuli M, Kohler S, Haile SR, Gouni-Berthold I et al. Low to moderate sugar-sweetened beverage consumption impairs glucose and lipid metabolism and promotes inflammation in healthy young men: A randomized controlled trial. *Am J Clin Nutr.* 2011;94:479–85. Epub 2011/06/17.
62. Aeberli I, Hochuli M, Gerber PA, Sze L, Murer SB, Tappy L et al. Moderate amounts of fructose consumption impair insulin sensitivity in healthy young men: A randomized controlled trial. *Diabetes Care.* 2013;36:150–6. Epub 2012/08/31.
63. Hallfrisch J, Reiser S, Prather ES. Blood lipid distribution of hyperinsulinemic men consuming three levels of fructose. *Am J Clin Nutr.* 1983;37(5):740–8. Epub 1983/05/01.
64. Reiser S, Powell AS, Scholfield DJ, Panda P, Fields M, Canary JJ. Day-long glucose, insulin, and fructose responses of hyperinsulinemic and nonhyperinsulinemic men adapted to diets containing either fructose or high-amylose cornstarch. *Am J Clin Nutr.* 1989;50(5):1008–14.
65. Morino K, Petersen KF, Shulman GI. Molecular mechanisms of insulin resistance in humans and their potential links with mitochondrial dysfunction. *Diabetes.* 2006;55(Suppl. 2):S9–15.
66. Jornayvaz FR, Shulman GI. Diacylglycerol activation of protein kinase cepsilon and hepatic insulin resistance. *Cell Metab.* 2012;15(5):574–84. Epub 2012/05/09.
67. DGAC. Report of the Dietary Guidelines Advisory Committee (DGAC) on the Dietary Guidelines for Americans, 2010. http://wwwcnppusdagov/DGAs2010-DGACReporthtm.
68. Cox CL, Stanhope KL, Schwarz JM, Graham JL, Hatcher B, Griffen SC et al. Consumption of fructose-but not glucose-sweetened beverages for 10 weeks increases circulating concentrations of uric acid, retinol binding protein- 4, and gamma-glutamyl transferase activity in overweight/obese humans. *Nutr Metab.* 2012;9(1):68. Epub 2012/07/26.
69. Mayes PA. Intermediary metabolism of fructose. *Am J Clin Nutr.* 1993;58(5 Suppl.):754S–65S.
70. Glantzounis GK, Tsimoyiannis EC, Kappas AM, Galaris DA. Uric acid and oxidative stress. *Curr Pharm Des.* 2005;11(32):4145–51. Epub 2005/12/27.
71. Lanaspa MA, Sanchez-Lozada LG, Choi YJ, Cicerchi C, Kanbay M, Roncal-Jimenez CA et al. Uric acid induces hepatic steatosis by generation of mitochondrial oxidative stress: Potential role in fructose-dependent and -independent fatty liver. *J Biol Chem.* 2012;287(48):40732–44. Epub 2012/10/05.
72. Lanaspa MA, Sanchez-Lozada LG, Cicerchi C, Li N, Roncal-Jimenez CA, Ishimoto T et al. Uric acid stimulates fructokinase and accelerates fructose metabolism in the development of fatty liver. *PLoS ONE.* 2012;7(10):e47948. Epub 2012/11/01.
73. Lanaspa MA, Cicerchi C, Garcia G, Li N, Roncal-Jimenez CA, Rivard CJ et al. Counteracting roles of amp deaminase and amp kinase in the development of fatty liver. *PLoS ONE.* 2012;7(11):e48801. Epub 2012/11/16.

74. Tapia E, Cristobal M, Garcia-Arroyo FE, Soto V, Monroy-Sanchez F, Pacheco U et al. Synergistic effect of uricase blockade plus physiological amounts of fructose-glucose on glomerular hypertension and oxidative stress in rats. *Am J Physiol Renal Physiol*. 2013;304:F727–36. Epub 2013/01/11.
75. Alzamendi A, Castrogiovanni D, Ortega HH, Gaillard RC, Giovambattista A, Spinedi E. Parametrial adipose tissue and metabolic dysfunctions induced by fructose-rich diet in normal and neonatal-androgenized adult female rats. *Obesity (Silver Spring)*. 2010;18(3):441–8. Epub 2009/08/22.
76. Gersch MS, Mu W, Cirillo P, Reungjui S, Zhang L, Roncal C et al. Fructose, but not dextrose, accelerates the progression of chronic kidney disease. *Am J Physiol Renal Physiol*. 2007;293(4):F1256–61. Epub 2007/08/03.
77. Kanuri G, Spruss A, Wagnerberger S, Bischoff SC, Bergheim I. Role of tumor necrosis factor alpha (tnfalpha) in the onset of fructose-induced nonalcoholic fatty liver disease in mice. *J Nutr Biochem*. 2011;22:527–34. Epub 2010/08/31.
78. Sanchez-Lozada LG, Mu W, Roncal C, Sautin YY, Abdelmalek M, Reungjui S et al. Comparison of free fructose and glucose to sucrose in the ability to cause fatty liver. *Eur J Nutr*. 2010;49(1):1–9. Epub 2009/07/25.
79. Dekker MJ, Su Q, Baker C, Rutledge AC, Adeli K. Fructose: A highly lipogenic nutrient implicated in insulin resistance, hepatic steatosis, and the metabolic syndrome. *Am J Physiol Endocrinol Metab*. 2010;299(5):E685–94. Epub 2010/09/09.
80. Cox CL, Stanhope KL, Schwarz JM, Graham JL, Hatcher B, Griffen SC et al. Circulating concentrations of monocyte chemoattractant protein-1, plasminogen activator inhibitor-1, and soluble leukocyte adhesion molecule-1 in overweight/obese men and women consuming fructose- or glucose-sweetened beverages for 10 weeks. *J Clin Endocrinol Metab*. 2011;96(12):E2034–8. Epub 2011/10/01.
81. Giltay EJ, Elbers JM, Gooren LJ, Emeis JJ, Kooistra T, Asscheman H et al. Visceral fat accumulation is an important determinant of PAI-1 levels in young, nonobese men and women: Modulation by cross-sex hormone administration. *Arterioscler Thromb Vasc Biol*. 1998;18(11):1716–22. Epub 1998/11/13.
82. Shimomura I, Funahashi T, Takahashi M, Maeda K, Kotani K, Nakamura T et al. Enhanced expression of PAI-1 in visceral fat: Possible contributor to vascular disease in obesity. *Nat Med*. 1996;2(7):800–3. Epub 1996/07/01.
83. Bruun JM, Lihn AS, Pedersen SB, Richelsen B. Monocyte chemoattractant protein-1 release is higher in visceral than subcutaneous human adipose tissue (AT): Implication of macrophages resident in the AT. *J Clin Endocrinol Metab*. 2005;90(4):2282–9. Epub 2005/01/27.
84. Bergheim I, Weber S, Vos M, Kramer S, Volynets V, Kaserouni S et al. Antibiotics protect against fructose-induced hepatic lipid accumulation in mice: Role of endotoxin. *J Hepatol*. 2008;48(6):983–92. Epub 2008/04/09.
85. Kavanagh K, Wylie AT, Tucker KL, Hamp TJ, Gharaibeh RZ, Fodor AA et al. Dietary fructose induces endotoxemia and hepatic injury in calorically controlled primates. *Am J Clin Nutr*. 2013;98(2):349–57. Epub 2013/06/21.
86. Thuy S, Ladurner R, Volynets V, Wagner S, Strahl S, Konigsrainer A et al. Nonalcoholic fatty liver disease in humans is associated with increased plasma endotoxin and plasminogen activator inhibitor 1 concentrations and with fructose intake. *J Nutr*. 2008;138(8):1452–5. Epub 2008/07/22.
87. Wei Y, Wang D, Topczewski F, Pagliassotti MJ. Fructose-mediated stress signaling in the liver: Implications for hepatic insulin resistance. *J Nutr Biochem*. 2007;18(1):1–9.
88. Wei Y, Wang D, Moran G, Estrada A, Pagliassotti MJ. Fructose-induced stress signaling in the liver involves methylglyoxal. *Nutr Metab (Lond)*. 2013;10(1):32. Epub 2013/04/10.
89. Lewis GF, Carpentier A, Adeli K, Giacca A. Disordered fat storage and mobilization in the pathogenesis of insulin resistance and type 2 diabetes. *Endocr Rev*. 2002;23(2):201–29.
90. Ferre P, Foufelle F. Hepatic steatosis: A role for de novo lipogenesis and the transcription factor Srebp-1c. *Diabetes Obes Metab*. 2010;12(Suppl. 2):83–92. Epub 2010/11/05.
91. Biddinger SB, Hernandez-Ono A, Rask-Madsen C, Haas JT, Aleman JO, Suzuki R et al. Hepatic insulin resistance is sufficient to produce dyslipidemia and susceptibility to atherosclerosis. *Cell Metab*. 2008;7(2):125–34. Epub 2008/02/06.
92. Brown MS, Goldstein JL. Selective versus total insulin resistance: A pathogenic paradox. *Cell Metab*. 2008;7(2):95–6. Epub 2008/02/06.
93. Sparks JD, Sparks CE, Adeli K. Selective hepatic insulin resistance, VLDL overproduction, and hypertriglyceridemia. *Arterioscler Thromb Vasc Biol*. 2012;32(9):2104–12. Epub 2012/07/17.
94. Christian P, Sacco J, Adeli K. Autophagy: Emerging roles in lipid homeostasis and metabolic control. *Biochim Biophys Acta*. 2013;1831(4):819–24. Epub 2013/01/01.

95. Fisher EA. The degradation of apolipoprotein B100: Multiple opportunities to regulate VLDL triglyceride production by different proteolytic pathways. *Biochim Biophys Acta*. 2012;1821(5):778–81. Epub 2012/02/22.
96. Sato R, Miyamoto W, Inoue J, Terada T, Imanaka T, Maeda M. Sterol regulatory element-binding protein negatively regulates microsomal triglyceride transfer protein gene transcription. *J Biol Chem*. 1999;274(35):24714–20.
97. Hussain MM, Shi J, Dreizen P. Microsomal triglyceride transfer protein and its role in Apob-lipoprotein assembly. *J Lipid Res*. 2003;44(1):22–32.
98. Yao Z, Wang Y. Apolipoprotein C-Iii and hepatic triglyceride-rich lipoprotein production. *Curr Opin Lipidol*. 2012;23(3):206–12. Epub 2012/04/19.
99. Sundaram M, Zhong S, Bou Khalil M, Zhou H, Jiang ZG, Zhao Y et al. Functional analysis of the missense Apoc3 mutation Ala23thr associated with human hypotriglyceridemia. *J Lipid Res*. 2010;51(6):1524–34. Epub 2010/01/26.
100. Qin W, Sundaram M, Wang Y, Zhou H, Zhong S, Chang CC et al. Missense mutation in Apoc3 within the C-terminal lipid binding domain of human Apoc-Iii results in impaired assembly and secretion of triacylglycerol-rich very low density lipoproteins: Evidence that Apoc-Iii plays a major role in the formation of lipid precursors within the microsomal lumen. *J Biol Chem*. 2011;286(31):27769–80. Epub 2011/06/17.
101. Chen M, Breslow JL, Li W, Leff T. Transcriptional regulation of the apoc-iii gene by insulin in diabetic mice: Correlation with changes in plasma triglyceride levels. *J Lipid Res*. 1994;35(11):1918–24. Epub 1994/11/01.
102. Nielsen S, Karpe F. Determinants of VLDL-triglycerides production. *Curr Opin Lipidol*. 2012;23(4):321–6. Epub 2012/05/24.
103. Krssak M, Falk Petersen K, Dresner A, DiPietro L, Vogel SM, Rothman DL et al. Intramyocellular lipid concentrations are correlated with insulin sensitivity in humans: A 1 h NMR spectroscopy study. *Diabetologia*. 1999;42(1):113–6.
104. Watt MJ, Hoy AJ. Lipid metabolism in skeletal muscle: Generation of adaptive and maladaptive intracellular signals for cellular function. *Am J Physiol Endocrinol Metab*. 2012;302(11):E1315–28. Epub 2011/12/22.
105. Samuel VT, Shulman GI. Mechanisms for insulin resistance: Common threads and missing links. *Cell*. 2012;148(5):852–71. Epub 2012/03/06.
106. Anderson EJ, Lustig ME, Boyle KE, Woodlief TL, Kane DA, Lin CT et al. Mitochondrial H_2O_2 emission and cellular redox state link excess fat intake to insulin resistance in both rodents and humans. *J Clin Invest*. 2009;119(3):573–81. Epub 2009/02/04.
107. Coen PM, Goodpaster BH. Role of intramyocelluar lipids in human health. *Trends Endocrinol Metab*. 2012;23(8):391–8. Epub 2012/06/23.
108. Tappy L, Mittendorfer B. Fructose toxicity: Is the science ready for public health actions? *Curr Opin Clin Nutr Metab Care*. 2012;15(4):357–61. Epub 2012/05/24.

20 Sugars, Fructose, Hypertension, and Kidney Disease

Laura Gabriela Sánchez Lozada, Magdalena Madero, Sirirat Reungjui, and Richard J. Johnson

CONTENTS

KEY POINTS

- Fructose raises blood pressure in animals and humans.
- The mechanism may relate to its ability to induce sympathetic nervous system activation, endothelial dysfunction, oxidative stress, and the generation of uric acid.
- Reduction of sugar intake in humans results in a reduction of blood pressure.
- Administration of fructose to animals results in glomerular hypertension, arteriolopathy, and tubolointestinal disease.
- Fructose administration accelerates chronic kidney disease in rats.
- Proximal tubular cells can also produce fructose via activation of the polyol pathway and endogenously produced fructose may have a role in experimental diabetic nephropathy and other models.

INTRODUCTION

Fructose is a monosaccharide found naturally in fruits and honey and is also a major constituent in added sugars, including sucrose and high-fructose corn syrup (HFCS). Fructose can also be produced in the gut by degradation of fructose polymers (fructans) by bacteria-containing fructanases. Finally, fructose can be generated from dietary sorbitol or from glucose by the polyol (aldose reductase-sorbitol dehydrogenase) pathway. Currently, the major dietary source of fructose is from added sugars, especially in the adolescent and young adult population. However, increasing evidence suggests that endogenously produced fructose may also be important in the pathogenesis of kidney disease. In this chapter, we will review the current evidence for fructose in driving hypertension and kidney disease.

FRUCTOSE AND HYPERTENSION

Primary (essential) hypertension is one of the most common diseases worldwide and affects over 70 million individuals in the USA. It was once uncommon, being present in only 5–10% of the population, but it has increased markedly over the last 100 years in association with western diet and culture [1]. While primary hypertension used to be rare in children, it has become increasingly observed in this population, especially among children who are obese and insulin-resistant. The increased frequency of hypertension carries significant morbidity, as hypertension remains the primary cause of stroke and heart failure, and the second most common cause of end-stage renal disease.

While fructose is known to have acute effects on blood pressure (BP), the role of fructose in driving primary hypertension in humans remains a very controversial topic. We will briefly summarize the studies that both support and argue against this hypothesis. Reviews on this topic are also available in Reference [2].

ANIMAL STUDIES

The administration of fructose to rats has been known to induce features of metabolic syndrome since the early 1950s [3]. One of the characteristic features is an increase in systemic BP, as documented by tail-cuff BPs, intra-arterial BP, and renal micropuncture measurements [4–7]. However, the gold standard for BP measurement in rodents is to place an intra-arterial pressure transducer that allows continuous BP in the conscious, nonsedated state [8]. Two studies subsequently reported that 24-h ambulatory BPs were normal in rats fed fructose despite these animals developing other features of metabolic syndrome [9,10]. It was, therefore, thought that the reason for this discrepancy may relate to the possibility that fructose may enhance sympathetic nervous system (SNS) responses that might lead to an increase in BP response with the handling that occurs with tail cuff or intra-arterial BP measurement, but not be as evident when animals are not being manipulated. Indeed, there is evidence that fructose stimulates SNS activity in rats [11]. More recently, studies using the 24-h intra-arterial BP monitoring system have documented that BP is elevated during the initial intake of fructose or sucrose compared to control animals and in some cases persists throughout the feeding period [12,13].

A variety of studies have investigated the mechanism(s) involved in fructose-induced hypertension in laboratory animals [2]. Recent studies suggest that the primary mechanism relates to the ability of fructose to increase intracellular and serum uric acid levels. These are summarized below.

Role of Uric Acid

Fructose is the only sugar that stimulates the production of uric acid within cells. This is because the first enzyme in fructose metabolism, fructokinase C, rapidly metabolizes fructose to fructose-1-phosphate in an unregulated manner. This results in the accumulation of AMP, which is metabolized by AMP deaminase to inosine monophosphate and eventually uric acid. Uric acid increases in cells that metabolize fructose (such as the hepatocyte) and then spills out into the circulation, peaking within 10–30 min [14,15].

Understanding the role of uric acid in hypertension in laboratory animals is complicated by the fact that rats, like most mammals, have much lower serum uric acid levels than humans. This is because most mammals express the enzyme uricase in their livers, which degrades uric acid, ultimately generating allantoin. Indeed, it is difficult to raise uric acid in rats unless uricase is inhibited. However, when rats were given the uricase inhibitor, oxonic acid, rats became hypertensive within several weeks [16]. Subsequently, numerous studies demonstrated that uric acid is a biologically active, proinflammatory substance, even when in soluble form. While it can function as an antioxidant in the extracellular environment [17,18], it is prooxidative within the cell, including in adipocytes, vascular smooth muscle cells, endothelial cells, cardiac fibroblasts, renal tubular cells, islet cells, and hepatocytes [19–25]. Oxidative stress is mediated in part by a stimulation of NADPH oxidase in the cytoplasm and mitochondria [19,21,22]. Uric acid can also generate radicals upon reaction with peroxynitrite [26].

Uric acid induces oxidative stress rapidly inside the cell and may have a key role in driving the biological actions of uric acid [23]. This includes the activation of mitogen-activated protein kinases, induction of nuclear transcription factors, and the production of chemokines (such as monocyte chemoattractant protein-1), vasoactive mediators (angiotensin II, thromboxane, and endothelin), inflammatory mediators (including C-reactive protein) including inflammasomes, and growth factors [27–30]. A decrease in NO also occurs, due to effects on uptake and metabolism of L-arginine, and scavenging by oxidants or uric acid itself [19,22,31–33]. Indeed, the initial hypertension induced by uric acid can be prevented by agents that block oxidative stress or the renin angiotensin system or that stimulate endothelial NO production [16,34,35].

While the acute effects of uric acid are mediated by vascular effects of uric acid itself, over time rats develop microvascular disease in their kidney, likely due to the direct stimulation of vascular smooth muscle cell proliferation [28,36]. The development of microvascular disease in the kidney results in some ischemia distally with the development of mild interstitial inflammation that alters the ability of the kidney to excrete salt [37]. Once microvascular disease develops in hyperuricemic rats, salt-sensitive hypertension develops and will persist even if the uric acid levels return to normal [38]. Thus, there appears to be two ways uric acid can induce hypertension, with the first being via direct effects on the vasculature and the second driven by subtle renal microvascular disease that is induced over time. Consistent with these observations, early studies in humans suggest that serum uric acid is highly associated with new onset hypertension [39], especially in adolescents, and pilot studies also support a role for uric acid in driving the hypertensive response [40,41].

As noted, fructose raises uric acid in rats, and the administration of high doses (60% fructose diet) increases serum uric acid and systemic BP (measured by tail cuff or by intra-arterial measurement under anesthesia) [4,5]. Fructose-fed rats also develop renal microvascular lesions similar to that observed with hyperuricemia [5,6]. Both the hypertension and renal microvascular disease can be prevented by lowering serum uric acid [4,5].

The fact that rodents express uricase can explain why high doses of fructose are needed to induce hypertension and metabolic syndrome in rats. Indeed, if uricase is inhibited, serum uric acid increases significantly more in response to fructose [42]. Furthermore, much lower doses of fructose are required to induce features of metabolic syndrome if uricase is inhibited in the rat [43]. In addition, female animals tend to have lower uric acid levels than male animals due to the uricosuric effects of estrogen, and, while not tested, this could provide an explanation for why female rats are relatively resistant to the effects of fructose [44].

Direct Vascular Effects

A key observation is that the administration of fructose to rats results in evidence for endothelial dysfunction, as noted by a decrease in urinary nitrites, and decreased vasodilation of renal and mesenteric arteries in response to acetylcholine [45–47]. Interestingly, the development of hypertension occurs several weeks after the development of endothelial dysfunction [47]. The mechanism may, in part, be due to suppression of production of nitric oxide (NO) by endothelial cells, as fructose reduces NO levels and transiently reduces eNOS expression in cultured endothelial cells [48] and eNOS activity in the aorta [49]. Moreover, overexpression of eNOS in vivo can block the development of hypertension in fructose-fed rats [50]. Fructose also has other negative effects on endothelium, such as stimulating production of leukocyte adhesion molecules (ICAM-1) [48] and blocking endothelium-derived hyperpolarizing factor [51]. A role for angiotensin II may also be involved in fructose-mediated hypertension, as blocking angiotensin II formation or action can restore eNOS activity [49], block oxidative stress in the blood vessels, and lower BP [52].

SNS Activation and Leptin

Fructose administration to mice has been shown to increase BP, in part, by activation of the SNS in the brain stem [13], and the rise of BP in fructose-fed animals can be blocked by chemical sympathectomy [53]. One potential mechanism by which they may occur is via fructose-mediated stimulation of leptin. Fructose-fed rats develop leptin resistance [54] and eventually postprandial leptin levels [55]. While leptin is best known for its role in mediating satiety, there is also increasing evidence that leptin may be an important mediator for hypertension in metabolic syndrome via its effects to induce SNS activation in the brain [56]. The ability of leptin to stimulate SNS activity occurs in both leptin-sensitive and -resistant states.

Relationship with Sodium Intake

The hypertension induced by fructose (or sucrose) is known to have an important relationship with salt intake, as the hypertension is much less evident on a low-salt diet, whereas it may be severe and persistent on a high-salt diet [57–59]. Fructose increases sodium absorption by the small bowel and also reduces urinary sodium excretion [59]. In addition, the ability of fructose to induce renal microvascular disease provides a mechanism for inducing salt-sensitive hypertension [37]. Furthermore, the presence of a high-salt diet with fructose results in a decrease in eNOS expression in the renal medulla [60] that may play a role in impairing sodium excretion in the setting of high BP.

HUMAN STUDIES

Does Fructose Increase Serum Uric Acid?

The animal studies suggest that fructose may cause hypertension primarily via the generation of uric acid. This raises the clinical question of whether fructose increases serum and intracellular uric acid. As mentioned earlier, the principal mechanism by which fructose raises uric acid is as a consequence of nucleotide turnover that occurs from the transient ATP depletion that occurs with fructose administration. Studies in humans show that this can occur with relatively small doses of fructose given orally [61]. Indeed, the administration of fructose to humans results in an acute rise in serum uric acid [62]. Clinically, the rise in uric acid can easily be demonstrated in the first 30–60 min following an oral fructose, sucrose, or HFCS challenge [63]. Subjects administered a high-fructose diet for 10 weeks also show higher uric acid levels over the 24-h period [64]. Over time, even fasting serum uric acid levels rise in humans fed diets high in fructose [65]. This may be due to a stimulation in uric acid synthesis from amino acid precursors [14,66] in addition to its effects on nucleotide turnover [15]. Epidemiological studies also link high-fructose intake, or intake of sugary soft drinks, with increased risk for elevated serum uric acid levels or gout, especially in men [67–69]. The association of soft drink intake, elevated serum uric acid, and hypertension has also been reported in adolescents [70]. In another study, fructose intake was associated with higher serum uric acid levels in boys [71]. In contrast, a study using US NHANES 1999–2004 databases could not find an association of fructose intake with uric acid levels [72].

A meta-analysis also concluded that short-term intake of fructose does not increase serum uric acid compared to control diets [73]. However, in most of these studies, the serum uric acid levels were determined after an overnight fast when serum uric acid would not be expected to be high in a short-term study [74,75]. The meta-analysis also included control groups that were fed sucrose (which also contains fructose) [73].

Does Fructose Raise BP in Humans?

Studies in animals suggest that the rise in BP with fructose is best observed during the time of fructose ingestion. Indeed, in humans, the administration of fructose results in an acute increase in BP that is not observed with glucose or water [74] (Table 20.1). Humans administered soft drinks containing sucrose or HFCS also show an immediate rise in BP associated with a rise in serum uric acid, and the BP rise is greater in humans given HFCS and is associated with higher serum uric acid and fructose levels [63]. We also administered high doses (200 g/day) of fructose to healthy men for a period of 2 weeks and noted a significant increase in both fasting serum uric acid and in 24-h ambulatory BP [75]. In this study, one-half of the subjects were randomized to receive allopurinol therapy, and in this group the rise in fasting serum uric acid was prevented and an increase in BP did not occur [75]. Although these studies provide strong evidence that fructose can raise BP in humans, other studies providing high-fructose diets could not show an increase in BP [76]. Indeed, a meta-analysis reported that fructose does not raise BP in short-term studies [77]. However, this study also suffers from similar methodologic issues [78,79] in that BP was typically measured only in the morning after an overnight fast when BP would not expect to be elevated in a short-term study. Thus, the data are convincing that the intake of fructose acutely increases BP in humans.

Is Fructose Intake Associated with Hypertension in Humans?

An important point with epidemiological studies is to consider fructose from added sugars differently from fructose from natural fruits. This is not because the fructose is different, but rather because natural fruits contain a variety of substances that can block the metabolic effects of fructose, including vitamin C, antioxidants, potassium, fiber, and other nutrients [45,80,81]. Epidemiological studies that evaluate total fructose intake (including fruits) may not show a relationship with hypertension [82], whereas this becomes readily evident when the analysis only evaluates the fructose content from added sugars [83].

Salt intake is also important to evaluate in subjects ingesting fructose from added sugars. One study in adolescents found that salt intake is higher in adolescents taking high-fructose diets, suggesting that some of the association of fructose-rich diets may be due to the higher salt intake [84]. However, as noted in the animal studies, the presence of high-salt diet may act synergistically with fructose to raise BP [58]. Indeed, one study found that the intake of fructose was independently associated with hypertension but this relationship was amplified in the presence of a high-salt diet [85].

The baseline serum uric acid level may also be important to be able to evaluate the relationship of fructose with BP. We had shown in experimental studies that uric acid regulates the expression of fructokinase and that pretreatment of cells with uric acid increases the ATP depletion in response to fructose [86]. A study of subjects with non-alcoholic fatty liver disease also showed that a higher baseline serum uric acid is associated with a greater depletion of hepatic ATP in response to fructose [87].

TABLE 20.1
Main Clinical and Epidemiological Studies of the Association Between Fructose and BP

Study	Study Design and Population	Follow Up	Independent Variable/Intervention	Outcome	Findings	Observations
Brown et al.	Randomized cross-over study ($n = 15$)	2 h	Water, fructose, and glucose intake	Raise in BP, heart rate, cardiac output, peripheral resistance	Fructose significantly increased BP	BP was not modified by glucose intake
Ha et al.	Meta-analyses 13 ($n = 352$) and 2 hypercaloric ($n = 24$) trials	Median follow-up of 4 weeks (range: 15.5 days to 10 weeks)	Fructose intake (in isocaloric or hypercaloric exchange for other carbohydrates)	BP	Isocaloric substitution of fructose for other carbohydrates did not adversely affect BP in humans	Less than half of the studies were randomly assigned, and BP was the primary outcome in only three of 15 studies. BP measurements were not postprandial, at which time the acute effects of fructose on BP are best shown
Perez-Pozo et al.	Randomized controlled trial ($n = 74$)	2 weeks	200 g of fructose intake with or without allopurinol	Metabolic syndrome components	High doses of fructose raise the BP and cause the features of metabolic syndrome	Lowering the uric acid level prevents the increase in mean arterial BP
Lee et al.	Randomized cross-over study ($n = 40$)	6 h	HFCS vs. sucrose sweetened beverages	Pharmacokinetics of fructose and acute metabolic and hemodynamic responses	HFCS raises BP more than sucrose-sweetened beverages	HFCS leads to greater fructose systemic exposure and significantly different acute metabolic effects
Forman et al.	Nurses' Health Study 1 ($n = 88{,}540$), Nurses' Health Study 2 ($n = 97{,}315$), and the Health Professionals Follow-up Study ($n = 37{,}375$)	20, 14, and 18 years, respectively	Fructose, vitamin C	Incident hypertension	Fructose and vitamin C are not associated with incident hypertension	Fructose accounted in the study included fruits that contain fiber, antioxidants, vitamin C

Jalal et al.	National Health and Nutrition Examination Survey ($n = 4528$)	Cross-sectional	Fructose intake	Hypertension	Increased fructose intake of ≥74 g/day independently and significantly associated with higher odds of elevated BP levels	Fructose content from added sugars
Brown et al.	International study of macro/micronutrients and BP ($n = 2696$)	Cross-sectional	Sugar-sweetened beverages, diet beverages, sugar intake	BP	SSB intake related directly to BP	Significant sugar–sodium interaction for individuals with above-median 24-h urinary sodium excretion, 2SD fructose intake was associated with systolic/diastolic BP differences
Chen	PREMIER Study ($n = 810$)	18 months	Behavioral Intervention Trial	BP	A reduction of 1 SSB serving per day in addition to reduced sugar intake was associated with significant reduction in BP	Findings persisted after adjustment for weight change over the follow-up time
Madero et al.	Randomized trial ($n = 131$) overweight subjects	6 weeks	Two energy-restricted diets—a very-low-fructose diet vs. a low natural fructose diet	Weight loss and MS parameters	Weight loss was significantly higher in the moderate natural fructose group than the low-fructose group	Both low-fructose diets resulted in significant BP lowering effect; however, diets were hypocaloric and this could have affected BP
Brymora et al.	Case series ($n = 28$), CKD cohort	6 weeks	Very-low-fructose diet	BP and inflammation	Significant reduction of BP was observed in the BP dipper group	Low-fructose diet was also associated with reduced high sensitivity C-reactive protein (hsCRP) and soluble intercellular adhesion molecule (sICAM)

Fructose-induced hyperuricemia is also greater in subjects with primary hypertension [88]. These observations could explain a recent study that found that fructose intake is associated with uric acid in boys, and uric acid is associated with hypertension, but fructose itself is not associated with BP [71].

Thus, the data strongly suggest that fructose intake, particularly from added sugars, is associated with hypertension and that these effects might best be observed in subjects with elevated serum uric acid levels and/or on a high-salt diet.

Does Reducing Fructose Intake Lower BP?

To date, there have been very few studies to investigate the effect of reducing fructose intake on BP. As noted in the animal studies, it is possible that chronic fructose intake may induce subtle renal injury that will perpetuate salt-sensitive hypertension even if fructose intake is reduced. Nevertheless, diets such as DASH are effective in lowering BP and are in essence a diet low in fructose from added sugars. In addition, one study reported that a reduction of one soft drink per day results in a net reduction in systolic BP of 2 mmHg and a 1 mm in diastolic BP after 18 months [89]. In another study by Madero et al. [90], a hypocaloric very-low-fructose diet and a hypocaloric low-fructose diet (fructose provided by fruits) for 6 weeks resulted in significant BP-lowering effect (8.7 mmHg in SBP and 5.6 mmHg in DPB). Since low-fructose diets also reduced body weight, this effect may have also contributed with the reduction in BP. Brymora et al. [91] also reported that a low-fructose diet reduced BP in subjects with CKD who had a "dipping pattern" of BP (i.e., whose BP tended to fall during sleep). In addition to BP lowering, a low-fructose diet may also improve mitochondrial density in the white blood cells of subjects with hypertension, suggesting an improvement in overall mitochondrial function [92].

SUMMARY: ROLE OF FRUCTOSE IN HYPERTENSION

In summary, experimental studies demonstrate that fructose can induce elevated BP, especially during fructose intake. The mechanism is driven likely, in part, by fructose-induced hyperuricemia, but there is also evidence that fructose may have direct effects on the vasculature and also may affect sodium absorption and excretion (Figure 20.1). In humans, fructose has also been shown to raise BP, in part by increasing intracellular and serum uric acid levels. Intake of fructose from added sugars is associated with hypertension in humans, and lowering fructose intake from added sugars results in a reduction in BP. Hence, these studies document an emerging role for fructose in being a contributor to elevated BP in humans.

FRUCTOSE AND KIDNEY DISEASE

There is also emerging interest in the role of fructose in chronic kidney disease as well as potentially being involved in kidney stones. We provide an overview below.

EXPERIMENTAL STUDIES

Fructose may be able to induce kidney disease via two different mechanisms, including by raising serum uric acid or by direct effects of fructose on the kidney. There is increasing evidence that both may be operative.

Fructose-Induced Hyperuricemia as a Cause of Kidney Disease

Our initial studies focused on the possibility that fructose may raise serum uric acid and that an elevation in serum uric acid might increase the risk for kidney disease. Indeed, we had found that increasing serum uric acid in rats caused renal microvascular disease that impaired renal

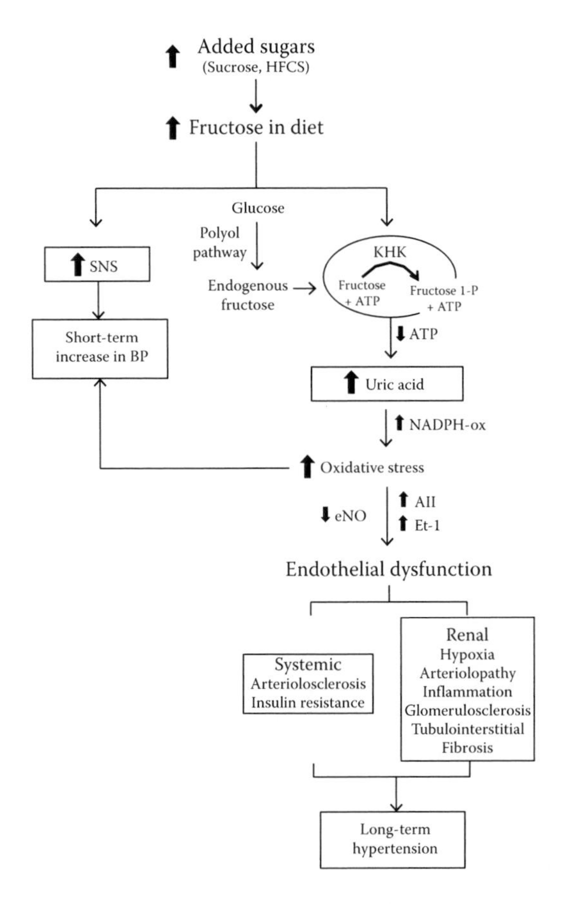

FIGURE 20.1 Proposed mechanism(s) by which fructose may cause hypertension and kidney disease. Key: AII, angiotensin II; ATP, adenosine triphosphate; Et-1, endothelin-1; eNO, endothelial nitric oxide; KHK, fructokinase; SNS, sympathetic nervous system.

autoregulation, resulting in increased transmission of systemic pressure to the glomerular capillaries in association with a reduction in renal blood flow [93]. Rats made chronically hyperuricemic developed glomerular hypertrophy and eventually glomerulosclerosis [94]. In rats with chronic kidney disease, raising serum uric acid caused persistent glomerular hypertension and accelerated the renal damage [27,95,96].

Similarly, we found that the administration of fructose to rats also caused a similar renal microvascular disease, with impaired autoregulation and glomerular hypertension, and that this could be prevented if the increase in serum uric acid was prevented with febuxostat [5]. The glomerular hypertension from fructose can be augmented if uricase is inhibited [43]. Long-term administration of fructose has also been reported to cause glomerulosclerosis in rats [97,98]. Similarly, a high-fructose intake was shown to accelerate chronic kidney disease in rats that was not observed with a similar diet high in glucose [99]. These data suggested that fructose may increase the risk for chronic kidney disease similar to an elevation in uric acid. This is potentially important as there is increasing evidence that uric acid may be a true risk factor for chronic kidney disease [100].

Direct Effects of Dietary Fructose on the Kidney

While fructose may induce its effects via systemic hyperuricemia, it is known that the metabolism of fructose by fructokinase results in ATP depletion, intracellular uric acid generation, and oxidative stress [21]. In particular, the proximal tubule is a rich source of fructokinase and can take up fructose from the urinary lumen via the transporter, Glut5 [101]. When proximal tubular cells metabolize fructose, there is ATP depletion, oxidative stress, and the release of chemokines, and this can be prevented if fructokinase is silenced [25]. Indeed, the administration of fructose to laboratory rats and mice can result in tubulointerstitial injury with prominent proximal tubular involvement [97,101,102]. The renal injury is associated with inflammation associated with the release of chemokines (monocyte chemoattractant protein-1) [101] and with the expression of the NOD-like receptor 3 (NLRP3) inflammasome [30]. These latter changes could be reversed by treatment with allopurinol [30]. Whether this is a consequence of lowering serum uric acid or intracellular uric acid within the proximal tubule is not known.

Endogenous Fructose and Renal Disease

Until now, we have discussed the role of fructose in hypertension and kidney disease solely from the standpoint of dietary fructose. Generally, there has been little discussion for a role for endogenously generated fructose in any disease state. However, fructose can be generated from glucose (fructoneogenesis) through the polyol pathway that involves conversion of glucose to fructose by aldose reductase followed by the metabolism of sorbitol to fructose by sorbitol dehydrogenase. In the proximal tubule, aldose reductase levels are normally low or absent, but the polyol pathway can be induced by increases in serum osmolarity, by hyperglycemia, and by ischemia. Currently, our group is studying models of kidney disease induced by diabetes or dehydration, and in preliminary studies we can show that mice lacking fructokinase show significant renal protection in these conditions [103] (and unpublished data). We suspect that the endogenous fructose-fructokinase pathway may have an important role in various kidney diseases. Thus, the stealth production of fructose may be yet another way for kidney disease and/or hypertension to develop.

HUMAN STUDIES

It has only been in the last few years that clinical studies have begun to evaluate the role of fructose in kidney disease. There are reports that sugary soft drinks increase the risk for albuminuria [104]. Sugar-sweetened drinks and hyperuricemia are also associated with the presence of chronic kidney disease but not with the progression of kidney disease [105,106]. Clearly more studies investigating this relationship are needed.

There has also been one study evaluating the effect of low-fructose diet in subjects with chronic kidney disease. In this study, there was no progression of kidney disease in either the control or treatment group, thus precluding any conclusion on the effect of this diet on renal function. However, the subjects given the low-fructose diet did show a reduction in circulating C-reactive protein. As mentioned earlier, those subjects with dipping BP ($n = 20$) showed a reduction in BP, whereas those subjects with nondipping BP ($n = 8$) did not [91].

While not the subject of this chapter, there is also increasing evidence that intake of sugary soft drinks is associated with increased risk for kidney stones [107]. This may relate to the fact that soft drink intake is greatest in hotter climates where dehydration is common, but also may relate to the ability of fructose to increase urinary oxalate [108]. As the prevalence of kidney stones is increasing worldwide, studies investigating the role of fructose in its pathogenesis are needed.

SUMMARY

Fructose is a simple sugar that is distinct from all other nutrients in its ability to cause ATP depletion and rapid nucleotide turnover. This process leads to the production of intracellular uric acid and oxidative stress that appears to have important effects on the vasculature and the kidney. Increasing evidence suggests that fructose may have a role in some subjects with hypertension and kidney disease. The major dietary sources are HFCS and sucrose. Further studies need to be performed to determine whether excessive intake of these added sugars may have a role in the current epidemic of hypertension and chronic kidney disease that is being observed throughout the world.

CONFLICTS OF INTEREST

R.J.J. is an inventor on patent applications from the University of Colorado (US2013/0195886 and US2013/0224218) related to blocking fructose metabolism in the treatment of kidney disease and metabolic syndrome. He is on the Scientific Advisory Board of Amway, the Scientific Board of XORT Therapeutics, and of Rivermend Health LLC. He has received research funding from Danone Research and Amway. R.J.J. and L.G.S.-L. are also members of Colorado Research Partners LLC that has an interest in developing therapeutic inhibitors for sugar metabolism. The other authors declared no competing interests.

REFERENCES

1. Johnson RJ, Titte S, Cade JR, Rideout BA, Oliver WJ. Uric acid, evolution and primitive cultures. *Semin Nephrol*. 2005;25(1):3–8.
2. Madero M, Perez-Pozo SE, Jalal D, Johnson RJ, Sanchez-Lozada LG. Dietary fructose and hypertension. *Curr Hypertens Rep*. 2011;13(1):29–35. Epub 2010/10/20.
3. Hill R, Baker N, Chaikoff IL. Altered metabolic patterns induced in the normal rat by feeding an adequate diet containing fructose as sole carbohydrate. *J Biol Chem*. 1954;209(2):705–16. Epub 1954/08/01.
4. Nakagawa T, Hu H, Zharikov S, Tuttle KR, Short RA, Glushakova O et al. A causal role for uric acid in fructose-induced metabolic syndrome. *Am J Physiol Renal Physiol*. 2006;290(3):F625–31.
5. Sanchez-Lozada LG, Tapia E, Bautista-Garcia P, Soto V, Avila-Casado C, Vega-Campos IP et al. Effects of febuxostat on metabolic and renal alterations in rats with fructose-induced metabolic syndrome. *Am J Physiol Renal Physiol*. 2008;294(4):F710–8.
6. Sanchez-Lozada LG, Tapia E, Jimenez A, Bautista P, Cristobal M, Nepomuceno T et al. Fructose-induced metabolic syndrome is associated with glomerular hypertension and renal microvascular damage in rats. *Am J Physiol Renal Physiol*. 2007;292(1):F423–9.
7. Hwang IS, Ho H, Hoffman BB, Reaven GM. Fructose-induced insulin resistance and hypertension in rats. *Hypertension*. 1987;10(5):512–6.
8. Kurtz TW, Griffin KA, Bidani AK, Davisson RL, Hall JE. Recommendations for blood pressure measurement in animals: Summary of an AHA scientific statement from the council on high blood pressure research, professional and public education subcommittee. *Arterioscler Thromb Vasc Biol*. 2005;25(3):478–9.
9. Brands MW, Garrity CA, Holman MG, Keen HL, Alonso-Galicia M, Hall JE. High-fructose diet does not raise 24-hour mean arterial pressure in rats. *Am J Hypertens*. 1994;7(1):104–9.
10. D'Angelo G, Elmarakby AA, Pollock DM, Stepp DW. Fructose feeding increases insulin resistance but not blood pressure in Sprague-Dawley rats. *Hypertension*. 2005;46(4):806–11.
11. Cunha TS, Farah V, Paulini J, Pazzine M, Elased KM, Marcondes FK et al. Relationship between renal and cardiovascular changes in a murine model of glucose intolerance. *Regul Pept*. 2007;139(1–3):1–4.
12. Roncal-Jimenez CA, Lanaspa MA, Rivard CJ, Nakagawa T, Sanchez-Lozada LG, Jalal D et al. Sucrose induces fatty liver and pancreatic inflammation in male breeder rats independent of excess energy intake. *Metabolism*. 2011;60(9):1259–70. Epub 2011/04/15.
13. Farah V, Elased KM, Chen Y, Key MP, Cunha TS, Irigoyen MC et al. Nocturnal hypertension in mice consuming a high fructose diet. *Auton Neurosci*. 2006;130(1–2):41–50.
14. Raivio KO, Becker A, Meyer LJ, Greene ML, Nuki G, Seegmiller JE. Stimulation of human purine synthesis de novo by fructose infusion. *Metabolism*. 1975;24(7):861–9. Epub 1975/07/01.
15. Maenpaa PH, Raivio KO, Kekomaki MP. Liver adenine nucleotides: Fructose-induced depletion and its effect on protein synthesis. *Science*. 1968;161(847):1253–4.
16. Mazzali M, Hughes J, Kim YG, Jefferson JA, Kang DH, Gordon KL et al. Elevated uric acid increases blood pressure in the rat by a novel crystal-independent mechanism. *Hypertension*. 2001; 38(5):1101–6.
17. Ames BN, Cathcart R, Schwiers E, Hochstein P. Uric acid provides an antioxidant defense in humans against oxidant- and radical-caused aging and cancer: A hypothesis. *Proc Natl Acad Sci USA*. 1981;78(11): 6858–62.

18. Kuzkaya N, Weissmann N, Harrison DG, Dikalov S. Interactions of peroxynitrite with uric acid in the presence of ascorbate and thiols: Implications for uncoupling endothelial nitric oxide synthase. *Biochem Pharmacol*. 2005;70(3):343–54.
19. Sautin YY, Nakagawa T, Zharikov S, Johnson RJ. Adverse effects of the classic antioxidant uric acid in adipocytes: NADPH oxidase-mediated oxidative/nitrosative stress. *Am J Physiol Cell Physiol*. 2007;293(2):C584–96. Epub 2007/04/13.
20. Corry DB, Eslami P, Yamamoto K, Nyby MD, Makino H, Tuck ML. Uric acid stimulates vascular smooth muscle cell proliferation and oxidative stress via the vascular renin-angiotensin system. *J Hypertens*. 2008;26(2):269–75.
21. Lanaspa MA, Sanchez-Lozada LG, Choi YJ, Cicerchi C, Kanbay M, Roncal-Jimenez CA et al. Uric acid induces hepatic steatosis by generation of mitochondrial oxidative stress: Potential role in fructose-dependent and -independent fatty liver. *J Biol Chem*. 2012;287(48):40732–44. Epub 2012/10/05.
22. Sanchez-Lozada LG, Lanaspa MA, Cristobal-Garcia M, Garcia-Arroyo F, Soto V, Cruz-Robles D et al. Uric acid-induced endothelial dysfunction is associated with mitochondrial alterations and decreased intracellular ATP concentrations. *Nephron Exp Nephrol*. 2012;121(3–4):e71–8. Epub 2012/12/14.
23. Yu MA, Sanchez-Lozada LG, Johnson RJ, Kang DH. Oxidative stress with an activation of the renin–angiotensin system in human vascular endothelial cells as a novel mechanism of uric acid-induced endothelial dysfunction. *J Hypertens*. 2010;28(6):1234–42. Epub 2010/05/21.
24. Cheng TH, Lin JW, Chao HH, Chen YL, Chen CH, Chan P et al. Uric acid activates extracellular signal-regulated kinases and thereafter endothelin-1 expression in rat cardiac fibroblasts. *Int J Cardiol*. 2010;139(1):42–9. Epub 2008/10/24.
25. Cirillo P, Gersch MS, Mu W, Scherer PM, Kim KM, Gesualdo L et al. Ketohexokinase-dependent metabolism of fructose induces proinflammatory mediators in proximal tubular cells. *J Am Soc Nephrol*. 2009;20(3):545–53.
26. Imaram W, Gersch C, Kim KM, Johnson RJ, Henderson GN, Angerhofer A. Radicals in the reaction between peroxynitrite and uric acid identified by electron spin resonance spectroscopy and liquid chromatography mass spectrometry. *Free Radic Biol Med*. 2010;49(2):275–81. Epub 2010/04/22.
27. Kang DH, Nakagawa T, Feng L, Watanabe S, Han L, Mazzali M et al. A role for uric acid in the progression of renal disease. *J Am Soc Nephrol*. 2002;13(12):2888–97.
28. Kang DH, Park SK, Lee IK, Johnson RJ. Uric acid-induced C-reactive protein expression: Implication on cell proliferation and nitric oxide production of human vascular cells. *J Am Soc Nephrol*. 2005;16(12):3553–62.
29. Kanellis J, Watanabe S, Li JH, Kang DH, Li P, Nakagawa T et al. Uric acid stimulates monocyte chemoattractant protein-1 production in vascular smooth muscle cells via mitogen-activated protein kinase and cyclooxygenase-2. *Hypertension*. 2003;41(6):1287–93.
30. Hu QH, Zhang X, Pan Y, Li YC, Kong LD. Allopurinol, quercetin and rutin ameliorate renal Nlrp3 inflammasome activation and lipid accumulation in fructose-fed rats. *Biochem Pharmacol*. 2012;84(1):113–25. Epub 2012/03/20.
31. Schwartz IF, Grupper A, Chernichovski T, Hillel O, Engel A, Schwartz D. Hyperuricemia attenuates aortic nitric oxide generation, through inhibition of arginine transport, in rats. *J Vasc Res*. 2011;48(3):252–60. Epub 2010/11/26.
32. Zharikov S, Krotova K, Hu H, Baylis C, Johnson RJ, Block ER et al. Uric acid decreases no production and increases arginase activity in cultured pulmonary artery endothelial cells. *Am J Physiol Cell Physiol*. 2008;295(5):C1183–90. Epub 2008/09/12.
33. Gersch C, Palii SP, Kim KM, Angerhofer A, Johnson RJ, Henderson GN. Inactivation of nitric oxide by uric acid. *Nucleosides Nucleotides Nucleic Acids*. 2008;27(8):967–78.
34. Sanchez-Lozada LG, Soto V, Tapia E, Avila-Casado C, Sautin YY, Nakagawa T et al. Role of oxidative stress in the renal abnormalities induced by experimental hyperuricemia. *Am J Physiol Renal Physiol*. 2008;295(4):F1134–41.
35. Sanchez-Lozada LG, Tapia E, Lopez-Molina R, Nepomuceno T, Soto V, Avila-Casado C et al. Effects of acute and chronic L-arginine treatment in experimental hyperuricemia. *Am J Physiol Renal Physiol*. 2007;292(4):F1238–44.
36. Mazzali M, Kanellis J, Han L, Feng L, Xia YY, Chen Q et al. Hyperuricemia induces a primary renal arteriolopathy in rats by a blood pressure-independent mechanism. *Am J Physiol Renal Physiol*. 2002;282(6):F991–7.
37. Rodriguez-Iturbe B, Johnson RJ. The role of renal microvascular disease and interstitial inflammation in salt-sensitive hypertension. *Hypertens Res*. 2010;33(10):975–80. Epub 2010/08/06.
38. Watanabe S, Kang DH, Feng L, Nakagawa T, Kanellis J, Lan H et al. Uric acid, hominoid evolution, and the pathogenesis of salt-sensitivity. *Hypertension*. 2002;40(3):355–60.

39. Feig DI, Johnson RJ. Hyperuricemia in childhood primary hypertension. *Hypertension*. 2003;42(3):247–52.
40. Feig DI, Soletsky B, Johnson RJ. Effect of allopurinol on blood pressure of adolescents with newly diagnosed essential hypertension: A randomized trial. *JAMA*. 2008;300(8):924–32.
41. Soletsky B, Feig DI. Uric acid reduction rectifies prehypertension in obese adolescents. *Hypertension*. 2012;60(5):1148–56. Epub 2012/09/26.
42. Stavric B, Johnson WJ, Clayman S, Gadd RE, Chartrand A. Effect of fructose administration on serum urate levels in the uricase inhibited rat. *Experientia*. 1976;32(3):373–4.
43. Tapia E, Cristobal M, Garcia-Arroyo FE, Soto V, Monroy-Sanchez F, Pacheco U et al. Synergistic effect of uricase blockade plus physiological amounts of fructose–glucose on glomerular hypertension and oxidative stress in rats. *Am J Physiol Renal Physiol*. 2013;304(6):F727–36. Epub 2013/01/11.
44. Song D, Arikawa E, Galipeau D, Battell M, McNeill JH. Androgens are necessary for the development of fructose-induced hypertension. *Hypertension*. 2004;43(3):667–72.
45. Reungjui S, Roncal CA, Mu W, Srinivas TR, Sirivongs D, Johnson RJ et al. Thiazide diuretics exacerbate fructose-induced metabolic syndrome. *J Am Soc Nephrol*. 2007;18(10):2724–31.
46. Kamata K, Yamashita K. Insulin resistance and impaired endothelium-dependent renal vasodilatation in fructose-fed hypertensive rats. *Res Commun Mol Pathol Pharmacol*. 1999;103(2):195–210.
47. Katakam PV, Ujhelyi MR, Hoenig ME, Miller AW. Endothelial dysfunction precedes hypertension in diet-induced insulin resistance. *Am J Physiol*. 1998;275(3 Pt 2):R788–92.
48. Glushakova O, Kosugi T, Roncal C, Mu W, Heinig M, Cirillo P et al. Fructose induces the inflammatory molecule Icam-1 in endothelial cells. *J Am Soc Nephrol*. 2008;19(9):1712–20.
49. Miatello R, Risler N, Gonzalez S, Castro C, Ruttler M, Cruzado M. Effects of enalapril on the vascular wall in an experimental model of syndrome X. *Am J Hypertens*. 2002;15(10 Pt 1):872–8.
50. Zhao CX, Xu X, Cui Y, Wang P, Wei X, Yang S et al. Increased endothelial nitric-oxide synthase expression reduces hypertension and hyperinsulinemia in fructose-treated rats. *J Pharmacol Exp Ther*. 2009;328(2):610–20. Epub 2008/11/15.
51. Katakam PV, Ujhelyi MR, Miller AW. EDHF-mediated relaxation is impaired in fructose-fed rats. *J Cardiovasc Pharmacol*. 1999;34(3):461–7.
52. Shinozaki K, Ayajiki K, Nishio Y, Sugaya T, Kashiwagi A, Okamura T. Evidence for a causal role of the renin–angiotensin system in vascular dysfunction associated with insulin resistance. *Hypertension*. 2004;43(2):255–62.
53. Verma S, Bhanot S, McNeill JH. Sympathectomy prevents fructose-induced hyperinsulinemia and hypertension. *Eur J Pharmacol*. 1999;373(2–3):R1–4.
54. Shapiro A, Mu W, Roncal C, Cheng KY, Johnson RJ, Scarpace PJ. Fructose-induced leptin resistance exacerbates weight gain in response to subsequent high-fat feeding. *Am J Physiol Regul Integr Comp Physiol*. 2008;295(5):R1370–5. Epub 2008/08/16.
55. Lee YC, Ko YH, Hsu YP, Ho LT. Plasma leptin response to oral glucose tolerance and fasting/re-feeding tests in rats with fructose-induced metabolic derangements. *Life Sci*. 2006;78(11):1155–62.
56. Hall JE, da Silva AA, do Carmo JM, Dubinion J, Hamza S, Munusamy S et al. Obesity-induced hypertension: Role of sympathetic nervous system, leptin, and melanocortins. *J Biol Chem*. 2010;285(23):17271–6. Epub 2010/03/30.
57. Johnson MD, Zhang HY, Kotchen TA. Sucrose does not raise blood pressure in rats maintained on a low salt intake. *Hypertension*. 1993;21(6 Pt 1):779–85. Epub 1993/06/01.
58. Vasdev S, Gill V, Parai S, Gadag V. Fructose-induced hypertension in Wistar-Kyoto rats: Interaction with moderately high dietary salt. *Can J Physiol Pharmacol*. 2007;85(3–4):413–21.
59. Singh AK, Amlal H, Haas PJ, Dringenberg U, Fussell S, Barone SL et al. Fructose-induced hypertension: Essential role of chloride and fructose absorbing transporters Pat1 and Glut5. *Kidney Int*. 2008;74(4):438–47.
60. Nishimoto Y, Tomida T, Matsui H, Ito T, Okumura K. Decrease in renal medullary endothelial nitric oxide synthase of fructose-fed, salt-sensitive hypertensive rats. *Hypertension*. 2002;40(2):190–4.
61. Bawden SJ, Stephenson MC, Marciani L, Aithal GP, Macdonald IA, Gowland PA et al. Investigating alterations in hepatic atp levels following fructose and fructose + glucose ingestion: A simple non-invasive technique to assess liver function using 31p Mrs. *Proc Intl Soc Mag Reson Med*. 2012;20:1369.
62. Stirpe F, Della Corte E, Bonetti E, Abbondanza A, Abbati A, De Stefano F. Fructose-induced hyperuricaemia. *Lancet*. 1970;2(7686):1310–1.
63. Le MT, Frye RF, Rivard CJ, Cheng J, McFann KK, Segal MS et al. Effects of high-fructose corn syrup and sucrose on the pharmacokinetics of fructose and acute metabolic and hemodynamic responses in healthy subjects. *Metabolism*. 2012;61(5):641–51. Epub 2011/12/14.
64. Cox CL, Stanhope KL, Schwarz JM, Graham JL, Hatcher B, Griffen SC et al. Consumption of fructose- but not glucose-sweetened beverages for 10 weeks increases circulating concentrations of uric acid,

retinol binding protein-4, and gamma-glutamyl transferase activity in overweight/obese humans. *Nutr Metab (Lond).* 2012;9(1):68. Epub 2012/07/26.

65. Reiser S, Powell AS, Scholfield DJ, Panda P, Ellwood KC, Canary JJ. Blood lipids, lipoproteins, apoproteins, and uric acid in men fed diets containing fructose or high-amylose cornstarch. *Am J Clin Nutr.* 1989;49(5):832–9.
66. Emmerson BT. Effect of oral fructose on urate production. *Ann Rheum Dis.* 1974;33(3):276–80.
67. Choi HK, Curhan G. Soft drinks, fructose consumption, and the risk of gout in men: Prospective cohort study. *BMJ.* 2008;336(7639):309–12.
68. Choi JW, Ford ES, Gao X, Choi HK. Sugar-sweetened soft drinks, diet soft drinks, and serum uric acid level: The third national health and nutrition examination survey. *Arthritis Rheum.* 2007;59(1):109–16.
69. Gao X, Qi L, Qiao N, Choi HK, Curhan G, Tucker KL et al. Intake of added sugar and sugar-sweetened drink and serum uric acid concentration in US men and women. *Hypertension.* 2007;50(2):306–12.
70. Nguyen S, Choi HK, Lustig RH, Hsu CY. Sugar-sweetened beverages, serum uric acid, and blood pressure in adolescents. *J Pediatr.* 2009;154(6):807–13. Epub 2009/04/21.
71. Bobridge KS, Haines GL, Mori TA, Beilin LJ, Oddy WH, Sherriff J et al. Dietary fructose in relation to blood pressure and serum uric acid in adolescent boys and girls. *J Hum Hypertens.* 2013;27(4):217–24. Epub 2012/09/14.
72. Sun SZ, Flickinger BD, Williamson-Hughes PS, Empie MW. Lack of association between dietary fructose and hyperuricemia risk in adults. *Nutr Metab (Lond).* 2010;7:16. Epub 2010/03/03.
73. Wang DD, Sievenpiper JL, de Souza RJ, Chiavaroli L, Ha V, Cozma AI et al. The effects of fructose intake on serum uric acid vary among controlled dietary trials. *J Nutr.* 2012;142(5):916–23. Epub 2012/03/30.
74. Brown CM, Dulloo AG, Yepuri G, Montani JP. Fructose ingestion acutely elevates blood pressure in healthy young humans. *Am J Physiol Regul Integr Comp Physiol.* 2008;294(3):R730–7.
75. Perez-Pozo SE, Schold J, Nakagawa T, Sanchez-Lozada LG, Johnson RJ, Lillo JL. Excessive fructose intake induces the features of metabolic syndrome in healthy adult men: Role of uric acid in the hypertensive response. *Int J Obes (Lond).* 2010;34(3):454–61. Epub 2009/12/24.
76. Stanhope KL, Schwarz JM, Keim NL, Griffen SC, Bremer AA, Graham JL et al. Consuming fructose-sweetened, not glucose-sweetened, beverages increases visceral adiposity and lipids and decreases insulin sensitivity in overweight/obese humans. *J Clin Invest.* 2009;119(5):1322–34. Epub 2009/04/22.
77. Ha V, Sievenpiper JL, de Souza RJ, Chiavaroli L, Wang DD, Cozma AI et al. Effect of fructose on blood pressure: A systematic review and meta-analysis of controlled feeding trials. *Hypertension.* 2012;59(4):787–95. Epub 2012/02/15.
78. Madero M, Lozada LG, Johnson RJ. Fructose likely does have a role in hypertension. *Hypertension.* 2012;59(6):e54; author reply e5–6. Epub 2012/05/02.
79. Johnson RJ, Nakagawa T, Sanchez-Lozada LG, Shafiu M, Sundaram S, Le M et al. Perspectives: Sugar, uric acid, and the etiology of diabetes and obesity. *Diabetes.* 2013;62(10):3307–15.
80. Vasdev S, Gill V, Parai S, Longerich L, Gadag V. Dietary vitamin E and C supplementation prevents fructose induced hypertension in rats. *Mol Cell Biochem.* 2002;241(1–2):107–14.
81. Hu QH, Wang C, Li JM, Zhang DM, Kong LD. Allopurinol, rutin, and quercetin attenuate hyperuricemia and renal dysfunction in rats induced by fructose intake: Renal organic ion transporter involvement. *Am J Physiol Renal Physiol.* 2009;297(4):F1080–91. Epub 2009/07/17.
82. Forman JP, Choi H, Curhan GC. Fructose and vitamin C intake do not influence risk for developing hypertension. *J Am Soc Nephrol.* 2009;20(4):863–71. Epub 2009/01/16.
83. Jalal DI, Smits G, Johnson RJ, Chonchol M. Increased fructose associates with elevated blood pressure. *J Am Soc Nephrol.* 2010;21(9):1543–9. Epub 2010/07/03.
84. He FJ, Marrero NM, MacGregor GA. Salt intake is related to soft drink consumption in children and adolescents: A link to obesity? *Hypertension.* 2008;51(3):629–34.
85. Brown IJ, Stamler J, Van Horn L, Robertson CE, Chan Q, Dyer AR et al. Sugar-sweetened beverage, sugar intake of individuals, and their blood pressure: International study of macro/micronutrients and blood pressure. *Hypertension.* 2011;57(4):695–701. Epub 2011/03/02.
86. Lanaspa MA, Sanchez-Lozada LG, Cicerchi C, Li N, Roncal-Jimenez CA, Ishimoto T et al. Uric acid stimulates fructokinase and accelerates fructose metabolism in the development of fatty liver. *PLoS One.* 2012;7(10):e47948. Epub 2012/11/01.
87. Abdelmalek MF, Lazo M, Horska A, Bonekamp S, Lipkin EW, Balasubramanyam A et al. Higher dietary fructose is associated with impaired hepatic adenosine triphosphate homeostasis in obese individuals with type 2 diabetes. *Hepatology.* 2012;56(3):952–60. Epub 2012/04/03.
88. Fiaschi E, Baggio B, Favaro S, Antonello A, Camerin E, Todesco S et al. Fructose-induced hyperuricemia in essential hypertension. *Metabolism.* 1977;26(11):1219–23.

89. Chen L, Caballero B, Mitchell DC, Loria C, Lin PH, Champagne CM et al. Reducing consumption of sugar-sweetened beverages is associated with reduced blood pressure: A prospective study among United States adults. *Circulation.* 2010;121(22):2398–406.
90. Madero M, Arriaga JC, Jalal D, Rivard C, McFann K, Perez-Mendez O et al. The effect of two energy-restricted diets, a low-fructose diet versus a moderate natural fructose diet, on weight loss and metabolic syndrome parameters: A randomized controlled trial. *Metabolism.* 2011;60(11):1551–9. Epub 2011/05/31.
91. Brymora A, Flisinski M, Johnson RJ, Goszka G, Stefanska A, Manitius J. Low-fructose diet lowers blood pressure and inflammation in patients with chronic kidney disease. *Nephrol Dial Transplant.* 2012;27(2):608–12. Epub 2011/05/27.
92. Hernández-Ríos R, Hernández-Estrada S, Cruz-Robles D, Hernández-Lobato S, Villalobos-Martín M, Johnson RJ et al. Low fructose and low salt diets increase mitochondrial DNA in white blood cells of overweight subjects. *Exp Clin Endocrinol Diabetes.* 2013;121(9):535–8.
93. Sanchez-Lozada LG, Tapia E, Avila-Casado C, Soto V, Franco M, Santamaria J et al. Mild hyperuricemia induces glomerular hypertension in normal rats. *Am J Physiol Renal Physiol.* 2002;283(5):F1105–10.
94. Nakagawa T, Mazzali M, Kang DH, Kanellis J, Watanabe S, Sanchez-Lozada LG et al. Hyperuricemia causes glomerular hypertrophy in the rat. *Am J Nephrol.* 2003;23(1):2–7.
95. Sanchez-Lozada LG, Tapia E, Santamaria J, Avila-Casado C, Soto V, Nepomuceno T et al. Mild hyperuricemia induces vasoconstriction and maintains glomerular hypertension in normal and remnant kidney rats. *Kidney Int.* 2005;67(1):237–47.
96. Sanchez-Lozada LG, Tapia E, Soto V, Avila-Casado C, Franco M, Zhao L et al. Treatment with the xanthine oxidase inhibitor febuxostat lowers uric acid and alleviates systemic and glomerular hypertension in experimental hyperuricaemia. *Nephrol Dial Transplant.* 2008;23(4):1179–85.
97. Kizhner T, Werman MJ. Long-term fructose intake: Biochemical consequences and altered renal histology in the male rat. *Metabolism.* 2002;51(12):1538–47.
98. Zaoui P, Rossini E, Pinel N, Cordonnier D, Halimi S, Morel F. High fructose-fed rats: A model of glomerulosclerosis involving the renin–angiotensin system and renal gelatinases. *Ann NY Acad Sci.* 1999;878:716–9. Epub 1999/07/23.
99. Gersch MS, Mu W, Cirillo P, Reungjui S, Zhang L, Roncal C et al. Fructose, but not dextrose, accelerates the progression of chronic kidney disease. *Am J Physiol Renal Physiol.* 2007;293(4):F1256–61.
100. Johnson RJ, Nakagawa T, Jalal D, Sanchez-Lozada LG, Kang DH, Ritz E. Uric acid and chronic kidney disease: Which is chasing which? *Nephrol Dial Transplant.* 2013;28(9):2221–8. Epub 2013/04/02.
101. Nakayama T, Kosugi T, Gersch M, Connor T, Sanchez-Lozada LG, Lanaspa MA et al. Dietary fructose causes tubulointerstitial injury in the normal rat kidney. *Am J Physiol Renal Physiol.* 2010;298(3):F712–20. Epub 2010/01/15.
102. Aoyama M, Isshiki K, Kume S, Chin-Kanasaki M, Araki H, Araki S et al. Fructose induces tubulointerstitial injury in the kidney of mice. *Biochem Biophys Res Commun.* 2012;419(2):244–9. Epub 2012/02/22.
103. Roncal-Jimenez CA, Ishimoto T, Lanaspa MA, Rivard C, Nakagawa T, Ejaz AA et al. Fructokinase activity mediates dehydration-induced renal injury. *Kidney Int.* 2014;86(2):294–302.
104. Shoham DA, Durazo-Arvizu R, Kramer H, Luke A, Vupputuri S, Kshirsagar A et al. Sugary soda consumption and albuminuria: Results from the National Health and Nutrition Examination Survey, 1999–2004. *PLoS One.* 2008;3(10):e3431.
105. Bomback AS, Derebail VK, Shoham DA, Anderson CA, Steffen LM, Rosamond WD et al. Sugar-sweetened soda consumption, hyperuricemia, and kidney disease. *Kidney Int.* 2010;77(7):609–16. Epub 2009/12/25.
106. Bomback AS, Katz R, He K, Shoham DA, Burke GL, Klemmer PJ. Sugar-sweetened beverage consumption and the progression of chronic kidney disease in the Multi-Ethnic Study of Atherosclerosis (MESA). *Am J Clin Nutr.* 2009;90(5):1172–8. Epub 2009/09/11.
107. Taylor EN, Curhan GC. Fructose consumption and the risk of kidney stones. *Kidney Int.* 2008;73(2):207–12. Epub 2007/10/12.
108. Taylor EN, Curhan GC. Determinants of 24-hour urinary oxalate excretion. *Clin J Am Soc Nephrol.* 2008;3(5):1453–60. Epub 2008/07/25.

21 Effect of Sugars on Markers of Cardiometabolic Disease

An Overview of Meta-Analyses

Viranda H. Jayalath, Vanessa Ha, Effie Viguiliouk, Vivian L. Choo, Adrian I. Cozma, Russell J. de Souza, and John L. Sievenpiper

CONTENTS

KEY POINTS

- Recent research has implicated fructose and fructose-containing sugars in the development of obesity, type 2 diabetes mellitus, and cardiovascular disease.
- Evidence supporting these adverse links originate primarily from animal models of fructose overfeeding, cross-sectional and ecological analyses, and some short-term human studies of fructose feeding at high-fructose doses
- High-quality evidence from randomized controlled trials, prospective cohorts, and systematic reviews and meta-analyses of these studies currently do not support any adverse relation of sugars with cardiometabolic markers of chronic disease, when fructose and fructose-containing sugars are compared to other carbohydrates under calorically matched conditions.

INTRODUCTION

Over the last 50 years, global sugar consumption patterns have increased in parallel with the increase in refined grain and sugar-sweetened beverage (SSB) products [1,2]. As reviewed in other chapters, added sugars—primarily sucrose and high-fructose corn syrup (HFCS)—have long been implicated in metabolic and cardiovascular disorders [3]. Recent attention has focused on the fructose moiety of sugars, buttressing a potential fructose-mediated role in exacerbating cardiometabolic risk factors including body weight, glycemic control, blood pressure, blood lipids, and hepatic function [2,4,5]. The effects of chronic, fructose-containing sugar consumption have even been likened to those of chronic alcoholism [5]. Likewise, several public health initiatives directed toward limiting sugar intake have been proposed, including taxing SSBs [6], SSB serving size restrictions in New York City [7], front-of-package warning labels similar to that on cigarette packages [8], and the use of a fructose index (similar to the glycemic index) to predict fructose-mediated cardiovascular disease (CVD) risk [9].

Despite the widespread health concerns regarding consumption of dietary sugars, fructose, in particular (as reviewed in other chapters), this chapter aims to discuss the limited high-quality meta-evidence supporting a specific role of fructose in this context. Ecological analyses and animal models of fructose overfeeding (>60% total energy, above twice the 95th percentile of fructose intake in humans) chiefly support fructose as a contributor to aggravating cardiometabolic parameters [2,4,10]. Ecological analyses have limited credibility beyond hypothesis generation due to the use of availability data and numerous unadjusted potential confounders. Animal models and human studies of fructose overfeeding are valuable for identifying biological plausibility (as outlined in other chapters) and act as useful disease models for pharmacological interventions. However, extrapolation of animal model conclusions to humans is limited owing to differences in comparative physiology and supraphysiological dosing. In addition, these lines of evidence neglect the dietary context—characterized by unhealthy diet and lifestyle choices—in which fructose-containing sugars are generally consumed: a context more associated with cardiometabolic diseases than fructose-containing sugars alone [11,12]. Both lines of evidence, alongside cross-sectional analyses, are considered lower-quality evidence by dietary guidelines and policy-makers.

Prospective cohort studies and randomized controlled trials, and systematic reviews and meta-analyses of each, constitute the highest level of evidence used to formulate dietary guidelines and public policy. Several prospective cohort studies and many (>50) controlled feeding trials have investigated the link between sugars and cardiometabolic disease risk factors (see Chapter 16). The interpretation of these levels of evidence has important design considerations. A distinction must be made between the three major feeding trial designs: isocaloric, hypercaloric, and hypocaloric. In isocaloric trials, fructose-containing sugars are compared with other sources of carbohydrate under calorically matched conditions (energy-matched comparisons), allowing the effect of the fructose-containing sugar to be isolated from that of energy. On the other hand, in hypercaloric and hypocaloric trials, calories from fructose-containing sugars are either added to or subtracted from background diets and compared with the background diets alone (energy-unmatched comparisons). Likewise, for prospective cohorts, a critical distinction must be made between energy-adjusted and energy-unadjusted models.

This chapter will critically review, chiefly through the use of high-quality systematic reviews and meta-analyses, the current clinical and epidemiological literature assessing the relationship between fructose-containing sugars and body weight, glycemic control, uric acid, blood pressure, blood lipids, hepatic function, and overall CVD risk.

SUGARS IN DIETARY GUIDELINES

Dietary modification of risk factors is the cornerstone of prevention of the five diet-related chronic diseases identified by the 2010 Dietary Guidelines for Americans, including CVD, hypertension, diabetes, cancer, and osteoporosis [13]. Although fructose has been related to the first four diseases, recommendations regarding acceptable levels of intake vary across major health organizations, focusing primarily on restricting consumption for managing serum lipids (Table 21.1). Only a few guidelines address the levels of acceptable fructose intake: 2013 American Diabetes Association (ADA) [14,15], 2004 European Association for the study of Diabetes (EASD) [16], 2013 Canadian Diabetes Association (CDA) [17], and the 2011 American Heart Association (AHA) [18].

TABLE 21.1
Recommended Dietary Modifications by Current Practice Guidelines

Guideline[a]	Macronutrient[b] (CHO:PRO:FAT % E)	Carbohydrate Quality	Fat Quality	Fibre	Cholesterol	Added Sugars	Fructose
General Medicine							
WHO/FAO 2003	55–75% CHO: 10–15% PRO: 15–30% FAT	Unrefined carbohydrates	SFA: <10% E TFA: <1% E PUFA: 6–10% E n-6 PUFA: 5–8% E n-3 PUFA: 1–2% E MUFA: by difference	>25 grams per day	<300 mg per day	<10% E	—
USDA 2010	45–65% CHO: 10–35% PRO: 20–35% FAT	Whole grains	SFA: <10% E TFA: minimize Replace SFA with MUFA/PUFA Minimize SFA/TFA	Males: 38 grams per day Females: 25 grams per day	<300 mg per day	Minimize	—
IOM	45–65% CHO: 10–35% PRO: 20–35% FAT	—	n-6 PUFA: 5–10%E n-3 PUFA: 0.6–1.2%E	Males: 30–38 grams per day Females: 21–25 grams per day	None recommended	<25% E	—
Overweight/Obesity							
AHA 2009	—			N/A		Women: <100 cal per day Men: <150 cal per day	N/A
Diabetes							
ADA 2008	≥130 grams per day CHO: 15–20% PRO	Whole grain foods, LGI	SFA: <7%E TFA: minimize Increase PUFA	14 grams per 1000 calories	<200 mg per day	Limit	Naturally occuring fructose, 3–4% energy
CDA 2013	45–60% CHO:15–20% PRO: <35% FAT	LGI	SFA: <7%E TFA: minimize PUFA: <10% E Replace SFA with MUFA, choose n-3 PUFA Often SFA and TFA: <10% E	25–50 grams per day	—	≤10% E	≤60 grams per day

continued

TABLE 21.1 (continued)
Recommended Dietary Modifications by Current Practice Guidelines

Guideline[a]	Macronutrient[b] (CHO:PRO:FAT % E)	Carbohydrate Quality	Fat Quality	Fibre	Cholesterol	Added Sugars	Fructose
EASD 2004	45–60% CHO: 10–20% PRO: <35% FAT	High fber, LGI	MUFA: <10–20%E PUFA: <10%E	40 grams per day	<300 mg per day	Diabetics: ≤50 grams per day normal: ≤10%E	—
Hypertension							
JNC7	Limit total fat intake	—	—	—	—	—	—
CHEP 2013	—	Increase whole grain	Limit SFA	Increase especially soluble fiber	Limit	≤5 Tablespoons per day	—
Dyslipidemia							
NCEP-ATP III	50–60% CHO: 15% PRO: 20–35% FAT	Increase complex CHO	SFA: <7% E PUFA: <10% E MUFA: <20% E	Total: 20–30 grams per day Soluble: 10–25grams per day	<200 mg per day	—	—
AHA 2011	TG 150–199 mg/dL: 50–60% CHO: 15% PRO: 25–35% FAT TG 200–499 mg/dL: 50–55% CHO: 15–20% PRO: 30–35% FAT TG ≥500 mg/dL: 45–50% CHO: 20% PRO: 30–35% FAT	—	SFA: <7% E; <5% E TF: avoid PUFA: 10–20% E MUFA: 10–20% E Omega –3: 0.5–1 grams per day; 1–2 grams per day	—	—	TG 150–199 mg/dL: <10% E TG 200–499 mg/dL: 5–10% E TG ≥500 mg/dL: <5% E	TG 150–199 mg/dL: <100g per day E TG 200–499 mg/dL: 5–100g per day TG ≥500 mg/dL: <50g per day
CCS 2012	—	—	SFA: <7% E Omega-3: 2–4 grams per day	Soluble fiber: 10 grams per day	<300 mg per day	Limit	—
Heart Health							
AHA 2006	25–35% FAT	—	SFA: <7 % E TF: <1 % E	High Fibre	<300 mg per day	Reduce	—

[a] AHA: American Heart Association; JNC7: Joint National Committee; CHEP: Canadian Hypertension Education Program; CCS: Canadian Cardiovascular Society; NCEP-ATP III: National Cholesterol Education Program- Adult Treatment Plan III; ADA: American Diabetes Association; CDA: Canadian Diabetes Association; EASD: European Association for the Study of Diabetes; WHO/FAO: World Health Organization/Food and Agricultural Organization; IOM: Institute of Medicine

[b] E: Energy, CHO: Carbohydrate, PRO: protein, SFA: Saturated Fatty Acid; TF: Trans Fat; MUFA: Monosaturated Fat Intake; PUFA: Polyunsaturated Fat Intake; TG: Triglycerides

Most dietary guidelines have instead focused on limiting total fructose-containing sugar consumption (Table 21.1). Guidelines for limiting total sugar consumption have addressed several factors of cardiometabolic risk, including glycemic control [14,16,17], management of serum lipids [18], weight control [13,14,16,19–21], and prevention of dental caries [21]. Despite these concerns, dose thresholds for fructose-containing sugars have been sparsely recommended: the CDA [17], AHA [18,20], and EASD guidelines [16] have proposed upper limits for fructose alone, while Joint World Health Organization (WHO)/Food and Agriculture Organization [21], and Canadian Hypertension Evaluation Program [22] have only recommended limiting total added sugars.

BODY WEIGHT AND OBESITY

A growing body of prospective cohort analyses has assessed the link between fructose consumption and body weight, with heterogeneous results. A WHO commissioned systematic review and meta-analysis synthesizing evidence from 16 cohorts of adults ($n = 289,614$) and 22 cohorts of children ($n = 29,219$) found no significant association between dietary sugar intake and change in body weight or other measures of adiposity [23]. A notable exception being SSB whose intake was significantly associated with markers of adiposity in adults, and overweight or obese children. These results are supported by a recent systematic review and meta-analysis assessing the relation between SSB consumption on body weight in 15 cohorts of children ($n = 25,745$) and seven cohorts of adults ($n = 174,252$) [24]. This study also reported a significant dose–response relationship: for each incremental increase in daily servings of SSBs consumed, an increase of 0.06 (95% CI: 0.02–0.10) unit in body mass index (BMI) and 0.22-kg (95% CI: 0.09–0.34 kg) body weight increases were observed in children and adults, respectively. Although these observational results provide a sound basis for concern, it is not possible to draw direct causal relationships between SSBs and body weight. SSB intake is only significantly related to changes in body weight under comparisons between extreme quantiles [23,24], at levels unreflective of added-sugar consumption patterns of the average American [1,25]. Individuals whose SSB consumption parallels these extreme intakes also tend to consume more energy, smoke more, and exercise less [26]. Moreover, a pooled analysis of three Harvard cohorts ($n = 120,877$) have demonstrated that body weight increases from one 12-oz SSB is similar to or less than other dietary contributors in which SSBs are collinear: unprocessed meat, French fries, processed meat, trans fat, boiled, baked, or mashed potatoes, and potato chips (Figure 21.1) [27]. Thus, one must be careful in ascribing too much culpability to SSBs. The weight gain associated with SSBs may be more related to an unhealthy dietary pattern for which SSBs are a marker, rather than the fructose-containing sugar itself.

High-quality evidence from randomized, controlled feeding trials further support these evidence. Consistently, findings suggest that weight gain appears to be driven by excess energy consumption, rather than any fructose-specific modality (Figure 21.2a). In a systematic review and meta-analysis of 37 randomized controlled feeding trials in 637 participants with a median fructose dose of 69.1-g/day (17% energy), isocaloric exchange of fructose was found to act no differently from other carbohydrates on body weight [28]. This effect persisted under positive, negative, or neutral energy balance conditions, as long as comparator diets were isocalorically matched with other carbohydrates. These findings in isocaloric trials have been replicated across other meta-analyses of fructose-containing sugars [23,29], suggesting that fructose does not act independently from its caloric contribution towards weight gain. Nevertheless, body weight increases are seen with fructose-containing sugars when baseline diets are supplemented with excess calories from fructose and compared to the baseline diet alone (Figure 21.2b) [23,28]. These hypercaloric trials have assessed fructose intake at extreme doses (>104 to 250 g/day, >18–97% energy) [23] unrepresentative of "real-world" dietary intakes [1]. Recently, considerable attention has focused on the weight-increasing potential of fructose-containing SSBs, the largest contributor of fructose in the North American diet [1]. A meta-regression analysis on five trials assessing the effects of SSBs reported a 0.2-kg proportional increase in body weight for every 20-oz. SSB consumed, over a 3–12-week period [30]. Similar trends are supported

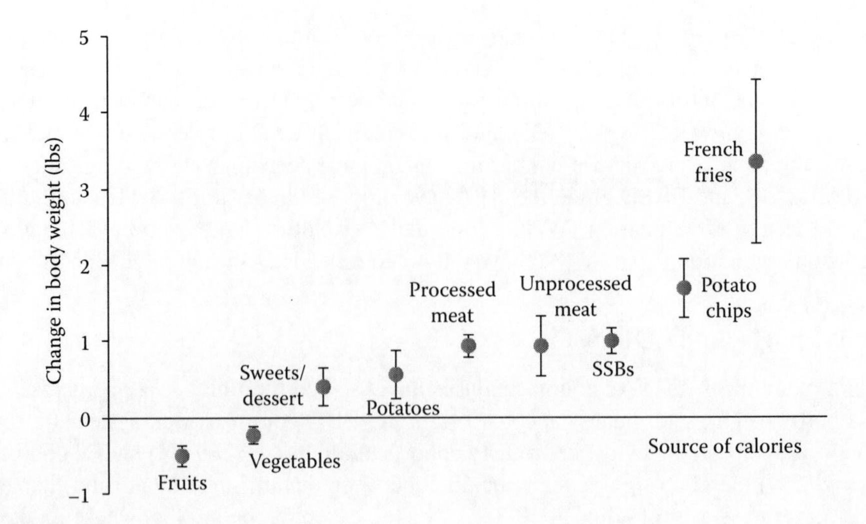

FIGURE 21.1 Relationship between increased dietary intakes and body weight change within a 4-year period: pooled data from 120,877 US men and women. Each red dot represented the multivariate-adjusted changes in body weight from increased dietary intake of specified food groups, and the vertical bars represent 95% confidence intervals. SSB: sugar-sweetened beverage. All relationships are $P \leq 0.001$. Adapted from Mozaffarian et al. [27].

by two recent meta-analyses of five and seven randomized controlled trials [24,31]. Despite the strong relationship between SSB-mediated energy supplementation trials and weight gain, its potential as an effective weight loss strategy is limited. In the same WHO commissioned meta-analysis, SSB-reduction interventions were successful in inducing weight loss in adults, but not children [23]. An updated systematic review of eight SSB-reduction trials also showed a non-significant effect on weight loss [31]. On the other hand, another recently published meta-analysis of five SSB-reduction trials in children showed a significant effect using fixed-effects models but not random effects models in the presence of significant heterogeneity [24,32]. One of the trials included in the two most recent meta-analyses [24,31] and another included in all three meta-analyses [23,24,31] examined 1- and 2-year postintervention follow-ups, respectively, to determine whether the weight loss seen during the intervention periods was sustainable [33,34]. Neither trial showed sustainable weight loss. Despite persistent reductions in SSB intake in the intervention group compared to the control group during the postintervention follow-up period in the one trial for which this information was available [33], there appeared to be a compensatory increase in the consumption of energy from other sources in the diet, leading to the observed lack of a body weight effect during the follow-up periods. Therefore, although SSB reduction may effectively reduce body weight in the short-term among some groups, the sustainability of this weight loss strategy over the long-term remains unclear.

Overall, isocaloric trials provide sound evidence that the body weight-modulating effects of fructose-containing sugars seen in hypercaloric and hypocaloric trials are mediated by its caloric contribution rather than properties inherent to fructose itself. However, in the absence of an alternative macronutrient comparator providing equal energy, disentangling the effects of sugary foods and beverages versus energy is complicated. Moreover, the relations between fructose-containing sugar intakes and dietary and lifestyle choices must not be overlooked.

GLYCEMIC CONTROL AND DIABETES

Since the late 1970s, a growing body of evidence has investigated fructose as an alternative sweetener for individuals with diabetes, largely owing to its low glycemic index [35] and early evidence of glycemic benefits from randomized trials [36].

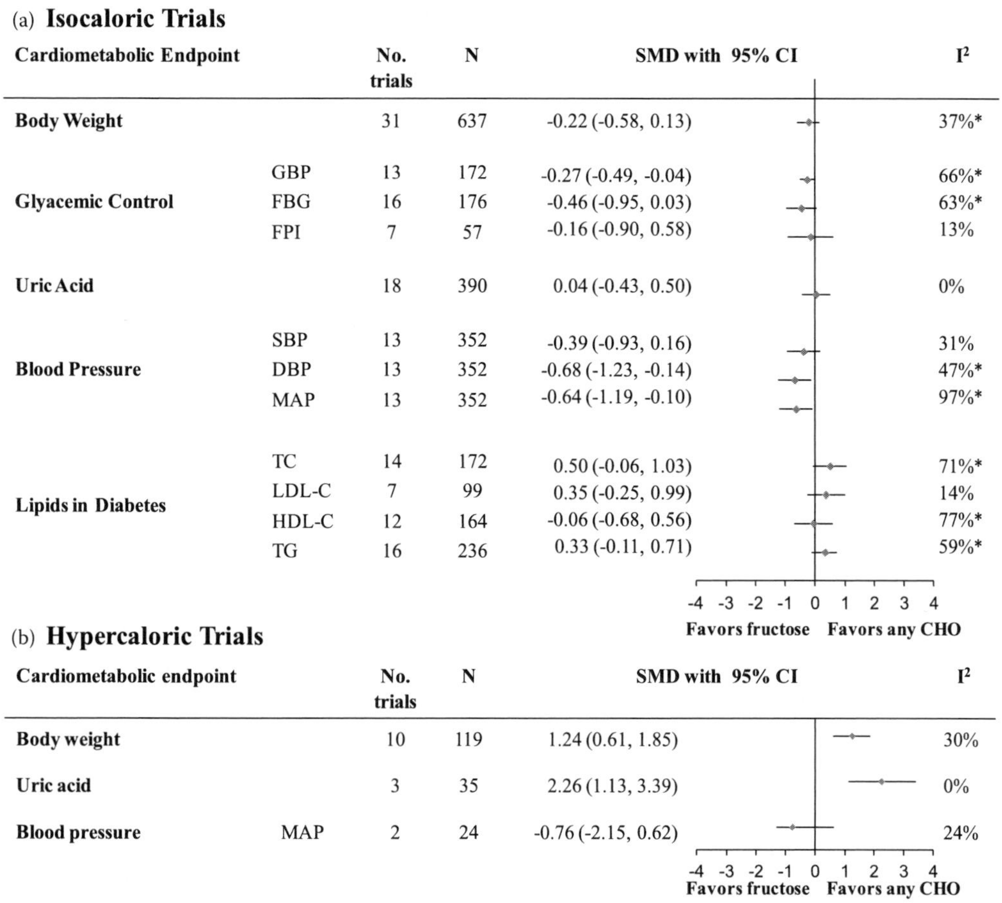

(a) **Isocaloric Trials**

Cardiometabolic Endpoint		No. trials	N	SMD with 95% CI	I²
Body Weight		31	637	-0.22 (-0.58, 0.13)	37%*
Glyacemic Control	GBP	13	172	-0.27 (-0.49, -0.04)	66%*
	FBG	16	176	-0.46 (-0.95, 0.03)	63%*
	FPI	7	57	-0.16 (-0.90, 0.58)	13%
Uric Acid		18	390	0.04 (-0.43, 0.50)	0%
Blood Pressure	SBP	13	352	-0.39 (-0.93, 0.16)	31%
	DBP	13	352	-0.68 (-1.23, -0.14)	47%*
	MAP	13	352	-0.64 (-1.19, -0.10)	97%*
Lipids in Diabetes	TC	14	172	0.50 (-0.06, 1.03)	71%*
	LDL-C	7	99	0.35 (-0.25, 0.99)	14%
	HDL-C	12	164	-0.06 (-0.68, 0.56)	77%*
	TG	16	236	0.33 (-0.11, 0.71)	59%*

-4 -3 -2 -1 0 1 2 3 4
Favors fructose Favors any CHO

(b) **Hypercaloric Trials**

Cardiometabolic endpoint		No. trials	N	SMD with 95% CI	I²
Body weight		10	119	1.24 (0.61, 1.85)	30%
Uric acid		3	35	2.26 (1.13, 3.39)	0%
Blood pressure	MAP	2	24	-0.76 (-2.15, 0.62)	24%

-4 -3 -2 -1 0 1 2 3 4
Favors fructose Favors any CHO

FIGURE 21.2 Forest plots of pooled effect estimates from a series of meta-analyses of controlled feeding trials of the effect of fructose on cardiometabolic biomarkers. In isocaloric trials (a), fructose was exchanged for other sources of carbohydrate; in hypercaloric trials (b), control diets were supplemented to provide excess energy from fructose and then compared with control diets alone. Summary estimates (diamonds) were derived from trial-level data that were pooled using generic inverse variance random-effects models. Each endpoint is represented as standardized mean differences (SMD) with pseudo-95% confidence intervals (CI). Asterisks indicate significant interstudy heterogeneity assessed by Cochran Q at a significance level of $P < 0.10$. TG: triglyceride; TC: total cholesterol; LDL-C: low-density-lipoprotein cholesterol; HDL-C: high-density-lipoprotein cholesterol; GBP: glycated blood protein; FBG: fasting blood glucose; FBI: fasting blood insulin; SBP: systolic blood pressure; DBP: diastolic blood pressure; MAP: mean arterial pressure. Adapted from Ha et al. [10].

Prospective cohort studies have found inconsistent associations between fructose-containing sugars and incident type 2 diabetes mellitus (T2DM). One cohort of 36,787 participants reported a significant protective association between total sugar intake and incident T2DM, a relationship partially explained by low-GI carbohydrates [37]. Conflicting results have been reported for individual sugars. Although one prospective cohort study found a significant diabetes risk reduction for sucrose [38], several cohorts have found no association with fructose or sucrose [37,39,40], and some have even found significant risk elevations with fructose [41,42]. In contrast, prospective cohorts assessing SSBs consistently suggest an increase in the risk of developing metabolic syndrome and T2DM. A systematic review and meta-analysis of 11 prospective cohorts in 310,819 participants found modest-yet-significant associations (pooled relative risk <1.30) between SSB intake and both incident T2DM and metabolic syndrome, when comparing the highest and lowest quantiles of SSB intake [43]. No relationship was observed, however, at levels of exposure equivalent at or below the 50th percentile for added sugar intake (49 g/day or 9.7% energy) in the USA [1]. These analyses were also complicated by evidence of significant unexplained inter-study heterogeneity. The heterogeneity may have partially related to the preferential inclusion of energy-unadjusted cohorts, combining both energy-adjusted and -unadjusted models in the meta-analysis. Although a meta-regression found no modification of association by adjusting for energy, this lack of adjustment significantly complicates interpretation of results. Additionally, adjustment for BMI, family history of diabetes, smoking, physical activity, and various other dietary factors associated with metabolic syndrome and diabetes varied among included cohorts. As high consumers of SSBs tend to have a Western dietary pattern, eat more calories, exercise less, and smoke more [13], incomplete correction for these potential confounders limit the interpretation of these results.

Conversely, controlled feeding trials support a beneficial effect of fructose on glycemic control (Figure 21.2a). Aside from fructose's low glycemic index, the glycemic benefits observed with fructose consumption may relate to a mechanism, whereby fructose upregulates glucokinase, increasing glycogen synthesis, decreasing hepatic glucogenesis, and improving the overall metabolic handling of glucose [44,45]. An earlier meta-regression analysis of eight trials reported a significant dose–response relationship in HbA1c reductions when fructose was exchanged isocalorically for other carbohydrates at doses below 100 g/day [39]. A more comprehensive systematic review and meta-analysis of 18 controlled feeding trials in 209 individuals with diabetes reported clinically meaningful HbA1c reductions approximating 0.53% when fructose was isocalorically exchanged for other carbohydrates at a median dose of 60 g/day [46]. Similar glycemic benefits have been observed with fruit sources of fructose in controlled feeding trials [47,48]. In a small systematic review and meta-analysis of six controlled feeding trials of 118 participants, catalytic fructose doses (22.5–36 g/day) at levels obtainable from fruits showed significant improvements in glycemic control, without adversely affecting other cardiometabolic parameters [49]. Other fructose-containing sugars and their corresponding effects on glycemic control are less consistent. With the exception of one small trial [50], the majority of controlled feeding trials assessing the effects of isocalorically exchanging sucrose (at intake up to 220 g/day or 44% energy) for other foods report harmful effects to glycemic parameters in people with and without diabetes [36,44,51–57]. Larger trials have failed to show consistent glycemic effects: neither the Carbohydrate Ratio Management in Europe National (CARMEN) diets nor the Pounds Lost trials reported any differences in glucose or insulin when comparing high versus low sugar intake interventions [58–60]. Even hypercaloric trials providing up to 9% of excess energy failed to show any adverse effects of sugars on glycemic control, in interventions up to 22 months [55,61,62].

Overall, these data indicate that fructose-containing sugars do not pose any harm for glycemic control and in fact fructose may even prove beneficial for individuals with diabetes [15]. Evidence from prospective cohorts investigating the associations between fructose-containing sugar intake and incident T2DM may be confounded by excess energy and poor lifestyle patterns and thus should be interpreted with caution.

URIC ACID AND HYPERURICEMIA

As outlined in detail in Chapters 19 and 20, fructose-induced increases in uric acid levels have been proposed as a driver of increased cardiometabolic disease risk through a nitric oxide-mediated mechanism [63]. The relationship between uric acid and fructose consumption has been evaluated by a few prospective analyses. No association was found between total fructose consumption from all dietary sources and incident hyperuricemia when comparing extreme levels of intake (≤6% vs. >11% energy) in a cohort of 9348 NHANES participants [64]. Two larger prospective analyses of total fructose intake reported significant increases in incident gout in both men and women, where men were at a considerably higher risk than women [65,66]. However, the lack of adjustment for meat intake in the male cohort and the loss of significance after adjustment for protein intake in females, both significant risk factors for gout [67], complicate the relationship between fructose intake and incident gout in these cohorts. Similar results are seen in prospective cohort analyses when comparing extreme quantiles of SSB intake [65,66,68]. A greater risk is again observed in men than women. In women, sugar-sweetened colas significantly increased gout risk, while other carbonated beverages with sugar did not [66]; it may be that these commonly consumed cola products are more representative of unhealthy dietary and lifestyle patterns and that this pattern may be contributing to the elevated gout risk more than the colas themselves [27,32,69].

High-quality controlled trials have failed to support these associations between fructose-containing sugars and uric acid, with effects seen only under excess energy conditions. In a systematic review and meta-analysis of 18 controlled feeding trials in 390 participants, fructose feeding (median dose = 94 g/day; range: 25–213 g/day; >95th percentile of intake) did not change uric acid levels when compared isocalorically to other carbohydrates (Figure 21.2a) [41]. Similar results yielded from an older meta-analysis with fructose doses <200 g/day [29]. Trials assessing the effect of sucrose on individuals with diabetes have also failed to show any aggravation of uric acid when compared to an isocaloric carbohydrate comparator [36,57]. Nevertheless, a systematic review and meta-analysis of three controlled feeding trials in 35 participants found a significant increase in serum uric acid when fructose provided excess calories (35% more calories, 215 g/day) than its comparator (Figure 21.2b).

Taken together, the results conclusively suggest uric acid-raising effects mediated by excess energy from fructose, and associations which may be confounded by poor lifestyle and dietary choices.

BLOOD PRESSURE AND HYPERTENSION

The relationship between fructose-containing sugar intake and blood pressure has been highly supported by animal and low-quality cross-sectional analyses [70] and is extensively reviewed in Chapter 20. A potential mechanism has been proposed wherein fructose depletes hepatic ATP and leads to downstream uric acid generation, subsequently generating oxidative stress in vascular smooth muscles, leading to endothelial dysfunction, and aggravating the renin–angiotensin pathway [70]. One trial that assessed the effects of allopurinol on lowering uric acid levels and metabolic syndrome features induced by extreme overfeeding with fructose (dose: 200 g/day or >2-fold the 95th-percentile for intake in the USA [1], providing 800 excess calories to the diet) has been repeatedly used to support this mechanism in humans [71]. Interpretation of this trial is complicated by the lack of a control group providing an equivalent amount of excess calories (800 kcal) from another macronutrient for comparison with the fructose group. In the absence of an isocaloric control group, it is impossible to conclude that any other form of carbohydrate similarly overfed would not result in the same increase in uric acid and subsequent rescue by allopurinol.

Higher-quality evidence from large-scale prospective cohort analyses and systematic reviews and meta-analyses of controlled feeding trials using appropriate control groups do not support this link. Prospective cohort analyses of the Nurses Healthy Study I and II (NHS-I and NHS-II) and the Health Professionals Follow-up Study (HPFS) reported no association between total fructose intake from all sources and incident hypertension, comparing the lowest to the highest levels of intake (≤6% to >14.3% energy) [72]. A small but significant protective association was even observed in NHS-I and HPFS, at the third quintile of intake (~9.5% energy, or ~50th percentile intake). This protective association may be related to fructose-containing sugar sources, as fruits, vegetables, and whole grains constituted a greater-than-average proportion of the diets among individuals in these cohorts [1,72], potentially conferring BP-protective effects [48,73]. Prospective cohort analyses of SSB intake relates differently to incident hypertension. The Coronary Artery Risk Development in Young Adults cohort, NHS-I, and NHS-II all showed modest-yet-significant increases in the risk of developing hypertension when comparing extreme quantiles of SSB intake, even after adjusting for fructose intake [26,74]. No association was observed in men (HPFS) [26]. In the absence of an association with total fructose, it is unclear how SSBs may exacerbate the risk of hypertension. A secondary analysis relating fructose from SSBs versus non-SSB sources found a significant risk elevation with SSB sources, but not with non-SSB sources [26]. A significant trend for risk reduction was even observed for fructose from non-SSB sources and incident hypertension in NHS-II [26]. Moreover, artificially sweetened beverages have been found to be significantly associated to the same degree with incident hypertension in NHS-I, NHS-II, and HPFS [26,75]. These epidemiological data suggest an SSB-hypertension axis independent of the fructose moiety of sugar. The elevated hypertension risk may relate to the lower satiety potential of SSBs, leading to increased energy intake, weight gain, and aggravation of cardiometabolic risk factors [26]. The risk may also relate to the collinearity that exists between SSBs and other aspects of an unhealthy lifestyle. High consumers of SSBs tend to consume more energy, smoke more, and exercise less [72]. High intakes of SSBs also correlate with high intakes of sweets and desserts, French fries, refined grains, and processed and red meats, each of which are independently related to weight gain [27] (Figure 21.1), and risk of T2DM [32,69,76]. These foods together characterize Western dietary patterns, which are more associated with cardiometabolic diseases than SSBs alone, even after adjusting for SSBs [11,12,76].

The lack of a BP-raising effect of fructose-containing sugars is supported by controlled feeding trials (Figure 21.2a). The effects of fructose on BP were found to be no different from other carbohydrates in a recent systematic review and meta-analysis of 13 isocaloric trials ($n = 352$) with a median fructose doses of 78.5 g/day (~90th percentile of intake) [77]. Significant reductions in diastolic BP and mean arterial BP were even observed in isocaloric trials. In two meta-analyzed hypercaloric trials ($n = 24$), however, a median fructose dose of 143 g/day (proving 18–25% excess energy than comparator) was found to significantly increase BP (Figure 21.2b), suggesting a mechanism mediated by excess energy [77]. Similar BP effects have been observed with other fructose-containing sugars. In the Pounds Lost trial, 811 adults were randomly assigned to four energy-matched weight loss diets emphasizing different macronutrients and found no difference in BP reductions under high and low carbohydrate conditions [59]. The effects of sucrose or sucrose-containing beverages on BP have been investigated in several additional trials, with mostly similar conclusions [44,51,78,79]. A few discrepancies do exist, however. One 6-month trial of 46 overweight individuals with metabolic syndrome reported a reduction in systolic blood pressure (SBP) with a low-fat, high-simple carbohydrate diet, compared to an energy matched low-fat, high-complex carbohydrate diet [78]. In contrast, another 6-month trial of 47 overweight individuals found a significant SBP-increasing effect with regular consumption of SSB compared to isocaloric semi-skim milk [80]. The interpretation of this result is complicated, however, as the study reported a significant change-from-baseline BP reduction for semiskim milk: a well-established relationship [73,81]; and no effect on change-from-baseline BP for SSBs. Thus, it is difficult to determine whether the observed effects were due to harmful effects of SSBs or beneficial effects of semiskim milk. Within the same trial and the Choose Healthy Options Consciously Everyday (CHOICE) trial, reducing calories from SSBs and replacing them with noncaloric beverages tended to decrease BP [80,82]. However, due to the relationship between calorie restriction, weight loss, and consequent BP reductions [59,83], disentangling the BP-lowering effect of a decrease in SSBs from that of a decrease in energy is difficult.

Taken together, the relationship between fructose-containing sugars and increases in BP and incident hypertension is tenuous. Increases appear to be mediated more by excess caloric intake and/or an unhealthy dietary pattern, rather than the sugars themselves.

BLOOD LIPIDS AND DYSLIPIDEMIA

Dietary guidelines recommend limiting fructose consumption due to its propensity to aggravate blood lipids [14,16–18] as reviewed in Chapter 19. Nevertheless, potential adverse effects on lipid profiles with fructose intake are only seen in controlled feeding trials at supraphysiological doses (>95th percentile of intake) and/or under hypercaloric feeding conditions (Figure 21.2a). A systematic review and meta-analysis of 16 controlled fructose feeding trials in 236 individuals with T2DM found no effect of fructose when isocalorically exchanged for other carbohydrates on fasting triglycerides (TG), LDL-C, HDL-C, and total cholesterol (TC) in overall analyses, but a significant TG-raising effect was observed at doses beyond >60 g/day in subgroup analyses [84]. Similarly, dose thresholds of >100 and >50 g/day were reported for fasting and postprandial TG, respectively, in a previous meta-analysis of 60 isocaloric trials in individuals with and without diabetes [85]. All of these thresholds exceed the current 50th percentile of fructose intake of Americans (49 g/day or 9.7% energy) [1]. On the other hand, intakes below 60 g/day have consistently shown no adverse effects on lipids [47,49,84]. The lack of any lipid-aggravating effects may relate to the inability of moderate fructose doses (<60 g/day) to stimulate hepatic de novo lipogenesis. Further analyses are necessary to better understand the implications of the TG-aggravating effects of high doses of fructose, and its relation to cardiometabolic disease risk. Unlike fructose, isocaloric exchange of sucrose does not appear to raise lipid parameters, irrespective of dose. With few exceptions [50,78], no significant differences in blood lipids were observed in trials where sucrose was isocalorically exchanged for other sources of energy up to 220 g/day, and for up to 22-month interventions, in individuals with and without diabetes [53–56,86–88]. SSBs, unlike sucrose, may confer TG-raising effects under isocaloric conditions under some limited circumstances. In a 6-month intervention trial, large intakes of SSBs (107 g/day sucrose) in isocaloric exchange for milk significantly increased TG [80].

A lack of effect has also been seen in ad libitum trials in which sugars are freely replaced with other carbohydrates. The CARMEN trial, a large-scale, well-powered controlled feeding trial of 316 participants found no change in blood lipids when comparing ad libitum high-sugar and high-complex carbohydrate diets, over 6 months [60].

In contrast with these results, lipid changes have been consistently reported in hypercaloric trials, in which fructose-containing sugars supplemented a diet with excess energy at high doses compared with the same diets where low-calorie sweeteners have replaced the sugars or the same diets alone (without the excess energy), and hypocaloric trials, in which the energy from existing sugars in the diet have been displaced by low-calorie sweeteners compared with the original diet containing the sugars. In one hypercaloric trial, diets supplemented with excess energy from large intakes of SSBs (107 g/day sucrose) significantly increased TG, compared with diets in which the energy from SSBs was displaced by low-calorie sweetened beverages or water over 6 months [80]. The reverse was seen in two other hypocaloric trials. Displacement of energy from sucrose using a low-calorie sweetener resulted in lower TG in both healthy [56] and hyperlipidemic participants [89].

Overall, fructose-containing sugars tend to have a TG-raising effect when consumed in excess in isocaloric trials. Moderate levels of consumption, however, do not seem to affect lipid parameters adversely under these same trial conditions. In the absence of an adequate macronutrient comparator supplementing or displacing the same amount of excess energy in the hypercaloric trials, it is difficult to exclude excess energy and extreme doses as the main culprit in mediating any adverse lipid effects of sugars.

LIVER HEALTH AND NONALCOHOLIC FATTY LIVER DISEASE

The relationship between fructose-containing sugar intake and nonalcoholic fatty liver disease (NAFLD) has recently received considerable attention from the scientific community. However, no prospective cohorts evaluating the association between fructose-containing sugar intake and incident NAFLD currently exist. Only lower-quality cross-sectional and retrospective studies have been reported, most of which support a positive association between fructose-containing sugars and NAFLD risk [90–92]. However, these same types of studies have also found positive associations with numerous factors which are equal or better predictors of the risk of developing NAFLD. These include increased caloric intake, total fat, total carbohydrate, animal protein, cholesterol, the n-6:n-3 polyunsaturated fatty acid ratios, and decreased dietary fiber intakes [93]. In the absence of high-quality prospective cohort studies, the reliability of these observational analyses in assessing the relationship between fructose-containing sugars and NAFLD risk is questionable.

A small number of controlled feeding trials have studied the effect of fructose on biomarkers of NAFLD. Short-term, isocaloric trials exchanging fructose for other carbohydrate sources have failed to show a harmful effect on liver biomarkers [94–96]. Conversely, hypercaloric feeding trials of fructose-sweetened beverages which supplemented background diets with 21–35% excess energy (104–220 g/day) reported elevations in both alanine aminotransferase (ALT) and intrahepatocellular lipids (IHCLs), markers of NAFLD [94,96–99]. Thus, the role of excess energy may play an important role in mediating the effects of fructose on NAFLD. Similar results have been reported for sucrose consumption. A 6-month randomized intervention in 46 participants found increases in IHCL when diets were hypercalorically supplemented with excess energy from 1-L/day of SSBs (430 calories, approximately 22% energy) in comparison to diets in which the energy from SSBs was displaced by low-calorie sweetened beverages or water. The same was true even where the SSBs were isocalorically substituted for milk [80]. Further research is necessary to determine whether SSBs will raise IHCL when isocalorically substituted for other drinks at levels representative of average US intakes.

These data suggest a signal for harm when fructose-containing sugars contribute excess energy to habitual diets or are substituted for milk, but not starch. Due to the scarcity of the available evidence, it is premature to draw conclusions regarding the effects of fructose-containing sugars on the risk of NAFLD.

CARDIOVASCULAR DISEASE

In the absence of large randomized trials assessing the effect of fructose-containing sugars on cardiovascular events, prospective cohort studies have failed to implicate fructose-containing sugars in the development of CVD. One cohort of 75,521 US women over a 10-year follow-up found no increase in CVD risk with sucrose or fructose intake comparing extreme quantiles of intake [100]. Similarly, another cohort examining total sugar intake in elderly Dutch males also reported no association with incident CVD [101]. Most prospective analyses have focused on SSBs and its relation with the incident CVD, with conflicting findings. A prospective analysis of 88,250 women in the NHS reported significant increases in the risk of developing coronary heart disease comparing the highest to the lowest level of SSB intake [102]. However, this analysis was not adjusted for total caloric intake, thus complicating the interpretation of these results. The relationship between SSB consumption and incidence of stroke is unclear. Prospective analyses of US women (n = 84,085), but not men (n = 43,371), reported significant increases in stroke risk when comparing the highest to the lowest quantiles of SSB intake [103]. Likewise, a Japanese cohort of 39,786 individuals analyzed over18 years found modest increases in the risk of ischemic stroke in women but not in men, when comparing the highest to the lowest quantiles of SSB intake [104]. The sex difference may be explained by differences in handling of carbohydrate quality. A recent systematic review and meta-analysis of 12 prospective cohorts found high-GI diets to be associated with increased risk for CVD in women, but not men [105]. Likewise, high SSB intakes may lower HDL-C and simultaneously increase triglycerides in women more than in men [106]. In addition, the associations are modest (relative risk <1.4), and no relationship exists at moderate intakes which are equivalent to the 50th percentile for intakes of added sugars in the USA [1].

The ability to draw conclusions regarding the relation of fructose-containing sugars with CVD risk is limited. The lack of an association with total sucrose or fructose, the differences in the associations for men and women, and the potential confounding of SSB analyses by unhealthy dietary and lifestyle factors remain important complicating factors.

CONCLUSIONS

Health concerns relating the consumption of fructose-containing sugars to cardiometabolic disease risk are chiefly founded in low-level evidence from animal models and ecological and cross-sectional studies. High-quality evidence from prospective cohorts and controlled feeding trials do not support these concerns. Prospective cohorts have not shown a significant relationship between sugars and weight gain, T2DM, hypertension, or CVD. The only reproducible disease risk elevating associations were reported with SSB intake, although these relations were not present at moderate levels of intake (~50th percentile of US intake). Moreover, these associations are highly subject to cofounding by other unhealthy dietary and lifestyle factors characteristic of a Western dietary pattern, which relates better with cardiometabolic risk than SSBs alone, even after adjustment for SSBs. Randomized controlled feeding trials are subject to the least confounding and are considered the highest level of evidence to inform public health policy and clinical practice guidelines. High-quality systematic reviews and meta-analyses of randomized controlled trials have found no adverse effects on measures of body weight, glycemic control, uric acid, blood pressure, blood lipids, and markers of NAFLD when representative doses of fructose-containing sugars are exchanged isocalorically for other sources of carbohydrate energy. Nevertheless, harmful effects on markers of cardiometabolic risk are observed when fructose-containing sugars are provided hypercalorically, or at supraphysiological doses, although not necessarily any more so than other sources of carbohydrate overfed at similar levels.

Additional high-quality studies are needed to assess the effect of fructose-containing sugars and the products sweetened with these sugars when freely replacing other sources of energy at "real-world" levels of exposure. In the absence of high-quality evidence supporting a unique link between fructose-containing sugars and markers of cardiometabolic diseases, the reduction of cardiometabolic disease risk should focus on modifying lifestyle factors and managing general overconsumption of highly palatable, energy-dense, nutrient-poor foods, including those high in refined carbohydrates and sugars.

CONFLICTS OF INTEREST

Vanessa Ha was funded by an Ontario Graduate Scholarship (OGS) and has received research support from the Canadian Institutes of Health Research (CIHR) and the World Health Organization (WHO) for work on a systematic review and meta-analysis of the relation of saturated fatty acids with health outcomes. She also received a travel award to attend the "Journey Through Science Day" hosted by PepsiCo and the New York Academy of Sciences (NYAS). Vivian Choo was funded by a 2013 summer Student Scholarship from the Canadian Sugar Institute (CSI). Adrian Cozma was funded by an OGS, CIHR Fredrick Banting and Charles Best Canada Graduate Scholarship, and Banting and Best Diabetes Centre (BBDC)-Novo Nordisk Studentship. He also received a travel award to attend the "Journey Through Science Day" hosted by PepsiCo and the NYAS. Russell J. de Souza has received research support from the CIHR, Calorie Control Council, Canadian Foundation for Dietetic Research (CFDR), and The Coca-Cola Company (investigator initiated, unrestricted). He has served as an external resource person to the WHO Nutrition Guidelines Advisory Group (NUGAG) and was the lead author of a systematic review and meta-analysis commissioned by the WHO of trans-fatty acids and health outcomes. The WHO paid for his travel and accommodation to attend NUGAG Meetings in Hangzhou, China, and Copenhagen, Denmark. John L. Sievenpiper has received research support from the CIHR, Calorie Control Council, The Coca-Cola Company (investigator initiated, unrestricted), Dr. Pepper Snapple Group (investigator initiated, unrestricted), Pulse Canada, and The International Tree Nut Council Nutrition Research & Education Foundation. He has received travel funding, speaker fees, and/or honoraria from the American Heart Association (AHA), American College of Physicians (ACP), American Society for Nutrition (ASN), National Institute of Diabetes and Digestive and Kidney Diseases (NIDDK) of the National Institutes of Health (NIH), Canadian Diabetes Association (CDA), Canadian Nutrition

Society (CNS), University of South Carolina, University of Alabama at Birmingham, Oldways Preservation Trust, Nutrition Foundation of Italy (NFI), Calorie Control Council, Diabetes and Nutrition Study Group (DNSG) of the European Association for the Study of Diabetes (EASD), International Life Sciences Institute (ILSI) North America, ILSI Brazil, Abbott Laboratories, Pulse Canada, CSI, Corn Refiners Association, World Sugar Research Organization, Dr. Pepper Snapple Group, and The Coca-Cola Company. He has consulting arrangements with Winston & Strawn LLP, Perkins Coie LLP, and Tate & Lyle. He is on the Clinical Practice Guidelines Expert Committee for Nutrition Therapy of both the Canadian Diabetes Association (CDA) and European Association for the study of Diabetes (EASD), as well as being on an ASN writing panel for a scientific statement on the metabolic and nutritional effects of fructose, sucrose, and HFCS. He is a member of the International Carbohydrate Quality Consortium (ICQC), an elected board member of the DNSG of the EASD, and an unpaid scientific advisor for the ILSI North America, Food, Nutrition, and Safety Program (FNSP). His wife is an employee of Unilever Canada. Viranda Jayalath and Effie Viguiliouk have no conflicts of interest to declare.

REFERENCES

1. Marriott BP, Cole N, Lee E. National estimates of dietary fructose intake increased from 1977 to 2004 in the United States. *J Nutr*. 2009;139(6):1228S–35S. Epub 2009/05/01.
2. Bray GA, Nielsen SJ, Popkin BM. Consumption of high-fructose corn syrup in beverages may play a role in the epidemic of obesity. *Am J Clin Nutr*. 2004;79(4):537–43. Epub 2004/03/31.
3. Yudkin J. *Pure, White, and Deadly: How Sugar is Killing Us and What We Can Do to Stop It*. London: Davis-Poynter, 1972.
4. Johnson RJ, Segal MS, Sautin Y, Nakagawa T, Feig DI, Kang DH et al. Potential role of sugar (fructose) in the epidemic of hypertension, obesity and the metabolic syndrome, diabetes, kidney disease, and cardiovascular disease. *Am J Clin Nutr*. 2007;86(4):899–906. Epub 2007/10/09.
5. Lustig RH, Schmidt LA, Brindis CD. Public health: The toxic truth about sugar. *Nature*. 2012;482(7383):27–9. Epub 2012/02/03.
6. Brownell KD, Farley T, Willett WC, Popkin BM, Chaloupka FJ, Thompson JW et al. The public health and economic benefits of taxing sugar-sweetened beverages. *N Engl J Med*. 2009;361(16):1599–605. Epub 2009/09/18.
7. Grynbaum MM. Will soda restrictions help new york win the war on obesity? *BMJ*. 2012;345:e6768. Epub 2012/10/12.
8. Association OM. Ontario Medical Association. Ontario's doctors call for urgent action to combat obesity epidemic. Ontario; 2012. https://www.oma.org/Mediaroom/PressReleases/Pages/ActiontoCombatObesityEpidemic.aspx. Retrieved: August 18, 2013.
9. Segal MS, Gollub E, Johnson RJ. Is the fructose index more relevant with regards to cardiovascular disease than the glycemic index? *Eur J Nutr*. 2007;46(7):406–17. Epub 2007/09/04.
10. Ha V, Jayalath VH, Cozma AI, Mirrahimi A, de Souza RJ, Sievenpiper JL. Fructose-containing sugars, blood pressure, and cardiometabolic risk: A critical review. *Curr Hypertens Rep*. 2013;15(4):281–97. Epub 2013/06/25.
11. Schulze MB, Fung TT, Manson JE, Willett WC, Hu FB. Dietary patterns and changes in body weight in women. *Obesity (Silver Spring)*. 2006;14(8):1444–53. Epub 2006/09/22.
12. Schulze MB, Hoffmann K, Manson JE, Willett WC, Meigs JB, Weikert C et al. Dietary pattern, inflammation, and incidence of type 2 diabetes in women. *Am J Clin Nutr*. 2005;82(3):675–84; quiz 714–5. Epub 2005/09/13.
13. Services USDoAaUSDoHaH. *Dietary Guidelines for Americans*, 7th Edition. Washington, DC: U.S. Government Printing Office; 2010.
14. Executive summary: Standards of medical care in diabetes—2011. *Diabetes Care*. 2011;34(Suppl. 1):S4–10. Epub 2011/01/14.
15. Evert AB, Boucher JL, Cypress M, Dunbar SA, Franz MJ, Mayer-Davis EJ et al. Nutrition therapy recommendations for the management of adults with diabetes. *Diabetes Care*. 2013;36(11):3821–42. Epub 2013/10/11.
16. Mann JI, De Leeuw I, Hermansen K, Karamanos B, Karlstrom B, Katsilambros N et al. Evidence-based nutritional approaches to the treatment and prevention of diabetes mellitus. *Nutr Metab Cardiovasc Dis*. 2004;14(6):373–94. Epub 2005/04/28.

17. Dworatzek PDAK, Gougeon R, Husein N, Sievenpiper JL, Williams SL. Canadian Diabetes Association 2013 Clinical Practice Guidelines for the Prevention and Management of Diabetes in Canada: Nutrition Therapy. *Can J Diabetes*. 2013;37:S45–55.
18. Miller M, Stone NJ, Ballantyne C, Bittner V, Criqui MH, Ginsberg HN et al. Triglycerides and cardiovascular disease: A scientific statement from the American Heart Association. *Circulation*. 2011;123(20):2292–333. Epub 2011/04/20.
19. Lichtenstein AH, Appel LJ, Brands M, Carnethon M, Daniels S, Franch HA et al. Diet and lifestyle recommendations revision 2006: A scientific statement from the American Heart Association Nutrition Committee. *Circulation*. 2006;114(1):82–96. Epub 2006/06/21.
20. Johnson RK, Appel LJ, Brands M, Howard BV, Lefevre M, Lustig RH et al. Dietary sugars intake and cardiovascular health: A scientific statement from the American Heart Association. *Circulation*. 2009;120(11):1011–20. Epub 2009/08/26.
21. Diet, nutrition, and the prevention of chronic diseases. *World Health Organ Tech Rep Ser*. 2003;916:i–viii, 1–149, backcover. Epub 2003/05/29.
22. Hackam DG, Quinn RR, Ravani P, Rabi DM, Dasgupta K, Daskalopoulou SS et al. The 2013 Canadian Hypertension Education Program Recommendations for blood pressure measurement, diagnosis, assessment of risk, prevention, and treatment of hypertension. *Can J Cardiol*. 2013;29(5):528–42. Epub 2013/04/02.
23. Te Morenga L, Mallard S, Mann J. Dietary sugars and body weight: Systematic review and meta-analyses of randomised controlled trials and cohort studies. *BMJ*. 2013;346:e7492. Epub 2013/01/17.
24. Malik VS, Pan A, Willett WC, Hu FB. Sugar-sweetened beverages and weight gain in children and adults: A systematic review and meta-analysis. *Am J Clin Nutr*. 2013;98(4):1084–102. Epub 2013/08/24.
25. Welsh JA, Sharma AJ, Grellinger L, Vos MB. Consumption of added sugars is decreasing in the United States. *Am J Clin Nutr*. 2011;94(3):726–34. Epub 2011/07/15.
26. Cohen L, Curhan G, Forman J. Association of sweetened beverage intake with incident hypertension. *J Gen Intern Med*. 2012;27(9):1127–34. Epub 2012/04/28.
27. Mozaffarian D, Hao T, Rimm EB, Willett WC, Hu FB. Changes in diet and lifestyle and long-term weight gain in women and men. *N Engl J Med*. 2011;364(25):2392–404. Epub 2011/06/24.
28. Sievenpiper JL, de Souza RJ, Mirrahimi A, Yu ME, Carleton AJ, Beyene J et al. Effect of fructose on body weight in controlled feeding trials: A systematic review and meta-analysis. *Ann Intern Med*. 2012;156(4):291–304. Epub 2012/02/22.
29. Livesey G. Fructose ingestion: Dose-dependent responses in health research. *J Nutr*. 2009;139(6):1246S–52S. Epub 2009/04/24.
30. Mattes RD, Shikany JM, Kaiser KA, Allison DB. Nutritively sweetened beverage consumption and body weight: A systematic review and meta-analysis of randomized experiments. *Obes Rev*. 2011;12(5):346–65. Epub 2010/06/08.
31. Kaiser KA, Shikany JM, Keating KD, Allison DB. Will reducing sugar-sweetened beverage consumption reduce obesity? Evidence supporting conjecture is strong, but evidence when testing effect is weak. *Obes Rev*. 2013;14(8):620–33. Epub 2013/06/08.
32. Fung TT, Rimm EB, Spiegelman D, Rifai N, Tofler GH, Willett WC et al. Association between dietary patterns and plasma biomarkers of obesity and cardiovascular disease risk. *Am J Clin Nutr*. 2001;73(1):61–7. Epub 2000/12/22.
33. Ebbeling CB, Feldman HA, Chomitz VR, Antonelli TA, Gortmaker SL, Osganian SK et al. A randomized trial of sugar-sweetened beverages and adolescent body weight. *N Engl J Med*. 2012;367(15):1407–16. Epub 2012/09/25.
34. James J, Thomas P, Kerr D. Preventing childhood obesity: Two year follow-up results from the Christchurch Obesity Prevention Programme in Schools (CHOPPS). *BMJ*. 2007;335(7623):762. Epub 2007/10/10.
35. Jenkins DJ, Wolever TM, Taylor RH, Barker H, Fielden H, Baldwin JM et al. Glycemic index of foods: A physiological basis for carbohydrate exchange. *Am J Clin Nutr*. 1981;34(3):362–6. Epub 1981/03/01.
36. Bantle JP, Laine DC, Thomas JW. Metabolic effects of dietary fructose and sucrose in types I and II diabetic subjects. *JAMA*. 1986;256(23):3241–6. Epub 1986/12/19.
37. Hodge AM, English DR, O'Dea K, Giles GG. Glycemic index and dietary fiber and the risk of type 2 diabetes. *Diabetes Care*. 2004;27(11):2701–6. Epub 2004/10/27.
38. Meyer KA, Kushi LH, Jacobs Jr. DR, Slavin J, Sellers TA, Folsom AR. Carbohydrates, dietary fiber, and incident type 2 diabetes in older women. *Am J Clin Nutr*. 2000;71(4):921–30. Epub 2000/03/25.
39. Colditz GA, Manson JE, Stampfer MJ, Rosner B, Willett WC, Speizer FE. Diet and risk of clinical diabetes in women. *Am J Clin Nutr*. 1992;55(5):1018–23. Epub 1992/05/01.
40. Janket SJ, Manson JE, Sesso H, Buring JE, Liu S. A prospective study of sugar intake and risk of type 2 diabetes in women. *Diabetes Care*. 2003;26(4):1008–15. Epub 2003/03/29.

41. Wang DD, Sievenpiper JL, de Souza RJ, Chiavaroli L, Ha V, Cozma AI et al. The effects of fructose intake on serum uric acid vary among controlled dietary trials. *J Nutr*. 2012;142(5):916–23. Epub 2012/03/30.
42. Montonen J, Jarvinen R, Knekt P, Heliovaara M, Reunanen A. Consumption of sweetened beverages and intakes of fructose and glucose predict type 2 diabetes occurrence. *J Nutr*. 2007;137(6):1447–54. Epub 2007/05/22.
43. Malik VS, Popkin BM, Bray GA, Despres JP, Willett WC, Hu FB. Sugar-sweetened beverages and risk of metabolic syndrome and type 2 diabetes: A meta-analysis. *Diabetes Care*. 2010;33(11):2477–83. Epub 2010/08/10.
44. Peterson DB, Lambert J, Gerring S, Darling P, Carter RD, Jelfs R et al. Sucrose in the diet of diabetic patients—Just another carbohydrate? *Diabetologia*. 1986;29(4):216–20. Epub 1986/04/01.
45. Hawkins M, Gabriely I, Wozniak R, Vilcu C, Shamoon H, Rossetti L. Fructose improves the ability of hyperglycemia per se to regulate glucose production in type 2 diabetes. *Diabetes*. 2002;51(3):606–14. Epub 2002/03/02.
46. Cozma AI, Sievenpiper JL, de Souza RJ, Chiavaroli L, Ha V, Wang DD et al. Effect of fructose on glycemic control in diabetes: A systematic review and meta-analysis of controlled feeding trials. *Diabetes Care*. 2012;35(7):1611–20. Epub 2012/06/23.
47. Jenkins DJ, Srichaikul K, Kendall CW, Sievenpiper JL, Abdulnour S, Mirrahimi A et al. The relation of low glycaemic index fruit consumption to glycaemic control and risk factors for coronary heart disease in type 2 diabetes. *Diabetologia*. 2011;54(2):271–9. Epub 2010/10/28.
48. Madero M, Arriaga JC, Jalal D, Rivard C, McFann K, Perez-Mendez O et al. The effect of two energy-restricted diets, a low-fructose diet versus a moderate natural fructose diet, on weight loss and metabolic syndrome parameters: A randomized controlled trial. *Metabolism*. 2011;60(11):1551–9. Epub 2011/05/31.
49. Sievenpiper JL, Chiavaroli L, de Souza RJ, Mirrahimi A, Cozma AI, Ha V et al. 'Catalytic' doses of fructose may benefit glycaemic control without harming cardiometabolic risk factors: A small meta-analysis of randomised controlled feeding trials. *Br J Nutr*. 2012;108(3):418–23. Epub 2012/02/23.
50. Coulston AM, Hollenbeck CB, Donner CC, Williams R, Chiou YA, Reaven GM. Metabolic effects of added dietary sucrose in individuals with noninsulin-dependent diabetes mellitus (NIDDM). *Metabolism*. 1985;34(10):962–6. Epub 1985/10/01.
51. Claesson AL, Holm G, Ernersson A, Lindstrom T, Nystrom FH. Two weeks of overfeeding with candy, but not peanuts, increases insulin levels and body weight. *Scand J Clin Lab Invest*. 2009;69(5):598–605. Epub 2009/04/28.
52. Blayo AFA, Rizkalla S, Bruzzo F, Slama G. Metabolic effects of daily intake of sucrose or fructose by diabetics for one year. *Med Nutr*. 1990;26(1):11–4.
53. Cooper PL, Wahlqvist ML, Simpson RW. Sucrose versus saccharin as an added sweetener in non-insulin-dependent diabetes: Short- and medium-term metabolic effects. *Diabet Med*. 1988;5(7):676–80. Epub 1988/10/01.
54. Jellish WS, Emanuele MA, Abraira C. Graded sucrose/carbohydrate diets in overtly hypertriglyceridemic diabetic patients. *Am J Med*. 1984;77(6):1015–22. Epub 1984/12/01.
55. Huttunen JK, Makinen KK, Scheinin A. Turku sugar studies. XI. Effects of sucrose, fructose and xylitol diets on glucose, lipid and urate metabolism. *Acta Odontol Scand*. 1976;34(6):345–51. Epub 1976/01/01.
56. Mann JI, Hendricks DA, Truswell AS, Manning E. Effects on serum-lipids in normal men of reducing dietary sucrose or starch for five months. *Lancet*. 1970;1(7652):870–2. Epub 1970/04/25.
57. Malerbi DA, Paiva ES, Duarte AL, Wajchenberg BL. Metabolic effects of dietary sucrose and fructose in type II diabetic subjects. *Diabetes Care*. 1996;19(11):1249–56. Epub 1996/11/01.
58. de Souza RJ, Bray GA, Carey VJ, Hall KD, LeBoff MS, Loria CM et al. Effects of 4 weight-loss diets differing in fat, protein, and carbohydrate on fat mass, lean mass, visceral adipose tissue, and hepatic fat: Results from the Pounds Lost Trial. *Am J Clin Nutr*. 2012;95(3):614–25. Epub 2012/01/20.
59. Sacks FM, Bray GA, Carey VJ, Smith SR, Ryan DH, Anton SD et al. Comparison of weight-loss diets with different compositions of fat, protein, and carbohydrates. *N Engl J Med*. 2009;360(9):859–73. Epub 2009/02/28.
60. Saris WH, Astrup A, Prentice AM, Zunft HJ, Formiguera X, Verboeket-van de Venne WP et al. Randomized controlled trial of changes in dietary carbohydrate/fat ratio and simple vs complex carbohydrates on body weight and blood lipids: The Carmen Study. The carbohydrate ratio management in European national diets. *Int J Obes Relat Metab Disord*. 2000;24(10):1310–8. Epub 2000/11/28.
61. Colagiuri S, Miller JJ, Edwards RA. Metabolic effects of adding sucrose and aspartame to the diet of subjects with noninsulin-dependent diabetes mellitus. *Am J Clin Nutr*. 1989;50(3):474–8. Epub 1989/09/01.
62. Chantelau EA, Gosseringer G, Sonnenberg GE, Berger M. Moderate intake of sucrose does not impair metabolic control in pump-treated diabetic out-patients. *Diabetologia*. 1985;28(4):204–7. Epub 1985/04/01.

63. Johnson RJ, Perez-Pozo SE, Sautin YY, Manitius J, Sanchez-Lozada LG, Feig DI et al. Hypothesis: Could excessive fructose intake and uric acid cause type 2 diabetes? *Endocr Rev*. 2009;30(1):96–116. Epub 2009/01/20.
64. Sun SZ, Flickinger BD, Williamson-Hughes PS, Empie MW. Lack of association between dietary fructose and hyperuricemia risk in adults. *Nutr Metab (Lond)*. 2010;7:16. Epub 2010/03/03.
65. Choi HK, Curhan G. Soft drinks, fructose consumption, and the risk of gout in men: Prospective cohort study. *BMJ*. 2008;336(7639):309–12. Epub 2008/02/05.
66. Choi HK, Willett W, Curhan G. Fructose-rich beverages and risk of gout in women. *JAMA*. 2010;304(20):2270–8. Epub 2010/11/12.
67. Choi HK, Atkinson K, Karlson EW, Willett W, Curhan G. Purine-rich foods, dairy and protein intake, and the risk of gout in men. *N Engl J Med*. 2004;350(11):1093–103. Epub 2004/03/12.
68. Bomback AS, Derebail VK, Shoham DA, Anderson CA, Steffen LM, Rosamond WD et al. Sugar-sweetened soda consumption, hyperuricemia, and kidney disease. *Kidney Int*. 2010;77(7):609–16. Epub 2009/12/25.
69. Pan A, Sun Q, Bernstein AM, Schulze MB, Manson JE, Willett WC et al. Red meat consumption and risk of type 2 diabetes: 3 cohorts of US adults and an updated meta-analysis. *Am J Clin Nutr*. 2011;94(4):1088–96. Epub 2011/08/13.
70. Johnson RJ, Sanchez-Lozada LG, Nakagawa T. The effect of fructose on renal biology and disease. *J Am Soc Nephrol*. 2010;21(12):2036–9. Epub 2010/12/01.
71. Perez-Pozo SE, Schold J, Nakagawa T, Sanchez-Lozada LG, Johnson RJ, Lillo JL. Excessive fructose intake induces the features of metabolic syndrome in healthy adult men: Role of uric acid in the hypertensive response. *Int J Obes (Lond)*. 2010;34(3):454–61. Epub 2009/12/24.
72. Forman JP, Choi H, Curhan GC. Fructose and vitamin C intake do not influence risk for developing hypertension. *J Am Soc Nephrol*. 2009;20(4):863–71. Epub 2009/01/16.
73. Appel LJ, Moore TJ, Obarzanek E, Vollmer WM, Svetkey LP, Sacks FM et al. A clinical trial of the effects of dietary patterns on blood pressure. Dash Collaborative Research Group. *N Engl J Med*. 1997;336(16):1117–24. Epub 1997/04/17.
74. Duffey KJ, Gordon-Larsen P, Steffen LM, Jacobs Jr. DR, Popkin BM. Drinking caloric beverages increases the risk of adverse cardiometabolic outcomes in the coronary artery risk development in young adults (CARDIA) study. *Am J Clin Nutr*. 2010;92(4):954–9. Epub 2010/08/13.
75. Winkelmayer WC, Stampfer MJ, Willett WC, Curhan GC. Habitual caffeine intake and the risk of hypertension in women. *JAMA*. 2005;294(18):2330–5. Epub 2005/11/10.
76. Halton TL, Willett WC, Liu S, Manson JE, Stampfer MJ, Hu FB. Potato and french fry consumption and risk of type 2 diabetes in women. *Am J Clin Nutr*. 2006;83(2):284–90. Epub 2006/02/14.
77. Ha V, Sievenpiper JL, de Souza RJ, Chiavaroli L, Wang DD, Cozma AI et al. Effect of fructose on blood pressure: A systematic review and meta-analysis of controlled feeding trials. *Hypertension*. 2012;59(4):787–95. Epub 2012/02/15.
78. Poppitt SD, Keogh GF, Prentice AM, Williams DE, Sonnemans HM, Valk EE et al. Long-term effects of ad libitum low-fat, high-carbohydrate diets on body weight and serum lipids in overweight subjects with metabolic syndrome. *Am J Clin Nutr*. 2002;75(1):11–20. Epub 2002/01/05.
79. Raben A, Vasilaras TH, Moller AC, Astrup A. Sucrose compared with artificial sweeteners: Different effects on ad libitum food intake and body weight after 10 wk of supplementation in overweight subjects. *Am J Clin Nutr*. 2002;76(4):721–9. Epub 2002/09/27.
80. Maersk M, Belza A, Stodkilde-Jorgensen H, Ringgaard S, Chabanova E, Thomsen H et al. Sucrose-sweetened beverages increase fat storage in the liver, muscle, and visceral fat depot: A 6-Mo randomized intervention study. *Am J Clin Nutr*. 2012;95(2):283–9. Epub 2011/12/30.
81. Soedamah-Muthu SS, Ding EL, Al-Delaimy WK, Hu FB, Engberink MF, Willett WC et al. Milk and dairy consumption and incidence of cardiovascular diseases and all-cause mortality: Dose–response meta-analysis of prospective cohort studies. *Am J Clin Nutr*. 2011;93(1):158–71. Epub 2010/11/12.
82. Tate DF, Turner-McGrievy G, Lyons E, Stevens J, Erickson K, Polzien K et al. Replacing caloric beverages with water or diet beverages for weight loss in adults: Main results of the choose healthy options consciously everyday (choice) randomized clinical trial. *Am J Clin Nutr*. 2012;95(3):555–63. Epub 2012/02/04.
83. Dansinger ML, Gleason JA, Griffith JL, Selker HP, Schaefer EJ. Comparison of the atkins, ornish, weight watchers, and zone diets for weight loss and heart disease risk reduction: A randomized trial. *JAMA*. 2005;293(1):43–53. Epub 2005/01/06.
84. Sievenpiper JL, Carleton AJ, Chatha S, Jiang HY, de Souza RJ, Beyene J et al. Heterogeneous effects of fructose on blood lipids in individuals with type 2 diabetes: Systematic review and meta-analysis of experimental trials in humans. *Diabetes Care*. 2009;32(10):1930–7. Epub 2009/07/14.

85. Livesey G, Taylor R. Fructose consumption and consequences for glycation, plasma triacylglycerol, and body weight: Meta-analyses and meta-regression models of intervention studies. *Am J Clin Nutr.* 2008;88(5):1419–37. Epub 2008/11/11.
86. Roberts AM. Effects of a sucrose-free diet on the serum-lipid levels of men in Antarctica. *Lancet.* 1973;1(7814):1201–4. Epub 1973/06/02.
87. Kaufmann NA, Poznanski R, Blondheim SH, Stein Y. Effect of fructose, glucose, sucrose and starch on serum lipids in carbohydrate induced hypertriglyceridemia and in normal subjects. *Isr J Med Sci.* 1966;2(6):715–26. Epub 1966/11/01.
88. Nikkila EA, Kekki M. Effects of dietary fructose and sucrose on plasma triglyceride metabolism in patients with endogenous hypertriglyceridemia. *Acta Med Scand Suppl.* 1972;542:221–7. Epub 1972/01/01.
89. Smith JB, Niven BE, Mann JI. The effect of reduced extrinsic sucrose intake on plasma triglyceride levels. *Eur J Clin Nutr.* 1996;50(8):498–504. Epub 1996/08/01.
90. Ouyang X, Cirillo P, Sautin Y, McCall S, Bruchette JL, Diehl AM et al. Fructose consumption as a risk factor for non-alcoholic fatty liver disease. *J Hepatol.* 2008;48(6):993–9. Epub 2008/04/09.
91. Abdelmalek MF, Lazo M, Horska A, Bonekamp S, Lipkin EW, Balasubramanyam A et al. Higher dietary fructose is associated with impaired hepatic adenosine triphosphate homeostasis in obese individuals with type 2 diabetes. *Hepatology.* 2012;56(3):952–60. Epub 2012/04/03.
92. Abid A, Taha O, Nseir W, Farah R, Grosovski M, Assy N. Soft drink consumption is associated with fatty liver disease independent of metabolic syndrome. *J Hepatol.* 2009;51(5):918–24. Epub 2009/09/22.
93. Mouzaki M, Allard JP. The role of nutrients in the development, progression, and treatment of nonalcoholic fatty liver disease. *J Clin Gastroenterol.* 2012;46(6):457–67. Epub 2012/04/04.
94. Silbernagel G, Machann J, Unmuth S, Schick F, Stefan N, Haring HU et al. Effects of 4-week very-high-fructose/glucose diets on insulin sensitivity, visceral fat and intrahepatic lipids: An exploratory trial. *Br J Nutr.* 2011;106(1):79–86. Epub 2011/03/15.
95. Aeberli I, Gerber PA, Hochuli M, Kohler S, Haile SR, Gouni-Berthold I et al. Low to moderate sugar-sweetened beverage consumption impairs glucose and lipid metabolism and promotes inflammation in healthy young men: A randomized controlled trial. *Am J Clin Nutr.* 2011;94(2):479–85. Epub 2011/06/17.
96. Ngo Sock ET, Le KA, Ith M, Kreis R, Boesch C, Tappy L. Effects of a short-term overfeeding with fructose or glucose in healthy young males. *Br J Nutr.* 2010;103(7):939–43. Epub 2009/11/26.
97. Le KA, Faeh D, Stettler R, Ith M, Kreis R, Vermathen P et al. A 4-wk high-fructose diet alters lipid metabolism without affecting insulin sensitivity or ectopic lipids in healthy humans. *Am J Clin Nutr.* 2006;84(6):1374–9. Epub 2006/12/13.
98. Le KA, Ith M, Kreis R, Faeh D, Bortolotti M, Tran C et al. Fructose overconsumption causes dyslipidemia and ectopic lipid deposition in healthy subjects with and without a family history of type 2 diabetes. *Am J Clin Nutr.* 2009;89(6):1760–5. Epub 2009/05/01.
99. Sobrecases H, Le KA, Bortolotti M, Schneiter P, Ith M, Kreis R et al. Effects of short-term overfeeding with fructose, fat and fructose plus fat on plasma and hepatic lipids in healthy men. *Diabetes Metab.* 2010;36(3):244–6. Epub 2010/05/21.
100. Liu S, Willett WC, Stampfer MJ, Hu FB, Franz M, Sampson L et al. A prospective study of dietary glycemic load, carbohydrate intake, and risk of coronary heart disease in US women. *Am J Clin Nutr.* 2000;71(6):1455–61. Epub 2000/06/06.
101. van Dam RM, Visscher AW, Feskens EJ, Verhoef P, Kromhout D. Dietary glycemic index in relation to metabolic risk factors and incidence of coronary heart disease: The Zutphen Elderly Study. *Eur J Clin Nutr.* 2000;54(9):726–31. Epub 2000/09/26.
102. Fung TT, Malik V, Rexrode KM, Manson JE, Willett WC, Hu FB. Sweetened beverage consumption and risk of coronary heart disease in women. *Am J Clin Nutr.* 2009;89(4):1037–42. Epub 2009/02/13.
103. Bernstein AM, de Koning L, Flint AJ, Rexrode KM, Willett WC. Soda consumption and the risk of stroke in men and women. *Am J Clin Nutr.* 2012;95(5):1190–9. Epub 2012/04/12.
104. Eshak ES, Iso H, Kokubo Y, Saito I, Yamagishi K, Inoue M et al. Soft drink intake in relation to incident ischemic heart disease, stroke, and stroke subtypes in Japanese men and women: The Japan Public Health Centre-Based Study Cohort I. *Am J Clin Nutr.* 2012;96(6):1390–7. Epub 2012/10/19.
105. Mirrahimi A, de Souza RJ, Chiavaroli L, Sievenpiper JL, Beyene J, Hanley AJ et al. Associations of glycemic index and load with coronary heart disease events: A systematic review and meta-analysis of prospective cohorts. *J Am Heart Assoc.* 2012;1(5):e000752. Epub 2013/01/15.
106. Matthews KA, Meilahn E, Kuller LH, Kelsey SF, Caggiula AW, Wing RR. Menopause and risk factors for coronary heart disease. *N Engl J Med.* 1989;321(10):641–6. Epub 1989/09/07.

22 Mechanisms of Nonalcoholic Fatty Liver Disease Induced by Dietary Sugars

Methods of Investigation

Qiong Hu and Elizabeth J. Parks

CONTENTS

KEY POINTS

- The development and identification of biomarkers for liver disease will allow larger-scale population studies of the impact of dietary sugars on nonalcoholic fatty liver.
- For medium-size, metabolic studies (sample sizes up to thousands of subjects), imaging techniques have advanced sufficiently to provide reproducible, noninvasive results of liver fat and fibrosis.
- The biochemical pathway of de novo lipogenesis is significantly elevated in nonalcoholic fatty liver disease and can be measured using stable, nonradioactive isotope administration.
- Research developments in the measurement of lipogenesis and fatty acid flux have shown that the timing of isotope labeling will influence the results.
- Advances in the use of isotopes, in combination with PET and CT, provide much promise in allowing real-time, in vivo measurements of lipid flux.
- Additional method development will be needed to assess the key outcome of liver fatty acid oxidation in vivo in humans.

INTRODUCTION

As described in other chapters, the intake of fructose in the diet has risen steadily over the past 30 years, as has the incidence of obesity and diabetes in the USA. One comorbidity associated with obesity and diabetes is nonalcoholic fatty liver disease (NAFLD) and recent observational studies have suggested a connection between dietary intake of fructose and NAFLD in children [1,2] and adults [3–5]. Given the strong interest in the metabolic causes of NAFLD, development of clinical research methods in this field has been expanding rapidly. The present paper will review methods for assessing liver metabolism in humans, with special reference to research techniques that can be used to assess metabolic changes when fructose-containing foods are consumed. Other chapters in this volume have reviewed the basic biochemical and metabolic fates of fructose in animals and humans. Here, we will consider the most recently identified research biomarkers that can be used for the detection of liver injury in fructose studies. Described next are methods for imaging liver fat and fibrosis and for measuring liver function using nuclear magnetic resonance spectroscopy. Lastly, we will provide an in-depth review of the use of stable isotopes to measure liver fatty acid flux and fructose effects on the process of hepatic de novo lipogenesis. Data from animal studies provide multiple molecular and biochemical mechanisms by which overconsumption of fructose leads to liver dysfunction. For the translation of these findings to human studies, the methods described herein hold much promise to allow the effects of fructose metabolism to be measured directly, noninvasively, and in vivo.

CURRENT BIOMARKERS AND TESTS FOR DIAGNOSIS OF NAFLD

Studies on the impact of fructose on metabolism performed in human studies with large sample sizes require accurate surrogate markers of liver physiology. As a result, although liver biopsy is the gold standard test for evaluating the nature and severity liver diseases [6,7], serum biomarkers have become the focus of recent research because of their noninvasiveness (low risk), potential for high reproducibility, and low cost. As shown in Table 22.1, among the biomarkers that have been associated with NAFLD, alanine transaminase (ALT), aspartate transaminase (AST), and the AST to ALT ratio are the most routinely measured indicators used to assess and predict hepatocellular damage and disease [8–10]. Westerbacka et al. [11] observed modestly strong, yet highly significant correlations between ALT and liver fat measured by proton magnetic resonance spectroscopy (^{1}H-MRS) for women ($r = 0.49$, $P < 0.0001$) and men ($r = 0.62$, $P < 0.0001$). Further, a study by Omagari et al. [12] of 1578 Japanese adults showed that serum ALT concentration not only indicated fatty liver at baseline, but also predicted a natural regression of fatty liver in adults whose ALT concentrations fell over the 7–8-year period. However, both Mofrad et al. [13] and Sorrentino et al. [14] have pointed out that NAFLD patients with steatohepatitis and advanced fibrosis may present with normal ALT values, and it is also acknowledged that plasma ALT concentrations are increased by other conditions such as alcohol intake [15], viral [16] and autoimmune hepatitis [17], and hepatotoxic medication [18,19].

Plasma AST is considered less specific than ALT in detecting liver disease [20]. Although AST concentration has received relatively less attention as an independent biomarker of NAFLD, Kotronen et al. [10] found it to independently predict higher liver fat in a group of diabetic and nondiabetic subjects (Table 22.1), and Gholam et al. [21] found that AST, when combined with the presence of diabetes, predicted nonalcoholic steatohepatitis (NASH). Moreover, Kotronen et al. [10] found that a low AST/ALT ratio independently predicted NALFD. Another liver function test commonly used as a marker of excess alcohol intake [22], gamma-glutamyltranspeptidase (GGT), was found by Tahan et al. (Table 22.1) as a marker for advanced fibrosis in NAFLD [23]. The major intermediate filament protein in the liver, cytokeratin 18 (CK-18), was first identified by Wieckowska et al. [24] to be an independent predictor for NASH. As shown in Table 22.1, CK-18 has been used to assess fibrosis and independently predict the presence of NASH in a large clinical trial with 139 adult patients with biopsy-proven NAFLD and 150 age-matched healthy controls [25]. In addition, CK-18 has a high accuracy for diagnosing NASH in children with fatty liver disease [26]. CC-chemokine ligand 2 (CCL-2), also known as monocyte chemotactic protein-1 (MCP-1; Table 22.1) has been shown to be elevated during the conversion from steatosis to NASH [27]. Page et al. [28] have shown that CCL-2 and HDLc levels together in multiple linear regression predicted advanced fibrosis in a study of 37 NAFLD patients. They have also shown that soluble Fas ligand (sFasL) levels were significantly higher in patients with fibrosis, suggesting sFasL as a key biomarker in need of further investigation (Table 22.1). Lastly, Tanaka et al. [29] demonstrated

TABLE 22.1
Summary of Routinely Used Biomarkers of Liver Function and Disease

Biomarkers	References	Research Subjects	Comments
		Protein/Enzymes	
ALT [11–14]	Westerbacka et al. [11]	132 nondiabetic, apparently healthy subjects (66 male, 66 female)	Serum ALT was moderately associated with liver fat in both women ($r = 0.49$, $P < 0.0001$) and men ($r = 0.62$, $P < 0.0001$)
	Omagari et al. [12]	1578 Japanese adults (1208 men and 370 women)	Serum ALT not only indicated fatty liver, but also predicted the natural regression of fatty liver
	Mofrad et al. [13]	386 patients with steatosis or steatohepatitis	51 patients of NAFLD or steatohepatitis with normal ALT values
	Sorrentino et al. [14]	80 obese subjects (BMI ≥ 35) with metabolic syndrome and normal liver enzyme test	Normal ALT levels can be found within a group of patients with varying degrees of NASH
AST [10]	Kotronen et al. [10]	359 nondiabetic and 111 type 2 diabetic subjects	Independently predicted liver fat content
AST and diabetes presence [21]	Gholam et al. [21]	97 obese subjects (BMI ≥ 40) undergoing Roux-en-Y gastric bypass surgery	A detection model incorporating AST and the presence of diabetes predicted NASH (sensitivity: 0.76; accuracy: 0.70)
AST/ALT [10]	Kotronen et al. [10]	359 nondiabetic and 111 type 2 diabetic subjects	Independently predicted NAFLD when the ratio was included as a factor in a calculated risk score
GGT [23]	Tahan et al. [23]	50 biopsy-proven NAFLD patients (24 male, 26 female)	Serum GGT levels predicted advanced fibrosis (AUROC = 0.74)
CK-18 [25,26]	Feldstein et al. [25]	139 biopsy-proven adult NAFLD patients and 150 age-matched controls	CK-18 independently predicted NASH (AUROC = 0.83)
	Feldstein et al. [26]	201 biopsy-proven NAFLD in children (age 10.7 ± 2.5)	CK-18 has high accuracy for diagnosing NASH in children (AUROC = 0.933)
CCL-2/MCP-1 [27]	Haukeland et al. [27]	47 histologically verified NAFLD patients and 30 matched healthy controls	CCL-2 is a significant predictor of disease activity in NAFLD ($P = 0.012$)
CCL-2/MCP-1 and HDLc [28]	Page et al. [28]	37 histologically proven NAFLD	CCL-2 with HDLc levels together in multiple logistic regression predicted advanced fibrosis ($P < 0.028$)
sFasL [28]	Page et al. [28]	37 histologically proven NAFLD	sFasL levels were higher in patients with fibrosis ($P < 0.015$)
Ferritin [29]	Tanaka et al. [29]	53 cryptogenic chronic hepatitis patients	Serum ferritin level (odds ratio 1.013, $P = 0.048$) may be a factor to discriminate NASH from cryptogenic chronic hepatitis
		Lipid Species and Related Metabolites	
Palmitoleic, oleic, γ-linolenic and dihomo-γ-linolenic acids	Puri et al. [30]	25 NAFLD, 50 NASH patients, and 50 lean normal controls	Levels of palmitoleic, oleic, γ-linolenic, and dihomo-γ-linolenic acids were increased in both NAFLD and NASH patients ($P < 0.01$)

continued

TABLE 22.1 (continued)
Summary of Routinely Used Biomarkers of Liver Function and Disease

Biomarkers	References	Research Subjects	Comments
Linoleic acid			Linoleic acid level was decreased in both NAFLD and NASH patients ($P < 0.05$)
5-HETE, 8-HETE, 15-HETE			Increased levels of 5-HETE, 8-HETE, and 15-HETE were associated with progression from normal to NAFLD to NASH
11-HETE [30]			11-HETE level was elevated in NASH patients only ($P < 0.01$)
TG 16:0, 18:0, 18:1 PC 18:1, 22:6 PC 20:4, ether linked 24:1 [31]	Orešič et al. [31]	679 obese or type 2 diabetes patients	These three lipids were found to be strongly associated with the diagnosis of NAFLD.

Abbreviations: ALT, alanine amino transferase; AST, aspartate transaminase; AUROC, area under receiver operating characteristic curve; CCL-2, CC-chemokine ligand 2; CK-18, Cytokeratin 18; GGT, gamma-glutamyltranspeptidase; HDL, high-density lipoprotein; HETE, hydroxy-eicosatetraenoic acid; MCP-1, monocyte chemotactic protein-1; NAFLD, nonalcoholic fatty liver disease; NASH, nonalcoholic steatohepatitis; PC, phosphatidylcholine; sFSL, soluable Fas ligand; TG, triacylglycerols; VLDL, very low-density lipoprotein.

that serum ferritin independently predicted NASH and may discriminate NASH from cryptogenic chronic hepatitis.

In recent years, scientists performing metabolomic analyses on plasma have identified several lipid species such as TG, phosphatidylcholine, or other related lipid metabolites to be associated with NAFLD. One molecule, in particular, 11(*S*)-hydroxy-eicosatetraenoic acid (11-HETE) was identified as an important indicator for NASH [30]. While most independent biomarkers identified so far hold great promise for use as noninvasive tests for NAFLD, these biomarkers each reflect different aspects of the pathology. Therefore, prediction of NAFLD and determination of the disease stage may be improved by combining one or more of these independent biomarkers. An excellent example of this is shown in Table 22.1, in which Orešič et al. [31] identified a serum metabolite signature comprising three lipid species which accurately allowed for the estimation of liver fat percentage. In addition, the composite biomarker was applied to a second group of subjects to validate its use in diagnosing NAFLD. The biomarker had a sensitivity of 69.1% and a specificity of 73.8% and was useful in predicting liver-TG reduction during a weight loss study.

Algorithm tools used for NAFLD/NASH diagnosis have also been developed by a number of groups. To develop a biomarker panel for the diagnosis of NASH, Younossi et al. [32] combined concentrations of CK-18, M30 and M65 (cleaved CK-18), adiponectin, and resistin. A group in France has also led the way in commercializing such tests, which include the SteatoTest [33], FibroTest [34], and the NashTest [35]. These panels utilize commonly measured patient characteristics (e.g., age, BMI, TG, ALT, AST/ALT) and mathematical equations to result in the diagnosis of NAFLD. The tests can be performed only in validated laboratories; for example, the results are calculated through the BioPredictive web site (http://www.biopredictive.com), and a score is obtained. An excellent review of the various biomarker and algorithm tests has been presented by Miller et al. [20]. With regard to clinical studies on the metabolic effects of fructose in healthy subjects and those with NAFLD, various concentrations of blood parameters (TG, nonesterified fatty acids, ferritin, etc.) have been used in adults [36,37] and children [2]. Much work is needed to validate these biomarkers for use in research.

However, in large population studies, in which a liver biopsy may not be appropriate (e.g., children, and those with early stages of disease), the indicators reviewed above can be readily used to test the effects of fructose. Given the large number of studies currently underway in this area, improvements in the use of biomarkers in liver research is expected in the very near future.

IMAGING TECHNIQUES FOR DIAGNOSIS OF NAFLD

Liver fat contents can be detected noninvasively using experimental imaging modalities such as ultrasound, computed tomography (CT), magnetic resonance imaging (MRI), and MRS. Excellent reviews on liver imaging techniques to quantify hepatic fat and to study NAFLD and NASH have been described in detail by Browning [38] and Ma et al. [39]. Clinical ultrasound is based on the reflection and attenuation of the sound beam by liver fat and is the first imaging modality used to assess liver abnormalities [38]. However, it can only qualitatively test for moderate or severe fatty infiltration [39]. While ultrasound may detect hepatic steatosis [40], it is unable to distinguish between NASH and other types of NAFLD [41]. Duplex Doppler ultrasonography, by determining the blood flow in the hepatic and portal vasculature [42], is used to enhance standard ultrasound and in patients with liver fatty infiltration [43] and cirrhosis [44,45], abnormal hepatic vein Doppler waveform has been observed. Newer technologies that supplement traditional ultrasonography include transient elastography for the detection of fibrosis [46,47] and contrast-enhanced ultrasonography to distinguish NAFLD from NASH [48]. These methods have been validated by comparison to biopsy analysis and are currently in use in many research studies.

Unenhanced CT (single-energy noncontrast CT) which generates a liver–spleen ratio is a technique which allows for the qualitative and semiquantitative evaluation for the presence of steatosis. The accumulation of fat results in a lower attenuation than the spleen, leading to a reduction of this ratio that diagnoses hepatic steatosis [39]. When the ratio is less than 1, it indicates the existence of moderate-to-severe fat accumulation [49]. Although contrast-enhanced CT can be used to stage fibrosis and determine the disease severity in chronic liver diseases [50,51], it is not able to differentiate steatosis from steatohepatitis [52]. On the other hand, MRI is one of the most sensitive methods to detect fatty infiltration of the liver [53]. Typically, MRI estimates the degree of fatty filtration by using chemical shift imaging which detects the difference in the precession frequencies between fat ($-CH_2$) and water ($-OH$) protons. Chemical shift imaging is able to accurately detect and quantify liver fat [53–55]. Recently, Mazhar et al. [56] found this technique to be sensitive and specific (sensitivity: 80%; specificity: 95%) in detecting mild-to-moderate liver fat. However, MRI is not capable of quantifying the absolute liver fat concentration. In a study of 30 patients with histopathologically proven NASH, Elias et al. [57] found that MRI findings of liver steatosis and fibrosis were moderately correlated with histopathologic grades of steatosis and fibrosis, respectively (steatosis: $r = 0.43$, $P < 0.05$; fibrosis: $r = 0.61$, $P < 0.001$). Contrast materials such as superparamagnetic iron oxide (SPIO) can be used to enhance MRI. Tomita et al. [58] performed SPIO-enhanced MRI in 19 NAFLD patients and reported a good correlation between histological NAFLD activity scores and the contrast agent (%T2 values) ($r = -0.58$, $P = 0.009$). A cutoff %T2 value of 32.5 predicted "definitive NASH" with a specificity and sensitivity of 72.7 and 87.5%, respectively. Another accurate but noninvasive method for assessment of fatty liver is MRS. Proton MRS has been demonstrated to be precise to measure the liver-TG content with a coefficient ≥ 0.90 [59,60]. A recent meta-analysis [61] comparing various imaging techniques with liver biopsy for evaluation of hepatic steatosis found that MRI and ^{1}H-MRS also perform better than ultrasound and CT for detecting disease grades, especially for mild disease (<30% steatosis). In addition to MRS, ^{31}P has been applied to study the cytosolic energy, glucose, and membrane phospholipid metabolism [62–64]. Earlier studies applied the ^{31}P-MRS technique to study fructose metabolism in the liver of healthy humans and animals [65,66] and concluded that dynamic ^{31}P-MRS was promising for the liver function evaluation. Although the imaging techniques discussed above are accurate and reproducible, they provide a snapshot of liver-TG content and cannot be used to understand intrahepatic metabolism in vivo.

Recent advances in the use of stable isotopes in humans have been made to test the impact of dietary and lifestyle factors on liver function and disease [67]. The methods that use stable isotope tracers to study fatty acid flux and fructose effects in the liver are discussed in the next section entitled "Isotopic Turnover Methods to Measure Fructose Effects in the Liver."

ISOTOPIC TURNOVER METHODS TO MEASURE FRUCTOSE EFFECTS IN THE LIVER

It is clear that fructose flux can increase the in vivo rate of fatty acid synthesis in a process termed de novo lipogenesis [68]. Data in animals are overwhelmingly clear (reviewed elsewhere in this volume) and numerous strong studies in humans have now shown that a bolus of fructose acutely stimulates the pathway of de novo lipogenesis [69,70]. Long-term consumption of fructose significantly stimulates lipogenesis and concurrently elevates plasma-TG concentrations in the fasting [71] and fed states [70,72]. However, the mechanism of the hypertriglyceridemia is complicated by the complexity of fatty acid sources, including lipogenesis, which contribute to TG synthesis in the liver. Over the past 10 years, a large body of literature has amassed to suggest that the de novo lipogenesis is chronically stimulated in subjects with conditions associated with hypertriglyceridemia, including those with obesity [69], insulin resistance [73], and diabetes [74,75]. Yet, conclusions about the direct contribution of lipogenesis from fructose to plasma TG elevations are impacted by a number of factors. With regard to methodology, de novo lipogenesis has been measured in plasma VLDL-TG fatty acids by labeling the pathway with heavy (deuterated) water or stably labeled acetate (fed or infused). We have shown that the level of newly made fatty acids in VLDL-TG mirrors that in liver [76]. Lipogenesis is frequently measured in units reflecting the percentage of the VLDL-TG palmitic acid that is derived from the lipogenic pathway. The percentage is used (as opposed to the absolute quantity of de novo palmitate in VLDL-TG) because the percentage reflects assembly of fatty acids into hepatic-TG and this value is unaffected by the turnover rate of these lipids when they are detected in plasma.

It is important to point out that the percentage of de novo fatty acids detected in VLDL-TG after isotope labeling will also depend on the length of time of isotope administration. Our laboratory [70,76–78] and others [74,79] have shown that a longer duration of labeling (>1–2 days) may be necessary to accurately assess lipogenesis in plasma TG of healthy subjects, possibly due to a delay in the movement of these fatty acids through intrahepatocyte storage pools before secreting out into plasma via VLDL-TG. Liver-TG is synthesized from a number of fatty acid sources including plasma FFA that clear to the tissue, dietary fatty acids, de novo synthesized fatty acids, and fatty acids stored in intracellular droplets. It appears that differences exist between the timing of the liver's usage of plasma FFA and de novo fatty acids for TG synthesis such that plasma FFA are immediately re-esterified when they enter the liver and move into a pool that is instantaneously used for TG synthesis and VLDL secretion [76]. For example, for many subjects, if an FFA isotope is infused beginning at 5:00 AM in the fasting state, this label will appear in VLDL-TG within 30 min, which is the estimated time for total assembly of a VLDL particle through the endoplasmic reticulum and Golgi in the liver. By contrast, it takes approximately 12 h of labeling with ^{13}C-acetate to achieve significant label of newly made fatty acids in the VLDL-TG pool in plasma. Thus, de novo fatty acids appear to be routed to a "delay pool" in the liver before being esterified into the TG pool used for VLDL synthesis. This delay is observed when either ^{13}C-acetate is infused or fed, or when oral dosing of deuterated water (D_2O) is used to label lipogenesis. The D_2O method involves giving research subjects multiple doses overnight to bring the body water pool up to steady enrichment followed by maintaining D_2O in drinking water the next day [80,81]. We have found that for subjects with fatty liver, daily dosing must continue for at least 5 days to achieve sufficient turnover of liver-TG pools to accurately measure lipogenesis in plasma VLDL-TG. Not only does the timing of the isotope administration impact the measurement of de novo lipogenesis, but also the timing of meals. Fasting levels of lipogenesis will be higher if subjects are administered isotopes concurrently with meal consumption, before the fasting measurement is made [70,77,78]. This suggests that if a delay pool does exist in the liver for newly made fatty acids, turnover of that pool is stimulated by food intake.

With regard to circadian rhythm, in a recent study in NAFLD patients, day-long measurements of lipogenesis showed peak levels between midnight and 2:00 AM [81] in agreement with studies in by Hudgins et al. [79] and Vedala et al. [74]. In the NAFLD patients, the peak level in TG-rich lipoproteins (VLDL and chylomicrons) was 24.1 ± 15.2% of palmitate [81], and this level then fell toward morning. In 10 of the 13 subjects, peak night-time values of de novo lipogenesis were above 35% of plasma lipoprotein-TG palmitate and in one subject, 60% of palmitate was derived from the de novo lipogenesis pathway [81]. When the fasting state is extended beyond 12 h, lipogenesis will continue to fall but patients with NAFLD exhibit poor suppression of the pathway even with an extended fast [81]. In these subjects, the intake of dietary sugars correlated with the extent of de novo lipogenesis (Lambert and Parks, Unpublished).

With respect to fructose intake increasing the content of liver fat, studies have given mixed results. In children with metabolic syndrome, fructose feeding was associated with elevations in liver-TG contents, but this effect has not been consistently observed in healthy lean subjects [82]. In this regard, more research is needed on the differing effects of fructose consumption in eucaloric diets versus when it is fed in excess of energy needs [83]. Research needs in the area of fructose's influence on metabolism and disease have been reviewed in a recent report from an NIH-sponsored consensus conference on the topic [83]. Theoretically, aside from stimulating fatty acid synthesis directly, fructose consumption can lead to elevations in plasma TG by two other mechanisms. If fructose is combined with glucose in an oral bolus, glucose's stimulation of insulin secretion could increase the production of enzymes for TG synthesis leading to greater TG concentrations than by just feeding fructose alone. Increased enzyme activity for TG synthesis, combined with dietary availability of fatty acids for esterification, or from adipose tissue flux can exaggerate the hypertriglyceridemia observed with diets high in sugars [84].

A third means by which fructose consumption can increase liver and plasma TG levels is through inhibition of fatty acid oxidation [85]. This effect is mediated by an intermediate in the fatty acid synthesis pathway, malonyl-CoA, which inhibits the transport of fatty acids into the mitochondria via carnitine-palmitoyl transferase [85]. Elegant studies by Frayn and coworkers demonstrated that in healthy subjects, dietary fatty acids were 40-fold less oxidized when fructose was present in just a single meal [86] or when it was consumed as a 3-day diet containing 53% of total energy from sugars compared to one with 32% of energy from sugars [87]. In addition to lower dietary fat oxidation, re-esterification of plasma FFA was also 2-fold higher. The effect of fructose to spare fatty acids from oxidation may even carry over from one meal to the next. Parks et al. studied healthy subjects consuming morning boluses of glucose (~75 g) or an equimolar mixture of 50:50 glucose:fructose on separate occasions. After both boluses, a standardized lunch was fed. When the glucose:fructose bolus was given in the morning, higher postlunch TG concentrations were observed compared to the postlunch TG concentrations after the glucose bolus [70].

If fructose consumption reduces the oxidation of fatty acids from the diet or from adipose tissue, it could be tested using combinations of imaging and isotope administration. Ravikumar et al. [88] used ^{13}C-labeled dietary fatty acids and performed MRS to demonstrate that diabetics cleared more of their dietary fat to liver compared to nondiabetic controls. Carpentier and colleagues [89] have developed an in vivo method using a positron-emitting fatty acid analog which is added to a meal and then tissue uptake of these dietary fatty acids is assessed by PET. They demonstrated that in muscles the absolute extraction of plasma FFA is similar between diabetics and healthy controls, despite the diabetics having greater plasma FFA concentrations [90]. This result would lead to greater availability of FFA for uptake in the liver. It is not known whether fructose fed concurrently would increase the retention dietary fat in the liver but it is possible that diabetics would be even more sensitive to the effects of fructose in causing NAFLD.

Given these developments in isotopic methods combined with imaging, one concept that can now be investigated is the impact of dietary fat consumed with and without fructose in individuals at risk for NAFLD. Thus, one hypothesis to be tested is that if fructose reduces liver fatty acid oxidation and increases re-esterification, then insulin-resistant individuals who clear more dietary lipid to liver would be more likely to store this lipid if the meal fat is consumed along with fructose. Many foods that contain high-fructose corn syrup can also be high in fat (i.e., jelly donuts, cakes, confectionaries). The effect of fructose to reduce fatty acid oxidation from any fatty acid source (dietary or endogenous) also suggests that liver-TG recycling should also increase as fatty acids liberated from intracellular TG droplets would be rechanneled back into synthesis. The relative impact of such substrate cycling is unknown.

FUTURE DIRECTIONS AND CONCLUSION

In summary, new clinical diagnostic and research methods have been employed to better define the level of disease in patients with suspected NAFLD. The predictive nature of biomarkers needs to be reproduced in new cohorts to strengthen their use and if any combination of biomarkers is going to be adopted for clinical practice, much more data are needed in comparison with liver biopsy data. For now, any changes in liver enzymes or in metabolomic analyses observed following fructose feeding in humans will be difficult to interpret. By contrast, the ability of newer imaging methods to quantitate changes in liver fat and fibrosis holds great promise in the study of liver metabolism. In future, MRI or MRS may become accepted clinical diagnostic tools for the measurement of liver-TG. By contrast, further innovations are needed in the in vivo use of isotopic molecules. In particular, no physiological method exists presently for the measurement of liver fatty acid oxidation without using hepatic artery and vein catheters. Quantifying liver fatty acid oxidation will be key to determining the impact of fructose feeding on inflammation and reactive oxygen species. Finally, since saturated fatty acids are the primary products of fructose-induced fatty acid synthesis in the liver [86,91], it may be that the cardiometabolic ramifications of fructose-induced elevations in de novo lipogenesis need to be compared to the results of consumption of dietary saturated fats. On very high fructose-containing diets, the quantity of palmitate made via hepatic de novo lipogenesis may still be less than the estimated quantity of preformed (dietary) palmitate that enters the liver, but it is currently unknown whether the local production of palmitate from dietary sugars can lead to downregulation of LDL receptors as shown for dietary saturated fatty acids [92]. The existence of intracellular compartmentalization of lipogenesis versus the route of trafficking of dietary fatty acids will be an important target for future investigation.

REFERENCES

1. Mager DR, Patterson C, So S, Rogenstein CD, Wykes LJ, Roberts EA. Dietary and physical activity patterns in children with fatty liver. *Eur J Clin Nutr*. 2010;64(6):628–35. Epub 2010/03/11.
2. Jin R, Le NA, Liu S, Farkas Epperson M, Ziegler TR, Welsh JA et al. Children with NAFLD are more sensitive to the adverse metabolic effects of fructose beverages than children without NAFLD. *J Clin Endocrinol Metab*. 2012;97(7):E1088–98. Epub 2012/05/01.
3. Assy N, Nasser G, Kamayse I, Nseir W, Beniashvili Z, Djibre A et al. Soft drink consumption linked with fatty liver in the absence of traditional risk factors. *Can J Gastroenterol*. 2008;22(10):811–6. Epub 2008/10/18.
4. Ouyang X, Cirillo P, Sautin Y, McCall S, Bruchette JL, Diehl AM et al. Fructose consumption as a risk factor for non-alcoholic fatty liver disease. *J Hepatol*. 2008;48(6):993–9. Epub 2008/04/09.
5. Abdelmalek MF, Suzuki A, Guy C, Unalp-Arida A, Colvin R, Johnson RJ et al. Increased fructose consumption is associated with fibrosis severity in patients with nonalcoholic fatty liver disease. *Hepatology*. 2010;51(6):1961–71. Epub 2010/03/20.
6. Bravo AA, Sheth SG, Chopra S. Liver biopsy. *N Engl J Med*. 2001;344(7):495–500. Epub 2001/02/15.
7. Saleh HA, Abu-Rashed AH. Liver biopsy remains the gold standard for evaluation of chronic hepatitis and fibrosis. *J Gastrointestin Liver Dis*. 2007;16(4):425–6. Epub 2008/01/15.
8. Nomura K, Yano E, Shinozaki T, Tagawa K. Efficacy and effectiveness of liver screening program to detect fatty liver in the periodic health check-ups. *J Occup Health*. 2004;46(6):423–8. Epub 2004/12/23.

9. Chang Y, Ryu S, Sung E, Jang Y. Higher concentrations of alanine aminotransferase within the reference interval predict nonalcoholic fatty liver disease. *Clin Chem*. 2007;53(4):686–92. Epub 2007/02/03.
10. Kotronen A, Peltonen M, Hakkarainen A, Sevastianova K, Bergholm R, Johansson LM et al. Prediction of non-alcoholic fatty liver disease and liver fat using metabolic and genetic factors. *Gastroenterology*. 2009;137(3):865–72. Epub 2009/06/16.
11. Westerbacka J, Corner A, Tiikkainen M, Tamminen M, Vehkavaara S, Hakkinen AM et al. Women and men have similar amounts of liver and intra-abdominal fat, despite more subcutaneous fat in women: Implications for sex differences in markers of cardiovascular risk. *Diabetologia*. 2004;47(8):1360–9. Epub 2004/08/17.
12. Omagari K, Takamura R, Matsutake S, Ichimura M, Kato S, Morikawa S et al. Serum alanine aminotransferase concentration as a predictive factor for the development or regression of fatty liver. *J Clin Biochem Nutr*. 2011;49(3):200–6. Epub 2011/12/01.
13. Mofrad P, Contos MJ, Haque M, Sargeant C, Fisher RA, Luketic VA et al. Clinical and histologic spectrum of nonalcoholic fatty liver disease associated with normal alt values. *Hepatology*. 2003;37(6):1286–92. Epub 2003/05/30.
14. Sorrentino P, Tarantino G, Conca P, Perrella A, Terracciano ML, Vecchione R et al. Silent non-alcoholic fatty liver disease—A clinical–histological study. *J Hepatol*. 2004;41(5):751–7. Epub 2004/11/03.
15. Liangpunsakul S, Qi R, Crabb DW, Witzmann F. Relationship between alcohol drinking and aspartate aminotransferase:alanine aminotransferase (Ast:Alt) ratio, mean corpuscular volume (Mcv), gamma-glutamyl transpeptidase (Ggt), and apolipoprotein A1 and B in the U.S. population. *J Stud Alcohol Drugs*. 2010;71(2):249–52. Epub 2010/03/17.
16. Ribeiro RM, Layden-Almer J, Powers KA, Layden TJ, Perelson AS. Dynamics of alanine aminotransferase during hepatitis C virus treatment. *Hepatology*. 2003;38(2):509–17. Epub 2003/07/29.
17. Miyake Y, Iwasaki Y, Terada R, Okamaoto R, Ikeda H, Makino Y et al. Persistent elevation of serum alanine aminotransferase levels leads to poor survival and hepatocellular carcinoma development in type 1 autoimmune hepatitis. *Aliment Pharmacol Ther*. 2006;24(8):1197–205. Epub 2006/10/04.
18. Amacher DE. Serum transaminase elevations as indicators of hepatic injury following the administration of drugs. *Regul Toxicol Pharmacol*. 1998;27(2):119–30. Epub 1998/07/22.
19. Amacher DE. A toxicologist's guide to biomarkers of hepatic response. *Hum Exp Toxicol*. 2002;21(5):253–62. Epub 2002/07/27.
20. Miller MH, Ferguson MA, Dillon JF. Systematic review of performance of non-invasive biomarkers in the evaluation of non-alcoholic fatty liver disease. *Liver Int*. 2011;31(4):461–73. Epub 2011/03/09.
21. Gholam PM, Flancbaum L, Machan JT, Charney DA, Kotler DP. Nonalcoholic fatty liver disease in severely obese subjects. *Am J Gastroenterol*. 2007;102(2):399–408. Epub 2007/02/22.
22. Whitfield JB. Serum gamma-glutamyltransferase and risk of disease. *Clin Chem*. 2007;53(1):1–2. Epub 2007/01/05.
23. Tahan V, Canbakan B, Balci H, Dane F, Akin H, Can G et al. Serum gamma-glutamyltranspeptidase distinguishes non-alcoholic fatty liver disease at high risk. *Hepatogastroenterology*. 2008;55(85):1433–8. Epub 2008/09/18.
24. Wieckowska A, Zein NN, Yerian LM, Lopez AR, McCullough AJ, Feldstein AE. In vivo assessment of liver cell apoptosis as a novel biomarker of disease severity in nonalcoholic fatty liver disease. *Hepatology*. 2006;44(1):27–33. Epub 2006/06/27.
25. Feldstein AE, Wieckowska A, Lopez AR, Liu YC, Zein NN, McCullough AJ. Cytokeratin-18 fragment levels as noninvasive biomarkers for nonalcoholic steatohepatitis: A multicenter validation study. *Hepatology*. 2009;50(4):1072–8. Epub 2009/07/09.
26. Feldstein AE, Alkhouri N, De Vito R, Alisi A, Lopez R, Nobili V. Serum cytokeratin-18 fragment levels are useful biomarkers for nonalcoholic steatohepatitis in children. *Am J Gastroenterol*. 2013;108(9):1526–31. Epub 2013/06/12.
27. Haukeland JW, Damas JK, Konopski Z, Loberg EM, Haaland T, Goverud I et al. Systemic inflammation in nonalcoholic fatty liver disease is characterized by elevated levels of Ccl2. *J Hepatol*. 2006;44(6):1167–74. Epub 2006/04/19.
28. Page S, Birerdinc A, Estep M, Stepanova M, Afendy A, Petricoin E et al. Knowledge-based identification of soluble biomarkers: Hepatic fibrosis in NAFLD as an example. *PLoS One*. 2013;8(2):e56009. Epub 2013/02/14.
29. Tanaka N, Tanaka E, Sheena Y, Komatsu M, Okiyama W, Misawa N et al. Useful parameters for distinguishing nonalcoholic steatohepatitis with mild steatosis from cryptogenic chronic hepatitis in the Japanese population. *Liver Int*. 2006;26(8):956–63. Epub 2006/09/07.
30. Puri P, Wiest MM, Cheung O, Mirshahi F, Sargeant C, Min HK et al. The plasma lipidomic signature of nonalcoholic steatohepatitis. *Hepatology*. 2009;50(6):1827–38. Epub 2009/11/26.

31. Orešič M, Hyötyläinen T, Kotronen A, Gopalacharyulu P, Nygren H, Arola J et al. Prediction of non-alcoholic fatty-liver disease and liver fat content by serum molecular lipids. *Diabetologia*. 2013;56(10):2266–74. Epub 2013/07/05.
32. Younossi ZM, Jarrar M, Nugent C, Randhawa M, Afendy M, Stepanova M et al. A novel diagnostic biomarker panel for obesity-related nonalcoholic steatohepatitis (NASH). *Obes Surg*. 2008;18(11):1430–7. Epub 2008/05/27.
33. Poynard T, Ratziu V, Naveau S, Thabut D, Charlotte F, Messous D et al. The diagnostic value of biomarkers (steatotest) for the prediction of liver steatosis. *Comp Hepatol*. 2005;4:10. Epub 2005/12/27.
34. Ratziu V, Massard J, Charlotte F, Messous D, Imbert-Bismut F, Bonyhay L et al. Diagnostic value of biochemical markers (fibrotest-fibrosure) for the prediction of liver fibrosis in patients with non-alcoholic fatty liver disease. *BMC Gastroenterol*. 2006;6:6. Epub 2006/03/01.
35. Poynard T, Ratziu V, Charlotte F, Messous D, Munteanu M, Imbert-Bismut F et al. Diagnostic value of biochemical markers (NASH test) for the prediction of non alcoholo steato hepatitis in patients with non-alcoholic fatty liver disease. *BMC Gastroenterol*. 2006;6:34. Epub 2006/11/14.
36. Abid A, Taha O, Nseir W, Farah R, Grosovski M, Assy N. Soft drink consumption is associated with fatty liver disease independent of metabolic syndrome. *J Hepatol*. 2009;51(5):918–24. Epub 2009/09/22.
37. Abdelmalek MF, Lazo M, Horska A, Bonekamp S, Lipkin EW, Balasubramanyam A et al. Higher dietary fructose is associated with impaired hepatic adenosine triphosphate homeostasis in obese individuals with type 2 diabetes. *Hepatology*. 2012;56(3):952–60. Epub 2012/04/03.
38. Browning JD. New imaging techniques for non-alcoholic steatohepatitis. *Clin Liver Dis*. 2009;13(4):607–19. Epub 2009/10/13.
39. Ma X, Holalkere NS, Kambadakone RA, Mino-Kenudson M, Hahn PF, Sahani DV. Imaging-based quantification of hepatic fat: Methods and clinical applications. *Radiographics*. 2009;29(5):1253–77. Epub 2009/09/17.
40. Saverymuttu SH, Joseph AE, Maxwell JD. Ultrasound scanning in the detection of hepatic fibrosis and steatosis. *Br Med J (Clin Res Ed)*. 1986;292(6512):13–5. Epub 1986/01/04.
41. Saadeh S, Younossi ZM, Remer EM, Gramlich T, Ong JP, Hurley M et al. The utility of radiological imaging in nonalcoholic fatty liver disease. *Gastroenterology*. 2002;123(3):745–50. Epub 2002/08/29.
42. Magalotti D, Marchesini G, Ramilli S, Berzigotti A, Bianchi G, Zoli M. Splanchnic haemodynamics in non-alcoholic fatty liver disease: Effect of a dietary/pharmacological treatment. A pilot study. *Dig Liver Dis*. 2004;36(6):406–11. Epub 2004/07/14.
43. Oguzkurt L, Yildirim T, Torun D, Tercan F, Kizilkilic O, Niron EA. Hepatic vein Doppler waveform in patients with diffuse fatty infiltration of the liver. *Eur J Radiol*. 2005;54(2):253–7. Epub 2005/04/20.
44. Bolondi L, Li Bassi S, Gaiani S, Zironi G, Benzi G, Santi V et al. Liver cirrhosis: Changes of Doppler waveform of hepatic veins. *Radiology*. 1991;178(2):513–6. Epub 1991/02/01.
45. von Herbay A, Frieling T, Haussinger D. Association between duplex Doppler sonographic flow pattern in right hepatic vein and various liver diseases. *J Clin Ultrasound*. 2001;29(1):25–30. Epub 2001/02/17.
46. Nahon P, Kettaneh A, Tengher-Barna I, Ziol M, de Ledinghen V, Douvin C et al. Assessment of liver fibrosis using transient elastography in patients with alcoholic liver disease. *J Hepatol*. 2008;49(6):1062–8. Epub 2008/10/22.
47. Yoneda M, Yoneda M, Mawatari H, Fujita K, Endo H, Iida H et al. Noninvasive assessment of liver fibrosis by measurement of stiffness in patients with nonalcoholic fatty liver disease (NAFLD). *Dig Liver Dis*. 2008;40(5):371–8. Epub 2007/12/18.
48. Iijima H, Moriyasu F, Tsuchiya K, Suzuki S, Yoshida M, Shimizu M et al. Decrease in accumulation of ultrasound contrast microbubbles in non-alcoholic steatohepatitis. *Hepatol Res*. 2007;37(9):722–30. Epub 2007/06/15.
49. Longo R, Ricci C, Masutti F, Vidimari R, Croce LS, Bercich L et al. Fatty infiltration of the liver. Quantification by 1 h localized magnetic resonance spectroscopy and comparison with computed tomography. *Invest Radiol*. 1993;28(4):297–302. Epub 1993/04/01.
50. Van Beers BE, Leconte I, Materne R, Smith AM, Jamart J, Horsmans Y. Hepatic perfusion parameters in chronic liver disease: Dynamic Ct measurements correlated with disease severity. *AJR Am J Roentgenol*. 2001;176(3):667–73. Epub 2001/02/27.
51. Hashimoto K, Murakami T, Dono K, Hori M, Kim T, Kudo M et al. Assessment of the severity of liver disease and fibrotic change: The usefulness of hepatic Ct perfusion imaging. *Oncol Rep*. 2006;16(4):677–83. Epub 2006/09/14.
52. Jacobs JE, Birnbaum BA, Shapiro MA, Langlotz CP, Slosman F, Rubesin SE et al. Diagnostic criteria for fatty infiltration of the liver on contrast-enhanced helical Ct. *AJR Am J Roentgenol*. 1998;171(3):659–64. Epub 1998/09/02.

53. Qayyum A, Goh JS, Kakar S, Yeh BM, Merriman RB, Coakley FV. Accuracy of liver fat quantification at MR imaging: Comparison of out-of-phase gradient-echo and fat-saturated fast spin-echo techniques—Initial experience. *Radiology*. 2005;237(2):507–11. Epub 2005/10/26.
54. Rofsky NM, Fleishaker H. Ct and MRI of diffuse liver disease. *Semin Ultrasound CT MR*. 1995;16(1):16–33. Epub 1995/02/01.
55. Pilleul F, Chave G, Dumortier J, Scoazec JY, Valette PJ. Fatty infiltration of the liver. Detection and grading using dual T1 gradient echo sequences on clinical MR system. *Gastroenterol Clin Biol*. 2005;29(11):1143–7. Epub 2006/03/01.
56. Mazhar SM, Shiehmorteza M, Sirlin CB. Noninvasive assessment of hepatic steatosis. *Clin Gastroenterol Hepatol*. 2009;7(2):135–40. Epub 2009/01/03.
57. Elias Jr. J, Jr., Altun E, Zacks S, Armao DM, Woosley JT, Semelka RC. MRI findings in nonalcoholic steatohepatitis: Correlation with histopathology and clinical staging. *Magn Reson Imaging*. 2009;27(7):976–87. Epub 2009/04/10.
58. Tomita K, Tanimoto A, Irie R, Kikuchi M, Yokoyama H, Teratani T et al. Evaluating the severity of nonalcoholic steatohepatitis with superparamagnetic iron oxide-enhanced magnetic resonance imaging. *J Magn Reson Imaging*. 2008;28(6):1444–50. Epub 2008/11/26.
59. Thomsen C, Becker U, Winkler K, Christoffersen P, Jensen M, Henriksen O. Quantification of liver fat using magnetic resonance spectroscopy. *Magn Reson Imaging*. 1994;12(3):487–95. Epub 1994/01/01.
60. Szczepaniak LS, Nurenberg P, Leonard D, Browning JD, Reingold JS, Grundy S et al. Magnetic resonance spectroscopy to measure hepatic triglyceride content: Prevalence of hepatic steatosis in the general population. *Am J Physiol Endocrinol Metab*. 2005;288(2):E462–E8.
61. Bohte AE, van Werven JR, Bipat S, Stoker J. The diagnostic accuracy of US, Ct, MRI and 1 h-MRS for the evaluation of hepatic steatosis compared with liver biopsy: A meta-analysis. *Eur Radiol*. 2011;21(1):87–97. Epub 2010/08/04.
62. Oberhaensli RD, Galloway GJ, Taylor DJ, Bore PJ, Radda GK. Assessment of human liver metabolism by phosphorus-31 magnetic resonance spectroscopy. *Br J Radiol*. 1986;59(703):695–9. Epub 1986/07/01.
63. Murphy DG, Bottomley PA, Salerno JA, DeCarli C, Mentis MJ, Grady CL et al. An in vivo study of phosphorus and glucose metabolism in Alzheimer's disease using magnetic resonance spectroscopy and pet. *Arch Gen Psychiatry*. 1993;50(5):341–9. Epub 1993/05/01.
64. Abrigo JM, Shen J, Wong VW, Yeung DK, Wong GL, Chim AM et al. Non-alcoholic fatty liver disease: Spectral patterns observed from an in vivo phosphorus magnetic resonance spectroscopy study. *J Hepatol*. 2014;60(4):809–15. Epub 2013 Nov 26.
65. Karczmar GS, Kurtz T, Tavares NJ, Weiner MW. Regulation of hepatic inorganic phosphate and ATP in response to fructose loading: An in vivo ^{31}P-NMR study. *Biochim Biophys Acta*. 1989;1012(2):121–7. Epub 1989/07/11.
66. Terrier F, Vock P, Cotting J, Ladebeck R, Reichen J, Hentschel D. Effect of intravenous fructose on the P-31 MR spectrum of the liver: Dose response in healthy volunteers. *Radiology*. 1989;171(2):557–63. Epub 1989/05/01.
67. Parks EJ, Hellerstein MK. Recent advances in liver triacylglycerol and fatty acid metabolism using stable isotope labeling techniques. *J Lipid Research*. 2006;47:1651–60.
68. Tappy L, Lê KA, Tran C, Paquot N. Fructose and metabolic diseases: New findings, new questions. *Nutrition*. 2010;26(11–12):1044–9.
69. Marques-Lopes I, Ansorena D, Astiasaran I, Forga L, Martinez JA. Postprandial de novo lipogenesis and metabolic changes induced by a high-carbohydrate, low-fat meal in lean and overweight men. *Am J Clin Nutr*. 2001;73(2):253–61. Epub 2001/02/07.
70. Parks EJ, Skokan LE, Timlin MT, Dingfelder CS. Dietary sugars stimulate fatty acid synthesis in adults. *J Nutr*. 2008;138(6):1039–46. Epub 2008/05/22.
71. Stanhope KL, Bremer AA, Medici V, Nakajima K, Ito Y, Nakano T et al. Consumption of fructose and high fructose corn syrup increase postprandial triglycerides, LDL-cholesterol, and apolipoprotein-B in young men and women. *J Clin Endocrinol Metab*. 2011;96(10):E1596–605. Epub 2011/08/19.
72. Stanhope KL, Schwarz JM, Keim NL, Griffen SC, Bremer AA, Graham JL et al. Consuming fructose-sweetened, not glucose-sweetened, beverages increases visceral adiposity and lipids and decreases insulin sensitivity in overweight/obese humans. *J Clin Invest*. 2009;119(5):1322–34. Epub 2009/04/22.
73. Schwarz JM, Linfoot P, Dare D, Aghajanian K. Hepatic de novo lipogenesis in normoinsulinemic and hyperinsulinemic subjects consuming high-fat, low-carbohydrate and low-fat, high-carbohydrate isoenergetic diets. *Am J Clin Nutr*. 2003;77(1):43–50. Epub 2002/12/25.

74. Vedala A, Wang W, Neese RA, Christiansen MP, Hellerstein MK. Delayed secretory pathway contributions to VLDL-triglycerides from plasma Nefa, diet, and de novo lipogenesis in humans. *J Lipid Res.* 2006;47(11):2562–74.
75. Wilke MS, French MA, Goh YK, Ryan EA, Jones PJ, Clandinin MT. Synthesis of specific fatty acids contributes to VLDL-triacylglycerol composition in humans with and without type 2 diabetes. *Diabetologia.* 2009;52(8):1628–37. Epub 2009/06/19.
76. Donnelly KL, Smith CI, Schwarzenberg SJ, Jessurun J, Boldt MD, Parks EJ. Sources of fatty acids stored in liver and secreted via lipoproteins in patients with nonalcoholic fatty liver disease. *J Clin Invest.* 2005;115(5):1343–51. Epub 2005/05/03.
77. Barrows BR, Parks EJ. Contributions of different fatty acid sources to very low-density lipoprotein-triacylglycerol in the fasted and fed states. *J Clin Endocrinol Metab.* 2006;91(4):1446–52. Epub 2006/02/02.
78. Timlin MT, Parks EJ. Temporal pattern of de novo lipogenesis in the postprandial state in healthy men. *Am J Clin Nutr.* 2005;81(1):35–42. Epub 2005/01/11.
79. Hudgins LC, Hellerstein MK, Seidman CE, Neese RA, Tremaroli JD, Hirsch J. Relationship between carbohydrate-induced hypertriglyceridemia and fatty acid synthesis in lean and obese subjects. *J Lipid Res.* 2000;41(4):595–604. Epub 2000/04/01.
80. Strawford A, Hoh R, Neese RA, Parks EJ, Turner S, Hellerstein MK. A placebo-controlled trial of the effects of combining megestrol-acetate with testosterone replacement therapy in AIDS-wasting syndrome. *J Amer Med Assoc.* 1999;281(14):1282–90.
81. Lambert JE, Ramos-Roman MA, Browning JD, Parks EJ. Increased de novo lipogenesis is a distinct characteristic of individuals with nonalcoholic fatty liver disease. *Gastroenterology.* 2014;146(3):726–35.
82. Bravo S, Lowndes J, Sinnett S, Yu Z, Rippe J. Consumption of sucrose and high-fructose corn syrup does not increase liver fat or ectopic fat deposition in muscle. *Appl Physiol Nutr Metab.* 2013;38(6):681–8.
83. Laughlin MR, Bantle JP, Havel PJ, Parks EJ, Klurfeld DM, Teff K et al. Clinical research strategies for fructose metabolism. *Adv. Nutr.* 2014;5:248–59.
84. Parks E, Hellerstein MK. Carbohydrate-induced hypertriacylglycerolemia: An historical perspective and review of biological mechanisms. *Amer J Clin Nutr.* 2000;71(2):412–33.
85. McGarry JD. Banting lecture 2001: Dysregulation of fatty acid metabolism in the etiology of type 2 diabetes. *Diabetes.* 2002;51(1):7–18.
86. Chong MF, Fielding BA, Frayn KN. Mechanisms for the acute effect of fructose on postprandial lipemia. *Am J Clin Nutr.* 2007;85(6):1511–20.
87. Roberts R, Bickerton AS, Fielding BA, Blaak EE, Wagenmakers AJ, Chong MF et al. Reduced oxidation of dietary fat after a short term high-carbohydrate diet. *Am J Clin Nutr.* 2008;87(4):824–31.
88. Ravikumar B, Carey PE, Snaar JE, Deelchand DK, Cook DB, Neely RD et al. Real-time assessment of postprandial fat storage in liver and skeletal muscle in health and type 2 diabetes. *Am J Physiol Endocrinol Metab.* 2005;288(4):E789–97. Epub 2004/12/02.
89. Labbe SM, Grenier-Larouche T, Croteau E, Normand-Lauziere F, Frisch F, Ouellet R et al. Organ-specific dietary fatty acid uptake in humans using positron emission tomography coupled to computed tomography. *Am J Physiol Endocrinol Metab.* 2011;300(3):E445–53. Epub 2010/11/26.
90. Labbe SM, Croteau E, Grenier-Larouche T, Frisch F, Ouellet R, Langlois R et al. Normal postprandial nonesterified fatty acid uptake in muscles despite increased circulating fatty acids in type 2 diabetes. *Diabetes.* 2011;60(2):408–15. Epub 2011/01/14.
91. Aarsland A, Chinkes D, Wolfe RR. Contributions of de novo synthesis of fatty acids to total VLDL-triglyceride secretion during prolonged hyperglycemia/hyperinsulinemia in normal man. *J Clin Invest.* 1996;98(9):2008–17.
92. Fox JC, McGill HCJ, Carey KD, Getz GS. In vivo regulation of hepatic LDL receptor MRNA in the baboon.: Differential effects of saturated and unsaturated fat. *J Biol Chem.* 1997;262:7014–20.

23 Dietary Sugars and Dental Health

Sára Karjalainen, Eva Söderling, and Adrian Lussi

CONTENTS

KEY POINTS

- Dietary sugars still play an important role in the etiology of dental caries, albeit the association between sucrose intake and caries is currently weaker than earlier.
- Another oral health problem, that is, dental erosion, is arising from increased consumption of sugary beverages.
- Fluoride reduces caries risk but has not been able to eliminate dental health problems completely.
- Daily use of sugar substitutes, xylitol, in particular, is a novel method to reduce the risk of caries.

INTRODUCTION

The harmful effect of sucrose on dental health has been discussed repeatedly during the last 30 years. According to contemporary research, the former strong association between sucrose intake and dental caries has weakened considerably. This is believed to be due to the generalized and widespread use of fluoride and fluoride products. In addition to caries, there is increased concern about a relatively new oral health problem arising from increased consumption of sugary beverages, that is, dental erosion. Most soft drinks, fruit juices, lemonades, and energy drinks are not only high in dietary sugars, but in addition they also contain organic and other acids. Frequent daily use of acidic drinks and juices may cause rapid erosion of enamel resulting in visible esthetic and functional harm to the dentition.

Fluoride reduces caries risk but has not been completely able to eliminate dental caries. More modern methods are needed to prevent caries among caries-prone individuals. Daily use of sugar substitutes, xylitol, in particular, is one example of a novel method to promote dental health and reduce the risk of caries.

This chapter reviews and highlights current knowledge on the links between dietary sugars and dental health as well as identifying priorities for future research.

DIETARY SUGARS AND THEIR ROLE IN THE DEVELOPMENT OF DENTAL CARIES

This chapter is restricted to review the effects of fermentable sugars in the oral cavity. These include disaccharides, such as sucrose, maltose, and lactose, and monosaccharides, such as glucose, fructose, and galactose. In animal studies, lactose and glucose syrups, common ingredients of soft drinks, have been found to be less cariogenic than sucrose [1,2]. Most sugary beverages, at least in the USA, contain high-fructose corn syrup which is chemically similar to invert sugar (50% fructose and 50% glucose). In a longitudinal study on preschool children, invert sugar was found slightly less cariogenic than sucrose [3]. Sugars can also be divided into intrinsic sugars found in fruits and vegetables, and free sugars which refer to all mono- and disaccharides added to food products.

The cariogenic effect of sugar-containing dietary products on dental health is mainly local and depends on many factors such as intake frequency and amount, consumption habits, and retention time, that is, the time the food product is retained in the oral cavity. In addition, individual's age, the density of his/her cariogenic oral flora, use of fluoride products, salivary flow rate, and oral clearance all affect the cariogenic impact.

Dental caries is defined as an infectious microbial disease that results in localized dissolution and destruction of enamel and dentine. In other words, caries is the result of repeated demineralizing episodes caused by organic acids produced by cariogenic species fermenting dietary sugars in the dental biofilm (dental plaque).

EFFECT OF DIETARY SUGARS ON CARIES-ASSOCIATED BACTERIA

The negative impact of dietary sugars on dental health is mediated by caries-associated bacteria in the dental biofilm. The oral cavity is an ideal habitat for many microorganisms. Several hundreds of species have been identified to thrive in the moist, warm, and favorable conditions of the human mouth, but only aciduric or acidogenic species such as mutans streptococci and lactobacilli are cariogenic [4]. Microbial colonization of the oral cavity starts from birth, and the number of species increases over time, especially following eruption of teeth [4–6]. The most diverse collection of microorganisms is found as biofilm on teeth. Dental biofilm contains early colonizers who are able to bind to saliva-coated tooth surfaces by the help of adhesion molecules. Some of the early colonizers such as *Streptococcus salivarius* and *S. sanguinis* are inert in relation to dental health. Some bacteria modify the microenvironment more suitable for later colonizers. Bacterial water-insoluble extracellular glucans and fructans grow the thickness of the biofilm and are dependent on high concentration of sucrose. These extracellular polymers enhance accumulation of mutans streptococci resulting in greater acid production immediately adjacent to the tooth surface. As byproduct of the glucan and fructan synthesis, cariogenic bacteria (mostly mutans streptococci and lactobacilli) in the biofilm start to produce lactic acid. The cariogenic mutans streptococci and lactobacilli can thrive in more acidic conditions than bacteria producing other organic acids such as propionic or butyric acid. Though other bacteria may also contribute to demineralization of enamel and dentine, this chapter is restricted to mutans streptococci and lactobacilli as their relation to caries has been studied most. As a result of exposure to sugar, the pH value of the biofilm covering the tooth surface may decrease to the point where demineralization of enamel can occur. This takes place around and below pH 5.5, which in the dental literature is called the "critical pH." A single oral sucrose rinse is known to cause an immediate drop in the pH of the biofilm below the critical pH followed by a slow return to baseline.

CARIES-RISK PERIODS AND SITES OF HUMAN TEETH

The outermost layer of a healthy sound enamel surface of any mature tooth has a higher concentration of fluoride than that of an unerupted or erupting tooth. Currently, it is believed that the uptake of fluoride ions is the result of an active exchange of minerals mediated by microbial accumulation covering the tooth surfaces during the most part of eruption [7]. Hence, newly erupted or erupting teeth of children and adolescents are more vulnerable to the harmful effects of excessive sucrose intake than fully erupted teeth. And indeed, the relationship between dietary sucrose and caries rises more steeply when newly erupted teeth are present in young children and adolescents. Further, high-risk periods occur later in life if salivary flow is reduced due to medications or radiation therapy of head and neck.

Differences in vulnerability between tooth surfaces may also occur: sites which encourage biofilm accumulation like fissures are at greater risk to become carious than surfaces that can be mechanically cleaned like proximal tooth surfaces or are continuously flushed by saliva like labial or palatal surfaces.

SUGAR INTAKE AND CARIES

The fact that frequent intake of sugary products with high sugar concentrations increases caries activity has been known for long but the association was experimentally shown in a 5-year longitudinal study [8]. Though some studies show that the amount of sugar intake is more important than frequency [2,9,10], the concept that frequency is more important is more generally accepted. However, a strong correlation exists between the two [2] and it is likely that in relation to caries both are potentially important. Nevertheless, when sugars are used in large amounts over protracted periods of time, caries scores are usually high. On the other hand, little decay is found in the absence of sugars, for example, among age cohorts born during war time [11], or among subjects unable to consume fructose or sucrose due to hereditary fructose intolerance [12]. Epidemiological studies further show that consumption of starchy staple foods and fresh fruit are associated with low levels of dental caries [13].

In European countries, a clear general trend of decreasing dental caries with only a minor decrease in total sugar consumption was found during the period between 1970 and 1980 [14]. It was concluded that the relationship between sugar consumption and caries is much weaker in the modern age of fluoride exposure than it used to be. However, children who consume a higher proportion of their total energy intake as sugars have even today more caries than children consuming less sugar [9,15,16]. The most recent review on sugar intake and caries demonstrates only a moderately significant relationship between sugar intake frequency and dental caries [17].

Instead of the former linear relationship between dietary sucrose and caries [18], the dose–response curve is currently believed to have a sigmoid shape: at levels of annual sugar consumption below 10 kg/person, the incidence of caries is acceptably low, between 15 and 35 kg/person, the incidence of caries increases more steeply, while beyond 35 kg/person, the curve flattens out [19]. Interpreted into practice, this could mean that the level of caries would be the same if the annual sugar consumption were 3–5 kg more than 35 kg/person, or in reverse, that a 3–5 kg decrease in annual sugar consumption would not automatically mean a decrease in caries incidence.

Using national averages of annual sugar consumption for research purposes may be misleading. Therefore, daily intake of sugars expressed as grams and proportions of total energy intake per day (*E*%) are preferred in current dietary studies. Evidence shows that when sugars consumption is <10*E*%, dental caries is low [13] but, sugar intake of adolescents can range between 17*E*% and 25*E*% [20,21]. The most recent WHO report on diet, nutrition, and prevention of chronic diseases recommend that the intake of free sugars should be limited to a maximum of no more than 10% of daily energy intake [22] and the frequency of consumption of foods and/or drinks containing free sugars should be limited to four times per day.

While the per capita consumption of sugar-containing products has been fairly stable during the last three decades, the consumption of sweets and soft drinks has increased, for example, in Sweden, Finland, and Australia [23–25]. Use of sucrose in developing countries is rapidly increasing to the levels reported by developed countries, and developing countries are currently major growth markets for the soft drink industry [26]. Consumption of high-sugar desserts and snacks may also be increasing in urban centers in some developing countries [26]. Caries remains a serious problem for disadvantaged individuals in many industrialized countries and is a rising problem in many developing countries [27]. Increasing urbanization and globalization have altered children's diets worldwide, promoting availability and access to processed foods and sweet drinks resulting in significant associations between sweet drink intake and caries experience [25].

RECOMMENDATIONS IN RELATION TO DENTAL HEALTH

Frequent (>4 times a day) and large (>10*E*%) amounts of sugar intake should be avoided.

Information and advice of sugar intake should be given for all parents of infants at maternity/well-baby clinics.

Sugar intake counseling at later ages should be given only for individuals at high caries risk.

Collaboration with schools and manufacturers of soft drinks and sweets should be built to reduce caries and erosion risk of adolescents.

EFFECT OF FLUORIDE

The generalized use of fluoride products is believed to be the reason why currently the relationship between sucrose intake and caries is weaker than before. Fluoride is a preventive agent that has been categorized as strongly cariostatic. Fluoride increases the resistance of teeth to sugar by raising the threshold of sugar intake at which caries progresses to cavitation and moves the dose–response curve to the right.

Although fluoride has had a profound effect on the level of caries progression, it is far from being a complete cure. It is unlikely that there is any concentration of fluoride that will eliminate caries completely. High-fluoride strategy cannot be followed in children to avoid risk of adverse effects due to overexposure to fluoride. Despite community water fluoridation, caries experience of 6- and 12-year-old children has increased since the mid to late 1990s in Australia which is believed to be due to the increased consumption of sweet drinks and bottled waters [25].

PRACTICAL IMPLICATIONS

Avoiding frequent sugar intake combined with toothbrushing twice a day with fluoridated toothpaste can generally be recommended for all dentate subjects commencing from early infancy. The feasible amount for toddlers is a thin smear of toothpaste, while a pea-size of toothpaste can be used for children of 6 years and above. Adolescents and adults, who no longer have developing teeth, nor any risk of overexposure to fluoride, may use larger amounts of toothpaste.

As sucrose intake habits modify the microbial composition of dental biofilm in early infancy, educating counseling and intervening is most important and cost-effective just before harmful sucrose intake habits are born. The recommended guidelines for parents of infants include: avoiding frequent consumption of juice and other sugar-containing drinks in the nursing bottle, discouraging the habit of a child sleeping with a bottle, promoting healthy eating patterns, limiting cariogenic foods to mealtimes, and avoiding sugar-containing snacks that are slowly eaten. Individual sugar intake counseling later in life is highly recommended for patients at high caries risk. Public should be made aware that consuming sweet drinks can have deleterious impact on dental health. Restricting sales of sweet drinks and sweet foods and instead providing healthy food and drinks for purchase in schools is important. Collaboration between public health authorities and manufacturers/distributors of soft drinks and sweets to support caries preventive programs is recommended.

In conclusion, controlling the consumption of sugar is still a justifiable part of caries prevention, however, not the only important aspect.

DIETARY ACIDS AND DENTAL HEALTH

Dental erosion has, for many years, been a condition of little interest to clinical dental practice or dental public health. It starts with softening of the outermost surface by (extrinsic or intrinsic) acids of different origins. This softened layer is vulnerable for abrasion and needs a long time (weeks to months) until it would be resistant against abrasive forces like that of toothbrushing. Only if a strong acidic insult is present, for example, after vomiting, will dental hard tissue dissolve without any abrasive forces involved. Thus, in most cases, overlapping between dental erosion and abrasion is present. Therefore, today the combination of these two processes that occurs in daily life is called erosive tooth wear.

Erosive tooth wear is becoming an increasingly important factor when considering the long-term health of the dentition. It is a condition in which many risk and protecting factors are involved. The interplay of chemical, biological, and behavioral factors is crucial and helps to explain why some individuals exhibit more erosion than others. Erosive tooth wear is not a new phenomenon. What is probably new is the increased attention to it since caries, the main "tooth disease," has been decreasing in many societies, although it is still much more spread compared to tooth wear. There is increasing evidence, from many studies, that excessive consumption of acidic drinks and foods poses a risk to dental hard tissues [28–35]. The prevalence of tooth wear and related risk factors in a sample of 3187 European adults was assessed in a recent study [36]. There were large differences between different countries with the highest levels of tooth wear observed in the UK. Important risk factors for tooth wear included heartburn or acid reflux, repeated vomiting, fresh fruits, and juice intake. In this adult sample, 29% had signs of tooth wear, making it a common feature in European adults.

Indeed, there is a trend toward increased consumption of acidic drinks and foods. In the year 2007, the worldwide annual consumption of soft drinks reached 552 billion liters, the equivalent of just under 83 L/person per year, and this was projected to increase to 95 L/person per year by 2012. However, the figure had reached an average of 212 L/person per year in the US already in 2009 [37]. The erosive potential of erosive agents, including acidic drinks or foodstuffs, depends on chemical factors (e.g., pH, calcium content, and buffering capacity). Biological factors, such as saliva, acquired pellicle, tooth structure, and positioning of the teeth in relation to soft tissues and tongue, are related to the pathogenesis of dental erosion. Furthermore, behavioral factors, including eating and drinking habits, regular exercise with dehydration and a decrease in salivary flow, excessive oral hygiene, and an unhealthy lifestyle (chronic alcoholism), are predisposing factors for dental erosion [38].

It is essential for medical personnel and patients to have a thorough knowledge of the erosive potential of popular dietary substances. Many drinks, foods, and medications, such as soft drinks, sports drinks, juices, salad dressings, candies, herbal teas, alcoholic drinks, vinegar, vitamin C tablets, etc., may be associated with the increase in erosion. Normally, soft drinks are mainly composed of filtered water, citric acid and/or phosphoric acid, artificial additives, and refined sugar. Thus, they offer limited nutritional benefit, but energy. Sports drinks, which are designed to replenish fluids lost during activity, typically contain water, electrolytes, acids, and sugar. Energy drinks are basically soft drinks that contain some forms of vitamins and other chemicals that boost energy for a very short span.

The erosive potential of certain drinks or foods can be estimated using the information in Table 23.1. The pH, calcium and fluoride contents, and the degree of softening (erosion) or hardening of the enamel surface when compared to baseline are given. In this study, enamel specimens were first immersed in 20 mL of freshly collected human saliva for 3 h to form the salivary pellicle. After immersion in the test solution for 2 min, the enamel samples were taken out of the respective solution and the hardness measurement was performed once again. Apple juice, soft drinks, energy drinks, sports drinks, juices, fruits, some medications, and alcoholic drinks caused statistically significant softening of enamel samples during this short immersion time of 2 min. Table 23.1 also shows that yoghurts, black tea, coffee, and mineral water without any acidic additives did not have a detrimental effect on enamel hardness. Flavored mineral water has, in contrast to plain mineral water, a high erosive potential that may not be recognized by consumers. This has some implication concerning dental health because the vast majority of the public is not aware of the erosive potential of these acidic drinks labeled as mineral water. Rose hip tea showed a distinct erosive potential.

In the context of judging the hardness numbers in Table 23.1, it has to be mentioned that decrease of hardness of some units (up to −5) will most probably not cause softening in vivo, because saliva may clear the substance very fast.

It is important to evaluate the different etiologic factors in order to identify persons at risk of erosion. Early detection of such risks is a prerequisite to initiating adequate preventive measures. The modern preventive strategy underlines the importance of training dentists to recognize early signs of erosive tooth wear. Only with these capabilities can dentists provide adequate care for patients. Often, patients themselves do not seek treatment until the condition is at an advanced stage, when teeth have become hypersensitive, or when esthetic appearance is affected. This is particularly true for patients who suffer from anorexia nervosa or bulimia. Dentin hypersensitivity is one possible sign of erosive tooth wear [38].

When dental erosion is detected by a dentist or when there are indications of an increased risk, a detailed patient assessment should be undertaken. All of the causes have to be taken into account. A very important part of the patient assessment is taking a case history. It is advisable to ask for a complete dietary intake for four consecutive days. The time of day and quantity of all ingested foods and beverages, including dietary supplements, should be recorded. Both weekdays and weekend days should be included, as dietary habits during weekends may differ considerably from those on weekdays. The dentist can determine the erosive potential of the different acidic food items and drinks, assess the frequency of ingestion during main meals and snacks, and then estimate the daily acid challenge. Erosion-protecting foods should also be considered.

Based on this information, preventive measures can be tailored to meet the specific needs of each patient. The data obtained from recording all foods and beverages consumed serve as a basis from which to reduce acid exposure and to change dietary habits accordingly. Consumption of acidic foods and beverages should be reduced and those that are taken should be consumed swiftly to reduce the time the products linger in the mouth. Slipping or sucking beverages through the front teeth are habits leading to increased risk of erosion. Adding calcium, phosphate, and/or fluoride ions, or calcium phosphate complexes, may decrease the erosive potential of some acidic beverages or fruit juices. Consuming modified beverages (e.g., orange juice with added calcium, sport drinks containing calcium or casein) is a simple but effective measure to prevent dental erosion [40]. In the case of intrinsic acid exposure, a causally determined systemic therapy should be initiated. Some recommendations [40] to reduce the risk of erosion are given in the adjacent text box.

TABLE 23.1
Erosive Potential of Different Beverages and Foodstuffs, pH, Calcium and Fluoride Content as Well as Change of Surface Microhardness (Vickers 50 mN) After 2 Min Incubation in Different Beverages and Foodstuffs

Tested Product	Important Erosive Ingredients	pH	[Ca] (mmol/L)	[F] (mg/L)	ΔSH_{2-0}
Soft drinks					
Coca-Cola	Phosphoric acid, flavors	2.5	1.1	0.22	−157
Coca-Cola light	Phosphoric acid, citric acid	2.6	0.8	0.22	−277
Fanta regular	Citric acid	2.7	0.5	0.04	−245
Ice tea classic	Citric acid	2.9	0.5	0.76	−84
Ice tea lemon	Citric acid	3.0	0.2	0.58	−86
Ice tea peach	Citric acid	2.9	0.1	0.53	−82
Pepsi Cola	Phosphoric acid, citric acid	2.4	0.3	0.04	−191
Pepsi Cola light	Phosphoric acid, citric acid	2.8	0.3	0.04	−180
Sports and energy drinks					
Gatorade	Citric acid	3.2	0.1	0.05	−125
Powerade	Malic acid, citric acid	3.7	0.3	0.21	−63
Red Bull	Citric acid, taurine	3.3	1.9	0.11	−89
Fruit juice					
Apple juice	Malic acid, oxalic acid	3.4	2.0	0.06	−145
Grapefruit juice	Citric acid	3.2	2.3	0.03	−153
Orange juice	Citric acid, malic acid	3.6	2.0	0.03	−60
Alcoholic drinks					
Beer	—	4.1	1.9	0.06	+1
Red wine	Malic acid, salicylic acid	3.4	1.3	0.07	−31
White wine	Malic acid, salicylic acid	3.6	1.3	0.27	−25
Medication					
Alka-Seltzer fizzy tablet	Acetylsalicylic acid, citric acid	6.2	2.1	0.08	−4
Aspirine-C fizzy tablet	Acetylsalicylic acid, vitamin C	5.5	2.0	0.08	−17
Neocitran	Vitamin C	2.9	4.6	0.09	−250
Yoghurt, milk					
Kiwi Tropicana	—	4.0	45.8	0.04	+7
Nature	—	3.9	43.3	0.04	+3
Mineral water					
Valser	—	5.6	9.9	0.60	−2
Valser Viva Lemon	Citric acid, herbs	3.3	9.8	0.63	−81
Tea and coffee					
Black tea	—	6.6	1.1	1.63	−1
Pepper mint	—	7.5	1.9	0.05	+1
Rose hip	Malic acids, tartaric acid	3.2	2.7	0.05	−181
Espresso	—	5.8	0.7	0.07	+4

Note: A positive ΔSH_{2-0} value denotes hardening of the surface, while a negative value represents softening (in part from [39]).

RECOMMENDATIONS TO REDUCE THE RISK OF EROSION

Reduce acid exposure by reducing the frequency (<4) and contact time of acids (main meals only).
Avoid acidic foods and drinks last thing at night.
Do not hold or swish acidic drinks in your mouth.
Avoid sipping, drink beverages swiftly, no sucking between teeth.
Choose calcium-enriched or modified (sports) drinks and foods with no or reduced erosive potential.
Be aware of acidic medicaments.
Chew tooth-friendly gum to stimulate saliva production and to reduce reflux.
When reflux is a problem: avoid reflux-inducing foods and beverages, such as wine, fatty foods (fried, etc.), tomatoes, coffee, black tea, chocolate.
Suspected gastroesophageal reflux: refer to gastroenterologist.
Anorexia/bulimia: initiate psychological or psychiatric treatment.

In addition to measures discussed above, it is sensible to instruct patients suffering from active erosive lesions about adequate dental hygiene. As a rule, teeth should be brushed immediately after eating. Other instructions should be recommended only if erosive processes are present or vomiting occurs. Recommendation to leave a time interval before brushing is no longer recommended. Dentifrice with low abrasiveness, soft toothbrushes, and gentle toothbrushing techniques are indicated.

The timing of toothbrushing in relation to tooth wear is still a matter of controversy. Some studies report a minimal protective capability of saliva in counteracting the acidic damaging effect. Others indicate that rehardening of the softened tooth surface is a process that takes a longer time. All these studies have used small sample sizes. In a large study sample, little evidence was found ($P = 0.088$) that postponing toothbrushing after breakfast had any effect on the degree of tooth wear. In contrary, delaying toothbrushing for up to 44 min was associated with more tooth wear, which is why postponing toothbrushing could not be considered protective [36]. Generally, dentists should not advise patients to delay toothbrushing after breakfast. Only if erosive processes are present or vomiting occurs, other instructions should be recommended by professionals, for example, toothbrushing and/or rinsing before acid intake. Toothbrushing before meals protects against caries and erosion [41,42].

SUGAR SUBSTITUTES AND DENTAL HEALTH WITH SPECIAL REFERENCE TO XYLITOL

Sugar substitutes, used to substitute sucrose, consist of carbohydrate monosaccharides such as glucose (dextrose) and fructose and disaccharides such as lactose and maltose. These carbohydrates are readily fermented in the dental biofilm (plaque) implicating that they are cariogenic. They have the same nutritive value as sucrose (4 cal/g).

The sugar alcohol or polyol sweeteners are also carbohydrates. Polyols such as erythritol, xylitol, and sorbitol occur in low amounts, for example, in fruits and plants (for formulas, see Figure 23.1). Most polyols are slowly fermented in dental biofilm but erythritol and xylitol show no acid production in dental biofilm. Polyols are used in sugar-free products to give bulk to the product. Except for erythritol, all polyols are laxative which restricts their daily consumption to 10–20 g/day. In most countries, polyols are given a lower nutritional value than that of sucrose.

For properties of the most common carbohydrate sweeteners, see Table 23.2. Sweetness value of intense sweeteners is several hundred times higher than that of sucrose. Most of the intense sweeteners are artificially produced, but stevioside occurs in the nature. Selected properties of the most common intense sweeteners are shown in Table 23.2.

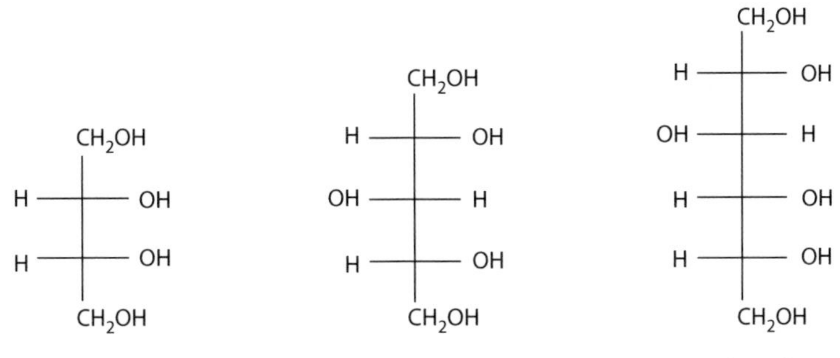

meso-erythritol
122.1

Xylitol
152.1

D-glucitol
sorbitol
182.2

FIGURE 23.1 Structures of the four-carbon erythritol, five-carbon xylitol, and six-carbon sorbitol. The molecular weight of each polyol is shown below the formula [43]. With permission from S. Karger AG, Basel.

TABLE 23.2
Properties of Common Sugars and Tooth-Friendly Sugar Substitutes

Sweetener	Natural Origin	Sweetness[a]	Acid Production in Dental Biofilm
Sugars			
Sucrose	Yes	1.0	High
Glucose	Yes	0.8	High
Fructose	Yes	1.5	High
Polyols			
Erythritol	Yes	0.8	No
Xylitol	Yes	1.0	No
Sorbitol	Yes	0.6	Low
Maltitol	No	0.9	Low
Lactitol	No	0.4	Low
Isomalt	No	0.5	Low
Intense sweeteners			
Aspartame	No	180	No
Saccharin	No	300	No
Sucralose	No	600	No
Acesulfame	No	200	No
Stevioside	Yes	200	No

[a] Sweetness of sucrose 1.0.

POLYOL SWEETENERS, MUTANS STREPTOCOCCI, AND DENTAL HEALTH

Mutans streptococci (MS) counts may not be important in healthy subjects but the early colonization of a child's teeth with MS is considered to increase the future caries risk of the child and high MS counts are a risk factor, for example, in xerostomic patients. In the existing clinical studies, sorbitol consumption neither decreases nor increases the MS counts (for review, see [44]). One study employing very high maltitol doses demonstrates a decrease in MS [45]. However, many studies have shown that xylitol consumption decreases MS (for review, see [46]). Some studies suggest that erythritol may also decrease MS [43].

Several mechanisms have been proposed to be responsible for the xylitol-dependent decrease in MS: growth inhibition with xylitol, elevated pH in the oral cavity acting against MS, a decrease in adhesive polysaccharides produced by MS. The xylitol-dependent decrease in MS appears to be both dose- and frequency-dependent [47]. Xylitol is not retained in the dental biofilm and is not an antimicrobial agent. Therefore, high enough doses and frequent exposure of oral microbiota are apparently needed for the desired "xylitol effects."

EFFECTS ON DENTAL BIOFILM

Considering that dental biofilm is an accepted risk factor of caries, while MS actually are not, surprisingly few studies have addressed the effect of polyols on dental biofilm. Biofilm models appear not to be optimal to study the effects of polyols [48].

TARGET GROUPS OF XYLITOL

Children with erupting teeth
Mothers/persons taking care of infants
Caries-active patients
Patients suffering from dry mouth
Patients with dental biofilm retention (mentally retarded patients, orthodontic patients with braces)

Several clinical studies on healthy subjects have demonstrated a decrease in the amount of dental biofilm in association with habitual xylitol consumption [44,46]. Chewing per se does not explain the decrease in dental biofilm since chewing gum base alone does not decrease the amount of dental biofilm. Sorbitol apparently neither decreases nor increases the amount of dental biofilm [29]. Xylitol dosages large and frequent enough to decrease MS counts also reduce the amount of dental biofilm. However, in the case of poor oral hygiene, the otherwise "effective" xylitol dosages do not seem to affect the amount of dental biofilm [49]. Thus "effective" doses of xylitol may not reduce dental biofilm or show other "xylitol effects" in subjects with exceptional oral conditions. The mechanism by which xylitol reduces dental biofilm can most probably be explained by the mechanisms behind the reduction of MS.

POLYOLS IN CLINICAL CARIES TRIALS

Clinical caries trials with sorbitol have been summarized by Mäkinen [43]. Sorbitol gum chewing can reduce caries occurrence when the gum is chewed for at least 20 min, however, then the "chewing effect" may be responsible for the result. In a recent trial, xylitol/maltitol and erythritol/maltitol lozenges showed no additional caries-preventive effect in low-caries conditions [50]. Of all polyols, by far the highest number of clinical trials has been published for xylitol.

CARIES TRIALS WITH XYLITOL

In the Turku Sugar Studies [51], in which the subjects were caries-active adults, all added sucrose in the diet was replaced with xylitol. Such a sugar substitution, though effective, is unrealistic. After that study all studies have dealt with partial substitution. In other words, sugar substitutes have been added to the normal diet usually in the form of candies or chewing gums. Very few caries trials have been conducted in adults. Recently, 21–80-year-old adults participated in a multicenter xylitol trial. Xylitol decreased caries occurrence on root surfaces but not on coronal surfaces [52].

Most clinical xylitol trials have been conducted on children. When looking at trials with caries occurrence as the outcome measure, a daily xylitol dose of 5 g or more appears to be effective in reducing caries occurrence [43,53]. The trials with low daily doses of xylitol showed no caries reduction. Interestingly, children with erupting teeth have benefited from the xylitol intervention most [54].

In most studies, xylitol was delivered in the form of chewing gums or slowly dissolving lozenges. With such products, the xylitol level in saliva stays elevated for several minutes. Chewing gums and lozenges are, however, not feasible delivery methods for infants. Giving xylitol to infants in the form of syrup [55] or in wipes [56] have decreased caries occurrence compared to control products. These methods being effective in delivering xylitol emphasize that xylitol works even without the involvement of saliva stimulation. Toothpastes with xylitol have received interest even though there are hardly any clinical studies to back up their effect. If toothpaste is used as recommended, the daily doses of xylitol will amount only to milligrams.

XYLITOL IN PREVENTION OF MS TRANSMISSION

Habitual xylitol consumption of mothers with high MS counts reduced the colonization of MS on the teeth of their children 5-fold at the age of 2 years [57]. This was reflected as a significant decrease of 70% in caries occurrence of their children when compared to the controls. A significant difference in caries occurrence was still to be detected when the children were 10 years old [58]. This finding has been confirmed by studies conducted with slightly different study designs in Sweden, Japan, and Estonia.

GUIDELINES FOR POLYOL USE FOR CARIES PREVENTION

There are several guidelines and recommendations concerning polyols in caries prevention. One among the most important is the xylitol recommendation of American Association of Paediatric Dentistry [59]. The most recent systematic review consistently concludes that habitual use of xylitol or polyol combination chewing gum/lozenges is an effective adjunct in caries prevention [60].

There are hundreds of publications on xylitol and oral health. Hence it is quite possible to draw clinical guidelines from these. According to the Finnish evidence-based guidelines for caries prevention [61], it is recommended that mothers of small children should use xylitol products (at least 5–6 g daily) especially if they are caries-active and that xylitol products (min. 5 g of xylitol) reduce the formation of caries when used daily after each meal.

Polyols, especially xylitol and possibly erythritol, offer a prevention method suitable for self-care but also population-based caries prevention programs. More clinical trials are, without doubt, needed but the already existing evidence supports the idea of using xylitol as an adjunct to other caries prevention methods. Especially, caries-active young mothers with infants, children with erupting teeth, and caries-risk patients should benefit from xylitol-based caries prevention.

MORE RESEARCH IS NEEDED ON

The influence of total sugar intake on the prevalence of dental decay in longitudinal study designs
Behavioral factors that influence sugar intake
The efficacy of dietary counseling and nutrition education on sugar intake
Caries-preventive effects of erythritol in randomized controlled trials
The mechanism of action of xylitol
The effects of xylitol consumption on oral microbiota other than MS

RECOMMENDATIONS OF FUTURE RESEARCH

Research on biological and behavioral factors that influence caries risk is needed. More studies are needed on the influence of the total sugar intake in relation to energy intake, the form in which it is consumed and the frequency of its consumption in relation to the prevalence of dental decay. Studies on nutrition education and counseling parents to reduce caries in children are needed. Preventive and oral health promotion programs should be planned and implemented for developing countries. Age-specific caries risk assessment tools with high sensitivity and specificity should be designed.

As caries-preventive polyols, erythritol and xylitol appear to be the most interesting. For erythritol, so far no clinical caries trials on its effects on dental health have been published. In spite of the abundant literature on xylitol, still more research is needed, for example, on the mechanisms of action. Also newer well-designed, placebo-controlled randomized controlled trials (RCTs) are still needed. Very few publications address possible synergistic effects of xylitol and other methods used in caries prevention. Apart from MS, hardly anything is known about the effects of xylitol consumption on oral microbiota.

REFERENCES

1. Grenby TH, Leer CJ. Reduction in 'smooth-surface' caries and fat accumulation in rats when sucrose in drinking water is replaced by glucose syrup. *Caries Res* 1974;8(4):368–72.
2. Rugg-Gunn AJ. Nutrition, diet and dental public health. *Community Dent Health* 1993;10(Suppl. 2):47–56.
3. Frostell G, Birkhed D, Edwardsson S. Effect of partial substitution of invert sugar for sucrose in combination with Duraphat treatment on caries development in preschool children. The Malmö study. *Caries Res* 1991;25(4):304–10.
4. Marsh PD, Nyvad B. The oral microflora and biofilms on teeth. In: Fejerskov O, Kidd E, Nyvad B, Baelum V, editors. Dental Caries, The Disease and its Clinical Management, 2nd ed. Oxford, UK; Iowa, USA; and Victoria, Australia: Blackwell Publishing; 2008.
5. Kirstilä V, Häkkinen P, Jentsch H, Vilja P, Tenovuo J. Longitudinal analysis of the association of human antimicrobial agents with caries increment and cariogenic micro-organisms: A two-year cohort study. *J Dent Res* 1998;77(1):73–80.
6. Meurman JH, Rytömaa I, Murtomaa H, Turtola L. Erupting third molars and salivary lactobacilli and *Streptococcus mutans* counts. *Scand J Dent Res* 1987;95(1):32–6.
7. Fejerskov O, Nyvad B, Kidd EAM. Pathology of dental caries. In: Fejerskov O, Kidd E, Nyvad B, Baelum V, editors. Dental Caries, The Disease and its Clinical Management, 2nd ed. Blackwell Publishing; 2008.
8. Gustafsson BE, Quensel CE, Lanke LS, Lundquist C, Grahnen H, Bonow BE, Krasse B. The Vipeholm dental caries study. The effect of different levels of carbohydrate intake on caries activity in 436 individuals observed for five years. *Acta Odontol Scand* 1954;11[3–4]:232–364.
9. Burt BA, Eklund SA, Morgan KJ, Larkin FE, Guire KE, Brown LO, Weintraub JA. The effects of sugars intake and frequency of ingestion on dental caries increment in a three-year longitudinal study. *J Dent Res* 1988;67(11):1422–9.
10. Szpunar SM, Eklund SA, Burt BA. Sugar consumption and caries risk in schoolchildren with low caries experience. *Commun Dent Oral Epidemiol* 1995;23(3):142–6.
11. Alanen P, Tiekso J, Paunio I. Effect of war-time dietary changes on dental health of Finns 40 years later. *Community Dent Oral Epidemiol* 1985; 13(5):281–4.
12. Newbrun E, Hoover C, Mettraux G, Graf H. Comparison of dietary habits and dental health of subjects with hereditary fructose intolerance and control subjects. *J Am Dent Assoc* 1980;101(4):619–26.
13. Moynihan P, Petersen PE. Diet, nutrition and the prevention of dental diseases. *Public Health Nutr* 2004;7(1A):201–26
14. Honkala E, Tala H. Total sugar consumption and dental caries in Europe—An overview. *Int Dent J* 1987;37(3):185–91.
15. Karjalainen S, Söderling E, Sewón L, Lapinleimu H, Simell O. A prospective study on sucrose consumption, visible dental biofilm and caries in children from 6 to 6 years of age. *Commun Dent Oral Epidemiol* 2001;29(2):136–42.

16. Ruottinen S, Karjalainen S, Pienihäkkinen K, Lagström H, Niinikoski H, Salminen M, Rönnemaa T, Simell O. Sucrose intake since infancy and dental health in 10-year-old children. *Caries Res* 2004;38(2):142–8.
17. Anderson CA, Curzon ME, Van Loveren C, Tatsi C, Duggal MS. Sucrose and dental caries: A review of the evidence. *Obes Rev* 2009;10(Suppl. 1):41–54.
18. Sreebny LM. Sugar availability, sugar consumption and dental caries. *Commun Dent Oral Epidemiol* 1982;10(1):1–7.
19. Sheiham A. Dietary effects on dental diseases. *Public Health Nutr* 2001;4(2B):569–91.
20. Burt BA, Pai S. Sugar consumption and caries risk: A systematic review. *J Dent Educ* 2001;65(10):1017–23.
21. Rugg-Gunn A, Adamson AJ, Appleton DR, Butler TJ, Hackett AF. Sugars consumption by 379 11–12-year-old English children in 1990 compared with results in 1980. *J Hum Nutr Diet* 2007;20(3):171–83.
22. World Health Organization. Diet, nutrition and the prevention of chronic diseases. Report of a Joint WHO/FAO Expert Consultation. *Geneva WHO Tech Rep Ser* 2003;916:105–18.
23. Birkhed D, Sundin B, Westin SI. Per capita consumption of sugar-containing products and dental caries in Sweden from 1960 to 1985. *Commun Dent Oral Epidemiol* 1989;17(1):41–3.
24. Nordblad A, Suominen-Taipale L, Rasilainen J, Karhunen T. Oral Health Care at Health Centres from the 1970s to the year 2000. National Research and Development Centre for Welfare and Health 2004, Report 278, 53 pp.
25. Lee JG, Brearley Messer LJ. Contemporary fluid intake and dental caries in Australian children. *Aust Dent J* 2011;56(2):122–31.
26. Ismail AI, Tanzer JM, Dingle JL. Current trends of sugar consumption in developing societies. *Commun Dent Oral Epidemiol* 1997;25(6):438–43.
27. Zero DT. Sugars—The arch criminal? *Caries Res* 2004;38(3):277–85.
28. Lussi A, Jäggi T, Schärer S. The influence of different factors on in vitro enamel erosion. *Caries Res* 1993;27(5):387–93.
29. Lussi A, Jaeggi T, Jaeggi-Schärer S. Prediction of the erosive potential of some beverages. *Caries Res* 1995;29(5):349–54.
30. Zero DT. Etiology of dental erosion—Extrinsic factors. *Eur J Oral Sci* 1996;104(2 Pt 2):162–77.
31. Parry J, Shaw L, Arnaud MJ, Smith AJ. Investigation of mineral waters and soft drinks in relation to dental erosion. *J Oral Rehabil* 2001;28(8):766–72.
32. Dugmore CR, Rock WP. Awareness of tooth erosion in 12 year old children and primary care dental practitioners. *Commun Dent Health* 2003;20(4):223–7.
33. Phelan J, Rees J. The erosive potential of some herbal teas. *J Dent* 2003;31(4):241–6.
34. Ehlen LA, Marshall TA, Qian F, Wefel JS, Warren JJ. Acidic beverages increase the risk of in vitro tooth erosion. *Nutr Res* 2008;28(5):299–303.
35. Hara AT, Zero DT. Analysis of the erosive potential of calcium-containing acidic beverages. *Eur J Oral Sci* 2008;116(1):60–5.
36. Bartlett D, Lussi A, West N, Bouchard P, Sanz M, Bourgeois D. Prevalence of tooth wear on buccal and lingual surfaces and possible risk factors in young European adults. *J Dent* 2013;41(11):1007–13.
37. Packer CD. Cola-induced hypokalaemia: A super-sized problem. *Int J Clin Pract* 2009;63(6):833–5.
38. Lussi A, Hellwig E, Ganss C, Jaeggi T. Buonocore memorial lecture. Dental erosion. *Oper Dent* 2009;34(3):251–62.
39. Lussi A, Megert B, Shellis RP, Wang X. Analysis of the erosive effect of different dietary substances and medications. *Br J Nutr* 2012;107(2):252–62.
40. Lussi A, Hellwig E, Jaeggi T. Dental erosion. Diagnosis, Risk Assessment, Prevention, Treatment. London: Quintessence Publishing; 2011, pp. 55–60.
41. Lussi A, Megert B, Eggenberger D, Jaeggi T. Impact of different toothpaste on the prevention of erosion. *Caries Res* 2008;42(1):62–7.
42. Wiegand A, Egert S, Attin T. Toothbrushing before or after an acidic challenge to minimize tooth wear? An in situ/ex vivo study. *Am J Dent* 2008;21(1):13–6.
43. Mäkinen KK. Sugar alcohol sweeteners as alternatives to sugar with special consideration of xylitol. *Med Princ Pract* 2011;20(4):303–20.
44. Maguire A, Rugg-Gunn AJ. Xylitol and caries prevention—Is it a magic bullet? *Br Dent J* 2003;194(8):429–36.
45. Ly KA, Riedy CA, Milgrom P, Rothen M, Roberts MC, Zhou L. Xylitol gummy bear snacks: A school-based randomized clinical trial. *BMC Oral Health* 2008;8:20.
46. Söderling E. Xylitol, mutans streptococci, and dental dental biofilm. *Adv Dent Res* 2009;21(1):74–8.
47. Milgrom P, Ly KA, Roberts MC, Rothen M, Mueller G, Yamaguchi DK. Mutans streptococci dose response to xylitol chewing gum. *J Dent Res* 2006;85(2):177–81.

48. Marttinen AM, Ruas-Madiedo P, Hidalgo-Cantabrana C, Saari MA, Ihalin RA, Söderling EM. Effects of xylitol on xylitol-sensitive versus xylitol-sensitive *Streptococcus mutans* strains in a three-species in vitro biofilm. *Curr Microbiol* 2012;65(3):237–43.
49. Merikallio MC, Söderling E. Xylitol as a dental biofilm-control agent in military conditions. *Mil Med* 1995;160(5):256–8.
50. Lenkkeri AM, Pienihäkkinen K, Hurme S, Alanen P. The caries-preventive effect of xylitol/maltitol and erythritol/maltitol lozenges: Results of a double-blinded, cluster-randomized clinical trial in an area of natural fluoridation. *Int J Paediatr Dent* 2011;22(3):180–90.
51. Scheinin A, Mäkinen KK, Ylitalo K. Turku sugar studies V. *Acta Odontol Scand* 1976;34(4):179–216.
52. Ritter AV, Bader JD, Leo MC, Preisser JS, Shugars DA, Vollmer WM, Amaechi NT, Holland JC. Tooth-surface-specific effects of xylitol: Randomized trial results. *J Dent Res* 2013;92(6):512–17.
53. Alanen P, Isokangas P, Gutmann K. Xylitol candies in caries prevention: Results of a field study in Estonian children. *Commun Dent Oral Epidemiol* 2000;28(3):218–24.
54. Hujoel PP, Mäkinen KK, Bennett CA, Isokangas P, Isotupa K, Paper Jr. DR, Mäkinen PL. The optimum time to initiate habitual gum chewing for obtaining long-term caries prevention. *J Dent Res* 1999;78(3):797–803.
55. Milgrom P, Ly KA, Tut OK, Mancl L, Roberts MC, Briand K, Gancio MJ. Xylitol pediatric oral syrup to prevent dental caries: A double-blind randomized clinical trial of efficacy. *Arch Pediatr Adolesc Med* 2009;163(7):601–7.
56. Zhan L, Cheng J, Chang P, Ngo M, Denbesten PK, Hoover CI, Featherstone JD. Effects of xylitol wipes on cariogenic bacteria and caries in young children. *J Dent Res* 2012;91(Suppl. 7):85S–95S.
57. Söderling E, Isokangas P, Pienihäkkinen K, Tenovuo J. Influence of maternal xylitol consumption on acquisition of mutans streptococci by infants. *J Dent Res* 2000;79(3):882–7.
58. Laitala ML, Alanen P, Isokangas P, Söderling E, Pienihäkkinen K. Long-term effects of maternal prevention on children's dental decay and need for restorative treatment. *Commun Dent Oral Epidemiol* 2013;41(6):534–40.
59. American Academy of Pediatric Dentistry, Council on Clinical Affairs. Policy on the use of xylitol in caries prevention. *Pediatr Dent* 2008–2009;30(Suppl.7):36–7.
60. Fontana M, Gonzáles-Cabebas C. Are we ready for definitive clinical guidelines on xylitol/polyol use? *Adv Dent Res* 2012;24(2):123–8.
61. Karies (hallinta) 10.2.2009. www.kaypahoito.fi

24 Dietary Sugars and Cancer Risk

Victoria J. Burley and Janet E. Cade

CONTENTS

KEY POINTS

- Around 30% of cancers in high-income countries could be prevented by improving dietary quality, maintaining a healthy body weight, and being physically more active.
- A number of theories exist as to how sugar could promote carcinogenesis. These are linked to insulin and insulin-like growth factor production, weight gain, transit time, and oxidative stress.
- Assessment of dietary sugar intakes in large epidemiological studies is challenging. Very few studies have differentiated between types of sugar; improved measures of dietary assessment are needed.
- The largest systematic reviews of diet and cancer conclude that evidence on sugar intake and cancer risk is limited.
- Case–control studies but not cohort studies have provided some evidence of positive relationships between sugar intake and cancer risk. Case–control studies are the weaker study design due to inherent limitations around recall bias.
- Colorectal cancer risk does not appear to be increased with intake of sugar, fructose, GI, or GL from the most recent systematic reviews on the topic. This is the cancer with the most evidence available on sugar intake in relation to risk.
- Endometrial cancer risk may be increased with higher intakes of sugar, CHO, and GL.
- One large cohort study has shown an increased risk of esophageal cancer with energy-adjusted sugar intake.

- For all other cancers, the evidence is inconclusive or does not suggest an effect of sugar on risk.

INTRODUCTION

In the USA, about 40% of the population will be diagnosed with some sort of cancer during their lifetime, according to cancer statistics provided by the Surveillance, Epidemiology, and End Results Program of the National Cancer Institute [1]. Rates of incidence and mortality for the most important cancer sites are shown in Figure 24.1. While it is generally accepted that different dietary factors are involved in either promoting or preventing cancers, the range of estimates for the proportion of cancers that may be attributed to diet and related lifestyle variables remains wide and varies by cancer site [2,3]. However, recent estimates suggest that around 30% of cancers in high-income countries may potentially be prevented by addressing dietary quality, through maintaining a healthy body weight, and through being physically active [4].

As reviewed in other chapters, consumption of dietary sugars is increasing worldwide [5], and in this chapter we will review the evidence of how this might contribute to risk of various cancers. Some attention has been given to the effects of sucrose, and a few studies have investigated the possible associations of fructose as well as glycemic index (GI) and glycemic load (GL) with cancer risk. It is plausible that diets, which are high in sugars, may promote carcinogenesis. A number of theories exist as to how sugar could promote carcinogenesis, although these are likely to be site-specific if a true relationship does occur. Sugar consumption may stimulate synthesis of insulin and insulin-like growth factor-I (IGF-I) [6], although other energy-containing nutrients would also have this effect. Insulin regulates energy metabolism and increases synthesis of IGF-1 and decreases a number of IGF-binding proteins [6]. This would lead to enhanced tumor development through promotion of cell proliferation and by inhibiting cell death. High sugar intake may promote weight

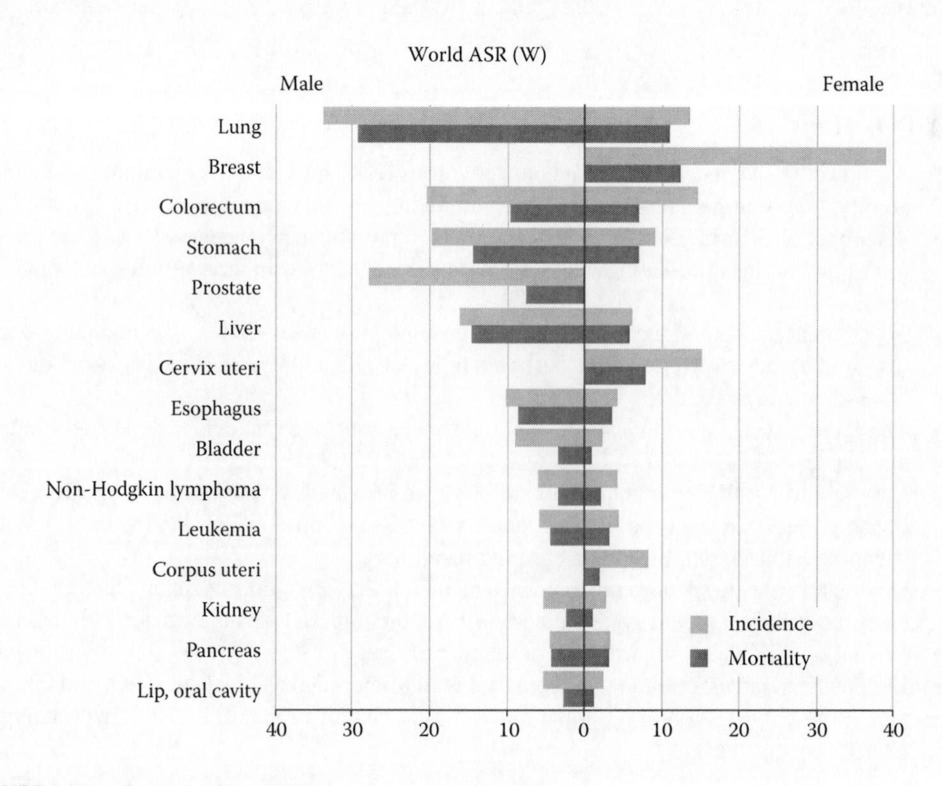

FIGURE 24.1 **(See color insert.)** Risks of cancer worldwide.

gain which is associated with a number of cancers [7]. Sucrose could increase mouth-to-anus transit time and increase the fecal concentration of secondary bile acids [8]; these compounds may have tumor-promoting capacity. Oxidative stress and associated metabolic abnormalities can be affected by carbohydrate intake along with other dietary components [9].

The largest systematic reviews of diet and cancer undertaken concluded that evidence on sugars and cancer risk was limited. The only potential relationship of note was that foods containing non-milk added sugars may increase risk of colorectal cancer [7]. It is particularly difficult to measure the effect of sugars on cancer risk because of inconsistency in the classification of sugars across studies. Dietary sugar assessments in most epidemiological studies are limited to food frequency questionnaires, which are subject to high degrees of measurement error. Urinary fructose has been used as a biomarker of sucrose intake [10], but has not been used in studies linking carbohydrate and cancer risk. An overview of epidemiological studies on carbohydrates and cancer concluded that data from prospective studies are too limited to be able to draw conclusions for an effect of sugars on cancer other than sucrose for colorectal, and perhaps lactose for ovarian cancer, with further research needed [8]. Case–control studies have provided some evidence of positive relationships between intake of dietary sugars and cancer risk [11,12]. However, inherent limitations of case–control study design, especially relating to potential bias in recall of diet, make the interpretation of findings difficult, especially when effects of dietary sugars on cancer may be small. Prospective cohort studies do not suffer from the same biases as case–control studies and have generally not seen positive associations between sugar intakes and cancer risks.

CANCERS OF THE DIGESTIVE TRACT

Cancers of the Mouth, Pharynx, and Larynx

Smoking and dietary factors are thought to be strongly implicated in the development of cancers that originate in the mouth and throat, through being in direct contact with inhaled or consumed carcinogens. Alcohol and smoking are considered the dominant risk factors, but the role of other dietary factors has also been explored in a considerable number of case–control studies and a more limited number of cohort studies [13]. The World Cancer Research Fund considered the evidence available up to 2007 and judged that there was a probable causal protective association between the consumption of nonstarchy vegetables, fruits, and carotenoid-rich foods. Few studies have investigated the relationship of these cancers with dietary sugars or sugar-rich foods.

One case–control study conducted in Italy and Switzerland investigated the relationship between foods groups, macronutrients, and laryngeal cancer in 527 incident cases and 1297 hospital controls [14,15]. Some evidence of reduced risk in individuals with greater consumption of total sugars was observed (OR 0.71, 95% CI 0.48–1.05) when comparing the lowest and highest consumption quintiles. However, there was some evidence of an increased risk with increasing consumption of sugars when analyzed as a food group (OR 1.55, 95% CI 1.04–2.13) when comparing the highest and lowest consumption quintiles. One cohort study has investigated the association between consumption of sugars and risk of cancer of the mouth and larynx. Tasevska et al. [16] explored the risk of 24 different malignancies in association with consumption of a range of different sugar exposures, including total sugars, sucrose, fructose, added sugars, added sucrose, and added fructose in the large NIH-AARP Diet and Health Study. Of more than 400,000 participants who were initially aged 50–71 years, 29,099 men and 13,355 women developed cancer after 7.2 years of follow-up. Oral cancer occurred in 547 men and 205 women and was found to be inversely associated with energy-adjusted added sucrose and added fructose intakes in men, but not in women. Overall, the highest consumers of total sugars, fructose, and sucrose had a 30% lower risk of oral cancer compared with the lowest consumers. No significant associations were observed, however, between dietary sugar consumption and risk of cancer of the larynx. Based on this limited body of evidence, there appears to be some suggestion of lower risk of cancers of the mouth and upper aerodigestive tract in people with higher sugar consumption. However, in both of these studies, multiple comparisons were undertaken, which increases the possibility that some of their findings may have occurred by chance.

Cancer of the Esophagus

Cancer of the esophagus is one of the most commonly occurring cancers worldwide, with higher rates among men (Figure 24.1). It confers a high mortality risk. There are two main types: adenocarcinoma and squamous cell carcinoma. Incidence rates of adenocarcinoma of the esophagus have increased markedly in higher-income countries in the last few decades, but rates of squamous cell carcinoma have remained relatively stable [17]. Tobacco smoking, particularly when combined with alcohol consumption, is a strong risk factor, and abdominal obesity is increasingly being recognized as an important driver for the rising incidence of adenocarcinoma of the esophagus [17]. From a dietary perspective, other than alcohol consumption and body fatness, for which the World Cancer Research Fund judged the evidence as "convincing," most studies have indicated lower risk of this cancer in people with dietary patterns incorporating greater amounts of nonstarchy vegetables, fruits, and foods rich in carotenoids and/or vitamin C [7]. In 2007, insufficient evidence was available upon which to base a judgment concerning the role of sugars and sugar-rich foods in the etiology of this cancer.

Since 2007, one cohort study has undertaken analyses exploring the role of carbohydrates in determining risk of cancers of the esophagus. In the NIH-AARP cohort study, adenocarcinoma of the esophagus was positively associated with consumption of energy-adjusted added sugars (HR 1.62, 95% CI 1.07–2.45) for Q5 versus Q1, although this association appears to be driven by the findings for men, since gender-specific analyses did not reveal an association in women [16].

One case–control study explored the relationship between dietary GI, GL, and risk of esophageal cancer [18]. For each 10-unit/day increase in GI, the odds of squamous cell esophageal cancer increased by 10% (OR 1.1, 95% CI 0.9–1.5), and for each 100-unit/day increment in GL, the odds were increased by 20% (OR 1.2, 95% CI 1.0–1.5). Similarly, in the NIH-AARP cohort study, no association was observed between dietary GI or GL for men and women combined; however, in men there was an elevation in risk in the highest quintile of dietary GI compared with the lowest (RR 1.50, 95% CI 1.10–2.05) [19]. However, case numbers in women were relatively small after just 7 years of follow-up. The authors of the NIH-AARP study indicate that the elevation in risk in men associated with increasing consumption of added sugars may be independent of body mass index, since omission of this variable from the analysis model did not materially influence the estimates of risk. They suggest that since there are parallels between the rising incidence of esophageal adenocarcinoma in the USA and consumption of high-fructose corn syrup-sweetened food and beverages, this finding is worthy of further investigation.

Gastric Cancers

Gastric cancer incidence has decreased worldwide over the last few decades, but it remains as one of the leading causes of cancer death around the world, particularly in males (see Figure 24.1). There is a marked disparity in incidence and mortality rates between richer and poorer regions of the world, with major reductions in higher-income countries relative to low- and middle-income regions [20]. Much of this reduction has been attributed to improvements in general nutrition, but also to improvements in living conditions and standards of hygiene which have lowered infection rates of *Helicobacter pylori*, one of the key causative agents of gastric adenocarcinomas occurring in the noncardia region of the stomach [21]. Interestingly, some research has suggested that hyperglycemia may act as a possible cofactor, increasing the gastric cancer risk of *H. pylori* infection and may increase the risk of developing gastric hyperplasia (a precursor of gastric cancer) [22,23].

There is a limited body of evidence concerning the potential impact of sugars and sugary foods on risk of gastric cancers. The World Cancer Research Fund in 2007 [7] was unable to draw any conclusions concerning the role of these dietary exposures due to the lack of studies at that time. Evidence is suggestive, however, that obesity, and, in particular, abdominal obesity may be associated with increased risk of stomach cancers occurring in the cardia, or upper region of the stomach, and there is therefore some potential for a link here with dietary sugar consumption [24].

Relatively few studies have explored the links between intake of dietary sugars and risk of stomach cancer. One Italian population-based case–control study reported some evidence of a reduction in risk in individuals consuming greater amounts of total dietary sugars [25]. This finding was somewhat at odds with earlier case–control studies that had suggested a positive association with dietary sugars or sugar-rich foods [26–28], but consistent with others that also demonstrated inverse associations [29]. Other case–control studies conducted in Europe and Canada have found no evidence of an association [25,30–32]. Generally, the results of case–control studies have been extremely inconsistent, possibly due to variations in dietary methodology, categorization of dietary sugars, adjustment for presence of *H. pylori* infection, and variation in location and subtype of stomach cancer within the studied population. The one cohort study that has published data on sugar consumption and gastric cancer risk found no evidence of an association [16].

In terms of dietary GI or GL, the evidence base is again rather limited. One case–control study conducted in Italy found no association with dietary GI, but participants in the highest category of GL experienced an elevation in risk of gastric cancer compared with those consuming low-GL diets (OR 1.94, 95% CI 1.47–2.55) [33]. One further hospital-based case–control study conducted in Serbia did not find an association with either dietary GI or GL [29]. Two cohort studies, conducted in Sweden and the USA, have investigated the role of dietary GI and GL in risk of stomach cancer [19,34]. Neither found any evidence of an association, although in both studies case numbers were relatively small. Collectively, evidence of a consistent robust association between gastric cancer risk and dietary sugar consumption or high-GI or -GL diets is lacking.

Cancers of the Colon and Rectum

Cancers in the colon and rectum are one of the most common types of cancer worldwide, with a relatively high associated mortality rate (Figure 24.1). There is considerable geographical variation in incidence rates globally, with many lower-income countries now experiencing rises in incidence, whilst in many higher-income regions, rates have tended to stabilize over the last few decades. In 2007, the World Cancer Research Fund judged that a number of dietary variables were "convincingly," or "probably" etiologically implicated in the development of colorectal cancer. In particular, red and processed meat, alcoholic drinks, and excessive body fatness were suggested to increase risk, whilst foods rich in dietary fiber, garlic, milk, and calcium were considered to be potentially protective [7].

With a more extensive evidence base than for other gastrointestinal cancers, some reviewers have suggested that colorectal cancer risk may be elevated in individuals consuming diets higher in total or added sugars. Based on results from five US and Canadian cohort studies, Key and Spencer [8] suggested that sucrose may elevate colorectal cancer risk, although none showed statistically significant associations. The World Cancer Research Fund (WCRF) also concluded that there was "limited suggestive evidence" that sugar is causally associated with colorectal cancer [7]. More recently, Galeone et al. [35] reviewed the literature on added sugars and risk of colorectal cancer and through meta-analysis, generated a pooled estimate of risk for eight case–control studies and one cohort study. The pooled estimate for the case–control studies indicated a 34% higher risk in the highest sugar consumers compared with the lowest (RR 1.34, 95% CI 1.07–1.70), although there was considerable heterogeneity around this estimate ($I^2 = 67\%$, $P = 0.002$), which suggests that interpretation should be cautious. The one cohort study they identified observed no association between dietary sugars (whether added or not) and risk of colorectal cancer in participants of the NIH-AARP study [16].

As part of the WCRF Continuous Update Project on colorectal cancer risk, Aune et al. [36] undertook update searches of the literature to October 2011 and were able to run meta-analyses of cohort studies that had provided risk estimates in association with sucrose and fructose consumption. The pooled estimates of risk for six and five studies, respectively, comparing highest and lowest consumers, were close to 1, and indicative of no association (sucrose RR 1.01, 95% CI 0.87–1.16 and fructose RR 1.01, 95% CI 0.87–1.27). Accordingly, the authors concluded that there is no evidence of an association between sucrose and fructose consumption and risk of colorectal cancer.

A number of reviews have been published on the relationship between dietary GI and GL and risk of colorectal cancer [35–38]. Using the superior dose–response meta-analysis approach, rather than comparison of high versus low consumption categories, Aune et al. [36] pooled the results of 12 cohort studies. The summary risk estimates indicated no association between either dietary GI (expressed per 10-unit/day increment RR 1.07, 95% CI 0.99–1.15, $I^2 = 39\%$) or GL (expressed per 50-unit/day increment RR 1.01, 95% CI 0.95–1.08, $I^2 = 47\%$) and risk of colorectal cancer.

It may be argued that a distinction should be made between sugars that are naturally occurring and those that have been "added," but the balance of evidence coming from the less-biased cohort studies would indicate that there is little evidence to support suggestions of an independent effect of dietary sugars, dietary GI or GL on colorectal cancer risk.

Pancreatic Cancer

Unlike some other cancer types, which have benefitted from improvements in detection and management in recent years, pancreatic tumors have remained one of the leading causes of cancer death in men and women around the world [39]. Cancers occurring in the pancreas tend to generate few early symptoms, get diagnosed rather late, and lead to poor survival times [40]. One of the key risk factors for cancer of the pancreas is type 2 diabetes, with a 1.5–2-fold increased risk [41]. It might, therefore, be hypothesized that modulations in glucose tolerance that could be induced through long-term consumption of diets rich in simple sugars or rapidly absorbed carbohydrates might be implicated in the development of this particular cancer and therefore warrant exploration as a modifiable factor for prevention.

Aune et al. [42] summarized the results of prospective cohort studies published up to September 2011 that had explored the relationship between dietary carbohydrates and risk of pancreatic cancer. Using a random-effects meta-analysis, the summary relative risk for each 25 g/day increment of dietary sucrose of 1.05 (95% CI 0.85–1.23) was indicative of no association. However, fructose intake was positively associated with risk of pancreatic cancer, with a 22% increased risk for each 25 g/day consumed (95% CI 8–37%). It is noteworthy that all seven cohort studies included in the meta-analysis were conducted in the USA, where soft drinks are generally sweetened with high-fructose corn syrup. The results of the NIH-AARP cohort analysis were not included in this meta-analysis, and in this US study, an inverse association was observed between consumption of added sucrose and added fructose and risk of pancreatic cancer, with some indication of a positive association with naturally occurring fructose (derived from fruits) [16]. Further cohort studies are warranted to tease apart inconsistencies between studies and the separate influences of total fructose, added fructose, and sugars derived from solid and liquid sources.

The relationship between dietary GI and GL and risk of pancreatic cancer has been summarized in two recent meta-analyses of cohort studies. Aune and colleagues undertook dose–response meta-analyses of nine cohort studies that were published before 2011. Neither GI nor GL was associated with risk of pancreatic cancer. Choi et al. [37] synthesized the results from the same number of cohort studies by using a random-effects meta-analysis comparing risk between highest and lowest consumers, rather than through the derivation of dose–response curves. Similar pooled estimates indicative of no association were reported.

HORMONE-DEPENDENT CANCERS

CANCERS OF THE FEMALE REPRODUCTIVE ORGANS

Cohort studies that have explored links between sugars and ovarian or endometrial cancer have focused on measurement of lactose or dairy products rather than total sugars. Lactose is a disaccharide that is found primarily in milk and milk products. Other foods may contain "hidden" lactose, such as breads or cereals. Lactose is converted by intestinal lactase to produce galactose and glucose.

A meta-analysis of three prospective cohort and 18 case–control studies found varying results. The case–control studies did not provide evidence of positive association between lactose and ovarian cancer risk. However, the cohort study results were consistent and showed significant positive associations between intakes of lactose, total dairy foods, and low-fat milk and risk of ovarian cancer. For a daily increment of 10 g lactose (approx. = 1 glass milk), the summary relative risk of ovarian cancer was 1.13 (95% CI 1.05–1.22) [43]. However, there was significant heterogeneity among results of all studies, which may affect the reliability of the findings, although no publication bias was evident. A pooled analysis of 12 prospective cohort studies found a weak, marginally significant positive association observed for lactose and ovarian cancer risk (pooled multivariate RR for 10 g/day increment of lactose, 1.04; 95% CI 0.99–1.08). Lactose intake was highly correlated with milk and calcium intake within this pooled analysis; those intakes were not associated with risk of ovarian cancer [44].

A large Canadian cohort study that followed up women for a mean of 16.4 years observed 264 incident ovarian cancer cases. They found no association between ovarian cancer risk and sugar intake, or for total carbohydrate or GI [45]. However, the large NIH-AARP study which was followed up for 7.2 years found that all sugars investigated (total and added sugars, fructose, and sucrose) were inversely associated with ovarian cancer risk [16] and this was not affected by adjusting for fruit intake. The authors suggest that their results may have been confounded or indicative of a particular dietary pattern.

High levels of circulating galactose have been postulated to be linked with increased risk of ovarian cancer. Galactose is formed from lactose and also found in dairy products, sugar beets, gums, and produced by the body. Galactose may impair ovarian feedback to the pituitary causing increased gonadotropin levels or by direct toxicity to the ovarian germ cells [43]. Case–control studies which have explored the relationship between galactose metabolism and risk of ovarian cancer have not found evidence to support this theory [46–48].

Endometrial cancer risk is linked to reproductive characteristics affecting hormone levels. Consumption of foods with high sugar content promotes insulin production, leading to obesity and potentially hyperinsulinemia. Insulin promotes cellular proliferation and tumor growth by acting directly on endometrial tissue. There are also insulin receptors in the endometrium [49]. Six cohort studies were included in a meta-analysis up to December 2011. A higher intake of total sugar, CHO, and GL were predictors of increased risk of endometrial cancer. The dose–response relative risk for 25 g/day additional sugar was 1.07 (95% CI 1.01–1.13) [50]. A systematic review and meta-analysis of four cohort and one case–control study published before December 2007 found an increased risk for endometrial cancer with higher GL consumption. Risk was increased further in obese women. No significant associations were observed for GI [51]. This implies that endometrial cancer risk may be linked more closely to blood glucose levels and hence insulin. In the European Prospective Investigation into Cancer (EPIC), there were no significant associations between major sugar-containing food groups and endometrial cancer risk. However, there was a slightly increased risk with total sugar consumption. On calibration of the results using 24-h recall values, there was a significantly higher risk associated with total sugar intakes (RR per 50 g/day 1.36, 95% CI 1.05–1.76) [52].

A similar size of effect was found in the Swedish Mammography Cohort. During 18.4 years of follow up in that cohort, 729 participants were diagnosed with incident endometrial cancer. Higher sucrose intake and consumption of sweet buns and cookies were significantly positively associated with increased risk [53].

A meta-analysis of diabetes-related cancers included five cohort studies that had examined endometrial cancer and GI/GL. The aim was to evaluate the hypothesis that GI or GL could predict cancer risk, particularly those cancers related to high levels of blood glucose or insulin. This review found that the highest category of GL intake was significantly associated with a 21% greater risk of developing endometrial cancer compared with the lowest category of intake (95% CI 1.07–1.37) [37].

Breast Cancer

Established risk factors for breast cancer are largely hormonal and reproductive factors. Risk among postmenopausal women is increased by obesity, probably because of relatively high estrogen production in obese women as a result of synthesis in adipose tissue from androgen precursors. Linking this to sugars intake, it is possible that high intakes of sucrose or high GL might increase risk by leading to obesity [8]. However, due to multicollinearity associated between sugars and other macronutrients, it is challenging to characterize risk as a result of sugars intake per se, and even more challenging to ascribe associations to one type of sugar over another. Other possible mechanisms have linked increasing blood glucose levels and measures of insulin resistance. This has been shown to increase risk of breast cancer in an Italian cohort [54]. However, circulating insulin and glucose levels were not predictive of future breast cancer incidence in a small US cohort, although there was a weak association with type 2 diabetes [55].

The World Cancer Research Fund systematic reviews of breast cancer and diet concluded that the evidence was limited regarding sugar, sucrose, sugary foods, and drinks so that no conclusion could be drawn [7]. Only a few cohort studies have explored sugar intakes in relation to breast cancer risk. No association was seen between sucrose and fructose intake in adolescents and risk of later breast cancer in the Nurses Health II cohort study [56]. There was also no association between any sugar (glucose, fructose, sucrose, maltose, lactose, or starch) and breast cancer risk in a Danish cohort of postmenopausal women. In addition, taking into account, tumor estrogen receptor status did not alter the results [57]. The Canadian National Breast Screening cohort also found no relationship between total sugar intake and risk of breast cancer [54].

Consumption of a high GI or GL diet could promote carcinogenesis by inducing hyperglycemia and hyperinsulinemia, linked to the IGF-1 system. A recent meta-analysis illustrated that IGF-1 levels were associated with premenopausal but not postmenopausal breast cancer risk [58]. However, a systematic review of 10 cohort studies and four case–control studies found no positive associations between GI or GL and risk of breast cancer [59]. A further systematic review including 13 cohort studies also found no relationship between GI or GL on risk of breast cancer [37]. The large European EPIC cohort found that overall GI, GL, and carbohydrate intakes were not related to breast cancer. However, there was a significant positive association in postmenopausal women who had estrogen receptor negative (ER–) breast cancer, comparing extreme quintiles of intakes for GL (HR Q5–Q1 1.36; 95% CI 1.02–1.82; $P_{trend} = 0.010$) and carbohydrate intake (HR Q5–Q1 1.41; 95% CI 1.05–1.89; $P_{trend} = 0.009$) [60]. Carbohydrate intake was also positively associated with ER– breast tumors in the E3N cohort of postmenopausal women [61]. The Swedish Mammography Cohort of 61,433 women found a weak positive association between GL but not GI or carbohydrate intake. In this cohort, stratification by estrogen and progesterone receptor status found statistically significant positive associations between GL, GI, and CHO intake for only ER + /PR– breast cancer [62]. It is not clear why there are inconsistencies in relation to hormone receptor status, and evidence to date is limited. GI and GL evaluate different aspects of total carbohydrate intake. GL uses the GI to estimate the impact of carbohydrate consumption taking into account the amount of carbohydrate that is consumed, assessing both the quality and quantity of dietary carbohydrate. GL and carbohydrate intake are correlated, although GL has been shown to be better than carbohydrate content of the diet to predict postprandial glycemia and insulin demand [63]. Nevertheless, caution is required when interpreting estimates of cancer rates linked to GI or GL since impact of total meal composition or meal preparation can affect results [8].

Prostate Cancer

Prostate cancer is the most common malignancy in men in high-income countries. It is a hormone-dependent cancer, and growth factors such as IGF-1 have been associated with risk of prostate cancer. Dietary carbohydrate may play a role in the etiology of this cancer through influences on the IGF-axis or insulin levels. One of the most potent stimulants for insulin production is carbohydrate consumption [64]. The IGF system is also influenced by genetic variation. IGF pathway genes were measured in >5500 Caucasian men and 5500 Caucasian women from the Breast and Prostate Cancer Cohort Consortium. Common genetic variation in the IGF-1 and SSTR5 genes do influence circulating levels although they explain only a small percentage of the variation in circulating IGF-I [65].

Epidemiological evidence linking sugars and prostate cancer is limited. The Malmo diet and cancer cohort found positive associations between intakes of cakes and biscuits and low-risk prostate cancer. However, there was no association between sucrose intake, or sweets and sugar intake and overall prostate cancer. Sugar-sweetened beverage intakes were associated with borderline increased risk of symptomatic prostate cancer [64]. The Prostate, Lung, Colorectal, and Ovarian Cancer Screening Trial did not find any associations between dietary CHO, GI, or GL [66]. A meta-analysis of three cohort studies, all from the USA, which had explored these exposures found no significant associations [37].

OTHER CANCERS

Limited evidence exists for sugar intake in relation to any other individual cancer type. The liver is exposed to high concentrations of insulin and IGF signaling. Deregulation of insulin-linked pathways may promote liver or bile duct cancer [67]. Total sugar intake in 477,206 participants in EPIC was positively associated with hepatocellular carcinoma (HR 1.43, 95% CI 1.17–1.74 per 50 g/day). Higher dietary CHO, GI, or GL was not associated with liver or biliary tract cancer [67]. In a Canadian case–control analysis, GI and GL were also not associated with liver cancer [32]. An Italian case–control study found significant positive trends between GI and GL and renal cell carcinoma [68].

A pooled analysis of the Nurses' Health Study and Health Professionals Follow-Up Study found that sugar-sweetened soda consumption was associated with increased risk of non-Hodgkin lymphoma. However, findings for men and women analyzed separately were inconsistent; men having increased risk but not women. Total and added sugars in the NIH-AARP study were positively associated with risk of leukemia in women but not in men [16].

Lung cancer may be influenced by diet, although smoking is by far the most important cause. Dietary patterns in men from the Netherlands Cohort Study on Diet and Cancer found that the pattern labeled "sweet foods" were inversely associated with lung cancer after multivariate adjustment (RR 0.80, 95% CI 0.70–0.90 per linear increment of 1 SD). This was unexpected; the higher intakes of monosaccharides, disaccharides, fruits, and lower consumption of alcohol associated with this pattern was not able to fully account for the protective effect [69]. Most research looking at diet and lung cancer has focused on fruits, vegetables, and related micronutrients, with little attention given to carbohydrates. No dietary effects on lung cancer have been established. Dietary factors and risk observed in studies are weak and may be due to residual confounding by smoking [8].

CONCLUSION

Despite a large amount of epidemiological research, the precise nature of the effect of sugar intake in the diet on risk of specific cancer types is still uncertain. Very few studies have differentiated between types of sugar, and improved measures of dietary assessment are needed. There is a limited amount of evidence linking reduced risk of mouth and upper aerodigestive cancer incidence with higher sugar intakes. However, risk of esophageal cancer is potentially increased with higher sugar intakes. The evidence around risk of sugar intake in relation to colorectal cancer incidence is more extensive but results are mixed leading to limited suggestive evidence of a role for sugar. Endometrial cancer risk may be increased with higher intakes of sugar, CHO, and GL. For other cancer types the evidence is inconclusive or does not suggest an effect of sugar. The link between sugar intake and obesity is one which is difficult to completely disentangle through adjustment for confounders. Although the epidemiological evidence linking sugars to cancer is mixed, there are potential mechanisms through which the two could be linked. Improved epidemiological methods which take account of all relevant confounders and have more robust measures of diet are needed.

REFERENCES

1. National Cancer Institute. SEER stat fact sheets: All cancer sites. 2013.
2. Danaei G, Vander Hoorn S, Lopez AD, Murray CJ, Ezzati M. Causes of cancer in the world: Comparative risk assessment of nine behavioural and environmental risk factors. *Lancet* 2005;366(9499):1784–93.
3. Parkin DM, Boyd L, Walker LC. The fraction of cancer attributable to lifestyle and environmental factors in the UK in 2010. *Br J Cancer* 2011;105(S2):S77–81.
4. World Cancer Research Fund. Cancer preventability estimates for food, nutrition, body fatness, and physical activity. 2013.
5. Popkin BM, Nielsen SJ. The sweetening of the world's diet. *Obes Res* 2003;11(11):1325–32.
6. Kaaks R, Lukanova A. Energy balance and cancer: The role of insulin and insulin-like growth factor-I. *Proc Nutr Soc* 2001;60(1):91–106.
7. World Cancer Research Fund/American Institute for Cancer Research. Food, nutrition, physical activity, and the prevention of cancer: A global perspective. Washington, DC: American Institute for Cancer Research; 2007.
8. Key TJ, Spencer EA. Carbohydrates and cancer: An overview of the epidemiological evidence. *Eur J Clin Nutr* 2007;61(Suppl. 1):S112–21.
9. Andersen CJ, Fernandez ML. Dietary strategies to reduce metabolic syndrome. *Rev Endocr Metab Disord* 2013;14(3):241–54.
10. Bingham S, Luben R, Welch A, Tasevska N, Wareham N, Khaw KT. Epidemiologic assessment of sugars consumption using biomarkers: Comparisons of obese and nonobese individuals in the European prospective investigation of cancer Norfolk. *Cancer Epidemiol Biomarkers Prev* 2007;16(8):1651–4.
11. Burley VJ. Sugar consumption and human cancer in sites other than the digestive tract. *Eur J Cancer Prev* 1998;7(4):253–77.
12. Burley VJ. Sugar consumption and cancers of the digestive tract. *Eur J Cancer Prev* 1997;6(5):422–34.
13. Lucenteforte E, Garavello W, Bosetti C, La VC. Dietary factors and oral and pharyngeal cancer risk. *Oral Oncol* 2009;45(6):461–7.
14. Bosetti C, La VC, Talamini R, Negri E, Levi F, Dal ML et al. Food groups and laryngeal cancer risk: A case–control study from Italy and Switzerland. *Int J Cancer* 2002;100(3):355–60.
15. Bosetti C, La VC, Talamini R, Negri E, Levi F, Fryzek J et al. Energy, macronutrients and laryngeal cancer risk. *Ann Oncol* 2003;14(6):907–12.
16. Tasevska N, Jiao L, Cross AJ, Kipnis V, Subar AF, Hollenbeck A et al. Sugars in diet and risk of cancer in the NIH-AARP Diet and Health Study. *Int J Cancer* 2012;130(1):159–69.
17. Lepage C, Drouillard A, Jouve JL, Faivre J. Epidemiology and risk factors for oesophageal adenocarcinoma. *Dig Liver Dis* 2013;45(8):625–9.
18. Augustin LS, Gallus S, Franceschi S, Negri E, Jenkins DJ, Kendall CW et al. Glycemic index and load and risk of upper aero-digestive tract neoplasms (Italy). *Cancer Causes Control* 2003;14(7):657–62.
19. George SM, Mayne ST, Leitzmann MF, Park Y, Schatzkin A, Flood A et al. Dietary glycemic index, glycemic load, and risk of cancer: A prospective cohort study. *Am J Epidemiol* 2009;169(4):462–72.

20. Bray F, Jemal A, Grey N, Ferlay J, Forman D. Global cancer transitions according to the Human Development Index (2008–2030): A population-based study. *Lancet Oncol* 2012;13(8):790–801.
21. Uemura N, Okamoto S, Yamamoto S, Matsumura N, Yamaguchi S, Yamakido M et al. *Helicobacter pylori* infection and the development of gastric cancer. *N Engl J Med* 2001;345(11):784–9.
22. Ikeda F, Doi Y, Yonemoto K, Ninomiya T, Kubo M, Shikata K et al. Hyperglycemia increases risk of gastric cancer posed by *Helicobacter pylori* infection: A population-based cohort study. *Gastroenterology* 2009;136(4):1234–41.
23. Jung MK, Jeon SW, Cho CM, Tak WY, Kweon YO, Kim SK et al. Hyperglycaemia, hypercholesterolaemia and the risk for developing gastric dysplasia. *Dig Liver Dis* 2008;40(5):361–5.
24. Crew KD, Neugut AI. Epidemiology of gastric cancer. *World J Gastroenterol* 2006;12(3):354–62.
25. Palli D, Russo A, Decarli A. Dietary patterns, nutrient intake and gastric cancer in a high-risk area of Italy. *Cancer Causes Control* 2001;12(2):2001.
26. Kaaks R, Tuyns AJ, Haelterman M, Riboli E. Nutrient intake patterns and gastric cancer risk: A case–control study in Belgium. *Int J Cancer* 1998;78(4):415–20.
27. La Vecchia C, Negri E, Decarli A, D'Avanzo B, Franceschi S. A case–control study of diet and gastric cancer in northern Italy. *Int J Cancer* 1987;40(4):484–9.
28. Tuyns AJ, Kaaks R, Haelterman M, Riboli E. Diet and gastric cancer: A case–control study in Belgium. *Int J Cancer* 1992;51(1):1–6.
29. Lazarevic K, Nagorni A, Jeremic M. Carbohydrate intake, glycemic index, glycemic load and risk of gastric cancer. *Central Eur J Public Health* 2009;17(2):75–8.
30. Lopez-Carrillo L, Lopez-Cervantes M, Ward MH, Bravo-Alvarado J, Ramirez-Espitia A. Nutrient intake and gastric cancer in Mexico. *Int J Cancer* 1999;83(5):601–5.
31. Lucenteforte E, Scita V, Bosetti C, Bertuccio P, Negri E, La VC. Food groups and alcoholic beverages and the risk of stomach cancer: A case–control study in Italy. *Nutr Cancer* 2008;60(5):577–84.
32. Hu J, La VC, Augustin LS, Negri E, de GM, Morrison H et al. Glycemic index, glycemic load and cancer risk. *Ann Oncol* 2013;24(1):245–51.
33. Augustin LSA, Gallus S, Negri E, La VC. Glycemic index, glycemic load and risk of gastric cancer. *Ann Oncol* 2004;15(4):581–4.
34. Larsson SC, Bergkvist L, Wolk A. Glycemic load, glycemic index and carbohydrate intake in relation to risk of stomach cancer: A prospective study. *Int J Cancer* 2006;118(12):3167–9.
35. Galeone C, Pelucchi C, La VC. Added sugar, glycemic index and load in colon cancer risk. *Curr Opin Clin Nutr Metab Care* 2012;15(4):368–73.
36. Aune D, Chan DS, Lau R, Vieira R, Greenwood DC, Kampman E et al. Carbohydrates, glycemic index, glycemic load, and colorectal cancer risk: A systematic review and meta-analysis of cohort studies. *Cancer Causes Control* 2012;23(4):521–35.
37. Choi Y, Giovannucci E, Lee JE. Glycaemic index and glycaemic load in relation to risk of diabetes-related cancers: A meta-analysis. *Br J Nutr* 2012;108(11):1934–47.
38. Mulholland HG, Murray LJ, Cardwell CR, Cantwell MM. Glycemic index, glycemic load, and risk of digestive tract neoplasms: A systematic review and meta-analysis. *Am J Clin Nutr* 2009;89(2):568–76.
39. Ferlay J, Soerjomataram I, Ervik M, Dikshit R, Eser S, Mathers C, Rebelo M, Parkin DM, Forman D, Bray, F. GLOBOCAN 2012 v1.0, Cancer Incidence and Mortality Worldwide: IARC CancerBase No. 11 [Internet]. Lyon, France: International Agency for Research on Cancer; 2013. Available from: http://globocan.iarc.fr, accessed on 02/08/2014.
40. Cartwright T, Richards DA, Boehm KA. Cancer of the pancreas: Are we making progress? A review of studies in the US Oncology Research Network. *Cancer Control* 2008;15(4):308–13.
41. Huxley R, Ansary-Moghaddam A, Berrington de GA, Barzi F, Woodward M. Type-II diabetes and pancreatic cancer: A meta-analysis of 36 studies. *Br J Cancer* 2005;92(11):2076–83.
42. Aune D, Chan DS, Vieira AR, Navarro Rosenblatt DA, Vieira R, Greenwood DC et al. Dietary fructose, carbohydrates, glycemic indices and pancreatic cancer risk: A systematic review and meta-analysis of cohort studies. *Ann Oncol* 2012;23(10):2536–46.
43. Larsson SC, Orsini N, Wolk A. Milk, milk products and lactose intake and ovarian cancer risk: A meta-analysis of epidemiological studies. *Int J Cancer* 2006;118(2):431–41.
44. Genkinger JM, Hunter DJ, Spiegelman D, Anderson KE, Arslan A, Beeson WL et al. Dairy products and ovarian cancer: A pooled analysis of 12 cohort studies. *Cancer Epidemiol Biomarkers Prev* 2006;15(2):364–72.
45. Silvera SA, Jain M, Howe GR, Miller AB, Rohan TE. Glycaemic index, glycaemic load and ovarian cancer risk: A prospective cohort study. *Public Health Nutr* 2007;10(10):1076–81.

46. Fung WL, Risch H, McLaughlin J, Rosen B, Cole D, Vesprini D et al. The N314D polymorphism of galactose-1-phosphate uridyl transferase does not modify the risk of ovarian cancer. *Cancer Epidemiol Biomarkers Prev* 2003;12(7):678–80.
47. Goodman MT, Wu AH, Tung KH, McDuffie K, Cramer DW, Wilkens LR et al. Association of galactose-1-phosphate uridyltransferase activity and N314D genotype with the risk of ovarian cancer. *Am J Epidemiol* 2002;156(8):693–701.
48. Merritt MA, Kotsopoulos J, Cramer DW, Hankinson SE, Terry KL, Tworoger SS. Duarte galactose-1-phosphate uridyl transferase genotypes are not associated with ovarian cancer risk. *Fertil Steril* 2012;98(3):687–91.
49. King MG, Chandran U, Olson SH, Demissie K, Lu SE, Parekh N et al. Consumption of sugary foods and drinks and risk of endometrial cancer. *Cancer Causes Control* 2013;24(7):1427–36.
50. Aune D, Navarro Rosenblatt D, Chan DSM, Vieira AR, Vieira R, Norat T. Dietary carbohydrates, glycemic index, glycemic load and endometrial cancer risk: A systematic review and meta-analysis of prospective studies. *Proc Nutr Soc* 2012;71:E170.
51. Mulholland HG, Murray LJ, Cardwell CR, Cantwell MM. Dietary glycaemic index, glycaemic load and endometrial and ovarian cancer risk: A systematic review and meta-analysis. *Br J Cancer* 2008;99(3):434–41.
52. Cust AE, Slimani N, Kaaks R, Van BM, Biessy C, Ferrari P et al. Dietary carbohydrates, glycemic index, glycemic load, and endometrial cancer risk within the European Prospective Investigation into Cancer and Nutrition cohort. *Am J Epidemiol* 2007;166(8):912–23.
53. Friberg E, Wallin A, Wolk A. Sucrose, high-sugar foods, and risk of endometrial cancer—A population-based cohort study. *Cancer Epidemiol Biomarkers Prev* 2011;20(9):1831–7.
54. Silvera SA, Jain M, Howe GR, Miller AB, Rohan TE. Dietary carbohydrates and breast cancer risk: A prospective study of the roles of overall glycemic index and glycemic load. *Int J Cancer* 2005;114(4):653–8.
55. Mink PJ, Shahar E, Rosamond WD, Alberg AJ, Folsom AR. Serum insulin and glucose levels and breast cancer incidence: The atherosclerosis risk in communities study. *Am J Epidemiol* 2002;156(4):349–52.
56. Frazier AL, Li L, Cho E, Willett WC, Colditz GA. Adolescent diet and risk of breast cancer. *Cancer Causes Control* 2004;15(1):73–82.
57. Nielsen TG, Olsen A, Christensen J, Overvad K, Tjonneland A. Dietary carbohydrate intake is not associated with the breast cancer incidence rate ratio in postmenopausal Danish women. *J Nutr* 2005;135(1):124–8.
58. Renehan AG, Harvie M, Howell A. Insulin-like growth factor (IGF)-I, IGF binding protein-3, and breast cancer risk: Eight years on. *Endocr Relat Cancer* 2006;13(2):273–8.
59. Mulholland HG, Murray LJ, Cardwell CR, Cantwell MM. Dietary glycaemic index, glycaemic load and breast cancer risk: A systematic review and meta-analysis. *Br J Cancer* 2008;99(7):1170–5.
60. Romieu I, Lazcano-Ponce E, Sanchez-Zamorano LM, Willett W, Hernandez-Avila M. Carbohydrates and the risk of breast cancer among Mexican women. *Cancer Epidemiol Biomarkers Prev* 2004;13(8):1283–9.
61. Lajous M, Boutron-Ruault MC, Fabre A, Clavel-Chapelon F, Romieu I. Carbohydrate intake, glycemic index, glycemic load, and risk of postmenopausal breast cancer in a prospective study of French women. *Am J Clin Nutr* 2008;87(5):1384–91.
62. Larsson SC, Bergkvist L, Wolk A. Glycemic load, glycemic index and breast cancer risk in a prospective cohort of Swedish women. *Int J Cancer* 2009;125(1):153–7.
63. Bao J, Atkinson F, Petocz P, Willett WC, Brand-Miller JC. Prediction of postprandial glycemia and insulinemia in lean, young, healthy adults: Glycemic load compared with carbohydrate content alone. *Am J Clin Nutr* 2011;93(5):984–96.
64. Drake I, Sonestedt E, Gullberg B, Ahlgren G, Bjartell A, Wallstrom P et al. Dietary intakes of carbohydrates in relation to prostate cancer risk: A prospective study in the Malmo Diet and Cancer cohort. *Am J Clin Nutr* 2012;96(6):01.
65. Gu F, Schumacher FR, Canzian F, Allen NE, Albanes D, Berg CD et al. Eighteen insulin-like growth factor pathway genes, circulating levels of IGF-I and its binding protein, and risk of prostate and breast cancer. *Cancer Epidemiol Biomarkers Prev* 2010;19(11):2877–87.
66. Shikany JM, Flood AP, Kitahara CM, Hsing AW, Meyer TE, Willcox BJ et al. Dietary carbohydrate, glycemic index, glycemic load, and risk of prostate cancer in the Prostate, Lung, Colorectal, and Ovarian Cancer Screening Trial (PLCO) cohort. *Cancer Causes Control* 2011;22(7):995–1002.

67. Fedirko V, Lukanova A, Bamia C, Trichopolou A, Trepo E, Nothlings U et al. Glycemic index, glycemic load, dietary carbohydrate, and dietary fiber intake and risk of liver and biliary tract cancers in Western Europeans. *Ann Oncol* 2013;24(2):543–53.
68. Galeone C, Pelucchi C, Maso LD, Negri E, Talamini R, Montella M et al. Glycemic index, glycemic load and renal cell carcinoma risk. *Ann Oncol* 2009;20(11):1881–5.
69. Balder HF, Goldbohm RA, van den Brandt PA. Dietary patterns associated with male lung cancer risk in the Netherlands Cohort Study. *Cancer Epidemiol Biomarkers Prev* 2005;14(2):483–90.

25 Dietary Sugars and Physical Performance

Asker E. Jeukendrup

CONTENTS

KEY POINTS

- Carbohydrate ingestion can improve performance during prolonged exercise (>2 h), but also during shorter higher-intensity exercise (~60 min).
- New proposed guidelines take into account the duration and intensity of exercise and advice is no longer restricted to the amount of carbohydrate, but also addresses type of carbohydrate. In general, smaller amounts of carbohydrate are recommended when exercise duration is shorter, and relatively high intakes are recommended for more prolonged and extreme exercise.
- There is a positive relationship between carbohydrate delivery (ingestion, digestion, absorption), exogenous carbohydrate oxidation, and exercise performance when the exercise is >2 h.
- Combinations of glucose and fructose (or other multiple transportable carbohydrates) have been shown to be most effective in increasing exogenous carbohydrate oxidation and exercise performance.

- The vast majority of sugars ingested during exercise are oxidized (70–90%) and carbohydrate ingestion is usually only a small percentage of the total energy expenditure in athletes (up to 25%).
- Since exercise is a major modulator of the metabolic fate of sugars, discussions on the effects of sugars should take into account physical activity.

INTRODUCTION

Especially in the context of exercise, it is important to define the term "sugars." The term typically refers to mono- and disaccharides including glucose, fructose, galactose, sucrose, maltose, lactose, and a few others. Sugars are a subcategory of carbohydrates, which also contain larger and more complex molecules. It is important to note that from a functional point of view, this subdivision is meaningless, as some of the complex molecules such as maltodextrins and amylopectin, for example, behave identical to glucose, whereas some of the simple sugars such as fructose behave quite differently. Therefore, in this chapter, we will not refer to the term sugar, but will use the term carbohydrate instead. Here we will discuss the effects of different types of carbohydrates on exercise metabolism and performance. This is also a plea to stop using terms such as simple and complex carbohydrates as these terms are confusing since some complex carbohydrates are metabolized much more rapidly than some simple sugars.

Both carbohydrate and fat are important energy sources during exercise. Carbohydrate is the main energy source when exercise intensities are relatively high and therefore essential for optimal performance in most competition settings. Fat stores are relatively large (even in a lean person there is enough for days of activity), whereas carbohydrate stores (in the muscle and liver) are small and may become depleted during 1–2 h of exercise. During exercise, carbohydrates are mobilized from their intramuscular and liver stores for energy production in the contracting muscle. Athletes employ strategies to optimize carbohydrate stores prior to exercise as well as topping up carbohydrate during prolonged activity.

The first report of carbohydrate use during long-distance runs dates back to around 520 BC. The athlete in this report is Pheidippides (539–490 BC), a Greek runner known for his 40-km run from the battlefield near Marathon to Athens to announce the Greek victory over Persia in the Battle of Marathon (490 BC). Although there is debate about whether Pheidippides actually ran this "marathon," it is pretty certain that he was an outstanding distance runner. Amongst many of his long runs, is a run from Athens to Sparta and back, a distance of at least 400 km in 3–4 days, during which he used figs as his main fuel. Figs are a good source of carbohydrate. According to the U.S. Department of Agriculture, a 60 g serving of dried, uncooked figs has 6 g of fiber and 29 g of sugar. A 60 g serving of fresh figs has 2 g of fiber and 10 g of sugar as well as 48 g of water.

Several centuries later in the 1920s, interesting observations were made by Levine et al. [1] during the Boston Marathon. They measured blood glucose in some of the participants of the 1923 Boston Marathon and observed that in most runners, glucose concentrations markedly declined after the race. The investigators suggested that low blood glucose levels were a cause of fatigue. To test that hypothesis, they encouraged several participants of the same marathon 1 year later to consume sugar (candy) during the race. This practice, in combination with a high-carbohydrate diet before the race, prevented hypoglycemia (low blood glucose) and significantly improved running performance (i.e., time to complete the race). Perhaps not the most robust study design, but interesting nevertheless.

In the 1960s, carbohydrate containing sports drinks started to be developed to deliver fluids to the athlete in order to prevent dehydration (but also energy in the form of sugars and other carbohydrates) [2]. In the 1980s, a number of studies demonstrated the ergogenic effects of carbohydrate intake during exercise [3–8]. These effects were initially reported during prolonged exercise (>2 h) but more recently, performance-enhancing effects have also been found during shorter-duration, higher-intensity exercise (30–60 min) [9–13] as well as skill sports where coordination, timing, and other cognitive tasks are an important component of performance [13–16]. This chapter will review the evidence that carbohydrates can enhance endurance performance and will discuss more recent findings on the effects of carbohydrates and in particular glucose and fructose during exercise. The metabolic fate of these sugars will be discussed as well as the mechanisms behind the ergogenic effects and some practical implications.

SUBSTRATE USE

At low-to-moderate exercise intensities, most energy can be obtained from oxidative phosphorylation of acetyl-CoA derived from both carbohydrate and fat (Figure 25.1). At higher exercise intensities, glycolysis is stimulated, and muscle glycogen is rapidly broken down to provide energy. Glucose is also mobilized from liver glycogen stores, transported to the muscle, and oxidized. At higher exercise intensities, fat oxidation is inhibited and fats play a less important role in energy provision. Fat oxidation in extreme cases (very prolonged exercise with depleted carbohydrate stores) has been reported to amount up to about 1 g/min but typically does not reach values above 0.5 g/min (2 kcal/min).

Body stores and maximal rates of adenosine triphosphate (ATP) resynthesis from different sources (phosphocreatine, carbohydrate, and lipid) are shown in Table 25.1. It is clear that fats cannot provide ATP at the same rate as carbohydrates. As such, carbohydrates are the most important energy source at exercise intensities above approximately 65% of maximal oxygen uptake (VO_2max). However, because body carbohydrate stores are relatively small, they may become depleted during exercise and this, as will be discussed below, can contribute to fatigue.

MUSCLE GLYCOGEN

Although noninvasive methods are available (nuclear magnetic resonance), the traditional method of quantifying muscle glycogen content is via muscle biopsy where a small amount of muscle is removed using a biopsy needle. The muscle sample is usually homogenized and the concentration of glycogen is described in terms of the number of "glucose or glucosyl units" per kg of tissue. Normal muscle glycogen concentrations at rest generally range from 60 to 150 mmol glucosyl units/kg wet

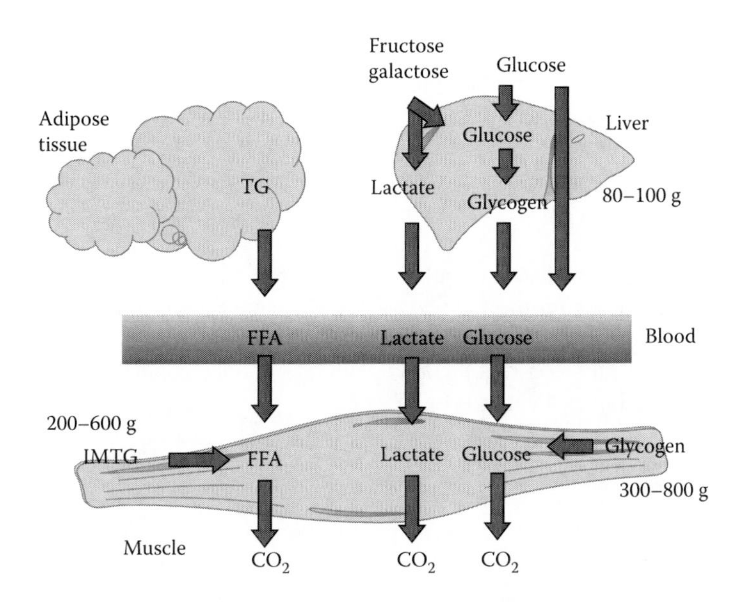

FIGURE 25.1 Substrate use during endurance exercise from different exogenous (fructose, galactose, glucose) and endogenous (adipose tissue triglyceride stores, muscle triglyceride stores, muscle and liver glycogen) sources.

TABLE 25.1
Body Stores and Maximal Rates of ATP Resynthesis from Different Sources

	Duration That Body Stores Can Theoretically Support Maximal Activity Using This Source Only	Max Rate of ATP Resynthesis (mmol ATP/kg ww/s)
PCr breakdown	10 s	2.25
Glycolysis (glycogen → lactate)	5–10 min	1.10
Glycogen oxidation	1–2 h	0.70
Glucose (from blood) oxidation	5–15 min	0.35
Fat oxidation	Days	0.25

weight (ww) or 250–650 mmol glucosyl units/kg dry weight (dw). The total amount of glycogen stored in an average athlete is equivalent to about 500–600 g. Glycogen both in muscles and liver is stored with about 3 g water for every gram of glycogen. Therefore, after a period of oral carbohydrate loading (a method regularly used by athletes where dietary carbohydrate intake is increased, leading up to competition), any additional weight gain will not be entirely due to the increased glycogen content alone, but also the presence of coincident water.

LIVER GLYCOGEN

Liver glycogen content depends on the nutritional state of the individual. For example, in the fed state, an adult liver weighing about 1.5 kg contains approximately 80 g of glycogen. Weight for weight, the liver contains more glycogen than does skeletal muscles. However, skeletal muscles represent by far the largest absolute glycogen store owing to the greater total body mass of skeletal muscles versus liver. After a number of days of high dietary carbohydrate intake, liver glycogen content can increase to about 100 g. Overnight fasting severely reduces total liver glycogen amounts (<20 g) [17]. This is because the main purpose of liver glycogen is to make sure blood glucose concentrations are maintained within a fairly narrow range (4–5 mmol/L). Liver glycogen stores are replenished after a meal but in the fasted state these stores will slowly decline as glucose is released into the circulation.

Acute fasting has no such effect on *muscle* glycogen stores. Muscle glycogen stores remain intact after an overnight fast. The main reason for this is that glucose, once inside the muscle cell, is phosphorylated to glucose-1-P (G-1-P) and the muscle does not contain enzymes to dephosphorylate G-1-P. Once glucose is in the muscle, it is trapped in the muscle and cannot return to the circulation. Muscle glycogen is used when the muscle contracts but its usage is minimal in resting conditions.

In the fasted state, glucose in the circulation is therefore derived predominantly from the liver (with a small contribution from the kidneys). After meal ingestion, glucose may also be derived from carbohydrate in that meal. When we refer to blood glucose as a substrate in this chapter, it is glucose derived from liver glycogen breakdown with or without a contribution of ingested carbohydrate, depending on timing of meal intake.

EXERCISE METABOLISM

Major shifts in substrate utilization occur in the transition from rest to exercise. Metabolism can be accelerated 10-fold, and carbohydrate and fat are rapidly mobilized from their respective storage sites. The relative contributions of carbohydrate and fat to energy production changes with exercise intensity and duration. For example, with transition from walking to running, substrate utilization shifts from oxidation of fatty acids with minor contributions from blood glucose to a large

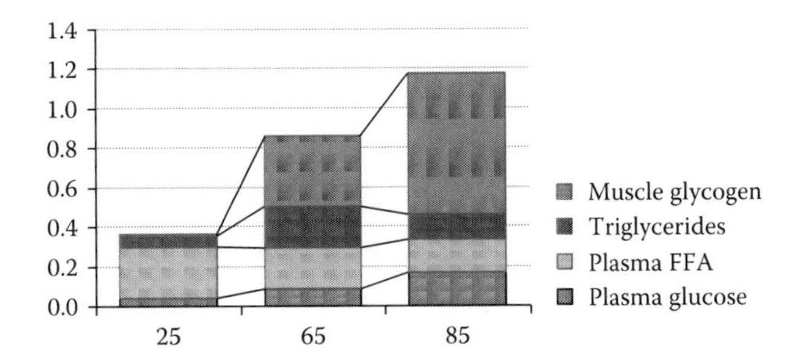

FIGURE 25.2 Substrate utilization during exercise at three different intensities (low intensity, 25% VO_2max; moderate intensity, 65% VO_2max; and high intensity, 85% VO_2max). It is clear that especially muscle glycogen plays an important role at moderate-to-high intensities. (Data from Romijn JA et al. *Am J Physiol.* 1993;265:E380–91.)

contribution of muscle glycogen and a reduced role of fatty acids (Figure 25.2). The recruitment of glycogen to support energy production during moderate to high-intensity exercise is necessary as this shift provides ATP at a rate sufficient to meet the higher energy demands of muscles at greater exercise intensity. Although there is an abundant store of fat in the body, fatty acids cannot be oxidized rapidly enough to support ATP production during heavy exercise. Nevertheless, during prolonged moderate-to-heavy exercise, muscle glycogen is degraded relatively quickly and the rate of fatty acid oxidation increases commensurately. The contribution of blood glucose increases [18] as well. If the exercise intensity increases further, muscle glycogen becomes the predominant fuel, blood glucose contributions increase, and fat metabolism is downregulated. The regulation of carbohydrate and fat metabolism is discussed in more detail in a number of reviews [19–21].

CAUSES OF FATIGUE DURING EXERCISE

Fatigue during exercise is a multifactorial process. Although in the vast majority of situations, no single factor causes muscle contraction to fail, low muscle glycogen content is consistently associated with exhaustion. Muscle glycogen breakdown during prolonged constant-pace exercise occurs more rapidly in type I than in type II skeletal muscle fibers. Nevertheless, at the point of fatigue, muscle glycogen concentrations are very low in both fiber populations. Individual fibers may selectively fail to contract due to insufficient ATP generation caused by local glycogen depletion. One of the main reasons for fatigue, however, is simply a drop in the rates of carbohydrate oxidation (from muscle glycogen and other sources). Fat oxidation is able to support exercise up to about 60–65% VO_2max. If an exercise intensity above that needs to be maintained, carbohydrate is required as a fuel to provide ATP at sufficient rates. If carbohydrate oxidation rates drop below a critical level and ATP cannot be resynthesized at high enough rates, muscle contraction will be negatively affected. At the same time, disturbances in energy status will send afferent signals to the brain. The brain integrates all feedback from the periphery (muscles and other tissues). Through the accumulated afferent feedback from these tissues (lactic acid, ADP, IMP, Pi, NAD+, low muscle glycogen, etc.), the brain is informed about the metabolic state of the muscle and when the number and intensity of these signals increases, the brain reduces motor output to these regions in an effort to reduce the negative afferent feedback.

Low blood glucose concentration, also known as hypoglycemia, is another contribution to fatigue during prolonged exercise. Blood glucose concentrations can decline in situations where exercise is prolonged enough to result in depletion of liver glycogen stores. Thus, without substrate, the liver can no longer sustain glucose production sufficient to maintain adequate blood glucose concentration. The resulting hypoglycemia reduces glucose supply to the brain, further contributing to fatigue. Athletes commonly refer to this metabolic situation as "hitting the wall" or "bonking." Usually at the same time, muscle glycogen is also reaching very low levels. Carbohydrate feeding during exercise is a simple way to maintain blood glucose concentration and prevent hypoglycemia.

CARBOHYDRATE INGESTION DURING EXERCISE AND PERFORMANCE

It has been known for some time that carbohydrate ingestion during exercise can increase exercise capacity and improve exercise performance [22,23]. In general, when compared with placebo ingestion during exercise longer than 2 h, carbohydrate feeding will prevent hypoglycemia, maintain high rates of carbohydrate oxidation, delay the onset of fatigue, reduce ratings of perceived exertion (RPE), and increase endurance capacity. Coyle et al. [4] demonstrated that blood glucose concentrations dropped to very low levels toward the end of exercise when subjects exercised at 70% to exhaustion over 3 h. However, when study participants were fed glucose during exercise, blood glucose concentrations and total carbohydrate oxidation rates were maintained, prolonging time to exhaustion by 1 h. In a follow-up study [6], cyclists exercised at 70% VO_2max until fatigue (170 min) on three occasions. During these trials, plasma glucose declined to very low concentrations (3 mmol/L) and respiratory exchange ratio (RER) fell from 0.87 to 0.81, indicating decreased carbohydrate use and increased fat utilization. After resting 20 min, the subjects attempted to continue exercise either [1] after ingesting a placebo, [2] after ingesting glucose polymers (3 g/kg), or [3] when glucose was infused intravenously ("euglycemic clamp"). Placebo ingestion did not restore euglycemia or RER. However, with glucose ingestion and infusion plasma glucose increased to ~5 mM and RER rose to 0.83. Plasma glucose and RER then fell gradually after carbohydrate ingestion but were maintained by glucose infusion. Most importantly, time to fatigue during this second exercise bout was significantly longer during the carbohydrate ingestion (26 min) or glucose infusion (43 min) compared with placebo (10 min).

These results have been confirmed by a large number of studies [8,24–28]. The ergogenic effects of carbohydrate ingestion have been discussed in more detail in a recent meta-analysis [29] as well as several comprehensive reviews [23,30,31]. It is clear that when carbohydrate is ingested, glycogen from the liver is "spared." Studies have shown that with very high carbohydrate intakes (3 g/min), hepatic glucose output can be completely blunted [32,33]. At lower carbohydrate intake rates, hepatic glucose output may not be completely blocked but it will be substantially reduced [32–34]. Muscle glycogen breakdown seems to be less affected by carbohydrate ingestion.

Since positive effects of carbohydrate feeding were typically seen during exercise lasting at least 2 h, it was believed for decades that the duration of exercise had to be at least 2 h for carbohydrate to demonstrate measurable impact on performance. However, more recent observations demonstrate that carbohydrate ingestion can improve exercise performance during shorter duration exercise of higher intensity (e.g., 1 h around 75% VO_2max). The mechanism behind these performance improvements with carbohydrate feeding during shorter duration, high-intensity exercise is completely different from the ergogenic effects during very prolonged exercise. In fact, no performance effect was observed during exercise at 75% VO_2max with intravenous glucose infusions in spite of accelerated tissue uptake of glucose [35]. This provides evidence that increasing glucose availability, as a substrate to the working muscle, has no effect during this type of activity. Interestingly, however, when subjects rinsed their mouth with a carbohydrate solution, this resulted in performance improvements [11] and these were similar to the improvements seen with carbohydrate ingestion. Therefore, there must be signals from the mouth to the brain that enable a greater power output and improved performance. There are numerous studies now that, on balance, show that this effect is real. These studies are reviewed in several recent papers [11,12,23,30,36]. This would suggest that the beneficial effects of carbohydrate feeding during exercise are not confined to its conventional metabolic advantage, but may also contribute to a more positive afferent signal capable of modifying motor output [37]. These effects are specific to carbohydrate and are independent of taste [38].

In summary, it is obvious that carbohydrate ingestion during exercise can enhance exercise performance. Effects have been demonstrated with intense exercise as short as 30 min and the ergogenic effects seem to be especially robust during very prolonged exercise (>2 h).

The mechanisms during prolonged exercise are of metabolic nature, whereas during shorter high-intensity exercise, where even a mouth rinse can be effective, the effects seem to be through afferent signals to the central nervous system.

EXPLANATION OF CARBOHYDRATE MOUTH RINSE PHENOMENON

It is known that whenever food or drink is placed in the mouth, taste receptor cells (TRCs) are stimulated, providing the first analysis of potentially ingestible food [39–41]. TRCs exist in groups of 50–100 in taste buds, which are distributed across different papillae of the tongue, soft palate, and epiglottis [42]. Electrical activity initiated by a taste cue is transmitted to gustatory neurons (cranial nerves VII, IX, and X) that innervate the taste buds [43,44]. This information converges on the nucleus of the solitary tract in the medulla and is subsequently relayed via the ventral posterior medial nucleus of the thalamus to the primary taste cortex, located in the anterior insula and adjoining frontal operculum, and the putative secondary taste cortex in the orbitofrontal cortex [39]. The primary taste cortex and orbitofrontal cortex have projections to regions of the brain, such as the dorsolateral prefrontal cortex, anterior cingulate cortex, and ventral striatum, which are thought to provide the link between gustatory pathways and the appropriate emotional, cognitive, and behavioral response [45,46]. The fact that many of these higher brain regions have been reported to be activated by oral carbohydrates and not nonnutritive sweeteners [38,47,48] may provide a mechanistic explanation for the positive effects of a carbohydrate mouth rinse on exercise performance. Thus, the actual sensing systems involved may be responding to carbohydrate or energy versus taste per se. To date, the receptors in the oral cavity that mediate these performance-related effects have not yet been identified and the exact role of various brain areas is not clearly understood. Further research is warranted to fully understand the separate taste transduction pathways for various types of carbohydrates and how these differ between mammalian species, particularly in humans. However, it has been convincingly demonstrated that carbohydrate is detected in oral cavity by unidentified receptors and this can be linked to improvements in exercise performance [11]. It appears that this effect is independent of the type of carbohydrate, although further confirmatory research is needed.

OPTIMIZING CARBOHYDRATE INTAKE RECOMMENDATIONS

It appears that in many situations some form of carbohydrate supplementation can have ergogenic effects. More recently, efforts have focused on optimizing the carbohydrate supply and to develop more specific recommendations for athletes in different sports and activities [36]. Evidence is accumulating that greater exogenous carbohydrate oxidation during prolonged exercise can result in better performance [23,49]. Therefore, research has aimed to identify carbohydrates that result in high exogenous carbohydrate oxidation rates [23]. Using stable isotope tracer techniques, the oxidation of ingested carbohydrate (exogenous carbohydrate oxidation) was investigated in a variety of carbohydrate types. It was concluded that carbohydrates could be separated into two different categories: those oxidized at rates up to 60 g/h (or 1 g/min) and others oxidized at lower rates (up to about 35 g/h or 0.6 g/min) (Table 25.2). The "faster" carbohydrates include glucose, maltose, sucrose, maltodextrins, and soluble starch. "Slower" carbohydrates are fructose, galactose, trehalose, isomaltulose, and insoluble starch. The main reasons for these lower oxidation rates include

1. Slower digestion (hydrolysis in the gut lumen)
2. Slower absorption
3. The necessity for conversion in the liver before oxidation by muscle

TABLE 25.2
Different Types of Carbohydrate According to Their Exogenous Carbohydrate Oxidation Rates

	Faster Carbohydrates	Slower Carbohydrates
Definition	Are oxidized at the highest possible rates when ingested during prolonged exercise	Are oxidized at lower rates when ingested during prolonged exercise
Oxidation rates	Up to 1 g/min	Up to 0.6 g/min
Examples	Glucose, maltose, sucrose, maltodextrins, amylopectin	Galactose, fructose, amylose, isomaltulose, trehalose
Digestion	No digestion needed: glucose Rapid: maltose, sucrose, maltodextrins, amylopectin	No digestion needed: fructose, galactose Slow: amylose, isomaltulose, trehalose
Main intestinal carbohydrate transporter	SGLT1 (glucose)	SGLT1 (galactose), GLUT5 (fructose)

Interestingly, the oxidation rate observed with consumption of "faster" carbohydrates can increase up to approximately 1 g/min but not higher [50]. Even when glucose was ingested at a rate of 3 g/min, the observed oxidation rate did not exceed 1 g/min [32]. This concept is reflected in guidelines published by the American College of Sports Medicine, which recommends intakes between 30 and 60 g of carbohydrate per hour for athletes during endurance exercise [51,52]. The upper limit of 60 g/h is a result of apparent maximal oxidation rates of carbohydrates at 1 g/min or 60 g/h.

In theory, possible reasons for the observed maximal oxidation rate limit during exercise include

1. Gastric emptying, digestion for di- and polysaccharides
2. Intestinal absorption
3. Extraction from the liver and storage
4. Uptake by the exercising muscle

It is unlikely that gastric emptying, extraction by the liver, or uptake by the muscle are limiting factors. However, there is evidence supporting the notion that intestinal absorption is the rate-limiting step and contributes most to the observed carbohydrate oxidation rate limit of 1 g/min [30,50]. The following section will discuss intestinal carbohydrate absorption in more detail.

ABSORPTION, DIGESTION, AND METABOLISM OF DIFFERENT SUGARS

The absorption of carbohydrates (mono- and disaccharides) may be passive or facilitated by intestinal transporters. A sodium-dependent glucose transporter called SGLT1 is the most abundant transporter in the intestine and transports glucose from the intestinal lumen across the apical membrane into the epithelial cells. Exit of glucose from the epithelial cells across the basolateral membrane is facilitated by GLUT2. SGLT1 appears to be saturated at a glucose intake around 60 g/h [12,23] and it is SGLT1 and not GLUT2 that appears limiting to exogenous carbohydrate oxidation.

Fructose is absorbed from the duodenum and jejunum through passive absorption as well as active transport by GLUT5, a transport protein located in the brush border membrane. Transport of fructose from the epithelial cell into the circulation is also facilitated by GLUT2.

The capacity of these intestinal transporters is not entirely clear. Textbooks state that the absorptive capacity for glucose is virtually unlimited, but studies during exercise suggest that no more than 60 g/h can be absorbed. GLUT5 seems to have a lower capacity than SGLT1 but this may depend on the conditions. Studies have demonstrated that fructose absorption increases in the presence of glucose. It is well known that fructose, when ingested on its own, is incompletely absorbed and can cause gastrointestinal distress (by promoting a hyperosmolar environment in the intestine). Malabsorption of fructose is reduced significantly in the presence of glucose.

The mechanism by which glucose facilitates the transport of fructose is not completely understood. Sucrose is a disaccharide composed of glucose and fructose. Absorption studies at rest show no differences between glucose and fructose ingested separately or as sucrose [53]. However, studies during exercise seem to demonstrate differences in oxidation rates between sucrose and equivalent amounts of glucose and fructose [23]. There is some evidence that sucrose may pass directly into the body as a disaccharide. Although an intestinal sucrose transporter has not been identified in humans and direct sucrose transfer to the circulation occurs in very small quantities in healthy individuals [54,55]. In addition to the SGLT1 and GLUT5 transport mechanism, there is evidence from animal studies that there might be sugar-induced trafficking of intracellular GLUT2 to the apical membrane which would facilitate both glucose and fructose transport (for review, see Reference 56) Recently, GLUT8 was also implicated in the regulation of mammalian intestinal fructose transport [57].

Most carbohydrates are hydrolyzed in the oral cavity, in the stomach, or intestinal lumen into their monosaccharide components and absorbed through SGLT1 with the exception of fructose and perhaps to a smaller degree sucrose. Once glucose is absorbed, it will be transported to the liver through the portal vein after which it will be delivered to various tissues including skeletal muscles. Fructose is essentially taken up by intestinal and liver cells and is rapidly and almost completely converted into triose-phosphates [58]. It appears that fructose is essentially converted into glucose and lactate in liver cells to be subsequently oxidized in extrahepatic tissues [59,60]. Increased blood lactate concentrations with fructose feeding during exercise suggest that a significant amount of fructose is converted into lactate [61–63]. Lactate is readily taken up by skeletal muscles and is an excellent substrate for oxidation. This will be discussed in more detail in the section on the metabolic fate of fructose.

GREATER OXIDATION OF MULTIPLE TRANSPORTABLE CARBOHYDRATES

Since a single carbohydrate source can only be oxidized at rates up to 1 g/min as a result of saturation of the intestinal transport system, the only way to increase total carbohydrate absorption is to engage different intestinal transporters simultaneously. Indeed, glucose ingested at a rate of >60 g/h in combination with an alternate carbohydrate (ex. fructose) dependent on a different transporter can result in observed oxidation rates that are well above 60 g/h [64]. A series of studies was conducted to characterize maximal oxidation rates with exogenous administration of various combinations of different carbohydrate (for reviews on this topic, see Refs. 12,13,23). In these studies, the rate of carbohydrate ingestion varied as well as type and combination of carbohydrate. All studies confirmed that simultaneous ingestion of multiple transportable carbohydrates resulted in higher oxidation rates than carbohydrate facilitated by a single transporter [22,23]. Up to 75% greater oxidation rates were observed in one study [65]. Interestingly, similar oxidation rates were detected when carbohydrates were administered as a gel [66] or low fat, low protein, low fiber energy bar [67] compared with a carbohydrate beverage.

MULTIPLE TRANSPORTABLE CARBOHYDRATES AND PERFORMANCE

There are several studies that link the increased exogenous carbohydrate oxidation rates observed with ingestion of multiple transportable carbohydrates to delayed fatigue and improved exercise performance. In one study, subjects ingested 1.5 g/min of glucose:fructose or glucose during 5 h of moderate intensity exercise and it was observed that the subjects' RPE was lower with the mixture of glucose and fructose than with glucose alone. Cyclists were also better able to maintain their cadence toward the end of 5 h cycling [68]. Rowlands et al. [69] confirmed these findings and reported reduced fatigue when ingesting a maltodextrin:fructose mix. It was also demonstrated that a glucose:fructose drink could improve exercise performance [70]. Cyclists exercised for 2 h on a cycle ergometer at 54% VO_2max during which they ingested either a carbohydrate drink or placebo and where then asked to perform a time trial that lasted approximately another 60 min. When the subjects ingested a glucose drink (at 1.8 g/min), they improved their power output by 9% (254 W vs. 231 W). However, when they ingested glucose:fructose, there was another 8% improvement of the power output over and above the improvement by glucose ingestion (275 W vs. 254 W). This is the first study to show that exogenous carbohydrate oxidation rates may be linked to performance and the first to demonstrate a clear performance benefit with glucose:fructose compared with glucose alone [70]. Others have since reported similar findings [71,72]. For example, Rowlands et al. [72] studied trained cyclists in mountain-bike races (average 141 min) and laboratory trials (94-min high-intensity intervals followed by 10 maximal sprints). Carbohydrate solutions (maltodextrin:fructose or glucose:fructose in 2:1 ratio) were ingested at a rate of, on average, 1.2 g carbohydrate/kg/h (or 95 g/h). The maltodextrin:fructose solution substantially reduced race time by 1.8% and abdominal cramps by 8.1 points on a 0–100 scale. After accounting for gastrointestinal discomfort, the effect of the maltodextrin:fructose solution on lap time was reduced by 1.1, suggesting that gastrointestinal discomfort explained part of the effect of maltodextrin:fructose on performance. In the laboratory, mean sprint power was enhanced by 1.4% with fructose–maltodextrin.

Performance benefits have generally be observed in studies that are 2.5 h or longer and effects start to become visible in the third hour of exercise [68]. When exercise duration is shorter, multiple transportable carbohydrates may not have the same performance benefits [73], but it must be noted that the effects are at least similar to other carbohydrate sources.

CARBOHYDRATE DURING EXERCISE AND PERFORMANCE: DOSE–RESPONSE

Very few well-controlled dose–response studies on carbohydrate ingestion during exercise and exercise performance have been published. Most of the older studies had serious methodological issues that made it difficult to establish a true dose–response relationship between the amount of carbohydrate ingested and performance. Until a few years ago, the conclusion seemed to be that you needed a minimum amount of carbohydrate (probably about 20 g/h based on one study) but it was generally assumed that there was no dose–response relationship [52].

More recently, however, evidence has been accumulating for a dose–response relationship between carbohydrate ingestion rates, exogenous carbohydrate oxidation rates, and performance. In one recent carefully conducted study, endurance performance and fuel selection were measured during prolonged exercise while ingesting glucose (15,30, and 60 g/h) [49]. Twelve subjects cycled for 2 h at 77% VO_2peak followed by a 20-km time trial. The results suggest a relationship between the amount of glucose ingested and improvements in endurance performance. The exogenous glucose oxidation rate increased with ingestion rate and it is possible that this is directly linked with, or responsible for, improved exercise performance.

A large-scale multicenter study by Smith et al. [74] also investigated the relationship between carbohydrate ingestion rate and cycling time trial performance to identify a range of carbohydrate ingestion rates that would enhance performance. In their study, across four research sites, 51 cyclists and triathletes completed four exercise sessions consisting of a 2-h constant load ride at a moderate to high intensity. Twelve different beverages (consisting of glucose:fructose in a 2:1 ratio) were compared, providing participants with 12 different carbohydrate doses raging from 10 to 120 g carbohydrate/h during the constant load ride. The carbohydrates used were multiple transportable carbohydrates (glucose:fructose). At all four sites, a common placebo that was artificially sweetened, colored, and flavored and did not contain carbohydrate was provided. The order of the beverage treatments was randomized at each site (3 at each site). Immediately following the constant load ride, participants completed a computer-simulated 20-km time trial as quickly as possible. The ingestion of carbohydrate significantly improved performance in a dose-dependent manner and the authors concluded that the greatest performance enhancement was seen at an ingestion rate between 60 and 80 g carbohydrate/h. Interestingly, these results are in line with an optimal carbohydrate

TABLE 25.3
Carbohydrate Intake Recommendations with Increasing Exercise Duration

Duration of Event	Carbohydrate Advised	Type of Carbohydrate
<30 min	No carbohydrate needed	
30–75 min	Small amounts of carbohydrate or a mouth rinse	Any type of carbohydrate
1–2 h	30 g/h	Glucose, sucrose, maltose, maltodextrin, or equivalent
2–3 h	60 g/h	Glucose, sucrose, maltose, maltodextrin, or equivalent
>2.5 h	Up to 90 g/h	A combination of glucose (60 g/h) and fructose (30 g/h)

intake proposed by a recent meta-analysis [75]. It is likely that once accustomed to higher intakes, the optimal intake during prolonged exercise may be closer to 90 g/h or even higher [12].

Based on the studies mentioned above, carbohydrate intake recommendation for more prolonged exercise can be formulated and are listed in newly proposed guidelines in Table 25.3.

CARBOHYDRATE INTAKE IN REAL-LIFE EVENTS

Relatively few studies have investigated how much carbohydrate athletes ingest during races and whether they meet the guidelines. In a study by Kimber et al. [76], the average carbohydrate intake during an Ironman distance triathlon was 1.0 g/kg BW/h in female triathletes and 1.1 g/kg BW/h in male triathletes. They achieved these carbohydrate intakes by ingesting very large amounts of carbohydrate during cycling (approximately 1.5 g/kg BW/h). Most of the intake occurred during the cycling leg where intake was almost three times as high as during the running leg. In male athletes, carbohydrate intake was positively correlated with finish time but this relationship could not be confirmed in females. A large study of endurance events by Pfeiffer et al. [77] demonstrated wide variation in carbohydrate intake reported by athletes between and within events, with highest intakes in cycling and triathlon events and lowest in marathons. In this study, it was also found that in Ironman races, carbohydrate intake was related to finish time with greater carbohydrate intake correlating to better performance. These findings appear to be in agreement with the recent dose–response studies by Smith et al. [49,78].

METABOLIC FATE OF FRUCTOSE

In the liver, fructose can be converted into glucose or lactate [58]. Fructose when ingested in combination with glucose or another type of carbohydrate with SGLT1-facilitated absorption will undergo hepatic metabolism to form lactate [58]. In all studies in which lactate concentrations are reported after the ingestion of fructose, plasma lactate concentrations rose rapidly after the ingestion of the carbohydrate. Lactate is an excellent substrate for the working muscle and it is believed that a large fraction of the ingested fructose in these studies was oxidized through conversion to lactate upon first pass through the liver [79]. It is clear from a number of studies that ingested carbohydrate is largely oxidized. The percentage of ingested carbohydrate oxidized is sometimes referred to as oxidation efficiency [22]. The oxidation efficiency depends on a number of factors including the amount of ingested carbohydrate, type of carbohydrate, and the duration of exercise. Typically 70–90% of ingested carbohydrate is oxidized during the exercise itself [22]. The remaining carbohydrate is likely to be oxidized in the postexercise period when metabolism is still elevated and/or used in liver and muscles to replenish the glycogen stores. There are studies demonstrating that fructose and galactose are preferentially used to restore liver glycogen stores, whereas glucose tends to be stored in the muscle [80]. In these studies, the different carbohydrates were ingested in relatively large quantities postexercise to aid recovery.

SUMMARY

In summary, recently there have been significant changes in the understanding of the role of carbohydrate metabolism during exercise. The new findings allow for more specific and more individualized advice with regard to carbohydrate ingestion during exercise. New proposed guidelines take into account the duration and intensity of exercise and advice is no longer restricted to the amount of carbohydrate, but also addresses type of carbohydrate. Recommendations presented in this review are derived mostly from studies with trained and well-trained athletes. Athletes who perform at absolute intensities that are lower will have lower carbohydrate oxidation rates and the amounts presented here should be adjusted (downwards) accordingly. Recommended carbohydrate intake can be achieved by consuming drinks, gels of low fat, low protein, and low fiber solid foods (bars) with selection determined by personal preference. Athletes can adopt a mix and match strategy to achieve their carbohydrate intake goals. However, carbohydrate intake should be balanced with a fluid intake plan and it must be noted that solid foods and highly concentrated carbohydrate solutions have been shown to reduce fluid absorption. Slowing of gastric emptying and absorption can be partly prevented by using multiple transportable carbohydrates and this is something the athlete should consider when developing their individualized nutrition strategy. Although more research is needed, it is highly recommended to train with a nutrition strategy that reduces the chance of gastrointestinal discomfort and increases absorptive capacity of the intestine. In combination with glucose, fructose stimulates rapid fluid and solute absorption in the small intestine and helps increase exogenous carbohydrate oxidation during exercise, an important response for improving exercise performance.

Since exercise is a major modulator of the metabolic fate of sugars, discussions on the effects of sugars should take into account physical activity.

CONFLICTS OF INTEREST

Asker E. Jeukendrup is an employee of the Gatorade Sports Science Institute, a division of Pepsi Co., Inc. The views expressed in this chapter are those of the authors and do not necessarily reflect the position or policy of Pepsi Co., Inc.

REFERENCES

1. Levine SA, Gordon B, Derick CL. Some changes in chemical constituents of blood following a marathon race. *JAMA*. 1924;82:1778–9.
2. Rovell D. *First in Thirst*. New York: Amacon; 2006.
3. Coyle EF, Coggan AR. Effectiveness of carbohydrate feeding in delaying fatigue during prolonged exercise. *Sports Med*. 1984;1:446–58.
4. Coyle EF, Coggan AR, Hemmert MK, Ivy JL. Muscle glycogen utilization during prolonged strenuous exercise when fed carbohydrate. *J Appl Physiol*. 1986;61(1):165–72.
5. Coggan AR, Coyle EF. Metabolism and performance following carbohydrate ingestion late in exercise. *Med Sci Sports Exerc*. 1989;21:59–65.
6. Coggan AR, Coyle EF. Reversal of fatigue during prolonged exercise by carbohydrate infusion or ingestion. *J Appl Physiol*. 1987;63(6):2388–95.
7. Mitchell JB, Costill DL, Houmard JA, Flynn MG, Fink WJ, Beltz JD. Effects of carbohydrate ingestion on gastric emptying and exercise performance. *Med Sci Sports Exerc*. 1988;20(2):110–5.
8. Murray R, Seifert JG, Eddy DE, Paul GL, Halaby GA. Carbohydrate feeding and exercise: Effect of beverage carbohydrate content. *Eur J Appl Physiol*. 1989;59:152–8.
9. Carter J, Jeukendrup AE, Mundel T, Jones DA. Carbohydrate supplementation improves moderate and high-intensity exercise in the heat. *Pflugers Arch*. 2003;446(2):211–9.
10. Carter JM, Jeukendrup AE, Jones DA. The effect of carbohydrate mouth rinse on 1-H cycle time trial performance. *Med Sci Sports Exerc*. 2004;36(12):2107–11.
11. Jeukendrup AE, Chambers ES. Oral carbohydrate sensing and exercise performance. *Curr Opin Clin Nutr Metab Care*. 2010;13(4):447–51. Epub 2010/05/11.

12. Jeukendrup AE, McLaughlin J. Carbohydrate ingestion during exercise: Effects on performance, training adaptations and trainability of the gut. *Nestle Nutr Inst Workshop Ser.* 2011;69:1–12; discussion 3–7. Epub 2012/02/04.
13. Jeukendrup A. The new carbohydrate intake recommendations. *Nestle Nutr Inst Workshop Ser.* 2013;75:63–71. Epub 2013/06/15.
14. Baker LB, Dougherty KA, Chow M, Kenney WL. Progressive dehydration causes a progressive decline in basketball skill performance. *Med Sci Sports Exerc.* 2007;39(7):1114–23. Epub 2007/06/29.
15. Dougherty KA, Baker LB, Chow M, Kenney WL. Two percent dehydration impairs and six percent carbohydrate drink improves boys basketball skills. *Med Sci Sports Exerc.* 2006;38(9):1650–8. Epub 2006/09/09.
16. Currell K, Conway S, Jeukendrup AE. Carbohydrate ingestion improves performance of a new reliable test of soccer performance. *Int J Sport Nutr Exerc Metab.* 2009;19(1):34–46. Epub 2009/05/01.
17. Nilsson LH, Hultman E. Liver glycogen in man: The effects of total starvation or a carbohydrate-poor diet followed by carbohydrate feeding. *Scand J Clin Lab Invest.* 1973;32:325–30.
18. van Loon LJ, Greenhaff PL, Constantin-Teodosiu D, Saris WH, Wagenmakers AJ. The effects of increasing exercise intensity on muscle fuel utilisation in humans. *J Physiol.* 2001;536(Pt 1):295–304.
19. Jeukendrup AE, Saris WHM, Wagenmakers AJM. Fat metabolism during exercise: A review. Part I: Fatty acid mobilization and muscle metabolism. *Int J Sports Med.* 1998;19(4):231–44.
20. Jeukendrup AE. Regulation of fat metabolism in skeletal muscle. *Ann NY Acad Sci.* 2002;967:217–35.
21. Jeukendrup AE. Modulation of carbohydrate and fat utilization by diet, exercise and environment. *Biochem Soc Trans.* 2003;31(Pt 6):1270–3.
22. Jeukendrup A. Carbohydrate feeding during exercise. *Eur J Sport Sci.* 2008;8(2):77–86.
23. Jeukendrup AE. Carbohydrate and exercise performance: The role of multiple transportable carbohydrates. *Curr Opin Clin Nutr Metab Care.* 2010;13(4):452–7. Epub 2010/06/25.
24. Neufer PD, Costill DL, Flynn MG, Kirwan JP, Mitchell JB, Houmard J. Improvements in exercise performance: Effects of carbohydrate feedings and diet. *J Appl Physiol.* 1987;62(3):983–8.
25. Hargreaves M, Costill DL, Coggan A, Fink WJ, Nishibata I. Effect of carbohydrate feedings on muscle glycogen utilisation and exercise performance. *Med Sci Sports Exerc.* 1984;16(3):219–22.
26. Coyle EF, Hagberg JM, Hurley BF, Martin WH, Ehsani AA, Holloszy JO. Carbohydrate feeding during prolonged strenuous exercise. *J Appl Physiol.* 1983;55(1):230–5.
27. Ivy JL, Miller W, Dover V, Goodyear LG, Sherman WM, Farrell S et al. Endurance improved by ingestion of a glucose polymer supplement. *Med Sci Sports Exerc.* 1983;15(6):466–71.
28. Bjorkman O, Sahlin K, Hagenfeldt L, Wahren J. Influence of glucose and fructose ingestion on the capacity for long term exercise in well trained men. *Clin Physiol.* 1984;4:483–94.
29. Vandenbogaerde TJ, Hopkins WG. Effects of acute carbohydrate supplementation on endurance performance: A meta-analysis. *Sports Med.* 2011;41(9):773–92. Epub 2011/08/19.
30. Jeukendrup AE. Carbohydrate intake during exercise and performance. *Nutrition.* 2004;20(7–8):669–77.
31. Cermak NM, van Loon LJ. The use of carbohydrates during exercise as an ergogenic aid. *Sports Med.* 2013;43(11):1139–55. Epub 2013/07/13.
32. Jeukendrup AE, Wagenmakers AJ, Stegen JH, Gijsen AP, Brouns F, Saris WH. Carbohydrate ingestion can completely suppress endogenous glucose production during exercise. *Am J Physiol.* 1999;276(4 Pt 1):E672–83.
33. Jeukendrup AE, Raben A, Gijsen A, Stegen JH, Brouns F, Saris WH et al. Glucose kinetics during prolonged exercise in highly trained human subjects: Effect of glucose ingestion. *J Physiol (Lond).* 1999;515(Pt 2):579–89.
34. Howlett K, Angus D, Proietto J, Hargreaves M. Effect of increased blood glucose availability on glucose kinetics during exercise. *J Appl Physiol.* 1998;84(4):1413–7.
35. Carter JM, Jeukendrup AE, Mann CH, Jones DA. The effect of glucose infusion on glucose kinetics during a 1-H time trial. *Med Sci Sports Exerc.* 2004;36(9):1543–50.
36. Jeukendrup AE. Nutrition for endurance sports: Marathon, triathlon, and road cycling. *J Sports Sci.* 2011;29(Suppl. 1):S91–9. Epub 2011/09/16.
37. Gant N, Stinear CM, Byblow WD. Carbohydrate in the mouth immediately facilitates motor output. *Brain Res.* 2010;1350:151–8. Epub 2010/04/15.
38. Chambers ES, Bridge MW, Jones DA. Carbohydrate sensing in the human mouth: Effects on exercise performance and brain activity. *J Physiol.* 2009;587(Pt 8):1779–94. Epub 2009/02/25.
39. Small DM, Bender G, Veldhuizen MG, Rudenga K, Nachtigal D, Felsted J. The role of the human orbitofrontal cortex in taste and flavor processing. *Ann NY Acad Sci.* 2007;1121:136–51. Epub 2007/09/12.
40. Bender G, Veldhuizen MG, Meltzer JA, Gitelman DR, Small DM. Neural correlates of evaluative compared with passive tasting. *Eur J Neurosci.* 2009;30(2):327–38. Epub 2009/07/21.

41. Chandrashekar J, Hoon MA, Ryba NJP, Zuker CS. The receptors and cells for mammalian taste. *Nature*. 2006;444(7117):288–94.
42. Scott TR, Plata-Salaman CR. Taste in the monkey cortex. *Physiol Behav*. 1999;67(4):489–511. Epub 1999/11/05.
43. Simon SA, de Araujo IE, Gutierrez R, Nicolelis MAL. The neural mechanisms of gustation: A distributed processing code. *Nat Rev Neurosci*. 2006;7(11):890–901.
44. Stapleton JR, Lavine ML, Wolpert RL, Nicolelis MA, Simon SA. Rapid taste responses in the gustatory cortex during licking. *J Neurosci*. 2006;26(15):4126–38. Epub 2006/04/14.
45. Kringelbach ML. Food for thought: Hedonic experience beyond homeostasis in the human brain. *Neuroscience*. 2004;126(4):807–19. Epub 2004/06/23.
46. Rolls ET. Sensory processing in the brain related to the control of food intake. *Proc Nutr Soc*. 2007;66(1):96–112. Epub 2007/03/09.
47. Frank GK, Oberndorfer TA, Simmons AN, Paulus MP, Fudge JL, Yang TT et al. Sucrose activates human taste pathways differently from artificial sweetener. *Neuroimage*. 2008;39(4):1559–69. Epub 2007/12/22.
48. Haase L, Cerf-Ducastel B, Murphy C. Cortical activation in response to pure taste stimuli during the physiological states of hunger and satiety. *Neuroimage*. 2009;44(3):1008–21. Epub 2008/11/15.
49. Smith JW, Zachwieja JJ, Peronnet F, Passe DH, Massicotte D, Lavoie C et al. Fuel selection and cycling endurance performance with ingestion of [^{13}C]glucose: Evidence for a carbohydrate dose response. *J Appl Physiol*. 2010;108(6):1520–9. Epub 2010/03/20.
50. Jeukendrup AE, Jentjens R. Oxidation of carbohydrate feedings during prolonged exercise: Current thoughts, guidelines and directions for future research. *Sports Med*. 2000;29(6):407–24.
51. Sawka MN, Burke LM, Eichner ER, Maughan RJ, Montain SJ, Stachenfeld NS. American College of Sports Medicine Position Stand. Exercise and fluid replacement. *Med Sci Sports Exerc*. 2007;39(2):377–90. Epub 2007/02/06.
52. Rodriguez NR, Di Marco NM, Langley S. American College of Sports Medicine Position Stand. Nutrition and athletic performance. *Med Sci Sports Exerc*. 2009;41(3):709–31. Epub 2009/02/20.
53. Gray GM, Ingelfinger FJ. Intestinal absorption of sucrose in man: Interrelation of hydrolysis and monosaccharide product absorption. *J Clin Invest*. 1966;45(3):388–98. Epub 1966/03/01.
54. Wallis GA, Wittekind A. Is there a specific role for sucrose in sports and exercise performance? *Int J Sport Nutr Exerc Metab*. 2013;23(6):571–83. Epub 2013/05/01.
55. Tasevska N, Runswick SA, McTaggart A, Bingham SA. Urinary sucrose and fructose as biomarkers for sugar consumption. *Cancer Epidemiol Biomarkers Prev*. 2005;14(5):1287–94. Epub 2005/05/17.
56. Kellett GL, Brot-Laroche E, Mace OJ, Leturque A. Sugar absorption in the intestine: The role of Glut2. *Annu Rev Nutr*. 2008;28:35–54. Epub 2008/04/09.
57. DeBosch BJ, Chi M, Moley KH. Glucose transporter 8 (Glut8) regulates enterocyte fructose transport and global mammalian fructose utilization. *Endocrinology*. 2012;153(9):4181–91. Epub 2012/07/24.
58. Mayes PA. Intermediary metabolism of fructose. *Am J Clin Nutr*. 1993;58(5 Suppl):754S–65S. Epub 1993/11/01.
59. Chandramouli V, Kumaran K, Ekberg K, Wahren J, Landau BR. Quantitation of the pathways followed in the conversion of fructose to glucose in liver. *Metabolism*. 1993;42(11):1420–3. Epub 1993/11/01.
60. Tappy L, Le KA. Metabolic effects of fructose and the worldwide increase in obesity. *Physiol Rev*. 2010;90(1):23–46. Epub 2010/01/21.
61. Jentjens RL, Achten J, Jeukendrup AE. High oxidation rates from combined carbohydrates ingested during exercise. *Med Sci Sports Exerc*. 2004;36(9):1551–8. Epub 2004/09/09.
62. Jentjens RL, Venables MC, Jeukendrup AE. Oxidation of exogenous glucose, sucrose, and maltose during prolonged cycling exercise. *J Appl Physiol*. 2004;96(4):1285–91.
63. Jentjens RL, Shaw C, Birtles T, Waring RH, Harding LK, Jeukendrup AE. Oxidation of combined ingestion of glucose and sucrose during exercise. *Metabolism*. 2005;54(5):610–8. Epub 2005/05/07.
64. Jentjens RL, Moseley L, Waring RH, Harding LK, Jeukendrup AE. Oxidation of combined ingestion of glucose and fructose during exercise. *J Appl Physiol*. 2004;96(4):1277–84.
65. Jentjens RL, Jeukendrup AE. High rates of exogenous carbohydrate oxidation from a mixture of glucose and fructose ingested during prolonged cycling exercise. *Br J Nutr*. 2005;93(4):485–92.
66. Pfeiffer B, Stellingwerff T, Zaltas E, Jeukendrup AE. Cho oxidation from a Cho gel compared with a drink during exercise. *Med Sci Sports Exerc*. 2010;42(11):2038–45. Epub 2010/04/21.
67. Pfeiffer B, Stellingwerff T, Zaltas E, Jeukendrup AE. Oxidation of solid versus liquid Cho sources during exercise. *Med Sci Sports Exerc*. 2010;42(11):2030–7. Epub 2010/04/21.
68. Jeukendrup AE, Moseley L, Mainwaring GI, Samuels S, Perry S, Mann CH. Exogenous carbohydrate oxidation during ultraendurance exercise. *J Appl Physiol*. 2006;100(4):1134–41.

69. Rowlands DS, Thorburn MS, Thorp RM, Broadbent S, Shi X. Effect of graded fructose coingestion with maltodextrin on exogenous ^{14}C-fructose and ^{13}C-glucose oxidation efficiency and high-intensity cycling performance. *J Appl Physiol.* 2008;104(6):1709–19. Epub 2008/03/29.
70. Currell K, Jeukendrup AE. Superior endurance performance with ingestion of multiple transportable carbohydrates. *Med Sci Sports Exerc.* 2008;40(2):275–81. Epub 2008/01/19.
71. Triplett D, Doyle JA, Rupp JC, Benardot D. An isocaloric glucose–fructose beverage's effect on simulated 100-km cycling performance compared with a glucose-only beverage. *Int J Sport Nutr Exerc Metab.* 2010;20(2):122–31. Epub 2010/05/19.
72. Rowlands DS, Swift M, Ros M, Green JG. Composite versus single transportable carbohydrate solution enhances race and laboratory cycling performance. *Appl Physiol Nutr Metab.* 2012;37(3):425–36. Epub 2012/04/04.
73. Hulston CJ, Wallis GA, Jeukendrup AE. Exogenous Cho oxidation with glucose plus fructose intake during exercise. *Med Sci Sports Exerc.* 2009;41(2):357–63. Epub 2009/01/08.
74. Smith JW, Zachwieja JJ, Horswill CA, Pascoe DD, Passe D, Ruby BC et al. Evidence of a carbohydrate dose and prolonged exercise performance relationship. *Med Sci Sports Exerc.* 2010;42(5):84.
75. Vandenbogaerde TJ, Hopkins WG. Monitoring acute effects on athletic performance with mixed linear modeling. *Med Sci Sports Exerc.* 2010;42(7):1339–44. Epub 2010/01/14.
76. Kimber NE, Ross JJ, Mason SL, Speedy DB. Energy balance during an ironman triathlon in male and female triathletes. *Int J Sport Nutr Exerc Metab.* 2002;12(1):47–62.
77. Pfeiffer B, Stellingwerff T, Hodgson AB, Randell R, Poettgen K, Res P et al. Nutritional intake and gastrointestinal problems during competitive endurance events. *Med Sci Sports Exerc.* 2012;44(2):344–51.
78. Smith JW, Pascoe DD, Passe DH, Ruby BC, Stewart LK, Baker LB et al. Curvilinear dose–response relationship of carbohydrate (0–120 g h^{-1}) and performance. *Med Sci Sports Exerc.* 2013;45(2):336–41. Epub 2012/09/13.
79. Lecoultre V, Benoit R, Carrel G, Schutz Y, Millet GP, Tappy L et al. Fructose and glucose co-ingestion during prolonged exercise increases lactate and glucose fluxes and oxidation compared with an equimolar intake of glucose. *Am J Clin Nutr.* 2010;92(5):1071–9. Epub 2010/09/10.
80. Decombaz J, Jentjens R, Ith M, Scheurer E, Buehler T, Jeukendrup A et al. Fructose and galactose enhance postexercise human liver glycogen synthesis. *Med Sci Sports Exerc.* 2011;43(10):1964–71. Epub 2011/03/17.
81. Romijn JA, Coyle EF, Sidossis LS, Gastaldelli A, Horowitz JF, Endert E et al. Regulation of endogenous fat and carbohydrate metabolism in relation to exercise intensity. *Am J Physiol.* 1993;265:E380–91.

26 Toward Evidence-Based Policies for Reduction of Dietary Sugars

Lessons from the Alcohol Experience

Laura A. Schmidt, Anisha I. Patel, Claire D. Brindis, and Robert H. Lustig

CONTENTS

KEY POINTS

- Obesity is not the only problem resulting from the overconsumption of added sugars. Metabolic syndrome, linked to the excess intake of added sugars, underlies most forms of chronic disease.

- Normal-weight people can experience metabolic syndrome. To the extent that added sugar overconsumption promotes metabolic disease, it poses a population-wide public health problem.
- Sugar and alcohol have parallels at multiple levels—they have metabolic, hedonic, cultural, and market similarities.
- Alcohol control provides an appropriate paradigm for reducing sugar consumption population-wide.
- Preconditions for the societal regulation of a substance include ubiquity, toxicity, abuse, and externalities. Added sugars meet all four.
- Public education and governmental guidelines alone are unlikely to alter consumption. Saturation of added sugars in the food supply must be addressed as well.
- The "iron law of public health policy" states that reductions in the availability of harmful substances will reduce their consumption, thereby reducing related health harms at the population level.
- Effective population-based strategies for reducing added sugar consumption include taxation, price controls, alteration of subsidies, regulation of sales and distribution, regulation of marketing and advertising, and subsidy withdrawal.

INTRODUCTION

Preceding chapters in this volume have reviewed data implicating the widespread availability and overconsumption of added dietary sugars as a determinant of chronic disease. By "overconsumption," we mean the consumption of added sugars (i.e., not those occurring naturally in foods such as fruits) beyond limits recommended by impartial scientific bodies such as the American Heart Association [1]. So far, public debate around the role of added sugars in health has targeted obesity and, to a lesser extent, dental disease. But a growing body of evidence suggests that obesity should not be the primary focus of concern. Metabolic syndrome, linked to the extended overconsumption of added sugars, is an underlying factor in most forms of chronic disease—diseases that are now the leading cause of death worldwide [2,3]. Some studies show that 20% of those deemed morbidly obese are metabolically healthy and will go on to have normal life spans [4,5]. Meanwhile up to 40% of normal-weight adults harbor metabolic perturbations typically seen in the obese and may manifest in metabolic syndrome, with its hallmarks being insulin resistance, hypertension, dyslipidemia, high cholesterol, and disproportionate waist circumstance [6,7].

Bench and clinical science findings on dietary sugars continue to be debated both in the halls of academe and by business enterprises that purvey sugary beverages and packaged foodstuffs [8–11]. There are legitimate concerns about *when* the science is solid enough that governments should act to reduce consumption of dietary sugars at the population level. And once government actors decide to intervene, there are further questions about precisely *how* to do so effectively, and particularly how to do so in ways that avoid substitution of sugar with other dietary components that are equally or even more detrimental to health [12].

Within US borders, these concerns, combined with industry lobbying, have thus far prevented meaningful policy changes that could substantially reduce intake of added dietary sugars population-wide [13]. This is ironic since Americans are among the most affected by the overconsumption of added sugars on a global basis, consuming on average nearly three times the dietary limit recommended by impartial expert panels [1]. Meanwhile, we are witnessing a global trend toward stricter regulation of sugar-laden foods and beverages. Fifteen countries, including Mexico most recently, have adopted sugar taxation regimes and more are currently deliberating [14]. At least one international bank has called for taxation as the most credible option for reducing the resultant health-care costs [15].

Even in the absence of meaningful policy change in America, the rising tide of scientific evidence has begun to shift the debate toward new concerns about metabolic disease, liver damage, and the potential addictive properties of added sugars [16]. This information is filtering through the medical community and down to individual consumers, leading to some changes in attitudes toward sugar. Thus, a recent report documents that 90% of physicians view dietary sugars as causative of diabetes and 65% view them as addictive [15]. Shifts in popular opinion have led to recent calls for stronger government intervention [17–19].

This chapter is motivated by an interest in promoting knowledge about evidence-based policy solutions to the health harms associated with the overconsumption of added sugars. Admittedly, this is challenging in the absence of a large body of public health evidence showing what does and does not work to prevent sugar-related health harms. Since the early 1970s, consumption of added sugars and related disease rates have precipitously climbed, leaving little time to accumulate all the evidence needed to advise policymakers. Given this, a useful strategy is to draw evidence from analogous or closely related public health issues where the evidence is vast and robust. So far, two substances have provided templates for such a regulatory framework: tobacco and alcohol. While tobacco provides a useful paradigm in some respects, it differs from sugar on several counts. Unlike sugar, tobacco is not a source of energy or nutrition, no amount of tobacco exposure is deemed safe, and its production and distribution channels are easily identified, that is, the tobacco market is concentrated in a few companies producing relatively few tobacco products. As elaborated below, we proffer that the alcohol paradigm is more immediately relevant to the debate surrounding dietary sugar policy.

Our goal is to first provide a bird's eye view of the alcohol literature and its relevance to sugar policy—one that will hopefully enable scientists and policymakers to better understand the connections between alcohol and sugar, both with respect to their health harms and policy solutions. Over the long history of alcohol policymaking, we have observed a gradual shift away from interventions solely directed towards changing individual health behaviors and toward those focused on the environment [20,21]. We argue that sugar policy should track the same pathway toward environmentally focused reforms. Hopefully, the world's 1500-year experience with controlling the harmful effects of alcohol overconsumption can allow us to truncate the process of political learning with respect to added sugars. Doing so will lead policymakers toward solutions focused on the food environment and toward policies that target marketing and availability—solutions that have proved successful with alcohol on a worldwide basis.

WHY IS ALCOHOL POLICY SO RELEVANT?

With respect to human health, as well as matters of public policy, there are important similarities between alcohol and dietary sugars. First, both are legal substances that have the built-in risk of producing potential health harms when overused. For both alcohol and sugar, particular patterns of overuse are important for short- and long-term health impacts. For alcohol, negative outcomes can be *acute*, such as binge drinking with its associated likelihood of acute health harms (e.g., respiratory depression, auto accidents, and other unintentional injuries). Alcohol overconsumption also has *chronic* impacts on health, such as long-term debilitating diseases including liver disease, heart disease, cancer, and dementia. While a majority of the health harms associated with added sugar overconsumption are chronic in nature, some acute harms have been observed, ranging from binge behavior to sugar-induced diabetic coma. Notably, many of the chronic health effects shared by sugar and alcohol involve elements of the metabolic syndrome, such as hypertension and dyslipidemia [22]. This comes as no surprise given that alcohol is obtained from the fermentation of sugars. Moreover, fructose, a common sugar, and alcohol are metabolized within the liver in a virtually identical fashion. It follows that their overconsumption would impact similar metabolic disease outcomes [23]. It should be noted that fructose and glucose have different effects on blood flow and in activating brain neural circuitry [24], such that their parallels with alcohol's effects will vary (see Chapter 15).

There are also neurobiological parallels between alcohol and sugar, including altered dopamine neurotransmission and reduced dopamine receptors suggestive of physical tolerance

[25,26]. Although not all scientists are convinced of the parallels, neuroimaging studies suggest that both sucrose and alcohol activate reward circuitry in the limbic region of the brain and that the pattern of activation is different from that of dietary fat [27]. This is taken by some as evidence that sucrose is capable of producing both reward and tolerance [28]. It has also been established that, particularly among women, there are common biological vulnerabilities to alcoholism and obesity and that the population prevalence of their co-occurrence is increasing over time due to the increased availability of highly palatable, sugary foods, and beverages [29].

Dietary sugars and alcohol also share important parallels in modern consumer societies, creating a basis for arguing that similar regulatory strategies would be appropriate. Both are highly profitable market commodities, with market shares and international trade driven by powerful, multinational corporations. Strategies for the marketing, sales, and distribution of alcohol bear striking similarities to those used by sugary beverage and food manufacturers. Furthermore, for both alcohol and added sugar, a disproportionate burden of the population-level health burden falls on low-socioeconomic, disenfranchised populations. This is, in part, due to deliberate targeting of low-income populations, as well as ethnic minority populations, with selective advertising and marketing.

NO ORDINARY COMMODITY

Today, many societies are debating the question of whether, like alcohol, heavy consumption of added sugars constitutes a significant threat to health that warrants government intervention—one that goes beyond sugar's known role in obesity. In modern liberal societies, personal choice and freedom are defining aspects of the political culture. This leads governments to be wary of encroachment into the personal lives of citizens. In the US, government sets a particularly high threshold on the use of regulatory control policies, confining intervention to only a few substances, including harmful addictive substances like alcohol as well as food additives proved to be carcinogenic. To justify intervention, health harms must be well documented, with clear evidence that overuse of the substance is disabling or causes premature mortality. In the US, many "personal responsibility" diseases only became public health crises after an accumulation of science demonstrated that everyone in the population was at risk. Examples include infectious diseases, such as syphilis, cholera, tuberculosis, and HIV; chemically induced diseases, such those attributable to tobacco, air pollution, and pesticides; nutritional diseases, such as vitamin deficiencies and endemic goiter; and "social" diseases, such as teen pregnancy and gun violence. If chronic metabolic diseases are similarly due to specific exposures, such as exposure to heavy doses of alcohol and added sugar, then these substances are more likely to qualify as public health concerns that warrant a governmental response.

In their seminal work, *Alcohol: No Ordinary Commodity*, Babor *et al.* [21] lay out specific criteria required before a substance qualifies for societal intervention. The phrase "ordinary commodity" derives from global debates over alcohol policy. Governments worldwide accept that alcohol constitutes a special case, as a market commodity, due to both its addictive properties and the health detriments of overconsumption. Consequently, structured interventions, such as price controls, taxation, and direct restrictions on availability, are used worldwide to regulate alcohol production and distribution. Indeed, early 2010 brought a U.N. World Health Assembly Resolution (WHA61.4) that promotes international public health regulations to counterbalance free market trade agreements fostering cross-border alcohol trade [30]. Growing evidence, from the molecular to the population levels, supports a similar rethinking of products laden with added sugar [31–33]. New evidence raises important questions about whether added sugar is just an "ordinary commodity," given its global overproduction and overconsumption, and its role in chronic metabolic disease. Babor et al. propose that four criteria must be met to justify government regulation of substance, all of which can be argued apply to added sugar:

Ubiquity

Every developed and developing country has manifested an increase in obesity prevalence alongside rising consumption of added sugars. This suggests some global environmental insult, particularly since the greatest increases in obesity prevalence have occurred in the youngest populations [34,35]. If obesity resulted from lack of willpower or aberrant behaviors, then one would expect high rates of success with behavioral interventions; yet results are underwhelming [36,37]. Furthermore, the prevalence of chronic or noncommunicable diseases (diabetes, heart disease, cancer, dementia) has increased worldwide concurrent with rising sugar consumption [38]. In America, 74% of packaged foods contain added sugar [39], thereby limiting consumer choice. As the price of dietary sugar has declined in recent decades, food manufacturers have taken advantage by adding more sugar to processed foods, so that it has taken the place of more expensive nutrients and acts to increase the shelf life of foods, thus decreasing depreciation.

Toxicity

It is taken as truism in the debate over obesity that dietary sugars are problematic because they constitute an abundant source of "empty calories." Indeed, the average American currently consumes 120 pounds of sugars per year or about three times the dietary limit put forth by the American Heart Association. A growing body of evidence shows that there are health effects due to heavy sugar consumption above and beyond its caloric equivalent. Thus, a recent study from the Centers for Disease Control and Prevention using the NHANES database has examined the relationship between cardiovascular mortality hazard risk and percent of calories as added sugars consumed. The authors demonstrate a parabolic curve with an inflection point at 15% of calories as added sugars; those approaching 30% of calories in added sugars exhibited a hazard ratio of three [40]. A recent prospective analysis of the European EPIC-Interact study found that sugary beverage consumption increased diabetes incidence by 29% exclusive of its total calories or body mass index [41]. Lastly, Basu et al. [42], using a global econometric analysis, showed that sugar availability predicted the prevalence of diabetes, exclusive of total calories, calories from other foodstuffs, aging, obesity, physical activity, or income. For every 150 calories per day in excess, diabetes prevalence increased 0.1%. If those 150 calories happened to come from a can of soda, diabetes prevalence increased by 1.1%.

The heavy consumption of one particular type of sugar, the monosaccharide fructose, adversely impacts human health, beyond and unrelated to its caloric equivalent, in many ways paralleling the health harms associated with alcohol overconsumption. Fructose (50% of table sugar and typically 55% of high-fructose corn syrup, although concentrations range up to 90%) is a specific cause of increased energy intake [43], weight gain [44], and metabolic syndrome [45]. As reviewed in Chapters 19 and 20, the hepatic metabolism of fructose qualitatively and quantitatively resembles that of alcohol, by promoting: (1) hypertension via uric acid production and lowering nitric oxide [46]; (2) dyslipidemia and hepatic steatosis through excessive *de novo* lipogenesis and defective lipid oxidation [47]; (3) skeletal muscle insulin resistance and oxidative stress [48]; (4) hepatic insulin resistance and inflammation; and (5) hyperglycemia via hepatic gluconeogenesis [22].

Abuse

As reviewed in Chapters 14 and 15, fructose acts on the brain to increase energy intake by: (1) lack of suppression of the hunger hormone ghrelin [43]; (2) by promoting high triglyceride levels, which prevent leptin transport signaling the brain to reduce caloric intake; (3) by promoting insulin resistance, which interferes with leptin signaling [49]; (4) by depleting hypothalamic malonyl-CoA, resulting in central nervous system starvation; and (5) altering dopamine signaling in the nucleus accumbens (the brain's reward center), making it more difficult for individuals to regulate consumption [50]. As with alcohol overconsumption, animal models demonstrate that prolonged, heavy sucrose use has the capability to decrease dopamine D_2 receptors in the reward center of the brain, thereby leading to increased sugar intake. Neuroimaging studies in humans demonstrate parallel evidence supporting the notion that this mechanism generalizes from animal to human models [51]. Furthermore, high sugar intake has been linked to reduced dopamine release in patients with metabolic syndrome so that affected patients must consume more sugar to achieve the same level of reward [52].

Externalities or Negative Impacts on Society

Certain substances not only harm the user, but also nonusers and the general public, thereby warranting regulation by governments. Evidence of harms produced by second-hand smoke and drinking-driving have provided strong arguments for tobacco and alcohol control, respectively. One argument that the food industry uses to prevent societal intervention on dietary sugars is the lack of an analogy to second-hand smoke or alcohol-related auto accidents. Currently, the downstream detriments of excessive sugar consumption are confined to economic losses, but these are quite substantial. It has been projected that Medicare will be bankrupt by 2026 as the health plan largely covering the high costs of end-state chronic diseases associated with metabolic syndrome. Private insurers in America pay an additional $2751 for health coverage related to obesity, whether the employee is obese or not. The Credit Suisse report [15] argues that the long-term economic, healthcare, and human costs of obesity now place the chronic effects of sugar overconsumption in the same category as alcohol and tobacco with respects to externalities [53,54].

HOW THE ALCOHOL EXPERIENCE INFORMS POLICY ON DIETARY SUGARS

We have thus far suggested that biological, hedonic, and societal similarities between dietary sugar and alcohol argue for a rethinking of the public policy status of added sugars and methods to reduce consumption for the public good. Given the long history of alcohol control, there exists a robust body of evidence related to the efficacy of policies implemented nationally and internationally to consider in shaping future sugar-related policy. At the outset, it is as important to review what has worked, as well as what has been shown to be not effective in the area of alcohol policy, and whether any such parallels are present in nutrition research.

Which Policies are Least Likely to Work and Why?

One of the most important findings from many decades of research on mitigating alcohol problems is that individually focused behavior change approaches tend to be less effective and cost-effective than regulatory controls on alcohol availability in the environment. Some of the strongest scientific consensus speaks to the lack of evidence on the effectiveness of school-based education programs. Despite being a mainstay of alcohol prevention for many decades, the worldwide evidence shows that school-based health education programs have little lasting impact on actual consumption behavior, although some may have short-term effects on knowledge and attitudes about drinking [21,55,56]. Individually focused medical approaches to treating alcohol abuse and dependence have a better record of efficacy and effectiveness. There is evidence that alcohol antagonist and agonist medications, and behavioral treatment approaches, can mitigate early- and late-stage alcohol dependence [57–59]. However, such "tertiary prevention" approaches are costly in comparison to "primary prevention" strategies aimed at reducing the overall availability of alcohol in the environment [60]. And while addiction treatment may be effective, it currently reaches less than 10% of the US population in need of care [61]. Treatment services are costly, with long waiting lists and usually require multiple episodes of care to achieve success [62].

Despite what we know from the alcohol experience, obesity and nutritional interventions in the US rely largely on individually focused strategies. And as with alcohol, the record of long-term success in individually focused obesity interventions leaves little cause for optimism [36,37,63]. In the US, a vast industry has sprung up for the treatment of end-state addiction and other alcohol use disorders. But the size and scope of this industry pales in comparison to the weight loss industry. And thus far, the majority of individually focused lifestyle interventions for weight loss have not proved effective long-term, with some evidence of producing significant iatrogenic harms, such as those resulting from "yo-yo dieting" [64]. In sum, most of the currently popular approaches—school-based health education and clinical treatments for end-state disease—have very little evidence supporting their efficacy and are not the strongest approaches for obesity prevention [56,62,65–67].

In the alcohol field, there are also some popular environmentally based interventions that appear to have only modest effectiveness. Government-sponsored media campaigns, including public service announcements and counter-advertising campaigns targeted against producer marketing messages, may have only modest effects with respect to alcohol [68]. Evidence from the US suggests that government labels warning consumers about the health effects of alcohol have little effect on total consumption, although they may have a limited effect on risky drinking patterns such as drinking-driving [69,70]. While econometric studies find some positive effects for alcohol advertising bans, studies of even short-term impacts on alcohol consumption behavior find no measureable effects [21]. Finally, regulations on the marketing and promotion of alcohol products have mainly targeted youth. Alcohol ads appear to have a cumulative effect that shapes young peoples' perceptions about alcohol by encouraging pro-drinking attitudes and greater consumption, but some of the most important advertising channels remain unregulated [71]. It should be noted that the record of success for counter-advertising and warning labels in tobacco prevention gives greater cause for optimism; more research is called for to ascertain how these approaches can be better put to use in other fields [72].

Voluntary agreements among alcohol manufacturers and distributors to control marketing, advertising, packaging, and sales restrictions have been tried repeatedly, but with little long-term success [21]. Often industries under attack propose voluntary regulatory agreements as a strategy to obviate the need for, or to at least postpone, outside governmental regulation. For this reason, these agreements are often symbolic, being written in ways that are not legally binding. Over time, even binding agreements break down and ultimately fail due to the lack of enforcement and monitoring [73]. Today, as manufacturers of sugary foods and beverages grow increasingly concerned about government intervention, proposals for industry self-regulation are becoming more common.

Historically, voluntary agreements within industry have focused on self-restrictions on alcohol marketing and advertising, particularly campaigns targeting young people [74]. After the repeated failure of voluntary codes, the US government banned alcohol advertising targeting young people, as well as all television advertising. But alcohol beverage company sponsorship at sporting and cultural events attended by young people remains a problem, and internet-based media channels are poorly regulated. Child-targeted media and advertising of high-sugar products is substantially more pervasive, particularly with regard to children's television programming [75–80]. In a 2003–2004 study of television advertisements aired during the most highly rated children's television programs, nearly 50% of the total calories in products advertised came from added sugars and 98% of cereal advertisements were for those high in added sugars [75]. A 2007 study showed that the average American child views 30,000 TV commercials annually marketing fast food or candy [81]. Of the 3.4 billion advertisements on children's web sites, 84% promote foods high in sodium, fat, or sugar [82]. Such advertising is associated with purchasing requests [83,84], as well as the intake of advertised foods and beverages [85–87].

Thus far, there are no US government bans on the marketing of products with high sugar content to children and, as with alcohol, industry-led voluntary agreements have not met with much success [88]. Producers of soft drinks and snack products have also promoted voluntary industry agreements to limit advertising and promotion to children in schools [89]. While studies report a trend of decreasing expenditures on television advertisements directed toward youth, there has been increased spending on advertising in other forms of media (e.g., cell phones, web, and social media) [90]. Although voluntary industry agreements may have led to a decrease in advertising of sweets and sugar-sweetened beverages over time [91], such agreements are limited only to the companies who voluntarily participate. In April 2011, a working group consisting of the Federal Trade Commission, the Food and Drug Administration, the Centers for Disease Control and Prevention, and the U.S. Department of Agriculture released preliminary recommendations for the nutritional quality of food marketed to children and adolescents, yet no upper limit for dietary sugars was discussed. Despite the voluntary nature of these guidelines, it is hoped that companies will feel pressure to comply with guidelines that encompass not only television advertising, but also other forms of multimedia advertising (e.g., web sites, online games, social media, movies) [92].

Which Policies are Most Likely to Work and Why?

Literature provides little evidence supporting the efficacy and cost-effectiveness of individually focused interventions, as well as industry voluntary agreements. While there is some evidence supporting the effectiveness of warning labels, counter-advertising and advertising restrictions, the effects tend to be modest at best. In contrast, there is strong, robust evidence supporting the effectiveness and cost-effectiveness of environmentally focused, market-based regulatory controls that impact the pricing, marketing, and distribution of alcohol, as well as sugar-laden, products [21,55,62,93–95].

All market-based policies build upon a premise that we call the *iron law of public health policy*. This argues that if societies wish to mitigate the harms caused by commodities with adverse health impacts, the best way to do so is by reducing the overall availability and the ease of accessing those products. In the large body of research on alcohol policy, the most effective, cost-effective, and unobtrusive public health interventions all share a common basis in the *iron law*. These include pricing strategies (such as taxation, direct price controls, and withdrawal of government crop subsidies), regulations on sales and distribution (e.g., bar open hours, restrictions on sales to minors) and ideally, the bundling of these interventions together to achieve more substantial impacts on the consumer environment. Virtually all are premised on the notion that by making alcohol—particularly in its most concentrated forms (e.g., spirits)—slightly harder to get and more costly to obtain, consumers will naturally curb their consumption of those products, thereby mitigating the adverse health impacts of overconsumption. We argue that, due to the similarities between alcohol and sugar, the *iron law* should apply not just to alcohol, but also to policies targeting the harmful effects of heavy sugar consumption.

STRATEGIES THAT WORK

Pricing Strategies

Taxation

Alcohol taxation, in the form of special excise duties, value-added taxes, and sales taxes, has proved worldwide among the most popular and effective ways to reduce overall per capita alcohol consumption, and in turn, alcohol-related health harms (for reviews, see [21,55,95–98]. If alcohol research offers no better lesson for policymaking around sugar, it is that even the relatively modest taxation of highly concentrated products—ideally greater than 20% of the product's price—offers a simple, effective policy option for addressing the growing population burden of sugar-related health harms. Taxation policies follow the economic law of supply and demand; adding a tax increases the price of the product such that consumers can afford to buy less, thereby reducing consumption.

Alcohol taxes are popular worldwide because they are relatively cheap and easy to collect and cause little market distortion [99]. Empirical studies show that alcohol taxation can have beneficial effects on both acute (e.g., injuries) and chronic (e.g., cirrhosis) health conditions—illnesses that disproportionately impact low socioeconomic status (SES) groups [100]. Time-series analyses show changes in population-based indicators of harm pursuant to changes in taxation levels. For instance,

Cook and Tauchen [101,102] compared US states that raised their liquor taxes to find significant reductions in heavy drinking, cirrhosis, motor vehicle accidents, and mortality (see also [103]). There is also evidence that alcohol taxes disproportionately impact youth and the heaviest drinkers in the population—groups at particularly high risk for alcohol-related harms [104].

In the US, public health promotion via food taxation has thus far been limited, although there is a longstanding tradition of taxing food products as a means to raise general revenues for local, state, and federal governments [89,105,106]. In contrast, the main thrust of alcohol taxation has been toward protecting public health. Thus, products are taxed on the basis of the harm they produce—a practice called "differential taxation" [94,107]. Domestically and internationally, highly concentrated alcohol products, such as spirits, tend to be taxed more heavily than less concentrated ones—in some cases, by a factor of 4 or even greater [93]. Careful studies in the Nordic countries underscore the public health benefits of this approach where, through careful tinkering with price controls and taxation, there have been demonstrable shifts in consumption toward lower alcohol-content products, such as light beer, with resultant reductions in alcohol-attributable harms [93,108].

As empirical evidence regarding the effects of sugar taxation remains more limited, it may be useful to borrow lessons from the tradition of alcohol taxation. One effective strategy for the differential taxation of added sugars would involve placing a per-gram tax on the amount of sugar added to products, or a tax rated by the proportion of calories from added sugars. While such a tax would ideally be applicable to the widest possible variety of processed food products to reduce consumption across the board, thus far, political discussions about sugar taxation have been limited to sugary drinks alone. Arguments over the efficacy of such a tax abound. Most current taxation proposals proffer a 10% tax, which would likely raise money for nutrition and health programs, but is unlikely to result in a salutary reduction in sugary beverage consumption. Econometric analyses, such as a new one from the UK, suggest that a 20% sales tax on sugary drinks would have measureable impacts on consumption—in the case of the UK, reducing consumption by 15%, which would manifest as a 1.3% reduction in obesity prevalence and 0.9% reduction in persons overweight [109].

Guidance from alcohol research indicates that a differential taxation approach could help to avoid some of the potential unintended consequences of taxation policies. On the one hand, it reduces incentives for producers and distributors to make changes in pricing and product content that could neutralize some benefits of the tax [110]. On the other hand, it would mitigate against potential problems with consumers substituting one sugar-laden product for another [55]. Experience shows that when alcohol tax regimes have proved too objectionable to the alcohol industry, tax increases are often neutralized by strategic changes in pricing by producers and sellers [110]. In such cases, taxation can reduce the consumption of one type of alcohol only to increase consumption of another. Similarly, product substitution can occur at the level of consumer choice. The potential for negative substitution clearly requires appropriate safeguards. In a study examining the association of state soft drink excise taxes, state soft drink sales, and beverage consumption, taxation led to decreased soft drink consumption among children and adolescents; however, consumption of other high-calorie beverages, such as fruit juice and whole milk, increased [111].

The limited literature on sugar taxation similarly suggests that if sugary foods and beverages are taxed heavily, without any changes in the price of unhealthy substitutes that do not contain added sugars, then consumers may simply substitute sugar-laden foods and beverages with equally calorically dense products, or artificially sweetened products, which have their own adverse health effects [112]. Ideally, taxation regimes will be accompanied by strategies that decrease the price of healthier food and beverage alternatives (e.g., whole fruits, vegetables, water) to counteract such a substitution effect [113].

Taxation policies for sugar must anticipate a common problem encountered with alcohol tax policies: the fact that they tend to be "regressive" taxes, that is, they tend to place a greater burden of cost on consumers with less disposable income [89,114,115]. Given the substantial socioeconomic disparities with both alcohol- and sugar-related health harms, one may question whether regressive taxation is not, in fact, in the broad public health interest [100]. The burden of chronic disease, after all, tends to be greatest in the lower social strata for alcohol, sugar, and chronic metabolic disease [116–118].

However, since the US has a strong tradition of consumer rights protection, regressive sugar taxes are likely to be seen as imposing unfair constraints on individual choice among economically disadvantaged groups (see [119]). By applying any proceeds from the tax to public health promotion programs serving lower-income groups targeted by industry, it is possible to balance out the regressive nature of the tax. In the case of sugar, tax revenues could be applied toward health care, park development and maintenance, children's sports programs, subsidies on fruits and vegetables, increased access to safe drinking water, and to commercial loan and development programs that encourage grocery stores and farmer's markets to relocate in underserved low-income communities, or "food deserts" [75,105,120]. One reason for the defeat of soda tax measures thus far is the concern that taxes from sugary beverages would go toward a general treasury where they are channeled into other general funding needs (e.g., cleaning highways, creating health profession schools, or programs), rather than being specifically earmarked for obesity and diabetes prevention or treatment [106].

Price Controls

In many places, alcohol taxation policies have been bolstered by the concentration of market power in government-controlled alcohol monopolies where it proves simple to place controls on price, production, import, and sales. This approach has been utilized in many US states and localities, as well as in parts of South America, Eastern Europe, and the Nordic countries. In such cases, government monopolies often use "differential pricing" to mark up the costs of more concentrated alcoholic beverages to discourage their use. By strategically positioning government-run stores on the outskirts of metropolitan areas, and prohibiting sales in grocery and corner stores, government monopolies are further able to create an environment that is less saturated by alcohol, thereby gently discouraging overconsumption. While it is difficult to imagine a government monopoly on sugary drinks or foods, analogous pricing strategies could be applied in government voucher programs, such as the Women, Infants, and Children Program (WIC) and the Supplemental Nutrition Assistance Program (SNAP; formerly known as Food Stamps), with the potential for similarly positive effects on health.

Subsidy Withdrawal

Crop subsidies for alcohol have been common on a worldwide basis, but many nation states have curtailed subsidization in the interest of promoting public health. Traditionally, there are two types of food crop subsidies: payments to farmers only when the price of the crop is low to keep them from going out of business, and payments to farmers based on performance, regardless of price. Subsidies for sugars in the US currently operate according to neither of these principles. Within the US sugar program, the USDA operates a complex loan program to guarantee sugar growers certain prices, which are enforced and enhanced using import barriers and domestic production controls [121].

Propping up markets for specific foodstuffs (such as sugar) with price subsidies causes market distortion and ultimately defies the *iron law of public health policy*. Ending the US sugar subsidy, on the other hand, would produce precisely those outcomes desired to protect public health—it would effectively raise the costs of sugar production, which would likely be passed on to consumers, thereby effectively raising the price of the most concentrated sugary foods and drinks. While the logic here seems sound, there are detractors who argue that such pricing effects could be rather limited [122]. To avoid exacerbating market distortion, termination of the USDA loan program would need to be accompanied by termination of the US corn subsidy, which artificially deflates the price of high-fructose corn syrup. A proposal to end these subsidies was debated in Congress as amendments to the Farm Bill of 2013. However, Congress ultimately took no action following heavy lobbying by industry trade groups.

In the absence of complete subsidy termination, a compromise would involve "differential subsidization." Here, instead of subsidizing corn and soy (commodity crops that are storable), government would subsidize the production of fresh fruits and vegetables. Promotion of high-fiber foods in US low-income food programs, such as through the WIC, SNAP, and the National School Lunch Program (NSLP), would be the most expedient places to begin. Differential subsidization is currently being applied to water in many parts of the US, as well as in the developing world [123], where inhabitants often have limited options for hydration due to the lack of readily accessible potable water.

Regulating Sales and Distribution

In addition to pricing strategies, some of the most effective means for limiting the volume of alcohol consumed—and to a lesser extent, risky patterns of drinking—involves making it less convenient to obtain alcohol at the point of sales. Once again, there is robust international evidence supporting the effectiveness of strategies that directly control alcohol availability, which include placing limits on opening hours or days for retail sales, regulating the placement and location of retail markets, the density of sales outlets within a particular community, and limits on who can legally purchase alcohol (for reviews, see [21,62,69,124,125]). Low SES communities in the US, for example, often have a higher density of alcohol beverage outlets due to weak enforcement of local and state zoning laws. Research has shown that reducing the density of retail alcohol outlets through stricter state licensing and zoning ordinances is associated with reductions in alcohol problems in these communities [126–128]. A reasonable parallel for added sugars would be to tighten licensing requirements on vending machines and snack bars that sell products with high concentrations of sugar in schools and workplaces. Implementation of such restrictions must be carefully regulated to avoid substitution of one sugar beverage for another by distributors [129]. In addition, states could apply zoning ordinances in ways that control the number of fast food outlets selling high-sugar foods and beverages in low SES communities, while providing incentives for the entry of grocery stores and farmer's markets that sell fruits and vegetables.

Albeit limited, there is already some evidence that such controls on distribution can be effective at reducing added sugars and unhealthy food consumption [130–132]. For example, many states and local jurisdictions have created policies to restrict the sales of sugar-sweetened beverages and high-sugar foods in schools. Although there is limited evidence regarding the impact of such sugar-related policies on childhood obesity [133], the literature suggests that these policies may be effective in decreasing access to and consumption of high-sugar foods and beverages [111,134–140].

Studies from schools provide an object lesson in how to best implement restriction on sales of unhealthy foods and beverages, not just in schools but also in workplaces and other public venues. Despite regulations, some studies suggest that there may not be full implementation of health-promoting food and beverage policies in schools [141–144], especially during celebrations and fundraisers [145,146]. Even when schools are adherent to nutrition policies, students may bring in unhealthy foods and beverages from home [139] or purchase unhealthy items off campus through corner stores or vendors [147]. Although many states and school districts limit sales of soda, flavored milks, 100% fruit juice and sports drinks, they may still be allowed, leading to problems with substitution [148]. In addition, a recent analysis of 5th and 8th grade children showed that consumption of soda declined during school hours, but total daily consumption was unaffected presumably due to consumption after school and at home [149].

All of this underscores the need for policymakers to think beyond regulating any particular environment, such as the school, to the wider context in which populations consume foods and beverages, including homes, worksites, parks, restaurants, corner stores, and food vendors [150]. Recent experience with school regulations also underscores the importance of careful enforcement.

THE NORDIC MODEL: BUNDLING POLICIES

Evidence from the field of alcohol control points to the *iron law of public health policy* and its call to reduce availability as a means of reducing alcohol consumption to improve public health. The value and importance of relying on policy development to reshape the environment in which individuals are expected to make appropriate behavioral choices is compelling. This goal can be achieved through a number of market-driven, environmental change strategies.

Each specific policy recommendation for alcohol (e.g., pricing, regulation of sales, and distribution) has the potential to make an environmental impact. The "Nordic Model of Alcohol Control" bundles more than one of these policy options together to achieve a more robust regulatory regime [93]. Most Nordic societies have struggled for generations with alcohol problems due to cultural patterns of "explosive drinking" whereby individuals tend to abstain from alcohol during the working week only to binge, largely on spirits, during "time out" on the weekends [151,152]. This pattern of drinking is associated with high rates of alcohol-related social harms, and high rates of intentional and unintentional injuries [62]. Prior to European Integration, most Nordic countries assumed governmental control over the production, supply, and distribution of alcoholic beverages. This allowed governments to manage the supply and distribution of alcohol by confining sales to government monopoly stores, applying controls at the point of distribution, as well as aggressive differential taxation schemes [93].

By combining or bundling multiple policy interventions known to be effective, some Scandinavian countries were able to bring about pronounced shifts in alcohol consumption and related problems population-wide, without resorting to all-out prohibition or more aggressive interventions that tend to be associated with unintended, negative consequences. The results of Sweden's bundled policy approach in the 1970s vividly demonstrates the effectiveness of policy bundling, where time-series analyses demonstrated dramatic declines in rates of alcohol-related admissions to hospitals (see Figure 26.1). It is unlikely that we will see chronic disease abatement until communities, states, and nations adopt a similarly comprehensive array of concurrent, synergistic policy strategies that fundamentally reshape their food environments.

CONCLUSION

Any successful regulatory approach to preventing the health harms associated with the overconsumption of dietary sugars must not just confront, but ideally balance, the complex and competing interests of consumers, government, and commercial interests, including producers, distributors, and retailers. The production and sale of alcohol, as with sugar, is an important economic activity that generates profits, jobs, tax dollars, and currency. Industrial producers and distributors face economic losses when consumption is reduced, thus placing public health goals at loggerhead with commercial interests. Meanwhile, government has its own competing interests. On the one hand, it is charged with protecting the economy, encouraging commodity exports, increasing its own tax base, and generating tariffs. On the other hand, governments are responsible for protecting public health, as well as financing the costs of chronic disease through pubic insurance programs like Medicare and subsidizing the costs of food through federal assistance programs for low-income populations. While these interests are not necessarily irreconcilable, understanding and balancing these personal–commercial–governmental alignments is essential for promoting effective regulatory regimes.

The political and economic barriers inherent in applying lessons learned from the alcohol experience to dietary sugar are significant, but not insurmountable. One barrier to policy change is the food industry itself. Virtually all food companies are now part of vast, publicly traded conglomerates that have a fiduciary responsibility to shareholders and are judged on 3-month profit cycles.

BOX 26.1 EFFECTS OF NORDIC ALCOHOL POLICY BUNDLING

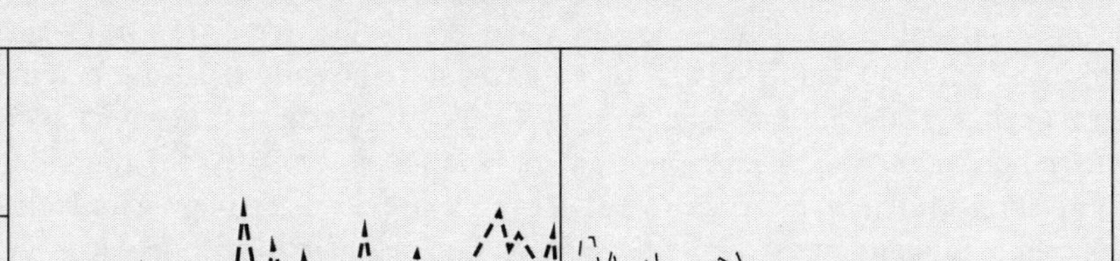

FIGURE 26.1 AAA-hospitalization rates per 100,000 aged 10–19 years. (Reprinted from Room R, editor. The effects of nordic alcohol policies: What happens to drinking and harm when alcohol controls change? Helsinki, Finland: Nordic Council for Alcohol and Drug Research, 2002, p. 121. With permission.)

In July 1977, Sweden passed a law that taxed medium-strength beer like strong beer and that limited the sales of medium beer to government-owned stores. Prior to that time, beer could be purchased in 11,550 grocery stores throughout Sweden. Sweden bundled a number of different control policies alongside, including reductions in the number of sales outlets, differential taxation, age restrictions on purchasing and confinement of spirit sales to government monopoly stores. The figure shows the time-series trend for hospitalizations due to alcoholism, alcohol intoxication, and alcohol psychosis throughout Sweden. The 1977 law reversed a trend in increased hospital admissions related to drinking in all age groups, but as shown here, particularly among younger people. The effects were particularly pronounced among young people because, given comparatively less disposable income to spend on alcohol, the price increase had a greater impact in discouraging consumption compared to adults.

This makes producers unlikely to change of their own volition, as experience with voluntary industry agreements has borne out. Yet food corporations are more likely to change if all members of the industry are made subject to the same rules, so that there is no competitive disadvantage. And as long as shareholders are made aware of corporate commitments to the social good, publicly traded corporations can legally pursue growth strategies that take public health into account—perhaps to their own "bottom-line" advantage by differentiating their firms as socially responsible. Approaches for sugar modeled on those proposed for salt reduction by the FDA and Institute of Medicine should be considered [153].

If there is any lesson to draw from the long story of alcohol control policy, it is an important cautionary tale. We have learned that highly aggressive, absolutist policy regimes—as evidenced by the US alcohol prohibition experiment from 1919 to 1933—are prone to unintended consequences that can undercut the ultimate success of any health policy project. Experience shows that aggressive restrictions on alcohol availability through prohibition and rationing can lower alcohol consumption and reduce alcohol-related morbidity, but often with adverse social side effects [21,154]. These included unintentionally stimulating the development of illegal markets that tend to push the population toward consumption of more concentrated forms of the product (e.g., spirits vs. wine), as well as problems of producer and consumer product substitution.

Parallels with our current epidemics of obesity and metabolic disease are striking and important. Rising rates of obesity and metabolic disease only began in the early 1970s as food manufacturers concerned about high fat levels in packaged, processed foods increased the content of dietary sugars in "low-fat" products to make them more palatable to the consumer. At the time, introduction of high-fructose corn syrup into the American marketplace provided enhanced economic competition in the packaged food industry, reducing the price of dietary sugars worldwide. It may very well be that the "solution" to reducing chronic disease risk—lowering the fat content of processed foods—was a key cause of rising sugar consumption, with all its ramifications for the increased risks of chronic disease via metabolic syndrome.

Such object lessons ultimately call for broad-based food policies that, while appreciating the problems associated with particularly harmful single food substances, such as added sugars, ultimately embrace the widest possible vision of a healthy food environment. To hold this broader vision means carefully analyzing and monitoring communities as they begin to implement a variety of local and state policy initiatives targeting added sugar consumption. And as has been true in the case in alcohol policy, bundled strategies will likely be needed to enable the types of comprehensive approaches that are key in changing our food environment.

ACKNOWLEDGMENTS

This research was supported by the UCSF Clinical and Translational Science Institute (CTSI), with funding from the National Center for Advancing Translational Sciences (NCATS) at the National Institutes of Health (NIH) (Grant Number UL1 TR000004). Prior versions of this manuscript were delivered by the primary author in oral presentations at the Annual Public Health Symposium at Washington University in St. Louis, MO, on April 11, 2009, and at the Annual Meeting of the Pediatric Academic Society in Vancouver, BC, on May 2, 2010. The authors are grateful for a prior critique by Dr. Steve Schroeder and for technical assistance by Ms. Juliana Fung in the manuscript's preparation. This chapter expands upon and develops themes previously raised in: Lustig RH, Schmidt LA, Brindis CD. Public Health: "The Toxic Truth About Sugar." *Nature*. 2012, 482 (February 2):27–9.

REFERENCES

1. Johnson RK, Appel LJ, Brands M, Howard BV, Lefevre M, Lustig RH et al. Dietary sugars intake and cardiovascular health, a scientific statement from the American Heart Association. *Circulation*. 2009;120(11):1011–20.
2. Moodie R, Stuckler D, Monteiro C, Sheron N, Neal B, Thamarangsi T et al. Profits and pandemics: Prevention of harmful effects of tobacco, alcohol, and ultra-processed food and drink industries. *Lancet*. 2013;381:670–9.
3. United Nations General Assembly. Political declaration of the high-level meeting of the general assembly on the prevention and control of non-communicable diseases. 2011.
4. Chan JM, Rimm EB, Colditz GA, Stampfer MJ, Willett WC. Obesity, fat distribution, and weight gain as risk factors for clinical diabetes in men. *Diabetes Care*. 1994;17:961–9.
5. McLaughlin T, Abbasi F, Cheal K, Chu J, Lamendola C, Reaven GM. Use of metabolic markers to identify overweight individuals who are insulin resistant. *Ann Int Med*. 2003;139:802–9.
6. Abbasi F, Chu JW, Lamendola C, McLaughlin T, Hayden J, Reaven GM et al. Discrimination between obesity and insulin resistance in the relationship with adiponectin. *Diabetes*. 2004;53(3):585–90.
7. Voulgari C, Tentolouris N, Dilaveris P, Tousoulis D, Katsilambros N, Stefanadis C. Increased heart failure risk in normal-weight people with metabolic syndrome compared with metabolically healthy obese individuals. *J Am Coll Cardiol*. 2011;58(13):1343–50.
8. Lustig RH. Fructose: It's alcohol without the "buzz". *Adv Nutr*. 2013;4:226–35.

9. Bray GA. Energy and fructose from beverages sweetened with sugar or high-fructose corn syrup pose a health risk for some people. *Adv Nutr.* 2013;4:220–5.
10. Rippe JM, Angelopoulos TJ. Sucrose, high-fructose corn syrup, and fructose, their metabolism and potential health effects: What do we really know? *Adv Nutr.* 2013;4:236–45.
11. White JS. Challenging the fructose hypothesis: New perspectives on fructose consumption and metabolism. *Adv Nutr.* 2013;4:246–56.
12. Katz DL. Perils of a sugar-coated scapegoat 2012. Available from: http://www.huffingtonpost.com/david-katz-md/sugar-diet_b_1553284.html.
13. Koplan JP, Brownell KD. Response of the food and beverage industry to the obesity threat. *JAMA.* 2010;304(13):1487–8.
14. Taylor AL, Parento EW, Schmidt LA. The increasing weight of regulation: Countries combat the global obesity epidemic. *Indiana Law J.* 2014;1:90.
15. Keating G, Natella S. Sugar: Consumption at a crossroads. *Credit Suisse*, 2013 September 2013.
16. Colbert JA, Adler JN. Sugar-sweetened beverages—Polling results. *New Engl J Med.* 2013;368(3):1464–6.
17. Academy of Medical Royal Colleges. Measuring up: The medical profession's prescription for the nation's obesity crisis. Academy of Medical Royal Colleges, 2013, http://www.aomrc.org.uk/doc_view/9673-measuring-up.
18. Waterfield B. Sugar is 'addictive and the most dangerous drug of the times'. *The Telegraph.* 17 September 2013.
19. Simopoulos AP, Bourne PG, Faergeman O. Bellagio report on healthy agriculture, healthy nutrition, healthy people. *J Nutrigenet Nutrigenom.* 2013;6(1):34–42.
20. Brunn K. Finland: The non-medical approach. 29th International Congress on Alcoholism & Drug Dependence. pp. 64–73.
21. Babor T, Caetano R, Casswell S, Edwards G, Geisbrecht N, Graham K et al. Alcohol: No ordinary commodity—Research and public policy. Oxford: Oxford University Press; 2003.
22. Lustig RH. Fructose: Metabolic, hedonic, and societal parallels with ethanol. *J Am Dietetic Assoc.* 2010;110(9):1307–21.
23. Room R, Rehm J. Alcohol and Non–Communicable Diseases—Cancer, Heart Disease and More. *Addiction.* 2011;106(1):1-2.
24. Page KA, Chan O, Arora J, Belfort-DeAguiar R, Dzuira J, Roehmholdt B et al. Effects of fructose vs glucose on regional cerebral blood flow in brain regions involved with appetite and reward pathways fructose consumption and weight gain. *JAMA.* 2013;309(1):63–70.
25. Colantuoni C, Rada P, McCarthy J, Patten C, Avena NM, Chadeayne A et al. Evidence that intermittent excessive sugar intake causes endogenous opioid dependence. *Obes Res.* 2002;10:478–88.
26. Garber AK, Lustig RH. Is fast food addictive? *Curr Drug Abuse Rev.* 2011;4:146–62.
27. Stice E, Burger KS, Yokum S. Relative ability of fat and sugar tastes to activate reward, gustatory, and somatosensory regions. *Am J Clin Nutr.* 2013;98(6):1377–84.
28. Ziauddeen H, Farooqi IS FP. Obesity and the brain: How convincing is the addiction model? *Nat Rev Neurosci.* 2012;13:279–86.
29. Grucza RA, Krueger RF, Racette SB, Norberg KE, Hipp PR, Bierut LJ. The emerging link between alcoholism risk and obesity in the United States. *Arch Gen Psychiatry.* 2010;67(12):1301.
30. Room R, Schmidt LA, Rehm J, Mäkela P. International regulation of alcohol. *BMJ.* 2008;337:a2364.
31. Brownell KD, Farley T, Willett WC, Popkin BM, Chaloupka FJ, Thompson JW et al. The public health and economic benefits of taxing sugar-sweetened beverages. *N Engl J Med.* 2009;361(16):1599–605.
32. Sturm R, Powell LM, Chriqui JF, Chaloupka FJ. Soda taxes, soft drink consumption, and children's body mass index. *Health Aff.* 2010;29(5):1052–8.
33. Bremer AA, Lustig RH. Effects of sugar-sweetened beverages on children. *Pediatr Ann.* 2012;41:26–30.
34. Ogden CL, Carroll MD, Curtin LR, Lamb MM, Flegal KM. Prevalence of high body mass index in US children and adolescents, 2007–2008. *JAMA.* 2010;303(3):242–9.
35. Ervin RB, Kit BK, Carroll MD, Ogden CL. Consumption of added sugar among U.S. children and adolescents, 2005–2008. NCHS data brief, no 87; Hyattsville, MD: National Center for Health Statistics, 2012.
36. Kamath CC, Vickers KS, Ehrlich A, McGovern L, Johnson J, Singhal V et al. Clinical review: Behavioral interventions to prevent childhood obesity: A systematic review and metaanalyses of randomized trials. *J Clin Endocrinol Metab.* 2008;93(12):4606–15.
37. McGovern L, Johnson JN, Paulo R, Hettinger A, Singhal V, Kamath C et al. Clinical review: Treatment of pediatric obesity: A systematic review and meta-analysis of randomized trials. *J Clin Endocrinol Metab.* 2007;93(12):4600–5.

38. Cecchini M, Sassi F, Lauer JA, Lee YY, Guajardo-Barron V, Chisholm D. Tackling of unhealthy diets, physical inactivity, and obesity: Health effects and cost-effectiveness. *Lancet*. 2010;376:1775–84.
39. Ng SW, Slining MM, Popkin BM. Use of caloric and noncaloric sweeteners in US consumer packaged foods, 2005–2009. *J Acad Nutr Diet*. 2012;112(11):1828–34.
40. Yang Q, Zhang Z, Gregg E, Flanders WD, Merritt R, Hu FB. Added sugar intake and cardiovascular disease mortality among US adults. *JAMA Intern Med*. 2014;174(4):516–24.
41. EPIC-Interact Consortium. Consumption of sweet beverages and type 2 diabetes incidence in European adults: Results from Epic-Interact. *Diabetologia*. 2013;56(7):1520–30.
42. Basu S, Yoffe P, Hills N, Lustig RH. The relationship of sugar to population-level diabetes prevalence: An econometric analysis of repeated cross-sectional data. *PLoS One*. 2013;8(2):e57873.
43. Teff KL, Grudziak J, Townsend RR, Dunn TN, Grant RW, Adams SH et al. Endocrine and metabolic effects of consuming fructose- and glucose-sweetened beverages with meals in obese men and women: Influence of insulin resistance on plasma triglyceride responses. *J Clin Endocrinol Metab*. 2009;94:1562–9.
44. Te Morenga L, Mallard S, Mann J. Dietary sugars and body weight: Systematic review and meta-analyses of randomised controlled trials and cohort studies. *BMJ*. 2012;346:e7492.
45. Rutledge AC, Adeli K. Fructose and the metabolic syndrome: Pathophysiology and molecular mechanisms. *Nutr Rev*. 2007;65(6):S13–23.
46. Perez-Pozo SE, Schold J, Nakagawa T, Sánchez-Lozada LG, Johnson RJ, Lillo JL. Excessive fructose intake induces the features of metabolic syndrome in healthy adult men: Role of uric acid in the hypertensive response. *Int J Obes*. 2009;34(3):454–61.
47. Abdelmalek MF, Suzuki A, Guy C, Unalp-Arida A, Colvin R, Johnson RJ et al. Increased fructose consumption is associated with fibrosis severity in patients with nonalcoholic fatty liver disease. *Hepatology*. 2010;51(6):1961–71.
48. Samuel VT. Fructose induced lipogenesis: From sugar to fat to insulin resistance. *Trends Endocrinol Metab*. 2011;22(2):60–5.
49. Lustig RH. Childhood obesity: Behavioral aberration or biochemical drive? Reinterpreting the first law of thermodynamics. *Nat Clin Pract Endocrinol Metab*. 2006;2(8):447–58.
50. Avena NM, Rada P, Hoebel BG. Evidence for sugar addiction: Behavioral and neurochemical effects of intermittent, excessive sugar intake. *Neurosci Biobehav Rev*. 2008;32(1):20–39.
51. Stice E, Spoor S, Bohon C, Small DM. Relation between obesity and blunted striatal response to food is moderated by Taqia A1 allele. *Science*. 2008;322:449–52.
52. Wang GJ, Logan J, Shumay E, Fowler J, Convit A, Dardo T et al. Peripheral insulin resistance affects brain dopaminergic signaling after glucose ingestion. Vancouver, BC: Society of Nuclear Medicine and Molecular Imaging; 2013. p. 29.
53. Finkelstein EA, Fiebelkorn IC, Wang G. National medical spending attributable to overweight and obesity: How much, and who's paying? *Health Aff*. 2003;W3:219–26.
54. Finkelstein EA, DiBonaventura M BS, Hale BC. The costs of obesity in the workplace. *J Occup Environ Med*. 2010;52:971–6.
55. Edwards G, Anderson P, Babor TF, Casswell S, Giesbrecht N, Godfrey C et al. Retail price influences on alcohol consumption, and taxation on alcohol as a prevention strategy. Alcohol policy and the public good. New York: Oxford University Press; 1994. pp. 109–213.
56. Battle KE, Brownell K. Confronting a rising tide of eating disorders and obestity: Treatment vs. prevention and policy. *Addictive Behav*. 1996;21(6):755–65.
57. Project Match Research Group. Matching alcoholism treatments to client heterogeneity: Project match posttreatment drinking outcomes. *J Stud Alcohol*. 1997;58:7–29.
58. McCarty D, McConnell KJ, Schmidt LA. Priorities for policy research on treatments for alcohol and drug use disorders. *J Subst Abuse Treat*. 2010;39(2):87–95.
59. Institute of Medicine. Broadening the base of treatment for alcohol problems. Washington, DC: National Academy Press; 1990.
60. Kendell RE, Suwaki H, Pacurucu-Castillo S, Poikolainen K, Tuyns A, Saxena S et al. An international debate: Alcohol policy and the public good. *Addiction*. 1995;90(2):181–203.
61. Schmidt L, Greenfield T, Mulia N. Unequal treatment: Racial and ethnic disparities in alcoholism treatment services. *Alcohol Res Health*. 2006;29(1):49–54.
62. Room R, Babor T, Rehrn J. Alcohol and public health. *Lancet*. 2005;365:519–30.
63. Shaw K, Gennat H, O'Rourke P, Del Mar C. Exercise for overweight or obesity. *Cochrane Database Syst Rev*. 2006(4):CD003817.
64. Brownell KD, Rodin J. Medical, metabolic, and psychological effects of weight cycling. *Arch Int Med*. 1994;154:1325–30.

65. Brownell KD, Farley T, Willett W, Popkin B, Chaloupka FJ, Thompson J. The public health and economic benefits of taxing sugar-sweetened beverages. *New Engl J Med.* 2009;361(16):1599–605.
66. Gonzalez-Suarez C, Worley A, Grimmer-Somers K, Dones V. School-based interventions on childhood obesity: A meta-analysis. *Am J Prev Med.* 2009;37(5):418–27. Epub 2009/10/21.
67. Walls HL, Peeters A, Proietto J, McNeil JJ. Public health campaigns and obesity—A critique. *BMC Public health.* 2011;11:136. Epub 2011/03/01.
68. Martin SE, editor. The effects of mass media on the use and abuse of alcohol. Rockville, MD: National Institute on Alcohol Abuse and Alcoholism; 1995.
69. Greenfield TK, Graves KL, Kaskutas LA. Alcohol warning labels for prevention: National survey results. *Alcohol, Health Res World.* 1993;17:67–75.
70. Greenfield TK, Johnson SP, Giesbrecht NA. The alcohol policy development process: Policy makers speak. American Public Health Association, Washington DC. November 15–19. 1998 (col. E536).
71. Atkin C, Neuendorf K, McDermott S. The role of alcohol advertising in excessive and hazardous drinking. *J Drug Educ.* 1983;13:313–23.
72. West R. What lessons can be learned from tobacco control for combating the growing prevalence of obesity? *Obesity Rev.* 2007;8(Suppl. 1):145–50.
73. Jernigan D. Thirsting for markets: The global impact of corporate alcohol. San Fafael, CA: Marin Institute for the Prevention of Alcohol and Other Drug Problems; 1997.
74. Jernigan DH. The global alcohol industry: An overview. *Addiction.* 2009;104:6–12.
75. Powell LM, Slater S, Mirtcheva D, Boa Y, Chaloupka FJ. Food store availability and neighborhood characteristics in the United States. *Prev Med.* 2007;44:189–95.
76. Adams J, Hennessy-Priest K, Ingimarsdottir S, Sheeshka J, Ostbye T, White M. Changes in food advertisements during 'prime-time' television from 1991 to 2006 in the UK and Canada. *Br J Nutr.* 2009;102(4):584–93. Epub 2009/02/27.
77. Colby SE, Johnson L, Scheett A, Hoverson B. Nutrition marketing on food labels. *J Nutr Educ Behav.* 2010;42(2):92–8.
78. Harrison K, Marske AL. Nutritional content of foods advertised during the television programs children watch most. *Am J Public Health.* 2005;95(9):1568–74.
79. Sutherland LA, Mackenzie T, Purvis LA, Dalton M. Prevalence of food and beverage brands in movies: 1996–2005. *Pediatrics.* 2010;125(3):468–74.
80. Mink M, Evans A, Moore CG, Calderon KS, Deger S. Nutritional imbalance endorsed by televised food advertisements. *J Am Diet Assoc.* 2010;110(6):904–10.
81. Kaiser Family Foundation. Food for thought: Television food advertising to children in the United States. 2007.
82. Ustjanauskas AE, Harris JL, Schwartz MB. Food and beverage advertising on children's web sites. *Pediatr Obesity.* 2013 July. doi: 10.1111/j.
83. Aktas Arnas Y. The effects of television food advertisement on children's food purchasing requests. *Pediatr Int.* 2006;48(2):138–45.
84. Chamberlain LJ, Wang Y, Robinson TN. Does children's screen time predict requests for advertised products? Cross-sectional and prospective analyses. *Arch Pediatr Adolesc Med.* 2006;160(4):363–8.
85. Koordeman R, Anschutz DJ, van Baaren RB, Engels RC. Exposure to soda commercials affects sugar-sweetened soda consumption in young women. An observational experimental study. *Appetite.* 2010;54(3):619–22.
86. Andreyeva T, Kelly IR, Harris JL. Exposure to food advertising on television: Associations with children's fast food and soft drink consumption and obesity. *Econ Hum Biol.* 2011;9(3):221–33.
87. Anschutz DJ, Engels RC, Van Strien T. Side effects of television food commercials on concurrent nonadvertised sweet snack food intakes in young children. *Am J Clin Nutr.* 2009;89(5):1328–33. Epub 2009/03/27.
88. Mello MM, Sutddert DM, Brennan TA. Obesity—The new frontier of public health law. *New Engl J Med.* 2006;354(24):2601–10.
89. Chriqui JF, Eidson SS, Bates H, Kowalczyk S, J CF. State sales tax rates for soft drinks and snacks sold through grocery stores and vending machines, 2007. *J Public Health Policy.* 2008;29:226–49.
90. Powell LM, Harris JL, Fox T. Food marketing expenditures aimed at youth: Putting the numbers in context. *Am J Prev Med.* 2013;45(4):453–61.
91. Powell LM, Szczypka G, Chaloupka FJ. Trends in exposure to television food advertisements among children and adolescents in the United States. *Arch Pediatr Adolesc Med.* 2010;164(9):794–802.
92. Neuman W. U.S. seeks new limits on food ads for children. *New York Times.* 28 April 2011.
93. Room R, editor. The effects of nordic alcohol policies: What happens to drinking and harm when alcohol controls change? Helsinki, Finland: Nordic Council for Alcohol and Drug Research; 2002.

94. Moore M, Gerstein D, editors. Alcohol and public policy: In the shadow of prohibition. Washington, DC: National Academy Press; 1981.
95. Osterberg E. Do alcohol prices affect consumption and related problems? In: Holder HD, Edwards G, editors. Alcohol and public policy: Evidence and issues. Oxford, UK: Oxford University Press; 1995. pp. 145–63.
96. Hurst W, Gregory E, Gussman T. International survey: Alcoholic beverage taxation and control policies. Ottawa, Canada: Brewers Association of Canada; 1997.
97. Wagenaar AC, Maldonado-Molina MM, Wagenaar BH. Effects of alcohol tax increases on alcohol-related disease mortality in Alaska: Time-series analyses from 1976 to 2004. *Am J Public Health*. 2009; 99(8):1464–70.
98. Godfrey C. Factors influencing the consumption of alcohol and tobacco: The use and abuse of economic models. *Br J Addiction*. 1989;84:1123–38.
99. Royal Colleges of Physicians. Alcohol and public health: The prevention of harm related to the use of alcohol. Medicine FoPH, editor. Hampshire, UK: Macmillan Education Ltd.; 1991.
100. Schmidt LA, Mäkelä P, Rehm J, Room R. Alcohol: Equity and social determinants. In: Blas E, Kurup AS, editors. Equity, social determinants, and public health programmes. Geneva: World Health Organization; 2010. pp. 11–30.
101. Cook PJ, Tauchen G. The effect of liquor taxes on heavy drinking. *Bell J Econ*. 1982;13:379–90.
102. Cook PA. The effect of liquor taxes on drinking, cirrhosis and auto fatalities. In: Moore M, Gerstein D, editors. Alcohol and public policy: In the shadow of prohibition. Washington, DC: National Academy Press; 1981. pp. 225–85.
103. Chaloupka FJ, Saffer H, Grossman M. Alcohol-control policies and motor-vehicle fatalities. *J Legal Stud*. 1993;22:161–86.
104. Chaloupka FJ, Grossman M, Saffer H. The effects of price on alcohol consumption and alcohol-related problems. *Alcohol Res Health*. 2002;26(1):22–34.
105. Caraher M, Cowburn G. Taxing food: Implications for public health nutrition. *Public Health Nutr*. 2005;8(8):1242–9.
106. Jacobson MF, Brownell K. Small taxes on soft drinks and snack foods to promote health. *Am J Public Health*. 2000;90(6):854–7.
107. Godfrey C. Price regulation. In: Robinson D, Maynard A, Chester R, editors. Controlling legal addictions. London: Macmillan and Eugenics Society; 1989. pp. 110–30.
108. Osterberg E, Karlsson T, editors. Alcohol policies in EU member states and Norway: A collection of country reports. Helsinki, Finland: STAKES; 2002.
109. Briggs ADM, Mytton OT, Kehlbacher A, Tiffin R, Rayner M, Scarborough P. Overall and income specific effect on prevalence of overweight and obesity of 20% sugar sweetened drink tax in UK: Ecomonic and comparative risk assessment modelling study. *Br Med J*. 2013;347:f6189. doi:10.1136/bmj.f6189.
110. Grunewald P, Treno A. Local and global alcohol supply: Economic and geographic models of community systems. *Addiction*. 2000;94(Suppl. 4):S537–49.
111. Fletcher JM, Frisvold D, Tefft N. Can soft drink taxes reduce population weight? *Contemp Econ Policy*. 2010;28:23–35.
112. Swithers SE. Artificial sweeteners produce the counterintuitive effect of inducing metabolic derangements. *Trends Endocrinol Metab*. 2013;24(9):431–41.
113. Waterlander WE, de Boer MR, Schuit AJ, Seidell JC, Steenhuis IH. Price discounts significantly enhance fruit and vegetable purchases when combined with nutrition education: A randomized controlled supermarket trial. *Am J Clin Nutr*. 2013;97(4):886–95.
114. Kuchler F, Tegene A, Harris JM. Taxing snack foods: Manipulating diet quality or financing information programs? *Rev Agric Econ*. 2005;27(1):4–20.
115. Leicester A, Windmeiger F. The ‘Fat Tax’: Economic incentives to reduce obesity. London: Institute for Fiscal Studies, 2004 Contract No.: 4.
116. Park YW, Zhu S, Palaniappan L, Heshka S, Carnethon MR, Heymsfield SB. The metabolic syndrome: Prevalence and associated risk factor findings in the US population from the Third National Health and Nutrition Examination Survey, 1988–1994. *Arch Intern Med*. 2003;163:427–36.
117. Kolsgaard ML, Andersen LF, Tonstad S, Brunborg C, Wangensteen T, Joner G. Ethnic differences in metabolic syndrome among overweight and obese children and adolescents: The Oslo Adiposity Intervention Study. *Acta Paediatr*. 2008;97(11):1557–63.
118. Dodd AH, Briefel R, Cabili C, Wilson A, Crepinsek MK. Disparities in consumption of sugar-sweetened and other beverages by race/ethnicity and obesity status among United States schoolchildren. *J Nutr Educ Behav*. 2013;45(3):240–9.

119. Byrd S. Civil rights and the 'Twinkie Tax': The 900-pound gorilla in the war on obesity. *Louisiana Law Rev*, 2004;65(1).
120. Skinner T, Miller H, Bryant C. The literature on the economic causes of and policy responses to obesity. *Acta Agric Scand Sect C*. 2005;2:128–37.
121. Edwards C. Why Congress should repeal sugar subsidy. CATO Institute Commentary; 2007, http://www.cato.org/publications/commentary/why-congress-should-repeal-sugar-subsidy.
122. Alston JM, Sumner DA, Vosti SA. Farm subsidies and obesity in the United States. Berkeley: University of California; 2007.
123. Ramirez SM, Stafford R. Equal and universal access? Water at mealtimes, inequalities, and the challenge for schools in poor and rural communities. *J Health Care Poor Underserved*. 2013;24(2):885–91.
124. Plant M, Single E, Stockwell T, editors. Alcohol: Minimizing the harm: What works? London, UK: Free Association Books Ltd.; 1997.
125. Hauritz M, Homel R, McIlwain G et al. Reducing violence in licensed venues through community safety action porjections: The Queensland experience. *Contemp Drug Probl*. 1998;25:511–51.
126. Gruenewald PJ, Remer L, Lipton R. Evaluating the alcohol environment: Community geography and alcohol problems. *Alcohol Res Health*. 2002;26(1):42–8.
127. Gruenwald P, Ponicki WR, Holder H. The realtionship of outlet densities to alcohol consumption: A times series cross-sectional analysis. *Alcoholism Clin Exp Res*. 1993;17:38–47.
128. Makela P, Tryggvesson K, Rossow I. Who drinks more or less when policies change? The evidence from 50 years of nordic studies. In: Room R, editor. The effects of nordic alcohol policies: What happens to drinking and harm when control systems change? Helsinki, Finland: Nordic Council for Alcohol and Drug Research; 2002. pp. 17–70.
129. Aubrey A. Mcdonald's says bye-bye to sugary sodas in happy meals. NPR; 2013; Available from: http://www.npr.org/blogs/thesalt/2013/09/26/226564560/mcdonalds-says-bye-bye-to-sugary-sodas-in-happy-meals.
130. French S, Jeffery RW, Story M, Breitlow KK, Baxter JS, Hanna P et al. Pricing and promotion effects on low-fat vending snack purchases: The Chips Study. *Am J Public Health*. 2001;91(1):112–7.
131. French S. Pricing effects on food choices. *Am Soc Nutr Sci*. 2003;133:841S–3S.
132. Reddy KS. Cardiovascular disease in non-western countries. *N Engl J Med*. 2004;350(24):2438–40.
133. Sanchez-Vaznaugh EV, Sánchez BN, Baek J, Crawford PB. 'Competitive' food and beverage policies: Are they influencing childhood overweight trends? *Health Affairs*. 2010;29(3):436–46.
134. Fox MK, Dodd AH, Wilson A, Gleason PM. Association between school food environment and practices and body mass index of US public school children. *J Am Diet Assoc*. 2009;109(2 Suppl):S108–17.
135. Briefel RR, Crepinsek MK, Cabili C, Wilson A, Gleason PM. School food environments and practices affect dietary behaviors of US public school children. *J Am Diet Assoc*. 2009;109(2 Suppl):S91–107.
136. Park S, Sappenfield WM, Huang Y, Sherry B, Bensyl DM. The impact of the availability of school vending machines on eating behavior during lunch: The youth physical activity and nutrition survey. *J Am Diet Assoc*. 2010;110(10):1532–6.
137. Johnson DB, Bruemmer B, Lund AE, Evens CC, Mar CM. Impact of school district sugar-sweetened beverage policies on student beverage exposure and consumption in middle schools. *J Adolesc Health*. 2009;45(3 Suppl):S30–7.
138. Woodruff SJ, Hanning RM, McGoldrick K. The influence of physical and social contexts of eating on lunch-time food intake among Southern Ontario, Canada, middle school students. *J Sch Health*. 2010;80(9):421–8.
139. Mendoza JA, Watson K, Cullen KW. Change in dietary energy density after implementation of the texas public school nutrition policy. *J Am Diet Assoc*. 2010;110(3):434–40.
140. Woodward-Lopez G, Gosliner W, Samuels SE, Craypo L, Kao J, Crawford PB. Lessons learned from evaluations of California's statewide school nutrition standards. *Am J Public Health*. 2010;100(11):2137–45.
141. Gaines AB, Lonis-Shumate SR, Gropper SS. Evaluation of Alabama public school wellness policies and state school mandate implementation. *J Sch Health*. 2011;81(5):281–7.
142. Whatley Blum JE, Beaudoin CM, O'Brien LM, Polacsek M, Harris DE, O'Rourke KA. Impact of Maine's statewide nutrition policy on high school food environments. *Prev Chronic Dis*. 2011;8(1):A19.
143. Samuels SE, Hutchinson KS, Craypo L, Barry J, Bullock SL. Implementation of California state school competitive food and beverage standards. *J Sch Health*. 2010;80(12):581–7.
144. Turner L, Chriqui JF, Chaloupka FJ. Classroom parties in United States elementary schools: The potential for policies to reduce student exposure to sugary foods and beverages. *J Nutr Educ Behav*. 2013;45(6):611–9.

145. Caparosa SL, Shordon M, Santos AT, Pomichowski ME, Dzewaltowski DA, Coleman KJ. Fundraising, celebrations and classroom rewards are substantial sources of unhealthy foods and beverages on public school campuses. *Public Health Nutr*. 2013;14:1–9.
146. Borradaile KE, Sherman S, Vander Veur SS, McCoy T, Sandoval B, Nachmani J et al. Snacking in children: The role of urban corner stores. *Pediatrics*. 2009;124(5):1293–8.
147. Storey M. The shifting beverage landscape. *Physiol Behav*. 2010;100(1):10–4.
148. Taber DR, Chriqui JF, Powell LM, Chaloupka FJ. Banning all sugar-sweetened beverages in middle schools: Reduction of in-school access and purchasing but not overall consumption. *Arch Pediatr Adol Med*. 2012;166:256–62.
149. Gittelsohn J, Kumar MB. Preventing childhood obesity and diabetes: Is it time to move out of the school? *Pediatr Diabetes*. 2007;8(Suppl. 9):55–69.
150. Schmidt L, Room R. Cross-cultural applicability in international classifications and research on alcohol dependence. *J Stud Alcohol*. 1999;60(4):448–62.
151. Room R, Janca A, Bennett L, Schmidgt L, Sartorius N. Who cross-cultural applicability research on diagnosis and assessment of substance use disorders: An overview of methods and selected results. *Addiction*. 1996;91(2):199–220.
152. Institute of Medicine. *Strategies to Reduce Salt Consumption in the United States*. Washington, DC: Institute of Medicine; 2010. ISBN 978-0-309-14805-4.
153. Moore MH, Gerstein DR, editors. Alcohol and public policy: Beyond the shadow of prohibition. Washington, DC: National Academy Press; 1981.

Index

I

O

P